Spatial Hearing and Auditory Perception

Spatial Hearing and Auditory Perception

Editor: Nora McDougal

AMERICAN
MEDICAL PUBLISHERS
www.americanmedicalpublishers.com

AMERICAN
MEDICAL PUBLISHERS
www.americanmedicalpublishers.com

Cataloging-in-Publication Data

Spatial hearing and auditory perception / edited by Nora McDougal.
p. cm.
Includes bibliographical references and index.
ISBN 979-8-88740-463-9
1. Directional hearing. 2. Auditory perception. 3. Space perception. 4. Hearing.
5. Auditory scene analysis. I. McDougal, Nora.
QP469 .S63 2023
612.85--dc23

American Medical Publishers,
41 Flatbush Avenue,
1st Floor, New York,
NY 11217, USA

ISBN 979-8-88740-463-9 (Hardback)

Contents

Contents

Preface

This book has been a concerted effort by a group of academicians, researchers and scientists, who have contributed their research works for the realization of the book. This book has materialized in the wake of emerging advancements and innovations in this field. Therefore, the need of the hour was to compile all the required researches and disseminate the knowledge to a broad spectrum of people comprising of students, researchers and specialists of the field.

Spatial hearing refers to an innate human ability, which enables the people to determine the direction of a sound source. In normal conditions, people can engage in spatial hearing effortlessly. People experience spatial hearing loss when they are unable to use spatial cues for determining the origin of sound in space. Auditory perception is the ability to receive and interpret information that reaches the ears. It is a multi-step process that includes detection, discrimination, identification, recognition and comprehension of the sound. There is a complex relation between age and the perception of sound source location. With the progression of age, hearing loss advances. This book includes some of the vital pieces of works being conducted across the world, on various topics related to spatial hearing and auditory perception. It will also provide interesting topics for research, which interested readers can take up. The book will serve as a valuable source of reference for graduate and post graduate students.

At the end of the preface, I would like to thank the authors for their brilliant chapters and the publisher for guiding us all-through the making of the book till its final stage. Also, I would like to thank my family for providing the support and encouragement throughout my academic career and research projects.

Editor

1

Anatomical limits on interaural time differences: an ecological perspective

William M. Hartmann* **and Eric J. Macaulay**

Psychoacoustics Laboratory, Department of Physics and Astronomy, Michigan State University, East Lansing, MI, USA

Correspondence:
William M. Hartmann, Department of Physics and Astronomy, Michigan State University, 567 Wilson Rd., East Lansing, MI 48824, USA
e-mail: hartmann@pa.msu.edu

Human listeners, and other animals too, use interaural time differences (ITD) to localize sounds. If the sounds are pure tones, a simple frequency factor relates the ITD to the interaural phase difference (IPD), for which there are known iso-IPD boundaries, 90°, 180°... defining regions of spatial perception. In this article, iso-IPD boundaries for humans are translated into azimuths using a spherical head model (SHM), and the calculations are checked by free-field measurements. The translated boundaries provide quantitative tests of an ecological interpretation for the dramatic onset of ITD insensitivity at high frequencies. According to this interpretation, the insensitivity serves as a defense against misinformation and can be attributed to limits on binaural processing in the brainstem. Calculations show that the ecological explanation passes the tests only if the binaural brainstem properties evolved or developed consistent with heads that are 50% smaller than current adult heads. Measurements on more realistic head shapes relax that requirement only slightly. The problem posed by the discrepancy between the current head size and a smaller, ideal head size was apparently solved by the evolution or development of central processes that discount large IPDs in favor of interaural level differences. The latter become more important with increasing head size.

Keywords: brainstem, evolution, binaural, sound localization, interaural time difference, spherical head model, rotation-azimuth transform

INTRODUCTION

More than 100 years ago, Lord Rayleigh pointed out that human listeners can make use of interaural time differences (ITD) to localize pure tones (Strutt, 1907). An example is illustrated by the functions in **Figure 1**, which represent the pressures at the two ears for a 1000-Hz tone. Here, the source of the tone is on the listener's right side so that the waveform in the right ear (red) starts before the waveform in the left (blue and dashed). As shown in region A, the ongoing wave in the right ear continues to lead the ongoing wave in the left. For instance, the positive-going zero crossing at time t_o in the left ear is preceded by a similar crossing in the right.

THE INTERAURAL PHASE PROBLEM

Rayleigh was quick to point out that there are practical limits to the utility of the ITD. When the azimuth increases enough that the interaural phase difference (IPD) becomes equal to 180°, the ongoing information from the ITD becomes totally ambiguous. As the azimuth increases further, and the IPD exceeds 180° (regions C and D), the ITD points to images with azimuths opposite to the actual source azimuth. Headphone experiments by Bernstein and Trahiotis (1985) have revealed just this kind of ambiguity. Thus, there is a 180° IPD limit on useful ITD cues. Region D is especially misleading—even dangerous. Although the source continues to be on the listener's right, the ongoing waveform indicates that the source is on the left—just as surely as it pointed to a source on the right in region A. In free-field listening, this misleading ongoing information actually dominates the (correct) onset information (Hartmann and Rakerd, 1989).

Sayers (1964) reported experiments indicating another IPD boundary of interest. As the ITD increases such that the IPD exceeds about 90° (region B), further increases in ITD cause the image to move back toward the midline. Also, in region B listeners sometimes lateralize images on the wrong side of the head. Yost (1981) similarly found frequent wrong-side lateralization in region B, and Elpern and Naughton (1964) showed that the maximum sensation of lateralization occurs for IPD = 90°. Thus, there is a 90° IPD limit on useful directional information from *changes* in the ITD, and the regions of ITD information are logically represented by IPD boundaries separated by 90° as shown in **Figure 1**.

Region E shows a confusion of yet another sort. Here, the ongoing waveforms are identical to those in region A, but the ITD in region E is larger by a full period of the tone (1000 μs). The same ongoing waveform corresponds to two different ITDs, indicating two different characteristic delays of the same sign, potentially associated with two different locations on the same side of the head.

It has been proposed that the IPD confusions noted here have been ameliorated by a binaural system that becomes insensitive to ITDs at high frequency. This idea will be called the "ecological interpretation," and the rest of this article will study its plausibility and possible modifications to it.

TRANSFORMATIONS

Because the IPD is the product of the ITD and the frequency of the tone, the IPD boundaries of **Figure 1** can be translated to ITD and frequency, as shown in **Figure 2**. These boundaries will be called "iso-IPD contours" or simply "IPD contours" or "IPD boundaries." The dashed horizontal line (HW) indicates the largest ITD that can be caused by the typical human head for sound sources in free field, sometimes called the Hornbostel–Wertheimer constant (von Hornbostel and Wertheimer, 1920). **Figure 2** shows it as the low-frequency limit of the head diffraction formula ITD = $(3a/v)\sin(90°) = 763\mu s$. Here a (8.75 cm) is the radius of the typical human head (Hartley and Fry, 1921; Algazi et al., 2001), and v (34,400 cm/s), is the speed of sound in room-temperature air.

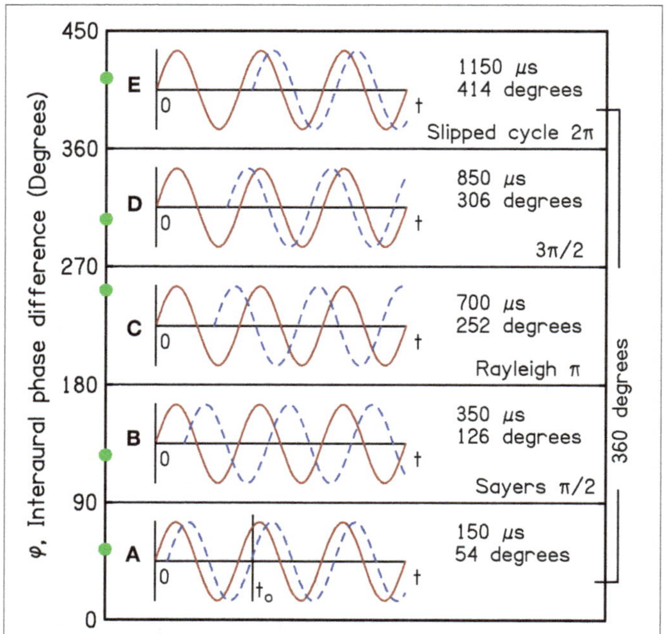

FIGURE 1 | Tones in the right ear (red) and left ear (blue and dashed) as functions of time and with particular interaural phase differences (IPD) as indicated on the vertical axis to illustrate different regions of IPD. The boundaries between regions, separated by 90°, are logically and perceptually important in sound localization.

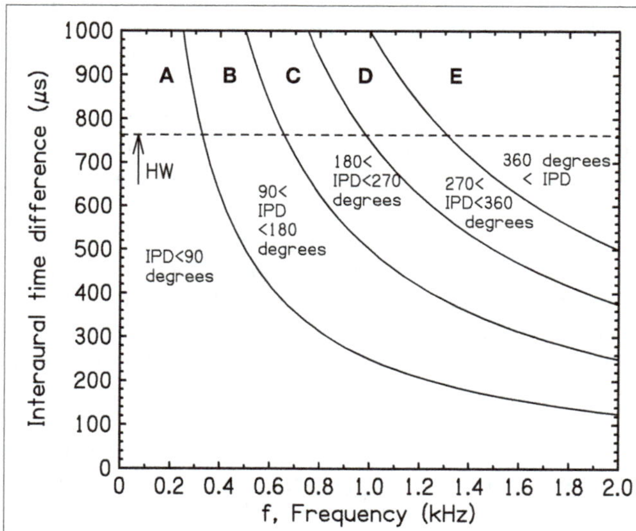

FIGURE 2 | Transformation of the iso-IPD boundaries in Figure 1 to a scale of frequency and interaural time difference (ITD). HW indicates the largest possible ITD for the average human head in free field.

Figure 2 shows that the iso-IPD contours, such as the 90° or 180° boundaries, are not important if the ITD is small or the frequency is low. Small ITDs occur in the real world when the azimuth of the source is small. Large ITDs, and large IPDs, occur when the source is off to the side of the listener. A representation in terms of source azimuth can be obtained by transforming the ITD axis in **Figure 2** to a scale of source azimuth, as shown in **Figure 3**.

SPHERICAL HEAD MODEL

The shaded regions in **Figure 3** are transformations to an azimuthal scale using a spherical head model (SHM). The iso-IPD contours separating the regions in **Figure 2** have become thin regions corresponding to different locations of the ears on the head.

SPHERICAL HEAD CALCULATIONS

The calculations for **Figure 3** were based on an exact mathematical treatment of the scattering of waves by a rigid sphere. Solutions to this scattering problem for plane wave incidence (infinite source distance) go back as far as Rayleigh (1896). A modern solution, which is a series of Legendre polynomials with frequency-dependent, complex spherical functions as coefficients, was given by Rschevkin (1963) and applied to interaural differences for a spherical head by Kuhn (1977). The spherical head calculation was generalized to finite source distance by Rabinowitz et al. (1993) and Duda and Martens (1998). In the limit of infinite source distance, the finite-distance solution

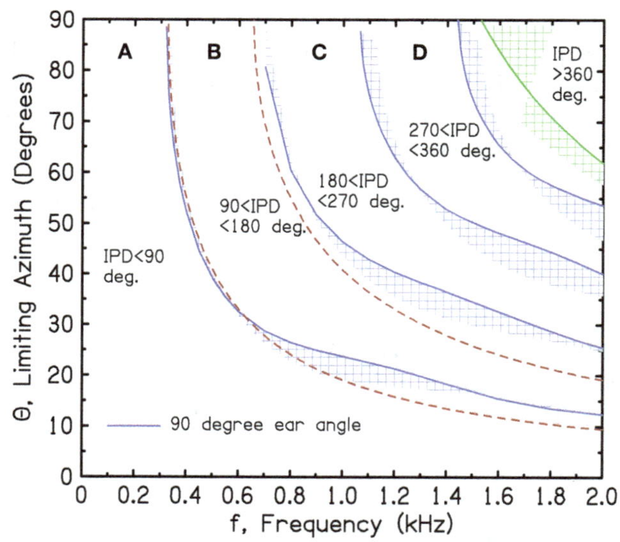

FIGURE 3 | Transforming the ITD axis in Figure 2 to an azimuthal axis using the spherical head diffraction model. The blue shaded regions are bounded by ear angles of 90° (solid blue line) and 110°. The green shaded region similarly shows the Woodworth model. The red dashed curves show the low-frequency limit of the spherical head model for IPDs of 90° and 180°.

reduces to Kuhn's result. Our **Figure 3** used the finite-distance solution with a source distance of 2 m to match experiment. However, there is actually very little difference between ITDs computed for a source at 2 m and a source at infinity. (The interaural level difference is much more sensitive to source distance.) The spherical head solution captures the important frequency dependence of the ITD that is also characteristic of human heads. The frequency dependence of the ITD for different azimuths, as plotted by Constan and Hartmann (2003) (their Figure 1), shows a significant drop in ITD between 400 and 2000 Hz.

The low-frequency limit, $(3a/v)\sin(\theta)$ generally underestimates the ITD at low frequency. For instance, Kuhn (1977) found that in order to match low-frequency KEMAR ITDs, it was necessary to increase the head radius from $a = 8.75$ to 9.3 cm. Kuhn tentatively attributed the apparent extra size to the pinnae, which would be indistinguishable from the bulk of the head when viewed with wavelengths corresponding to low frequencies. Fortunately, all the frequencies of interest in the current article are greater than 600 Hz, and in this range, the SHM ITD agrees better with measurements on human listeners. The high-frequency limit of the SHM is the creeping wave solution known as the Woodworth model (Woodworth, 1938). In this limit ITDs are smaller than in the low-frequency limit, with the decrease depending on the azimuth. For small azimuths, the high-frequency limiting ITD is 33% smaller than the low-frequency limit. At the other extreme, an azimuth of 90°, the high-frequency ITD is only 14% smaller.

The shaded contours in **Figure 3** arise from a range of assumptions about the angle of the listener's ears with respect to the forward direction. The boundaries indicated with solid blue lines correspond to an ear angle of 90°; the other edges of the shaded regions correspond to 110°. Thus, the contours are centered on an ear angle of 100°, as suggested by Blauert (1997) and used by Duda and Martens (1998) and by Treeby et al. (2007). For comparison, we note that Hartley and Fry (1921) suggested that the human ear is 97.5°.

The red, dashed lines represent the low-frequency (f) limit of the azimuth (Θ) for a spherical head with radius a: $\Theta = \arcsin[v/(6fa)]$ for the 180° IPD limit and $\Theta = \arcsin[v/(12fa)]$ for the 90° IPD limit.

As expected, the low-frequency limit agrees with the exact formula for a 90° ear angle near 400 Hz and departs from the exact formula as the frequency increases. The green, shaded region at high frequency shows the 360° IPD contour from the Woodworth model, which is only valid at high frequency. The calculations for ear angles between 90° and 110° were made using formulas for the Woodworth model from Aaronson and Hartmann (2014). This latter article shows that unless the frequency is very high, the Woodworth formula underestimates the ITD. That is why, for every frequency, an especially large azimuth is required to produce a given IPD—in this case, an IPD of 360°.

SPHERICAL HEAD ARRAY MEASUREMENTS

The spherical head calculations in **Figure 3** were tested against measurements of frequency and azimuth that targeted IPDs of interest. Measurements were made in an anechoic room (7.7 × 6.4 × 3.6 m) (IAC 107840) using an array of 13 loudspeaker sources (Minimus 3.5) spaced by 7.5° and located 2 m away from a binaural receiver. The array was a single quadrant (0–90°) to the right of the receiver. The receiver was a rigid spherical shell (Shapemaster, Ogden, IL) with a radius of 8.75 cm made of 6-mm PETG (glycol-modified polyethylene terephthalate) and mounted on a microphone stand 117 cm off the wire grid floor, the same height as the array sources. The forward direction of the sphere was defined by a laser beam through the center of the sphere. Two small holes were drilled at 90° from the forward direction to accommodate the ends of the probe tubes (0.95 mm O.D.) of Etymotic ER-7c probe microphones. (Etymotic Research, Elkgrove Village, IL). Therefore, the simulated ear angles were 90°. Signals from the microphones were first amplified with the associated probe-tube-compensating Etymotic preamplifier, and then given another 40 dB of gain before conversion to digital form by a DD1 two-channel 16-bit analog-to-digital converter (Tucker-Davis Technologies, Alachua, FL). Because the frequency of the signal was exactly known, it was possible to use matched filtering to process half-second samples of the digitized signals and to extract precise IPDs.

Estimates for the target IPD boundaries of 90°, 180°, 270°, and 360° are shown in **Figure 4**. They were determined by setting the frequency to successive values and measuring IPDs for the 13 sources. Then, source azimuths for the target IPD boundaries were interpolated from the measured IPDs. The interpolation procedure required the assumption that the IPD-azimuth relationship was smooth and locally linear. **Figure 4** shows that the interpolated azimuths agree reasonably well with the solid lines at the tops of the shaded regions, as expected for a 90° ear angle.

SPHERICAL HEAD ROTATION MEASUREMENTS

Because of our concern with the interpolated array measurements over 7.5° and with inadvertent scattering from the array structure

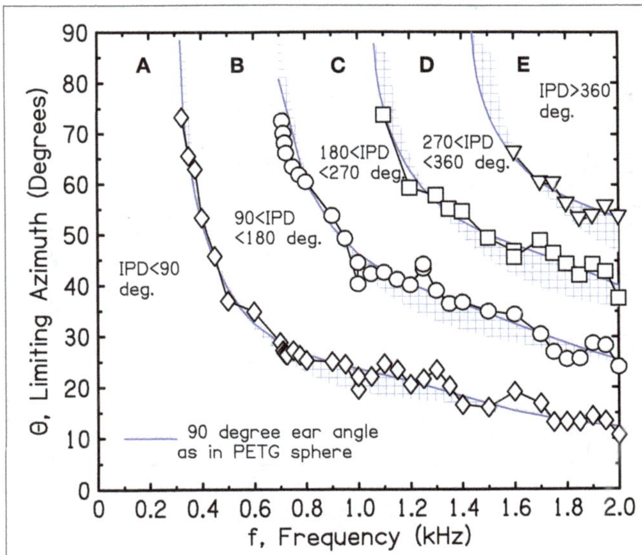

FIGURE 4 | Measured values of frequency and azimuth that lead to IPDs of 90°, 180°, 270°, and 360° (diamonds, circles, squares, triangles, respectively) for a perfect sphere. Values were interpolated from measurements using a source array in one quadrant.

itself, we repeated the IPD boundary measurements on the sphere using only a single loudspeaker source, 3 m from the sphere, in the anechoic room. The different source azimuths were obtained by rotating the sphere with its microphone stand using a calibrated rotating table on the wire grid floor. To make measurements, the sphere was rotated to a desired azimuth, and the frequency was varied to hit a targeted IPD. Thus, the procedure involved no interpolation. Unfortunately, the microphone stand could not be made perfectly vertical. To compensate, the measurements were made four times, rotating through 90° in all four quadrants with the expectation that the effect of the wobble would be mostly canceled in the average. The averages with standard deviations over the four rotations are shown in **Figure 5**. Again, the symbols lie close to the solid line for the 90° ear angle. In the end, the good agreement between the calculations and the measurements from both the array and the rotated head suggest good correspondence between the SHM and free-field reality for the IPDs of interest.

Figures 2–5 show that when the frequency is low, the IPD is within the most useful region, namely region A—0° to 90°. So long as the frequency is less than a critical value where the 90° iso-IPD contour intersects the top axis, region A applies for all azimuths, 0–90°. The SHM and our measurements agree that this critical frequency is well approximated by the low-frequency limit of the model, $v/(12a)$ or 328 Hz. Similarly, the IPD completely avoids the ambiguous 180° boundary and region C only if the frequency is less than 328 × 2 or 655 Hz. As the frequency increases beyond this value, the ambiguity and the misinformation provided by the ITD start to occur at ever smaller values of the azimuth. An important conclusion to be drawn from **Figures 2–5** is that both the 180° and the 90° iso-IPD boundaries are exceeded for tones with frequencies that are *not particularly high* and for azimuths that are *not particularly large*. The boundaries would appear to be real problems for the use of ITD cues in real-world sound localization.

HUMAN ITD SENSITIVITY

Because ITD information becomes increasingly misleading as the frequencies and azimuths increase, there would be survival value in a binaural system that becomes insensitive to ITD at moderately high frequency. Such a system would defend its owner from dangerous localization cues that could lead to mislocalization. In fact, there is unequivocal evidence that fine-structure ITD sensitivity disappears at about 1500 Hz. The upper limit of ITD sensitivity was explored by Zwislocki and Feldman (1956) and by Klumpp and Eady (1956), who found an upper limit of 1300 Hz. Mills (1958) found a limit of 1400 Hz, and Nordmark (1976) found 1430 Hz.

The most detailed exploration of the frequency dependence of ITD sensitivity was recently made by Brughera et al. (2013), paying particular attention to the high-frequency limit. The procedures in that work were approved by the Michigan State University institutional review board, and informed consent was obtained from all subjects. That exploration used a two-interval forced-choice task in which a tone led in one ear by the ITD on the first interval and led in the other ear by the ITD on the second. The difference between the two intervals, ΔITD (twice the ITD on each interval) is plotted in **Figure 6**. The thresholds in **Figure 6** show a broad minimum between 700 and 1000 Hz indicating the frequency region of greatest sensitivity. They show a sharp rise above 1200 Hz. Brughera et al. found that some listeners were sensitive to the ITD at 1400 Hz, but all listeners found it impossible to detect the ITD at 1450 Hz, in good agreement with Nordmark.

The shaded rectangle in **Figure 6** between 700 and 1000 Hz indicates the frequency range of greatest sensitivity to ITD. The

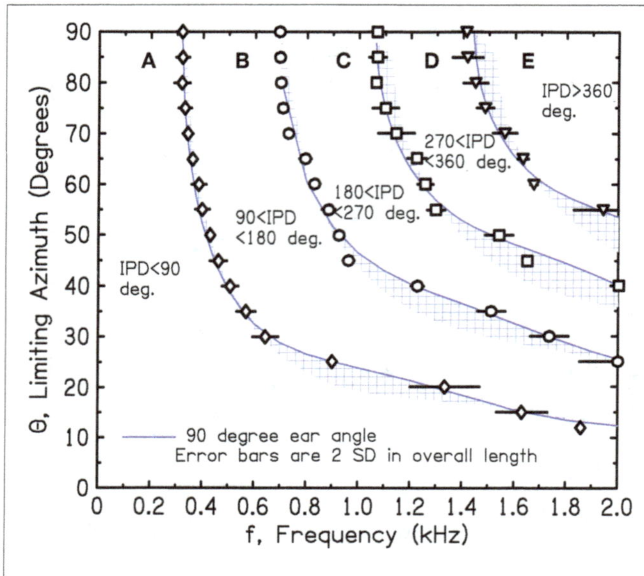

FIGURE 5 | Measured values of frequency and azimuth that lead to IPDs of 90°, 180°, 270°, and 360° for a perfect sphere. Values were measured in four quadrants using a single source and rotating the sphere. The average of the four is shown together with an error bar two standard deviations in overall length.

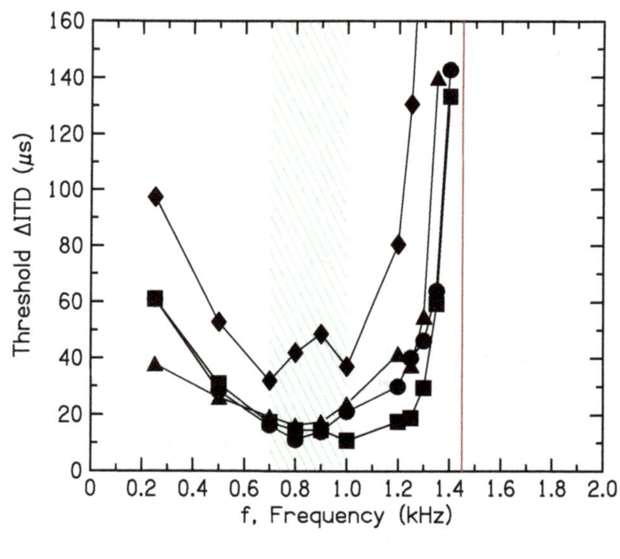

FIGURE 6 | Threshold interaural time differences as a function of frequency for four listeners measured by Brughera et al. (2013). The shaded rectangle indicates the frequency region of greatest sensitivity. The vertical solid line shows the brick wall.

vertical line in **Figure 6** at 1450 Hz indicates the upper limit. Because we are unaware of any experiment indicating ITD sensitivity for a tone with a frequency greater than 1450 Hz, the rest of this article will refer to the boundary at 1450 Hz as the "brick wall." It is striking that the frequency difference between the top of the region of greatest sensitivity and the brick wall is considerably less than an octave. It is an unusually sharp transition.

The loss of ITD sensitivity for sine tones above 1450 Hz is consistent with other binaural phenomena, such as binaural beats, which indicate a loss of interaural phase sensitivity near this frequency (Perrott and Nelson, 1969). Although the binaural masking level difference (MLD) is a more complicated effect, there is evidence of a similar limit in a dozen experiments cited by Durlach (1972), where the MLD as a function of frequency shows a discontinuity in slope near 1500 Hz (Durlach Figure 4).

The loss of phase sensitivity at the brick wall appears to be specifically a binaural phenomenon. There is good reason to believe that phase locking is maintained in the human auditory system for considerably higher frequencies. A low estimate for the loss of phase locking (between 2 and 3 kHz) comes from mistuned harmonic detection experiments (Hartmann et al., 1990). A high estimate (8 kHz) comes from frequency difference limen experiments (Moore and Ernst, 2012). Intermediate estimates (4–5 kHz) come from musical pitch experiments (e.g., Oxenham et al., 2011) or from assuming that phase locking in humans is similar to the auditory nerve of cat (Johnson, 1980). Apparently there is an especially low limit for the human binaural system. But although the lowpass character must follow the initial stage of binaural interaction, it is not certain where it originates. The neural modeling by Brughera et al. (2013), based on cat and gerbil physiology, identified the superior olive complex in the brainstem as the origin of the low limit. Whether the limit occurs in the superior olive or in the inferior colliculus, it is not unreasonable to focus on the brainstem and to conjecture that the limit represents an evolutionary adaptation of the brainstem to ITD values of negative utility as seen in **Figures 2–5**.

THE ECOLOGICAL INTERPRETATION

An ecological interpretation for the high-frequency limits of ITD sensitivity has often been proposed. Rayleigh (Strutt, 1907) argued that it was unlikely that listeners could localize sounds based only on ITD when the frequency was much above 512 Hz because the maximum delay across the head (about 800 μs) would lead to an IPD close to 180°. In 1909, Rayleigh (Strutt, 1909) also remarked on the 90° IPD boundary, leading to an even lower estimate for the maximum frequency for useable ITD. Yost and Hafter (1987) noted that delaying a 1666-Hz tone by a head width would be equivalent to no delay at all (region E). The 2005 review of binaural hearing by Stern et al. (2005) similarly suggested that the upper limit of ITD utility should be set by the size of the head. Moore's introduction to human hearing (1997) also noted the correspondence between the ambiguity of the ITD cue and the distance between the ears. Taking a somewhat different direction, Blauert (1997) argued that the head size establishes an upper limit of about 630 μs on useful ITDs. Schnupp et al. (2011) argued similarly, applying the same principle to all animals. Carlile (1996) noted that the only unambiguous tones are those with wavelength less than twice the head radius. Calculations by Harper and McAlpine (2004) showed that the optimum array for coding of cross-correlation in IPD-frequency space is mainly a function of an animal's head size.

As shown in **Figures 2–5**, the azimuths for the boundaries IPD = 90° and 180° are rapidly varying functions of frequency in the large azimuth regime. As shown in **Figure 6**, the ITD sensitivity also has a rapid frequency dependence. According to the ecological interpretation (EI), these regions of changing sensitivity ought to be sensibly related. **Figure 7** repeats the spherical head regions from **Figure 3**, and also repeats the region of greatest ITD sensitivity and the brick wall from **Figure 6**. **Figure 7** shows that the relationship is far from sensible.

As shown by the dotted lines in **Figure 7**, for the 180° boundary, the EI would assert that the binaural system has become insensitive to 1450-Hz tones because the IPD exceeds 180°, leading to wrong-sided images, whenever the azimuth is greater than 33°. By contrast, the binaural system has remained highly sensitive to 1000-Hz tones because they are more reliable. They lead to wrong-sided images only when the azimuth is greater than 45°. The problem with this picture is that the difference of only 12° of azimuth is hardly adequate motivation for a system to develop such a sharply tuned frequency response as the human binaural ITD system evidently has.

The corresponding analysis for the 90° iso-IPD contour (not shown in the figure) is even more disappointing. According to the EI, the binaural system rejects ITD information from a 1450-Hz tone because this tone leads to perceived images that move in directions opposite to reality when the azimuth is greater than 14°. By contrast, the binaural system maintains sensitivity to ITD information at 1000 Hz because it leads to misleading directional information only when the azimuth is greater than 24°. Again, the difference of only 10° seems to be a poor reason to evolve an ITD

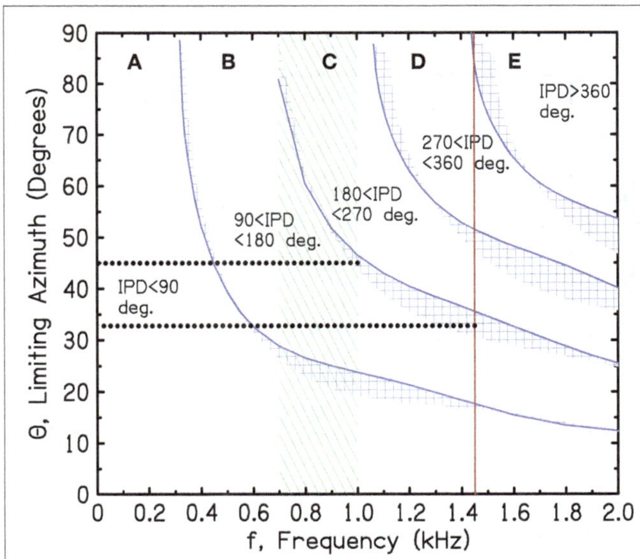

FIGURE 7 | Sensitivity regions from Figure 6 together with model boundaries for the IPD regions from Figure 3. The dotted lines refer to the argument in the text against the ecological interpretation given present-day human head sizes.

with a sharp frequency cutoff. Given the poor correspondence between the IPD boundaries and the limits of ITD sensitivity, one is tempted to abandon the ecological interpretation, at least in the quantitative detail presented here. Perhaps evolutionary pressures are actually responsible for the anomalously low cutoff frequency of ITD sensitivity, but then evolution stopped too soon and didn't get the cutoff quite low enough.

There is an alternative ecological theory, however, that leads to quantitatively good correspondence. The theory assumes that while the brainstem was evolving, and the medial superior olive and projections to it were developing, the head size was considerably smaller than the current human head. **Figure 8** is a repeat of **Figure 7** except that it makes the *small-head hypothesis*, assuming that the head is 50% smaller than our present-day human heads—a factor of 2 in diameter.

In **Figure 8** the upper limit of ITD sensitivity at 1450 Hz essentially eliminates the confusing ITDs in regions C, D, and E from contributing to sound localization. Only tones with an IPD less than the 180° iso-IPD contour can contribute. In another benefit, the most sensitive region between 700 and 1000 Hz extends to source azimuths as large as 60°. For the 90° iso-IPD contour, ITD information for 1450-Hz tones would be rejected because it leads to an incorrect sense of motion when the azimuth is greater than 27°. The confusing 90° iso-IPD contour does not enter the region of greatest ITD sensitivity until the azimuth has reached 40° (up from 23°). Therefore, a binaural system that developed to optimize ITD coding for a head diameter that is half as large appears to make sense acoustically. It makes some sense in evolutionary terms too because the brainstem is old brain, whereas the head expanded over very recent times to accommodate the neocortex.

A factor of two in diameter, however, may be extreme. Over the past 3.2 million years the brain size has expanded by a factor of 3 (Lynn, 1990). The cube root of 3 is 1.44 suggesting a head diameter that was 30% smaller than present day. Making the head

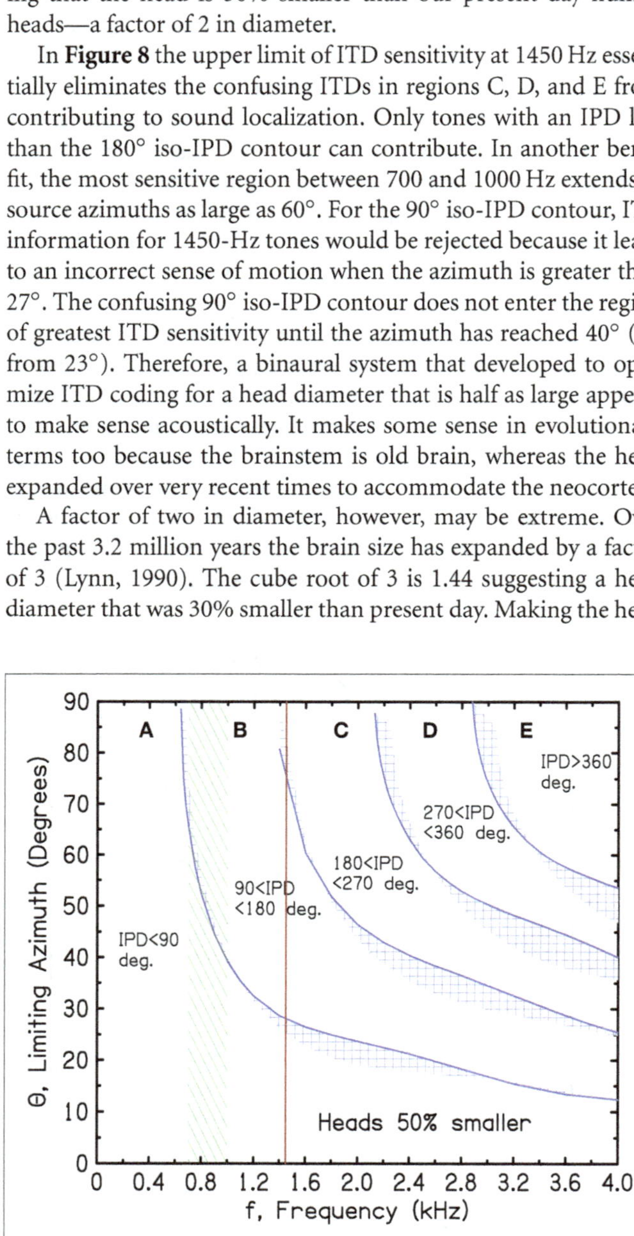

FIGURE 8 | Same as Figure 7 for a head diameter that is half as large as present-day human heads.

diameter 30% smaller (not shown in the figures) confers some advantages. Then the brick wall at 1450 Hz totally eliminates the most dangerous region, region D, for all azimuths.

The small-head hypothesis carries with it the assumption that the binaural properties of the brainstem have not greatly changed since the origin of homo with rapidly growing heads. That assumption can certainly be challenged because there is evidence that the binaural system changes—even in a single individual, even over a brief time. Evidence for changeable binaural processing is found in studies of development and plasticity. Experiments by Shinn-Cunningham et al. (1998), in which human auditory spatial maps were altered by feedback, or experiments by Hofman et al. (1998), where maps were altered by plugging one ear, show at least partial adaptation to new conditions. It is possible though that short-term accommodations such as these are entirely the result of cortical plasticity, revealing nothing about the brainstem. Concerning the brainstem itself, auditory brainstem response (ABR) experiments, as described in the review by Tzounopoulos and Kraus (2009), indicate plasticity in the brainstem that is both synaptic and intrinsic. The intrinsic plasticity shows changes at a fundamental biochemical level—a likely origin for the ITD brick wall. If brainstem plasticity appears on the time scale of a brief experiment or the development of a single individual, it seems unlikely that the binaural system would be resistant to ecological pressures for a few million years.

In contrast to the plasticity argument above, we conjecture that the binaural system, once adjusted for the ITDs available with small heads, did not change over evolutionary times because evolution found an alternative way to solve the problem of misleading ITDs, namely by using interaural level differences (ILD), which grew to be substantial as the head grew.

Calculations within the SHM show that the ILD is adequate to solve the problem in regions B, C, and D of **Figure 7**. Along the 90° iso-IPD contour (limit of region B), the ILD is greater than 2 dB except for the lowest frequencies, below 500 Hz. Even at the lowest frequencies the ILD is greater than 2 dB if the source is closer than 2 m. Along the 180° iso-IPD contour (limit of region C), the ILD is always greater than 3.5 dB and usually is much larger. ILDs of these magnitudes are adequate for human listeners to localize on the correct side of the head especially because the ITD cues are weak in these regions. Region D is somewhat more problematical. There, misleading ITD cues can be strong, and the correct ILDs along the 270° iso-IPD contour from 1100 to 1500 Hz are only slightly larger than along the 180° contour, partly because the relevant azimuths become large enough to involve the acoustical bright spot (Macaulay et al., 2010). Although region D, with strong, but wrong, ITD cues, represents more of a problem than region C, it is possible for the misleading ITD cues in both regions to be overcome at a higher level by a process that discounts ITD cues by contravening ILD cues.

The ILD does not solve the confusion problem in region E, where both the ITD and the ILD point in the same direction, and the ITD points to a secondary azimuth. However, **Figure 7** (current head size) shows that region E is perfectly eliminated by the brick wall at 1450 Hz.

KEMAR MEASUREMENTS

The experimental approach to the ecological interpretation using the spherical head (section 2) was consistent with historical approaches from the time of Rayleigh to the present. It probably applies to human heads better than to the other mammals that are frequently studied. It is possible, however, that the properties of real human heads might differ from the (SHM) in some important way with consequences for the theory. To obtain measurements of the IPD boundaries that are more realistic, we used a KEMAR manikin (large ears). As for the perfect sphere, we made two different measurements in the anechoic room, one with the 2-m array of 13 sources and the other with a rotating receiver and a single source. The sources were again at ear height.

Tones of fixed frequency were reproduced by the sources, and were recorded by the Etymotic ER-11 microphones within the KEMAR head and associated electronics. The recordings were again processed by matched filtering to obtain IPDs.

ARRAY MEASUREMENTS

The source azimuths leading to 90° and 180° IPDs were determined by linear interpolation within the 2-m array for a series of tone frequencies. The results are shown in **Figure 9** by circles and diamonds, which follow a smooth descending pattern except for prominent bumps near 1.3 kHz. We noted that a frequency of 1.3 kHz is close to the brick wall.

We suspected that the bumps were due to reflections from the manikin torso, and to test that idea we separated the head from the torso and mounted it on a microphone stand. However, the bumps persisted—somewhat changed in shape but at about the same frequencies. We next questioned the microphone system intrinsic to the KEMAR, and as a check on that system, we replaced it by probe microphones in the KEMAR ear canals (Etymotic ER-7c with associated electronics). The measurements with the alternative system almost perfectly reproduced those made with the KEMAR microphone system, including the bumps.

Because the bumps in the iso-IPD contours were observed in all our KEMAR head configurations and not observed in the array measurements using the perfect sphere, we tentatively concluded that the bumps near 1.3 kHz were caused by diffraction by the KEMAR head itself. However, the interpolated measurements from the array make assumptions about the smoothness of the contours, and those assumptions might not hold for a complicated head structure.

ROTATING KEMAR MEASUREMENTS

To check the measurements made with the array, we used a single loudspeaker 3 m away from the KEMAR, as for the rotated sphere measurements. We obtained different source azimuths by rotating the KEMAR with its mounting pole as an axis. However, unlike the sphere, the axis of rotation did not pass through the center of the head (COH). To relate angles of rotation to source azimuths, we developed the mathematics in Appendix, which solves the problem in principle. The KEMAR has a "+" sign on the top of its cranium and we took that point to be the COH for all measurements. The perpendicular distance from that point to the axis of rotation is 2 cm. As shown in the Appendix, the rotation-azimuth transformation depends on the ratio of this distance to the source distance, in this case a ratio of 2/300. With this value, the formula in the Appendix leads to an angular discrepancy of 0.5°, an error that can be ignored for our purposes.

Figure 10 shows the iso-IPD contours with mean and standard deviation measured across the two frontal quadrants. **Figure 11** shows the same for the two back quadrants. Although the details

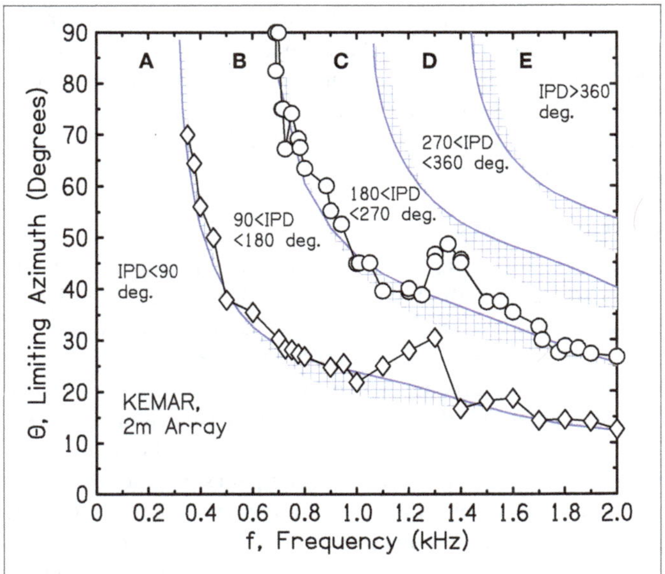

FIGURE 9 | Measured values of frequency and azimuth that lead to IPDs of 90° and 180° for a KEMAR manikin. Values were interpolated from measurements using a source array in one quadrant to the right of the manikin.

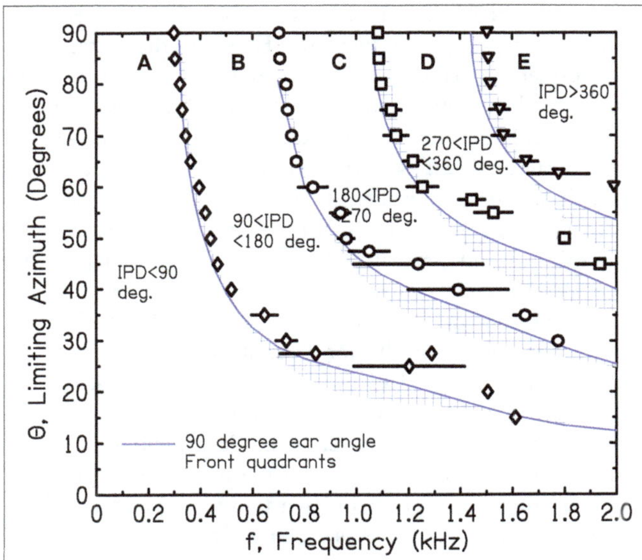

FIGURE 10 | Measured values of frequency and azimuth for IPDs of 90°, 180°, 270°, and 360° for a rotated KEMAR manikin. Values were measured in left and right quadrants in *front* of the head using a single source. The average of the two quadrants is shown together with an error bar two standard deviations in overall length. Long error bars indicate regions of non-monotonic IPD.

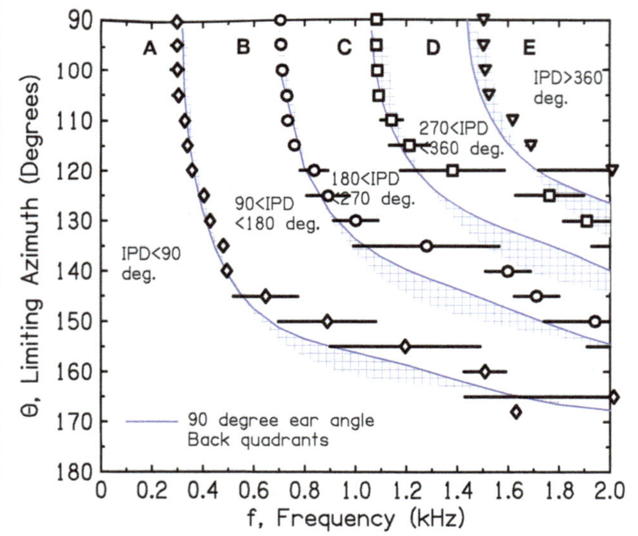

FIGURE 11 | Measured values of frequency and azimuth for IPDs of 90°, 180°, 270°, and 360° for a rotated KEMAR manikin. Values were measured in left and right quadrants in *back* of the head using a single source. The average of the two quadrants is shown together with an error bar two standard deviations in overall length. Long error bars indicate regions of non-monotonic IPD.

of the plots are not identical to **Figure 9**, the overall shape is the same, and the bumps for the 90° and 180° iso-IPD boundaries occur at the same frequencies. **Figures 10, 11** also show that the bumps occur at higher frequencies for the higher iso-IPD boundaries. The iso-IPD boundary measurements are similar for sources in front of the head (**Figure 10**) and sources behind the head (**Figure 11**). Some of the error bars seem rather long, especially as the frequency increases. However, these error bars don't represent actual errors. Instead, they represent regions of frequency and azimuth where the IPDs are not monotonic functions and oscillate around the boundary value. These badly-acting regions became evident as we rotated the head and varied the frequency. It also became evident that the disagreements between **Figures 9** and **10** owe much to the failure of the assumptions of smoothness and linearity which limit the accuracy of the interpolated values in **Figure 9**.

Our measurements have not been able to identify the feature of the head that is responsible for the mid-frequency bumps. The bumps occur at frequencies that are too low to be attributed to detailed anatomical features such as the pinnae. It is possible that they result from the overall elliptical shape of the head. **Figures 9–11** show that the effect of the bumps is to push the iso-IPD contours to somewhat higher frequencies and azimuths. Therefore, the useful region A is expanded in azimuth-frequency space. **Figures 10, 11** show that the region that is both allowed by the 1450-Hz brick wall and outside the misleading IPD region C is expanded by 5° or 10° of azimuth by the bumps. Alternatively one can observe that the frequency of the 180° IPD boundary for a given azimuth is increased. For instance, for an azimuth of 45° the boundary increases from about 1 to 1.2 kHz, which is in the right direction to agree better with the frequency of the brick wall.

DISCUSSION

THE PROBLEM

A central element of the Duplex Theory of sound localization is that ITDs in the fine structure of the sound cease to be informative once the frequency has exceeded a certain limit. The localization error measurements by Stevens and Newman (1936) have been interpreted (even recently) as indicating that the limiting frequency is 3000 Hz. However, 3000 Hz is far too high. The brick wall, which sets an upper limit for any use of ITD fine structure, is lower by a full octave. A limiting value of 1.5 kHz was suggested by Sandel et al. (1955), and this limit approximately agrees with the highest frequency for which ITD sensitivity can be measured (Brughera et al., 2013). The high-frequency limit has frequently been associated with the onset of ambiguities in the IPD caused by the rather large size of the human head. Attributing the high-frequency limit to the head size is the "ecological interpretation" (EI). Because the loss of fine-structure ITD sensitivity near 1.5 kHz is dramatically rapid, it is natural to look for a cause, and the EI provides one. However, to date, arguments for the EI have been quantitatively imprecise. The present article includes model calculations and experiments that make the statement of the EI more quantitative and precise. The calculations and experiments focused especially on critical iso-IPD boundaries where perceptions change. The calculations were all done with the spherical head diffraction model. An advantage of this model is that in the limit of an infinite source distance (plane wave incidence) the ITD and ILD depend only on the product of the frequency and head radius. Therefore, computations for a human listener at 500 Hz are the same as the computations at 1000 Hz for an animal with a head that is half the human size.

An initial comparison between ITD sensitivity and the iso-IPD boundaries offered little support for the EI. The brick-wall frequency of 1450 Hz is so high that many tones fall into the confusing region C where the IPD is greater than 180°. Tones with azimuths as small as 35° could be confusing like that, and much of the region of greatest ITD sensitivity falls into IPD region C when the azimuth is greater than 55°. The EI could be rescued by assuming that the frequency limits of the binaural system were established when heads were only half the diameter of present day human heads.

TONES EXPERIMENTS

In addition to asking whether an ecological connection actually exists between the frequency dependence of ITD sensitivity and the size of the head, one can also ask whether it is reasonable *even to expect* such a connection to exist. In the context of this paper, the frequency dependence corresponds to steady-state sine tones, but the sounds that are relevant in nature rarely meet those criteria. Therefore, one can question the value of our measurements and discussion depending on sine tones. However, the tonotopic organization of the auditory system means that different frequency regions contribute individually to an overall percept, and it is not unreasonable to characterize the influences from the regions by their responses to sine tones. For instance, specific contributions attributable to individual tonal components were demonstrated in experiments by Dye (1990). Similarly, ILD and ITD weighting functions measured by Macpherson and

Middlebrooks (2002) for lowpass and high-pass noise bands agreed with expectations based on sine tones. The use of sine tones in an ecological context can be justified by recognizing the significance of tonotopic regions and frequency limits for those regions.

A second objection to an ecological perspective based on sine tones comes from the importance of transient sounds, both in nature and in sound localization. Unlike the phase ambiguities that occur with periodic sounds, there is no physical ambiguity for transients whatever the ITD. *A priori*, there is no ecological reason for limiting the frequency range of ITD sensitivity if sound source location is determined by the interaural delays for transients. However, apparently the properties of the binaural system have not evolved to deal optimally with transient sounds. Although transients, as typified by clicks, contain timing information that spans the entire frequency range of hearing, most of that information appears to be wasted. Experiments with filtered clicks (Yost et al., 1971) show that the ITD information in clicks is not available above 1500 Hz—the same as for sine tones. Shepard and Shepard and Colburn (1976) found that ITD discrimination for clicks is not better than for 500-Hz sine tones. Klumpp and Eady (1956) studied ITD discrimination for tones, noise bursts, and clicks and found that discrimination was worst for clicks. Hartmann and Rakerd (1989) showed that the interaural parameters for a sine tone dominate a sharp onset transient for the tone unless room reflections cause the interaural parameters to be unreliable (Franssen effect). Therefore, although transient sounds would appear to provide useful, consistent information across the entire audible spectrum, they have evidently not guided the evolution of the human binaural system. In summary, despite the impoverished nature of sine-tone stimuli, it is necessary to take experiments using sine tones seriously in assessing the limitations of binaural hearing in the real world.

OTHER SPECIES

An ecological approach to binaural hearing would be incomplete without consideration of species other than our own. Other species raise several problems. First, relating ITDs to azimuths using the SHM is less justifiable. The SHM, and its Woodworth model limit, assume a perfect sphere with featureless ears at antipodes on the equator. These four assumptions are approximately realized for human heads. They are not realized for most of the several dozen mammals for which ITDs have been measured and compared with anatomy where the ears are on the top of the head. For such animals, interaural properties depend on details of the pinnae much more than for humans. Tollin and Koka (2009) noted that the height of the pinnae in cat is almost equal to the head diameter. Koka et al. (2008) found that the pinnae make a significant contribution to ILD, at 10 kHz, but pinnae are not important for humans at the anatomically scaled frequency of 2 kHz. The ITDs measured on adult chinchilla by Lupo et al. (2011) were a factor of 2 larger than predicted by the SHM. Although the ears of the marmoset are not on top of the head, they are much larger compared to head size than for human (Slee and Young, 2010).

Beyond such technical matters, a comparable approach to other animals would require comparing available ITDs or head size to binaural perception. Animal perception can be inferred from behavioral experiments, especially sound localization tasks, but mere localization is not enough. It is also necessary to know that the localization is mediated by ITD in order to arrive at comparisons equivalent to our human study.

By observing structure in the frequency dependence of the localization performance of chinchillas, Heffner et al. (1994) inferred a frequency of 2.8 kHz for the upper limit of ITD utility. This frequency leads to an IPD of 180° when the ITD is about 180 μs. This ITD can be translated into azimuth given the plot for the adult chinchilla by Jones et al. (2011). Altogether, the data indicate that sources with azimuths greater than 60° will produce IPDs greater than 180°, and thus in confusing region C. Therefore, chinchillas can be expected to face the same ITD confusions as human listeners. However, Jones et al. also note that infant chinchillas have heads that are smaller by 50%, and Tollin and Koka (2009) found the same for cats. As for humans, such a reduction in head size causes all available ITDs to fall into useful IPD regions, and the large-IPD problem goes away.

A remarkable graph in a chapter by Heffner and Heffner (2003) shows a plot of the highest frequency at which binaural phase sensitivity has been observed against the maximum ITD allowed by the anatomy. The plot shows 12 animals including human. The plot has a strong negative slope—the larger the maximum available ITD, the lower the frequency limit for useable ITD. Drawing a line on this plot corresponding to an IPD of 180°, shows that with only two exceptions, all the animals are sensitive to frequencies and ITDs such that the IPD exceeds 180° (region C). The two exceptions are for the smallest animals, least weasel and kangaroo rat.

Tollin and Koka (2009) have noted that for cats, chinchillas, and humans the head diameter increases by about a factor of two from infancy (or the onset of hearing) to adulthood. Assuming that this rule applies to all the animals on the plot one can replot the points corresponding to available ITDs that are reduced by 50%. Then all the remaining 10 animals, except for two, experience only IPDs in the useful regions A and B. The exceptions are the horse and the domestic pig. Included with humans in the region where a 50% reduction in head size eliminates confusion, are Jamaican and Egyptian fruit bats, chinchilla, cat, Japanese and pig-tailed macaques, horse, and cow. Therefore, the observed binaural sensitivity appears to be appropriate for most of the animals in infancy and not in adulthood.

CONCLUSION

Ultimately, the calculations and measurements in this article have not solved the problem posed by the disconnect between the brick wall, where human sensitivity to ITD fine structure vanishes, and current human head sizes. They have brought greater quantitative precision to the discussion. The ecological interpretation, which attributes the vanishing of ITD sensitivity to head size was shown to fail unless the frequency limits of the brainstem evolved when the head was considerably smaller than current adult human heads. Alternatively, the small head hypothesis may apply to infancy and development. If the limits of binaural processing in the brainstem were fixed during infancy, the ecological interpretation of ITD sensitivity would again be supported. Although plasticity experiments suggest that the brainstem might easily have evolved or developed to accommodate a larger head size, it is possible that there was and is no pressing need for such a change because the problem posed by the disconnect could be solved at a higher level where ITD and ILD cues are combined. The ability of higher levels to switch between several spatial maps in real time given changing circumstances, even in ferrets (Keating et al., 2013), indicates a plasticity that relieves lower levels from the need to adapt.

ACKNOWLEDGMENTS

Measurements used a computer program originally written by Prof. Brad Rakerd. We are grateful to Dr. Rickye Heffner, and to Oxford colleagues, especially Dr. Nicol Harper, for useful conversations. This work was supported by the AFOSR, grant 11NL002.

REFERENCES

Aaronson, N. L., and Hartmann, W. M. (2014). Testing, correcting, and extending the Woodworth model for interaural time difference. *J. Acoust. Soc. Am.* 135, 818–823. doi: 10.1121/1.4861243

Algazi, V. R., Avendano, C., and Duda, R. O (2001). Estimation of a spherical head model from anthropometry. *J. Audio Eng. Soc.* 49, 472–497.

Bernstein, L. R., and Trahiotis, C. (1985). Lateralization of low-frequency complex waveforms: the use of envelope-based temporal disparities. *J. Acoust. Soc. Am.* 77, 1868–1880. doi: 10.1121/1.391938

Blauert, J. (1997). *Spatial Hearing; The Psychophysics of Human Sound Localization*, revised edn. Cambridge, MA: MIT Press, 143.

Brughera, A., Dunai, L., and Hartmann, W. M. (2013). Human interaural time difference thresholds for sine tones: the high-frequency limit. *J. Acoust. Soc. Am.* 133, 2839–2855. doi: 10.1121/1.4795778

Carlile, S. (1996). "The physical and psychophysical basis of sound localization," in *Virtual Auditory Space: Generation and Applications*, ed S. Carlile (Austin, TX: R.G. Landes Co). doi: 10.1007/978-3-662-22594-3

Constan, Z. A., and Hartmann, W. M. (2003). On the detection of dispersion in the head-related transfer function. *J. Acoust. Soc. Am.* 114, 998–1008. doi: 10.1121/1.1592159

Duda, R. O., and Martens, W. L. (1998). Range dependence of the response of a spherical head model. *J. Acoust. Soc. Am.* 104, 3048–3058. doi: 10.1121/1.423886

Durlach, N. I. (1972). "Binaural signal detection - equalization and cancellation theory," in *Foundations of Modern Auditory Theory*, Vol. 2, ed J. Tobias (New York, NY: Academic Press), 369–462.

Dye, R. H. (1990). The combination of interaural information across frequencies: lateralization on the basis of interaural delay. *J. Acoust. Soc. Am.* 88, 2159–2170. doi: 10.1121/1.400113

Elpern, B. S., and Naughton, R. F. (1964). Lateralizing effects of interaural phase differences. *J. Acoust. Soc. Am.* 36, 1392–1393. doi: 10.1121/1.1919215

Harper, N. S., and McAlpine, D. (2004). Optimal neural population coding of an auditory spatial cue. *Nature* 430, 682–686. doi: 10.1038/nature02768

Hartley, R. V. L., and Fry, T. C. (1921). The binaural localization of pure tones. *Phys. Rev.* 18, 431–442. doi: 10.1103/PhysRev.18.431

Hartmann, W. M., McAdams, S., and Smith, B. K. (1990). Matching the pitch of a mistuned harmonic in an otherwise periodic complex tone. *J. Acoust. Soc. Am.* 88, 1712–1724. doi: 10.1121/1.400246

Hartmann, W. M., and Rakerd, B. (1989). Localization of sound in rooms IV - the Franssen effect. *J. Acoust. Soc. Am.* 86, 1366–1373. doi: 10.1121/1.398696

Heffner, H. E., and Heffner, R. S. (2003). "Audition," in *Handbook of Research Methods in Experimental Psychology*, ed S. Davis (Hoboken, NJ: Blackwell), 413–440. doi: 10.1002/9780470756973.ch19

Heffner, R. S., Heffner, H. E., Kearns, D., Vogel, J., and Koay, G. (1994). Sound localization in chinchillas. I: left/right discrimination. *Hear. Res.* 80, 247–257. doi: 10.1016/0378-5955(94)90116-3

Hofman, P. M., Van Riswick, J. G. A., and Van Opstal, A. J. (1998). Relearning sound localization with new ears. *Nat. Neurosci.* 1, 417–421. doi: 10.1038/1633

Johnson, D. H. (1980). Applicability of white noise nonlinear system analysis to the peripheral auditory system. *J. Acoust. Soc. Am.* 68, 876–884. doi: 10.1121/1.384826

Jones, H. G., Koka, K., Thornton, J. L., and Tollin, D. J. (2011). Concurrent development of the head and pinnae and the acoustical cues to sound location in a precocious species the Chinchilla (*Chinchilla lanigera*). *J. Assoc. Res. Otolaryngol.* 12, 127–140. doi: 10.1007/s10162-010-0242-3

Keating, P., Dahmen, J. C., and King, A. J. (2013). Context-specific reweighting of auditory spatial cues following altered experience during development. *Curr. Biol.* 23, 1291–1299. doi: 10.1016/j.cub.2013.05.045

Klumpp, R. B., and Eady, H. R. (1956). Some measurements of interaural time difference thresholds. *J. Acoust. Soc. Am.* 28, 859–860. doi: 10.1121/1.1908493

Koka, K., Read, H. L., and Tollin, D. J. (2008). The acoustical cues to sound location in the rat: measurements of directional transfer functions. *J. Acoust. Soc. Am.* 123, 4297–4309. doi: 10.1121/1.2916587

Kuhn, G. F. (1977). Model for the interaural time differences in the azimuthal plane. *J. Acoust. Soc. Am.* 62, 157–167. doi: 10.1121/1.381498 (Note that there is diffuse sound field work in J. Acoust. Soc. Am. by Kuhn.)

Lupo, J. E., Koka, K., Thornton, J. L., and Tollin, D. J. (2011). The effects of experimentally induced conductive hearing loss on spectral and temporal aspects of sound transmission through the ear. *Hear. Res.* 272, 30–41. doi: 10.1016/j.heares.2010.11.003

Lynn, R. (1990). The evolution of brain size and intelligence in man. *Hum. Evol.* 5, 241–244. doi: 10.1007/BF02437240

Macaulay, E. J., Hartmann, W. M., and Rakerd, B. (2010). The acoustical bright spot and mislocalization of tones by human listeners. *J. Acoust. Soc. Am.* 127, 1440–1449. doi: 10.1121/1.3294654

Macpherson, E. A., and Middlebrooks, J. C. (2002). Listener weighting of cues for lateral angle: the duplex theory of sound localization revisited. *J. Acoust. Soc. Am.* 111, 2219–2236. doi: 10.1121/1.1471898

Mills, A. W. (1958). On the minimum audible angle. *J. Acoust. Soc. Am.* 30, 237–246. doi: 10.1121/1.1909553

Moore, B. C. J. (1997). *Introduction to the Psychology of Hearing*, 4th edn. San Diego, CA: Academic Press, 215.

Moore, B. C. J., and Ernst, S. M. A. (2012). Frequency difference limens at high frequencies: evidence for a transition from a temporal to a place code. *J. Acoust. Soc. Am.* 132, 1542–1547. doi: 10.1121/1.4739444

Nordmark, J. O. (1976). Binaural time discrimination. *J. Acoust. Soc. Am.* 60, 870–880. doi: 10.1121/1.381167

Oxenham, A. J., Micheyl, C., Keebler, M. V., Loper, A., and Santurette, S. (2011). Pitch perception beyond the traditional existence region of pitch. *Proc. Natl. Acad. Sci. U.S.A.* 108, 7629–7634. doi: 10.1073/pnas.1015291108

Perrott, D. R., and Nelson, M. A. (1969). Limits for the detection of binaural beats. *J. Acoust. Soc. Am.* 46, 1477–1481. doi: 10.1121/1.1911890

Rabinowitz, W. M., Maxwell, J., Shao, Y., and Wei, M. (1993). Sound localization cues for a magnified head: implications from sound diffraction about a rigid sphere. *Presence* 2, 125–129.

Rayleigh, J. W. S. (Strutt, J. W.) (1896) *The Theory of Sound*, Vol. II, Dover edn. London, UK: Macmillan, 272.

Rschevkin, S. N. (1963) *A Course of Lectures on the Theory of Sound* Trans. P. E. Doak). New York, NY: Pergamon Press; McMillan, MSU lib QC225R9513 1963. [Copies in Main, Physics, and Eng. (derives diffraction on a sphere, useful for HRTF.)]

Sandel, T. T., Teas, D. C., Feddersen, W. E., and Jeffress, L. A. (1955). Localization of sound from single and paired sources. *J. Acoust. Soc. Am.* 27, 842–852. doi: 10.1121/1.1908052

Sayers, B. McA. (1964). Acoustic image lateralization judgements with binaural tones. *J. Acoust. Soc. Am.* 36, 923–926. doi: 10.1121/1.1919121

Schnupp, J., Nelken, I., and King, A. (2011) *Auditory Neuroscience, Making Sense of Sound*. Cambridge, MA: MIT Press, 177–186.

Shepard, N. T., and Colburn, H. S. (1976). Interaural time discrimination of clicks: dependence on interaural time and intensity differences. *J. Acoust. Soc. Am. (abst)* 59, S23. doi: 10.1121/1.2002500

Shinn-Cunningham, B. G., Durlach, N. I., and Held, R. M. (1998). Adapting to supernormal auditory localization cues. I. Bias and resolution. *J. Acoust. Soc. Am.* 103, 3656–3666. doi: 10.1121/1.423088

Slee, S. J., and Young, E. D. (2010). Sound localization cues in the marmoset monkey. *Hear. Res.* 260, 96–108. doi: 10.1016/j.heares.2009.12.001

Stevens, S. S., and Newman, E. B. (1936). The location of actual sources of sound. *Am. J. Psych.* 48, 297–306. doi: 10.2307/1415748

Stern, R. M., Wang, DeL., and Brown, G. J. (2005). "Binaural sound localization," in *Auditory Scene Analysis*, eds DeL. Wang and G. J. Brown (New York, NY: Wiley), 149.

Strutt, J. W. (1907). On our perception of sound direction. *Phil. Mag.* 13, 214–232. doi: 10.1080/14786440709463595

Strutt, J. W. (1909). On our perception of the direction of sound. *Proc. Roy Soc.* 83, 61–64. doi: 10.1098/rspa.1909.0073

Tollin, D. J., and Koka, K. (2009). Postnatal development of sound pressure transformations by the head and pinnae of the cat: binaural characteristics. *J. Acoust. Soc. Am.* 126, 3125–3136. doi: 10.1121/1.3257234

Treeby, B. E., Paurobally, R. M., and Pan, J. (2007). The effect of impedance on interaural azimuth cues derived from a spherical head model. *J. Acoust. Soc. Am.* 121, 2217–2226. doi: 10.1121/1.2709868

Tzounopoulos, T., and Kraus, N. (2009). Learning to encode timing: mechanisms of plasticity in the auditory brainstem. *Neuron* 62, 463–469. doi: 10.1016/j.neuron.2009.05.002

von Hornbostel, E. M., and Wertheimer, M. (1920). Über die Wahrnehmung der Schallrichtung, (On the perception of the direction of sound). *Sitzungsber. Akad. Wiss. (Berl.)* 20, 388–396.

Woodworth, R. S. (1938) *Experimental Psychology*. New York, NY: Holt. 520–523.

Yost, W. A. (1981). Lateral position of sinusoids presented with interaural intensive and temporal differences. *J. Acoust. Soc. Am.* 70, 397–409. doi: 10.1121/1.386775

Yost, W. A., and Hafter, E. R. (1987). "Lateralization," in *Directional Hearing*, eds W. A. Yost and G. Gourevitch (New York, NY: Springer), 56. doi: 10.1007/978-1-4612-4738-8

Yost, W. A., Wightman, F. L., and Green, D. M. (1971). Lateralization of filtered clicks. *J. Acoust. Soc. Am.* 50, 1526–1531. doi: 10.1121/1.1912806

Zwislocki, J., and Feldman, R. S. (1956). Just noticeable differences in dichotic phase. *J. Acoust. Soc. Am.* 28, 860–864. doi: 10.1121/1.1908495

APPENDIX

ROTATION-AZIMUTH TRANSFORM

The azimuth of a source with respect to an observer is an angle in the horizontal plane, as viewed from overhead. It is measured clockwise from the forward direction (determined by the nose) and extends through a full 360°, −180° to +180°. The azimuth angle occurs at the intersection of a line in the forward direction and a line that includes the center of the head (COH) and the source. The azimuth can be increased, for example by 30°, by moving the source location clockwise by 30° along a circle centered on the COH. Alternatively, the azimuth can be increased by 30° by leaving the source location fixed and rotating the head counterclockwise. However, this counterclockwise rotation of the head is not a rotation of 30°. That is because the axis of rotation for a human head, attached in the usual way to the human neck, does not pass through the COH. The purpose of this section is to show how to compensate for a discrepancy such as this. It develops the rotation-azimuth transformation.

The critical assumptions made in this treatment are (1) that the axis of rotation is vertical (perpendicular to the horizontal plane of the sources) and (2) that the extended line from the nose to the COH intersects the axis of rotation. The latter assumption is the "colinear assumption."

Summary

The essential geometry is shown in **Figure A1**. The source is initially in the forward direction. The rotation of the head from the forward direction is angle ϕ. The resulting source azimuth is θ. The relationship between ϕ and θ depends on b, the distance from the axis of rotation to the COH, and it depends on r, the distance from the axis of rotation to the source. It does not depend on b and r separately, but only on the ratio, $\rho = b/r$, where ρ must be less than 1. There is a three step process for determining θ from ϕ:
(1) Compute θ as

$$\theta = \arctan\left[\frac{\sin\phi}{\rho + \cos\phi}\right]. \qquad (1)$$

Because r is positive, ratio ρ has the same sign as directed distance b. If the axis of rotation lies between the COH and the nose (**Figure A1A**), then b is positive, and the magnitude of θ is less than the magnitude of ϕ. If the COH lies between the axis of rotation and the nose (**Figure A1B**) then b is negative, and the magnitude of θ is greater than the magnitude of ϕ. Because $\sin\phi/\cos\phi = \tan\phi$, it is evident that in the limit of a very distant source ($\rho = 0$) Equation (1) leads to $\theta = \phi$.
(2) Realize that ϕ and θ must both have the same sign. If Equation (1) causes θ to have a sign opposite to ϕ then add 180° to the computed value of θ. This is the correct way to deal with the ambiguity caused by the principal value range of the arctangent.
(3) If θ turns out to be greater than 180°, bring θ into the range from −180° to +180° by subtracting 360°.

This three-step procedure is adequate for all possible rotations, positive and negative. **Figure A2** shows the transformation between head rotation angle ϕ and the resulting source azimuth θ for two values of ρ, 0.2 and 0.8. The latter value corresponds to a source that is very close to the head, but it is included here because it illustrates mathematical asymmetries in the transformation that are not so apparent for small values of ρ such as 0.2.

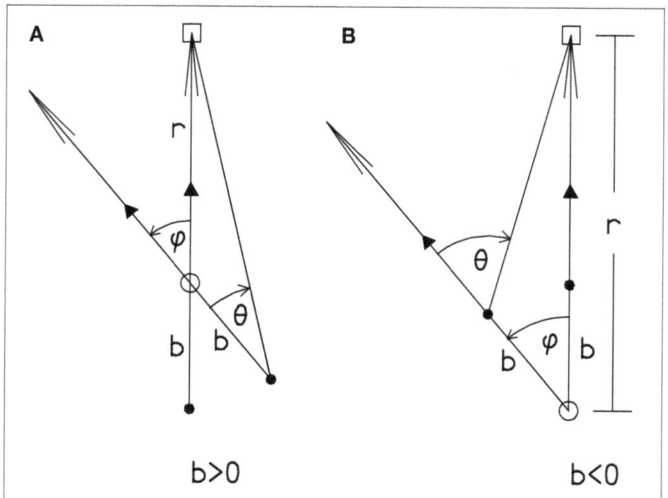

FIGURE A1 | The source of sound, indicated by the square, is fixed in space. The head is shown in two orientations, defined by the arrows indicating the forward directions. Consistent with the definition of the forward direction, the arrow passes through the nose (triangle) and the COH (black dot). Because of the colinear assumption, it also passes through the axis of rotation shown by the open circle. In case **(A)** the center of the head is behind the axis of rotation so that b and ρ are positive. In case **(B)** the center of the head is in front of the axis of rotation so that b and ρ are negative. Equation (1) and the three steps apply to both cases. The directed arcs show the positive directions for θ and ϕ.

Details of the transformation

All angles are measured from the forward direction. The forward direction is the directed line from the COH to the

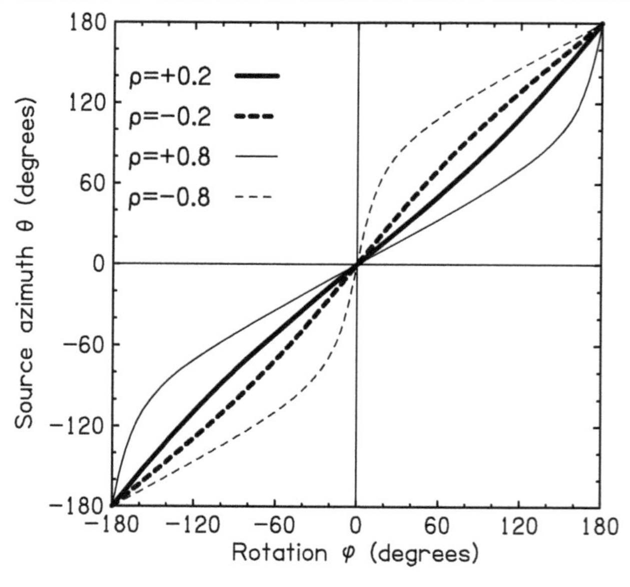

FIGURE A2 | Example calculation of the azimuth as a function of the head rotation angle for $\rho = \pm 0.2$ (heavy line) and $\rho = \pm 0.8$ (light line) for all possible values of the rotation.

nose. The source azimuth θ is positive clockwise (as seen from the top) so that sources with positive azimuth are to the right of the observer. Consistent with this convention, the convention for the sign of the head rotation ϕ is positive counterclockwise—again putting a source to the right of the observer.

We define the COH as a point in the real head chosen so that the diffraction around the head is best approximated by the diffraction by a sphere centered on that point. The COH does not depend on the location of the ears. In general, a line drawn between the ears (the interaural axis) will not necessarily pass through the COH.

Equation (1) for azimuth θ comes from solving the triangle shown in **Figure A1** using the sine law so that

$$\frac{\sin\theta}{r} = \frac{\sin(\theta - \phi)}{b}. \tag{2}$$

The arctangent formula is a simplification of this result from the sine law.

2

Auditory/visual distance estimation: Accuracy and variability

Paul W. Anderson*[1] *and Pavel Zahorik*[1,2]

[1] *Department of Psychological and Brain Sciences, University of Louisville, Louisville, KY, USA*
[2] *Division of Communicative Disorders, Department of Surgery, School of Medicine, University of Louisville, Louisville, KY, USA*

Correspondence:
Pavel Zahorik, Division of Communicative Disorders, Department of Surgery, School of Medicine, University of Louisville, MDA Building, Suite 220, 627 S. Preston Street, Louisville, KY 40292, USA
e-mail: pavel.zahorik@louisville.edu

Past research has shown that auditory distance estimation improves when listeners are given the opportunity to see all possible sound sources when compared to no visual input. It has also been established that distance estimation is more accurate in vision than in audition. The present study investigates the degree to which auditory distance estimation is improved when matched with a congruent visual stimulus. Virtual sound sources based on binaural room impulse response (BRIR) measurements made from distances ranging from approximately 0.3 to 9.8 m in a concert hall were used as auditory stimuli. Visual stimuli were photographs taken from the participant's perspective at each distance in the impulse response measurement setup presented on a large HDTV monitor. Participants were asked to estimate egocentric distance to the sound source in each of three conditions: auditory only (A), visual only (V), and congruent auditory/visual stimuli (A+V). Each condition was presented within its own block. Sixty-two participants were tested in order to quantify the response variability inherent in auditory distance perception. Distance estimates from both the V and A+V conditions were found to be considerably more accurate and less variable than estimates from the A condition.

Keywords: spatial hearing, sound localization, distance perception, multimodal, virtual sound

INTRODUCTION

Within the field of human sound localization, the perception of sound source distance has received relatively little scientific study compared to the perception of sound source direction. This is surprising given that the perception of distance is at least as important as direction for conveying important spatial information about our surroundings, such as locating or avoiding auditory objects under conditions when visual information may be ineffective or unavailable. Although generally less is known about auditory distance perception (ADP) than directional perception, it is clear that ADP results in both highly variable judgments (Zahorik et al., 2005) as well as systematic judgment biases (Zahorik, 2002a), especially when compared to directional localization performance, which is comparatively accurate and consistent (Middlebrooks and Green, 1991). In terms of judgment bias, there appears to be general consensuses across a variety of studies and listening conditions that far distances are underestimated while closer distances are overestimated (Zahorik et al., 2005). These results are seemingly at odds with our everyday experience of auditory space that appears to be consistent and relatively accurate. One possible explanation for this discrepancy is that in many everyday situations, ADP may be influenced by additional spatial information provided by other sensory modalities, such as vision. The goal of the current study is to better understand how visual input may influence both bias and variability in ADP.

Visual influences on the apparent direction of a sound source are well-known: The superior spatial resolution of vision dominates, or "captures," the less precise directional information input through the auditory modality. This effect, which underlies the ventriloquist's illusion, can influence sound sources separated from visual targets by as much as 55° (Thurlow and Jack, 1973). It also appears to be strengthened by temporal synchrony between auditory and visual targets (Jack and Thurlow, 1973), but is unaffected by either attention to the visual distracter or feedback provided to the participant (Vroomen and de Gelder, 2004).

Visual capture also appears to function in the distance dimension. For example, Gardner (1968) demonstrated a form of visual capture, he termed "The Proximity-Image Effect," in which the nearest visible sound source is mistakenly chosen by listeners to be the actual sound source. Mershon et al. (1980) later discovered that the presence of a visual stimulus does not always elicit an underestimation of the physical distance of a sound source, as Gardner's (1968) data suggest. They found that when an occluded sound source was located closer to listeners than a visible dummy loudspeaker, listeners would overestimate the distance of the sound source as being located at the more distant dummy loudspeaker. Taken together, the results from these two studies clearly demonstrate that the presence of plausible visual targets can influence ADP and that under the appropriate circumstances, this influence results in reduced ADP accuracy.

Under other circumstances, visual information can improve ADP accuracy. For example, Zahorik (2001) demonstrated that ADP accuracy in a reverberant environment improves when listeners have the opportunity to view multiple possible sound sources prior to making judgments. Two groups of listeners were tasked with judging the apparent distance to sound sources along a loudspeaker array. One group was able to view the entire loudspeaker array, and the second group was blindfolded throughout the experiment. Distance judgments provided by the group who were able to view the loudspeaker array were more accurate than judgments from the auditory-only group. Similar conclusions were drawn in a study performed by Calcagno et al. (2012) in which visual cues in the form of LEDs were either present or absent during an ADP task in a dark room. Their setup involved a mobile loudspeaker that was moved along a track between trials and LEDs that were placed at standard intervals along the track. When LEDs were present listeners were informed of the distance to the LEDs prior to the task. Results showed that auditory distance judgments were more accurate when the LEDs were present.

Visual information can also affect the variability of ADP. Results from Zahorik (2001) found ADP variability was reduced in the presence of visual information. However, Calcagno et al. (2012) did not observe a reduction in variability in the presence of visual cues. The reason for these contradictory results may arise from the methodologies used in the two studies. In Zahorik (2001) visual information included information about the room and all possible locations of the loudspeakers. On the other hand, Calcagno et al.'s (2012) listeners were limited in their visual information to LEDs in a dark room. Therefore, more reliable visual distance information in Zahorik (2001) may have led to less variable distance judgments.

Perhaps more interesting are the potential causes of large ADP variability in the absence of visual information. Few studies have explicitly examined this issue given the experimental demands of collecting datasets of sufficient size to reliably quantify ADP variability. Such variability may be conceptualized as originating from at least two sources: one related to the judgments/percepts within a single listener, and one related to differences in judgments/percepts between listeners. Past studies of ADP have not been designed to measure these sources of variability independently. Instead they typically have concentrated on a single source of variability. For example, some ADP studies have utilized a large number ($n = 80$–200) of listeners (Mershon and King, 1975; Mershon and Bowers, 1979; Mershon et al., 1989), but tested relatively few source distances and/or few repetitions per distance. Such designs limit investigation of ADP variability within individual listeners. Other studies (Coleman, 1968; Ashmead et al., 1995; Zahorik, 2002a) have tested greater numbers of source distances with many repetitions at each distance, but at the cost of evaluating fewer individual subjects overall ($n = 6$–9). Zahorik et al. (2005) reanalyzed the results from Zahorik (2002a) to assess ADP judgment variability and found that distance judgments for a sound source may vary between 20 and 60% of the source distance. However, given the relatively small number of listeners evaluated, it is difficult to know how these results may generalize to the population as a whole.

The present study was motivated by gaps in knowledge surrounding the interaction of vision and audition in the distance domain as well as the inherent judgment variability associated with ADP. To assess the degree to which ADP is improved when an auditory stimulus is matched with a congruent visual stimulus, participants judged egocentric distance to a virtual sound source in three conditions: auditory only (A), visual only (V), and congruent auditory/visual stimuli (A+V). Virtual auditory space techniques (Wightman and Kistler, 1989) were used for distance simulation, in order to allow for simple and rapid switching between source distances throughout the experiment. Although based on past results (Zahorik, 2001), it is expected that congruent visual stimuli will result in ADP judgments that are more veridical and less variable, the present study design allows for precise quantification of these variability reduction effects and offers improved generalization to the normal-hearing population as a whole.

MATERIALS AND METHODS

PARTICIPANTS

There were a total of 62 (41 female) participants, ranging in age from 18 to 46 ($M = 22.82$). Five participants were removed from analysis: Four because of concerns about their understanding of the task, and due to concerns about self-reported hearing status. All participants had normal hearing based on either self-reports ($n = 30$) or pure-tone audiometric screening ($n = 32$) at 25 dB HL from 250 to 8000 Hz. Informed consent was obtained from all participants prior to data collection, and participants were awarded either monetary compensation or course credit for their participation. All procedures in this study involving human subject participants were approved by the University of Louisville Institutional Review Board (IRB).

AUDITORY STIMULI

Binaural room impulse responses (BRIRs) were measured from 11 logarithmically-spaced distances ranging from 0.3048 to 9.7536 m at 0° azimuth in a 558-seat concert hall (Margaret Comstock Concert Hall, University of Louisville). The hall had a broadband reverberation time (T_{60}) of 1.9 s (ISO-3382, 1997). The auditorium was a complex shape with sloping floors and moveable "clouds" in the ceiling. It had a total volume of approximately 5225 m^3 (28.956 × 16.9164 × 10.668 m; L × W × H). All BRIR measurements were made with a KEMAR manikin (G.R.A.S. Type 45BM), with IEC711 ear-canal simulators (G.R.A.S. RA0045) and large pinnae (G.R.A.S. KB1060/1) at a fixed location near the edge of the performance stage, facing away from audience seating. The sound source, a high-quality 2-way co-axial loudspeaker (Beyma 8BX) mounted in a sealed 13.5-l cabinet, was moved across the stage to manipulate distance. BRIRs were estimated using Maximum Length Sequence (MLS) system identification techniques (Rife and Vanderkooy, 1989). The MLS signal was 2.73 s in duration (17-th order MLS), sampled at 48 kHz with 24-bit resolution. Five repetitions of this signal were presented and averaged to improve signal-to-noise ratio (SNR), which was <35 dB (0.2–20 kHz) at 9.7536 m.

All BRIR measurements were post-processed to compensate for the response characteristics of the measurement loudspeaker as well as the presentation headphones (Beyerdynamic DR-990 Pro) when coupled to the head. Because residual noise in the measured BRIRs can be easily detectable following virtual sound source synthesis, an additional time-windowing procedure was used to further improve SNR in the BRIRs. The procedure was based on that described by Zahorik (2002a). Briefly, the BRIR was first divided into 30 frequency bands (1/3-octave bandwidth, Gaussian shape) and an energy-decay curve was computed for each band using reverse integration. A straight line was then fit to the decay curve in dB/s over an energy range of −5 to −35 dB. This fit was then used to derive an exponentially-decaying time window for each frequency band. The time windows were then applied in each band, and the results summed across bands. This procedure was effective at improving SNR particularly in the later portions of the BRIR. The source signal for virtual synthesis was a 100 ms sample of Gaussian noise.

VISUAL STIMULI

Visual stimuli were digital photographs of the measurement loudspeaker taken from the position of the head of the KEMAR manikin (see **Figure 1**). The camera/lens combination (Nikon D70/Tokina f4 12 mm focal length) produced nearly a 90° field of view. The resulting images (2000 × 3008 pixels) were displayed on a high-quality large screen HDTV (either 46 or 40 in. diagonal). The viewing angle was approximately 51° at the participant's location.

PROCEDURE

The entire experiment took place in a double-walled sound proof booth (Acoustic Systems, Austin, TX). Participants were asked to estimate egocentric distance to the sound source in each of the three conditions: A, V, and A+V. Participants had the opportunity to play the auditory stimulus multiple times before entering their distance judgment. Once the stimulus was played a distance judgment could be entered at any time. Therefore, some listeners may have only had one exposure to the stimulus on a given trial while other listeners may have had multiple exposures on a given trial (data on the number of times a participant listened to the stimulus were not recorded). In the V and A+V conditions the visual stimulus was present for the entire duration of the trial.

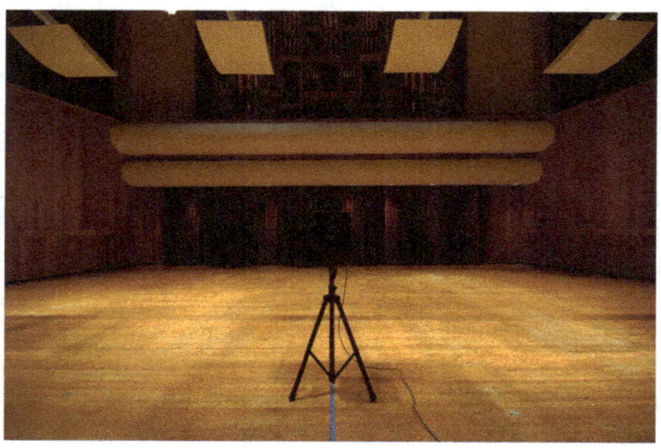

FIGURE 1 | Visual stimulus example. A photograph of the measurement loudspeaker was taken at each distance from where the KEMAR mannequin was placed during BRIR measurement at the front of the stage. In the V and A+V conditions a photograph was presented on a large flat screen HDTV and the participant provided a distance judgment to the sound source. In this example, the measurement loudspeaker is placed 2.44 m in front of the camera in Comstock Hall.

Judgments were input using a computer keyboard. Participants had the option of using units of either meters or feet. All judgments were required to be precise to two decimal places, and responses in feet were transformed to meters prior to all data analysis. Listeners were instructed to reserve a response of zero for a percept of inside the head locatedness (Blauert, 1997, p. 132). Most participants ($n = 45$), provided judgments in all three conditions. Each condition was tested within its own block of trials, which included 10 judgments for each of the 11 source distances, for a total of 110 judgments. The order of blocks was counterbalanced, and the order of trials within each block was randomized. An additional set of listeners ($n = 17$), participated only in the A condition and contributed 30 judgments for each of the 11 source distances for a total of 330 judgments. The data from this group of listeners were collected to increase the sample of auditory distance judgments, since we were interested in the amount of intra-subject variability inherent in ADP. Feedback was not provided to the participants. MATLAB software (Mathworks Inc., Natick, MA) was used for stimulus presentation and data collection.

DATA ANALYSIS

Following methods used in previous ADP and VDP studies (Da Silva, 1985; Sedgwick, 1986; Zahorik, 2001, 2002a; Zahorik et al., 2005), power functions of the following form were fit (least-squares criterion) to the geometric means in each condition: $\hat{y}_r = k\Phi_r^a$ ($\hat{y}_r$ = perceived distance, k = constant, a = power-law exponent, Φ_r = target source distance). The fit parameters, k and a, were used as measures of judgment accuracy. The exponent indicates the amount of non-linear compression ($a < 1$) or expansion ($a > 1$) in the function. The constant indicates the amount of linear compression ($k < 1$) or expansion ($k > 1$) in the function. The exponent and constant parameters are equivalent to slope and intercept respectively when perceived distance and physical distance are represented in logarithmic coordinates. Residual error from the fitted functions as well as the proportion of variance accounted for by the fitted function (R^2) were used to describe both between-subject and within-subject response variability. Measures of accuracy and variability were compared between conditions using independent samples t-tests with Bonferroni correction. Independent samples t-tests were used because not all subjects were tested in all conditions. Intra-subject variability was evaluated using independent t-tests comparing listeners in the A condition who performed 10 judgments per distance vs. those who performed 30 judgments per distance. Reliability of distance judgments across conditions was analyzed by computing the Pearson correlations across conditions for the fit parameters and R^2 values. All analyses were performed using MATLAB (Mathworks Inc., Natick, MA), except for the t-tests, which were performed using SPSS (IBM Corp., Armonk, NY).

RESULTS

Distance estimation results for a single representative participant (Code QAD) are shown in **Figures 2A–C** for the A, V, and A+V conditions respectively. Dots indicate the raw distance judgments provided by the participant (y), while the open circles represent the geometric mean ($\bar{y}$) for each distance. The function fits for

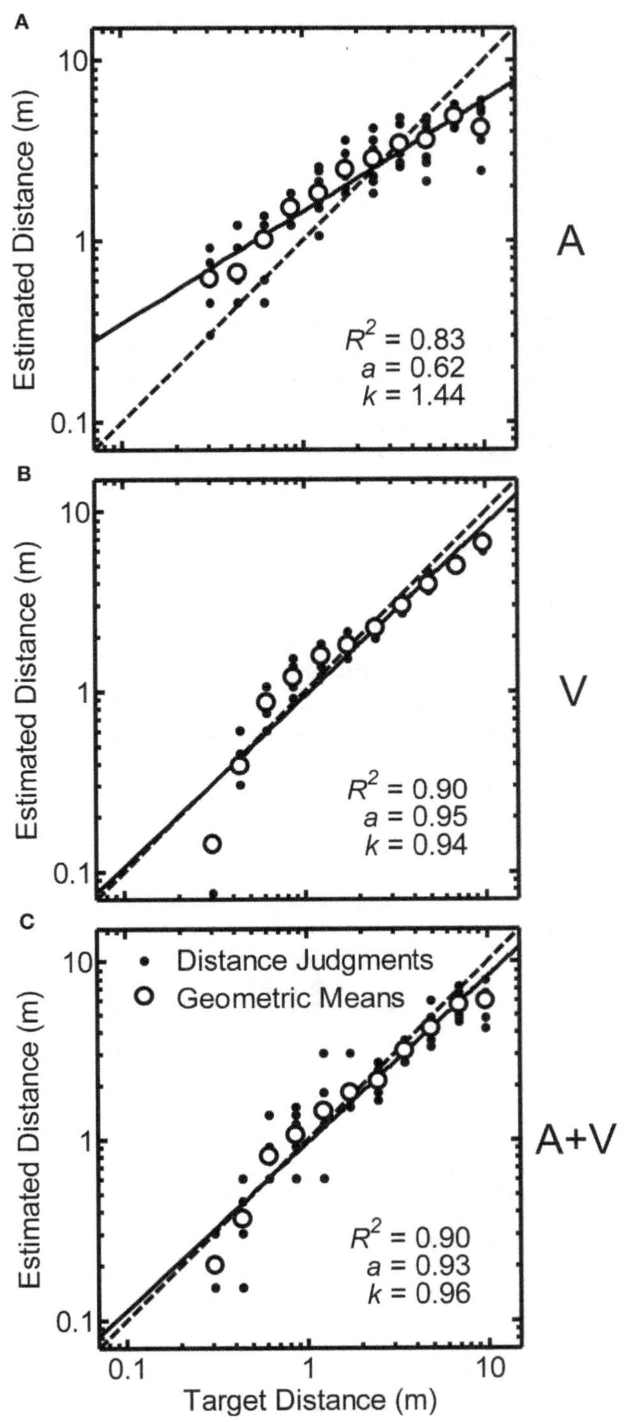

FIGURE 2 | Data from a single representative participant (code QAD) for auditory ("A," panel A), visual ("V," panel B), and auditory/visual ("A+V," panel C) conditions plotted on logarithmic axes. Dots show raw distance judgments (y): 10 replications/distance. Open circles indicate geometric means ($\bar{y}$) for each target distance. Data from each condition were fit with a power function ($\hat{y}$; solid line) of the form $\hat{y}_r = k\Phi_r^a$ ($\hat{y}_r$ = perceived distance, k = constant, a = power-law exponent, Φ_r = target source distance). Fit parameters and the proportion of variability accounted for by the fit (R^2) are shown in each panel. Perfectly accurate performance is indicated by the dotted line in each panel.

each condition are plotted as a solid line ($\hat{y}$), and the diagonal dotted line represents a perfectly accurate relationship between target distance and estimated distance (i.e., $a = 1$, $k = 1$). Each panel includes the fit parameters (a and k) and proportion of variability accounted for by the fit (R^2). Consistent with previous studies on both auditory (Zahorik et al., 2005) and visual distance estimation (Da Silva, 1985; Sedgwick, 1986), power functions appear to be good fits to the data, although the distance judgments are more accurate and less variable in the conditions with visual stimuli for this participant, as evidenced by the increase in R^2 and the facts that a and k are closer to 1.

Identical analyses were conducted for all remaining participants in each of the three stimulus conditions. Any distance judgments of "zero" were noted and removed from all subsequent analyses. Of most interest were zero responses in the A condition, since listeners were instructed to only provide a judgment of zero when the stimulus was perceived as located "inside the head." Only 0.25% of all judgments in the A condition were zero, indicating that the virtual sound sources were perceived as being localized outside the head in the vast majority of cases.

The distributions of R^2 values across all participants are displayed in **Figures 3A–C** for the A, V, and A—V conditions respectively. Because the histograms have a slightly negative skew, both the mean ± one standard deviation and median (interquartile range) are included in each panel along with the number of participants in each condition. High R^2 values indicate that power functions were good fits to the data and support the validity of the calculated power function fit parameters. The R^2 values were generally lower without visual input. The mean R^2 value for the A condition ($M = 0.638$, $SD = 0.216$) was significantly lower than the mean R^2 value for both the V ($M = 0.874$, $SD = 0.170$) and A+V ($M = 0.836$, $SD = 0.184$) conditions, as demonstrated by independent-samples t-tests with Bonferroni correction [A vs. V: $t_{(105)} = -6.085$, $p < 0.0003$; A vs. A+V: $t_{(105)} = -4.979$, $p < 0.0003$; V vs. A+V conditions: $t_{(88)} = 1.012$, $p > 0.945$]. Overall, these results suggest that power functions were relatively good fits to the data, but slightly less good for the A condition.

Exponents from the power function fits provide information about the amount of non-linear compression in the distance judgments. **Figures 4A–C** display histograms of the exponent values across all participants for the A, V, and A+V conditions respectively. Each panel includes the mean ± one standard deviation, the median (and interquartile range), and the number of participants in each condition. Considerable inter-subject variability may be noted. Using independent-samples t-tests with Bonferroni correction, it was determined that the exponents in the A condition ($M = 0.614$, $SD = 0.299$) were significantly lower than the exponents for both the V condition ($M = 0.916$, $SD = 0.267$) and A+V condition ($M = 0.874$, $SD = 0.271$) indicating greater compression in the A condition [A vs. V: $t_{(105)} = -5.398$, $p < 0.0003$; A vs. A+V: $t_{(105)} = -4.612$, $p < 0.0003$; V vs. A+V conditions: $t_{(88)} = 0.755$, $p > 0.999$]. One-sample t-tests were also performed to determine whether the exponents in each condition were different from a value of one, which corresponds to no compression. Exponents in all three conditions were significantly less than one [A: $t_{(61)} = -10.150$, $p < 0.0001$; V: $t_{(44)} = -2.082$, $p < 0.043$; A+V: $t_{(44)} = -3.115$,

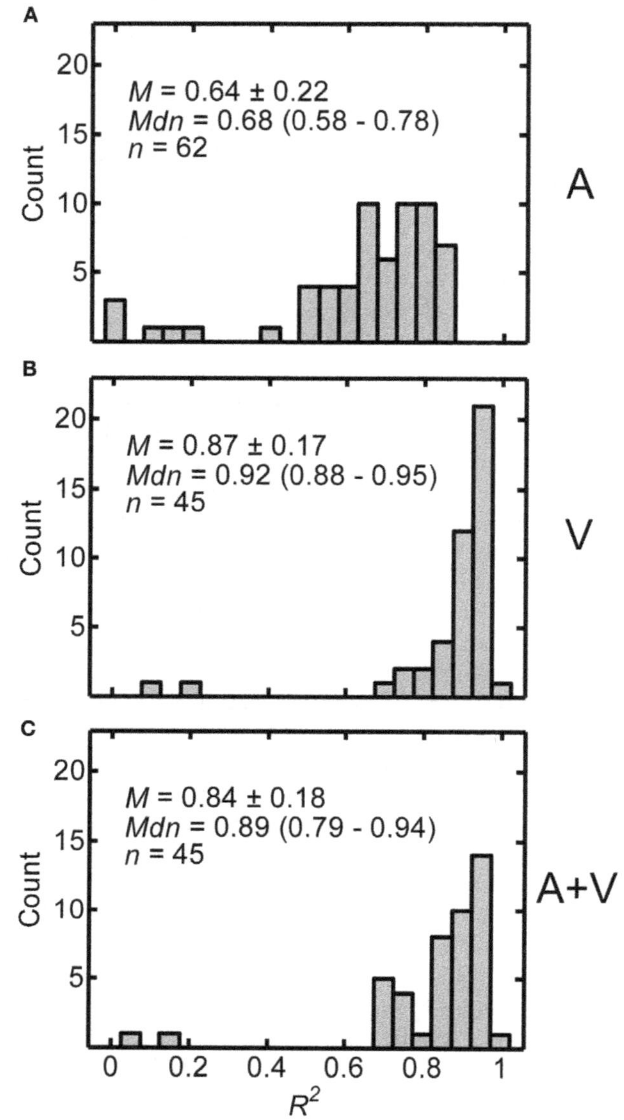

FIGURE 3 | Distributions of R^2 values from the power function fits for A (A), V (B), and A+V (C) conditions across participants. Each panel includes the following summary statistics: mean, $M \pm$ one standard deviation, median, *Mdn* (interquartile range), and number of participants, *n*, in each condition.

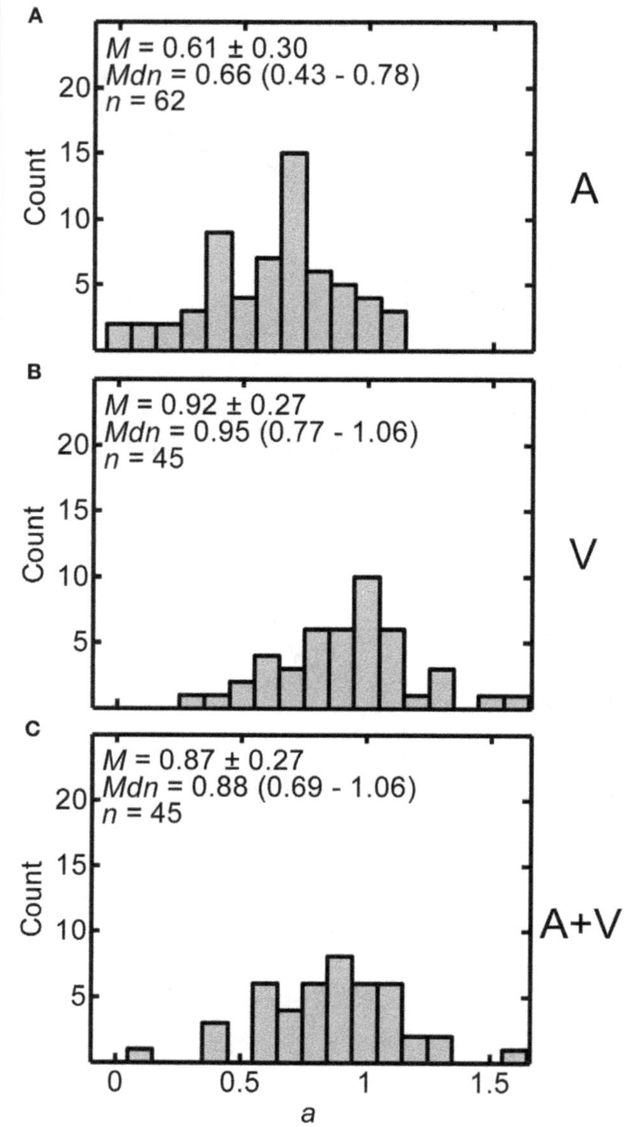

FIGURE 4 | Distributions of exponents (*a*) from power fits for all participants in A (A), V (B), and A+V (C) conditions. Each panel includes the following summary statistics: mean, $M \pm$ one standard deviation, median, *Mdn* (interquartile range), and number of participants, *n*, in each condition.

$p < 0.003$], indicating exponential compression in all conditions.

Constant values from the fits provide information about the amount of linear compression/expansion of the function. **Figures 5A–C** display histograms of the distributions of constant values across participants in the A, V, and A+V conditions respectively. The histograms are positively skewed, so both the mean $\pm$ one standard deviation and median (interquartile range) are included in each panel. Each panel also includes the number of participants in each condition. As in **Figure 4**, considerable inter-subject variability may be noted. Based on independent *t*-tests with Bonferroni correction, the constants in the A condition ($M = 2.217$, $SD = 1.992$) were significantly greater than constants in either the V ($M = 1.281$, $SD = 0.801$) or A+V conditions ($M = 1.383$, $SD = 0.912$). Overall, these results suggest that near distances are more overestimated in the A condition than in the V or A+V condition. The V and A+V conditions were not significantly different from each other [A vs. V: $t_{(85.359)} = 3.343$, $p < 0.003$; A vs. A+V: $t_{(90.815)} = 2.904$, $p < 0.015$; V vs. A+V: $t_{(88)} = -0.559$, $p > 0.999$]. One-sample *t*-tests confirmed that constants in all three conditions were greater than one [A: $t_{(61)} = 4.810$, $p < 0.0001$; V: $t_{(44)} = 2.356$, $p < 0.023$; A+V: $t_{(44)} = 2.816$, $p < 0.007$], indicating overestimation for distances less than 1 m in all conditions.

In order to assess the intra-subject variability of distance judgments, residuals from the power function fits for each

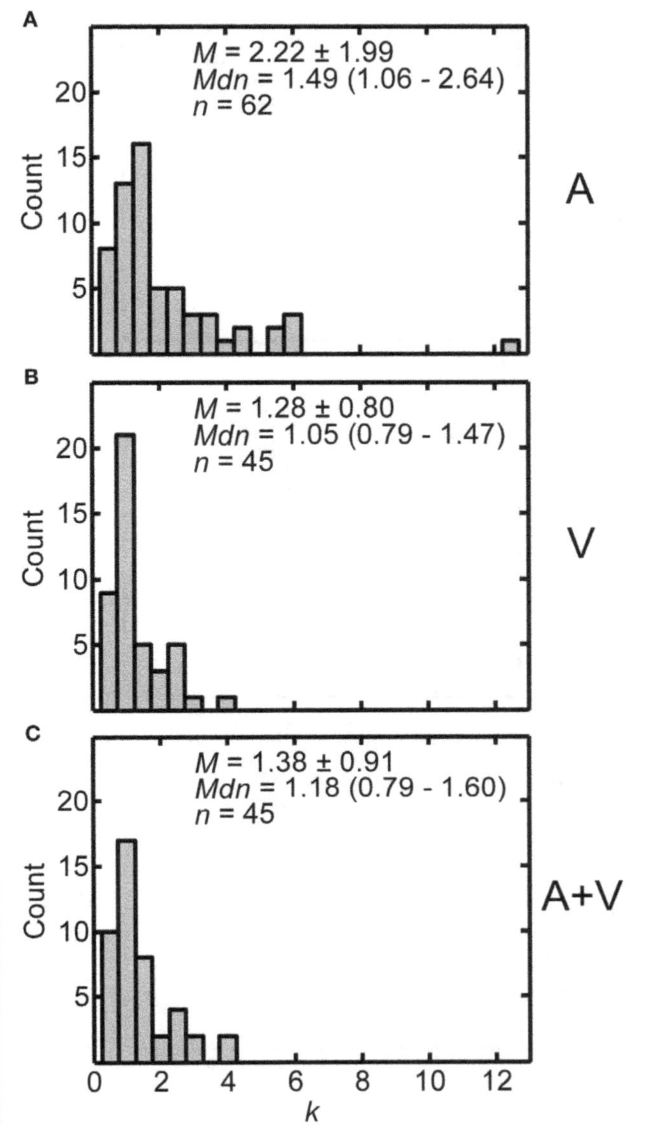

FIGURE 5 | Distributions of constants (k) from power fits for all participants in the A (A), V (B), and A+V (C) conditions. Each panel includes the following summary statistics: mean, M ± one standard deviation, median, *Mdn* (interquartile range), and number of participants, n, in each condition.

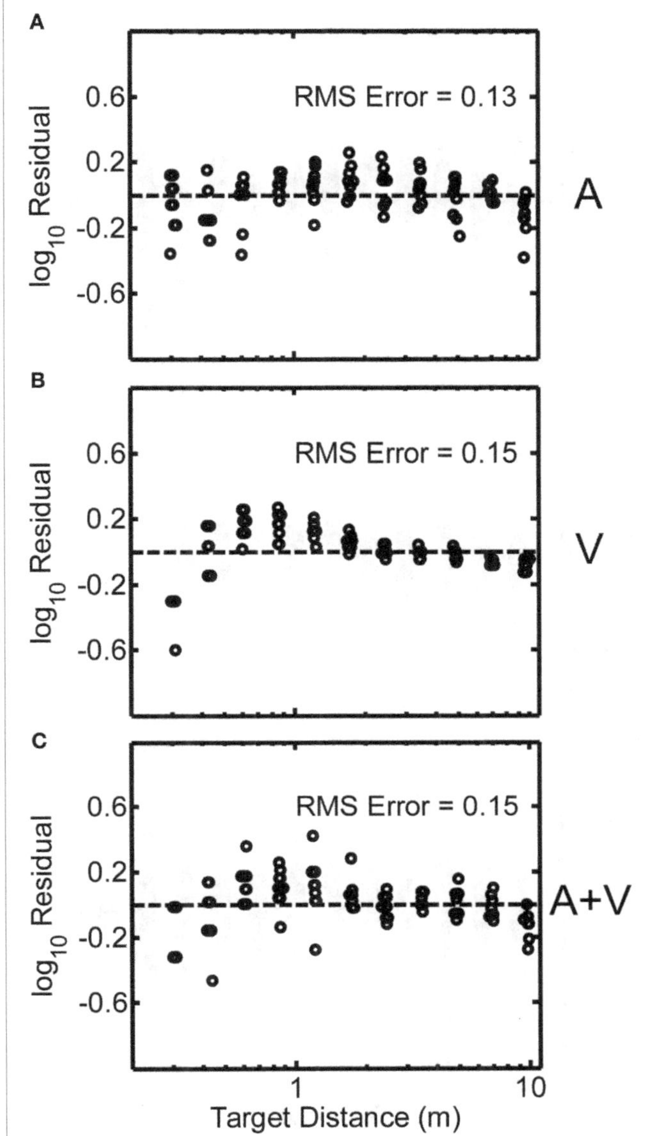

FIGURE 6 | Log-transformed residuals from the power function fit for a single representative participant (code QAD, see Figure 2) for the A (A), V (B), and A+V (C) conditions. RMS error across all distances is indicated in each panel. Small random jitter was added to the target distances on the x-axis for visualization purposes.

participant were analyzed for each condition. Such analyses allow the judgment variability explained by the power function fit to be removed from the data. What remains is an estimate of judgment error independent of the power-law relationship. **Figures 6A–C** display the log-transformed residuals plotted as a function of target distance in the A, V, and A+V conditions respectively for a representative participant (code QAD, see **Figure 2**). The RMS error listed in each panel is a measure of average deviation of the responses from the best-fitting power function, and was computed as the square-root of the mean squared deviation of the log-transformed residuals from zero. Although **Figure 6B** shows the log-transformed residuals decreasing in variability with increasing distance, this pattern is not generally representative of all participants in the study.

Log-transformed residuals pooled across all participants in the study are shown in **Figures 7A–C**. These residuals represent error remaining after power functions were fit to the individual subject data. Overall, the spread of the residuals was relatively homogeneous as a function of source distance, which indicates that judgment error was relatively independent of source distance. This was the rationale for our residual RMS error metric, which averages over all source distances. We also examined the distributions of the log-transformed residuals across all target distances. **Figures 8A–C** display normal-probability plots of the

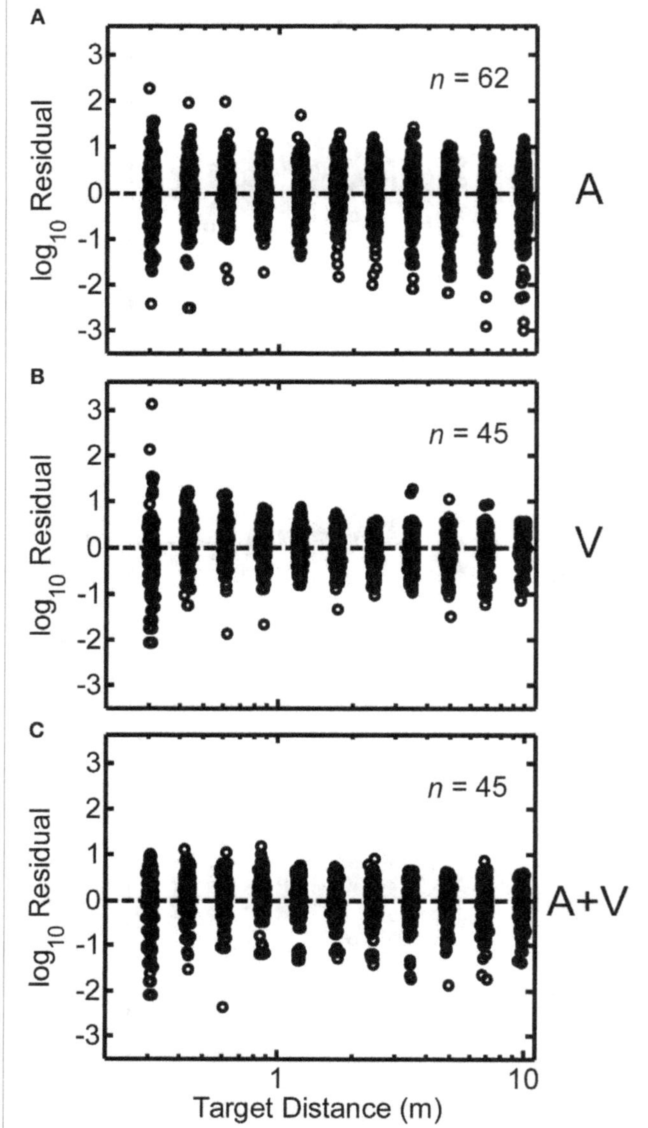

FIGURE 7 | Same as Figure 6, except results from all participants are shown. Each panel includes the number of participants per condition. Note that the spread of the residuals is relatively homogeneous as a function of distance.

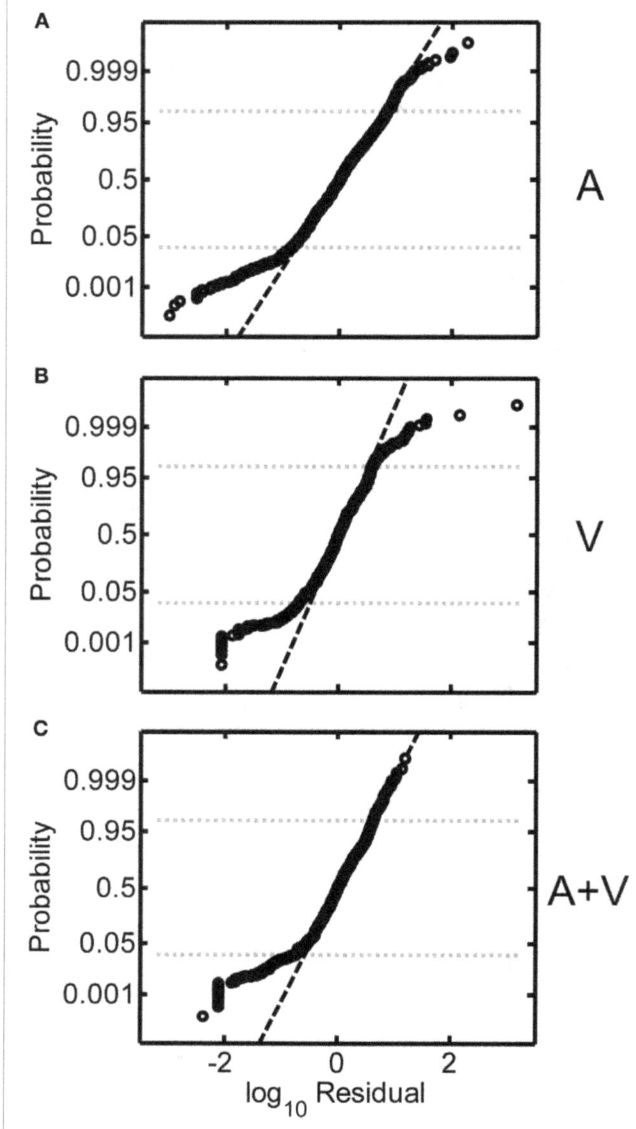

FIGURE 8 | Normal-probability plots of the log-transformed residuals (all participants) for the A (A), V (B), and A+V (C) conditions. The dashed diagonal line in each panel indicates normally distributed data. Probability values of 0.025 and 0.975 are shown for reference.

log-transformed residuals collapsed across distance for the A, V, and A+V conditions respectively. The dashed diagonal line in each panel indicates a normal distribution. In all three conditions, it may be observed that the distributions of the log-transformed residuals are very close to normal over a large range of probability values (0.025 and 0.975 are indicated by the dotted lines). Although very extreme values ($p < 0.025$ or $p > 0.0975$) do appear to deviate somewhat from normality, these distribution results are overall consistent with the notion that the underlying internal representation of distance and distance errors are logarithmically spaced (Zahorik, 2002b).

Distributions of RMS error in the A, V and A+V conditions are displayed in **Figures 9A–C** respectively. Each panel includes the following summary statistics: mean ± one standard deviation, median (interquartile range), and number of participants in each condition. The average RMS error for the A ($M = 0.226$, $SD = 0.111$) condition was significantly greater than both the V ($M = 0.152$, $SD = 0.108$) and A+V ($M = 0.163$, $SD = 0.086$) conditions. The V and A+V conditions were not significantly different from each other based on independent samples t-tests with Bonferroni correction. [A vs. V: $t_{(105)} = 3.440$, $p < 0.003$; A vs. A+V: $t_{(105)} = 3.190$, $p < 0.006$; V vs. A+V: $t_{(88)} = -0.523$, $p > 0.999$]. These results indicate that when visual stimuli were present, the distance estimates within individual subjects were less variable.

To evaluate the sensitivity of the power function fit procedures to the number of judgments available, fit parameters and

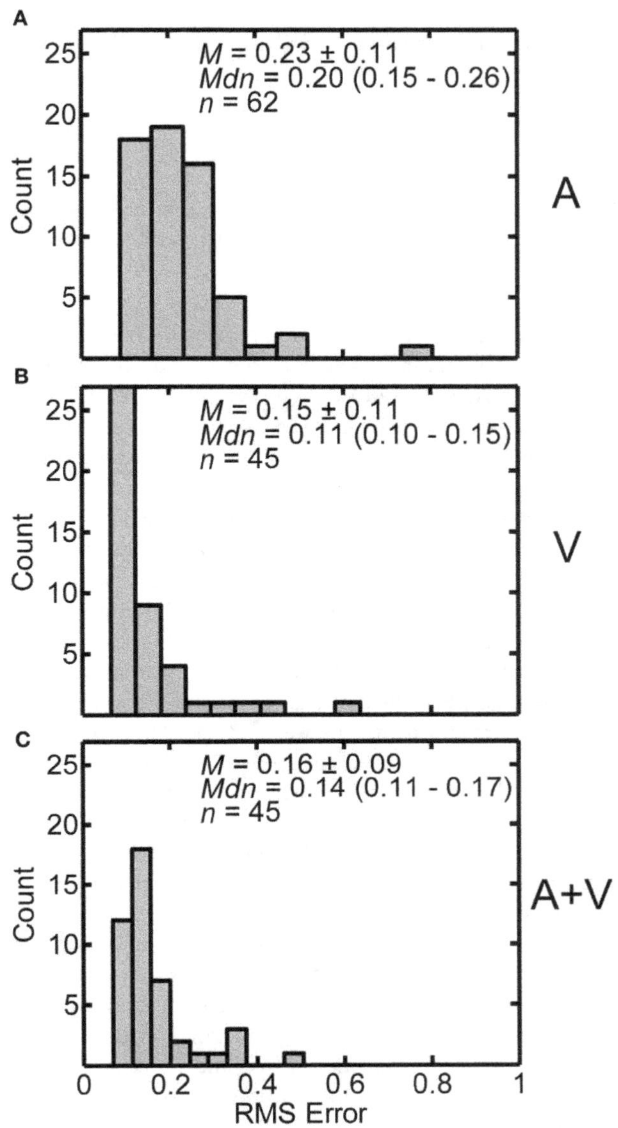

FIGURE 9 | Distributions of RMS errors from the power function fits from individual participants in the A (A), V (B), and A+V (C) conditions. Each panel includes the following summary statistics: mean, $M \pm$ one standard deviation, median, *Mdn* (interquartile range), and number of participants, *n*, in each condition.

R^2 values were compared between participants who performed 10 judgments per distance (a: $M = 0.649$, $SD = 0.259$; k: $M = 2.267$, $SD = 2.098$; R^2: $M = 0.650$, $SD = 0.208$) and a subset of participants who performed 30 judgments per distance (a: $M = 0.588$, $SD = 0.274$; k: $M = 2.130$, $SD = 1.694$; R^2: $M = 0.635$, $SD = 0.201$). Independent t-tests found no statistically significant difference between the two groups for either fit parameter or R^2 [a: $t_{(60)} = 0.802$, $p > 0.426$; k: $t_{(60)} = 0.240$, $p > 0.811$; R^2: $t_{(60)} = 0.246$, $p > 0.806$]. These results indicate that 10 judgments per distance is sufficient to reliably estimate the distance psychophysical function.

In order to assess reliability of distance judgments across the three stimulus conditions, correlations between power function fit parameters and statistics were computed. R^2 values in all three conditions were positively correlated [A and V: $r_{(43)} = 0.660$, $p < 0.001$; A and A+V: $r_{(43)} = 0.674$, $p < 0.001$; V and A+V: $r_{(43)} = 0.922$, $p < 0.001$]. This indicates that if a participant's power function fit was good in one condition then it was likely also a good fit in the remaining conditions. Exponents between all three conditions were also significantly positively correlated [A and V: $r_{(43)} = 0.537$, $p < 0.001$; A and A+V: $r_{(43)} = 0.557$, $p < 0.001$; V and A+V: $r_{(43)} = 0.896$, $p < 0.001$]. This indicates that participants with greater amounts of power-function compression, for example, display this trait consistently across stimulus conditions. Similar positive correlations were also observed for the fitted constant values [A and V: $r_{(43)} = 0.422$, $p < 0.004$; A and A+V: $r_{(43)} = 0.343$, $p < 0.021$; V and A+V: $r_{(43)} = 0.885$, $p < 0.001$].

DISCUSSION

Overall, the results from this study indicate that the presence of visual information improves the accuracy of distance judgments by making the relationship between target distance and judged distance more linear and reducing both inter- and intra-subject variability. These conclusions are based on the results of power function fits to the data in each of the three presentation conditions (A, V, A+V). The decision to fit our data with power functions was based on past reviews of both ADP (Zahorik et al., 2005) and VDP (Da Silva, 1985; Sedgwick, 1986) that used similar methods. Zahorik et al. (2005) fit power functions to 84 datasets from 21 past ADP articles. Da Silva (1985) summarized power function exponents for various visual distance perception studies. **Table 1** compares R^2 values and fit parameters (mean $\pm$ one standard deviation) from these reviews of past ADP (Zahorik et al., 2005) and VDP studies (Da Silva, 1985), with those from the current study. The summary of VDP exponents only includes studies in which full-cue conditions were used. R^2 values across all conditions and past ADP studies were generally high, which indicates that power function fits were good fits to both past and present data. Exponent and constant parameters from the fitted functions, which provide information about the amount of non-linear and linear compression/expansion of the functions, were, in most cases, similar between past and present studies. The mean exponent from the Zahorik et al. (2005) review was similar (within one standard deviation) to that observed in our A condition. Likewise for the V and A+V conditions, the mean exponents were similar (within one standard deviation) to the mean exponent resulting from Da Silva's (1985) summary. The constant values for the A condition were somewhat higher than reported by Zahorik et al. (2005). Evaluation of these differences is complicated by the fact that the variability of the constant values from the current investigation is much greater. This may be due to variability between subjects in their usage of the response scale that lacked a fixed anchor point. Because the Zahorik et al. (2005) dataset was based on average results from different studies, issues such as this that are related to individual subject variability were minimized, which may have also accounted for the somewhat higher average R^2 values they reported. Despite differences in sources of variability between studies, the fit parameters and R^2 values are all in relative agreement. All are within one standard deviation of each other.

Table 1 | Summary of results from past reviews of auditory and visual distance perception studies along with results from the current study.

Data source	A Condition	V Condition	A+V Condition	(Zahorik et al., 2005)—Audition	(Da Silva, 1985)—Vision
a	0.61 ± 0.30	0.92 ± 0.27	0.87 ± 0.27	0.54 ± 0.21	0.99 ± 0.13
k	2.22 ± 1.99	1.28 ± 0.80	1.38 ± 0.91	1.32 ± 0.75	
R^2	0.64 ± 0.22	0.87 ± 0.17	0.84 ± 0.18	0.91 ± 0.13	

Power function fit parameters (a and k) and R^2 (mean ± one standard deviation) are included from each study, except Da Silva (1985) which only provided a summary of exponent, a, values. Results from Zahorik et al. (2005) summarize data from 21 auditory studies. Results from Da Silva (1985) summarize data from 28 vision studies with full depth cues.

Another way to evaluate judgment biases beyond the analysis of the power function fit parameters is to determine the crossover point at which overestimation of close source distances switches to underestimation of farther source distances. This crossover point is the distance at which no bias occurs. Increasing or decreasing either fit parameter moves the crossover point further or closer respectively. Research in vision suggests that the crossover point may be related to a specific distance tendency (SDT; Gogel, 1969), which is the perceived distance of an object reported by participants under conditions with minimal distance cues. Mershon and King (1975) suggested that SDT can also be applied to ADP, given demonstrated tendencies for sounds to be localized toward the crossover point. Specifically, target distances located beyond the crossover point are perceived as closer, and therefore nearer to the crossover point. Conversely sound sources closer than the crossover point are localized farther away, which is again nearer to the crossover point. Mershon and King (1975) also hypothesize that SDT for auditory sources is strongly influenced by the reverberation level of a room. Hence, rooms with similar reverberation characteristics should produce similar SDTs.

In the current study, the crossover point for the A condition was approximately 3.23 m, based on the median exponent and constant parameters from the power function fits. This crossover point is greater than reported by Zahorik et al. (2005) dataset, which was approximately 1.9 m. Because the exponent values were similar in the two studies, it may be concluded that this crossover point discrepancy is caused primarily by the difference in the power function constant parameters. Following Mershon and King's (1975) hypothesis that SDT is related to reverberation level, it seems plausible that these differences in constant values might be linked to differences in the acoustical properties of the rooms used in the two studies. Although the acoustic environments across the data sets analyzed in Zahorik et al. (2005) varied widely, it is likely that the concert hall environment used in the current study had greater amounts of reverberation than the average room in Zahorik et al. (2005) dataset. Greater amounts of reverberation are known to produce greater distance judgments (Mershon and King, 1975), and therefore perhaps greater constant parameters in the power function fits, which in turn produce a more distant SDT. Such conclusions need to be approached cautiously, however, given the large individual variability observed in the constant values, as previously discussed. For VDP, Gogel (1969) found that visual context was necessary to localize visual targets away from the SDT. Reverberation level in ADP may provide the context necessary for sound sources to appear displaced from the SDT.

The observation that distance judgment biases observed in the A+V condition were much lower than the A condition, and nearly identical to those observed in the V condition, we take as evidence of a degree of visual capture in the distance dimension. This result is very similar to the well-known visual capture effects for discrepancies in the angular separation between auditory and visual targets—also known as the "Ventriloquist Effect." It has been demonstrated that a visual stimulus can bias localization of the auditory sound source when the two are as much as 30° apart in the horizontal plane (Jack and Thurlow, 1973) and 55° in the vertical plane (Thurlow and Jack, 1973). This is a large effect. It is more than an order of magnitude larger than the minimum audible angle that is detectable between two sound sources separated in horizontal angle, which is between 1° and 4° on the median plane (Mills, 1958). Strong visual capture effects have been previously observed in the distance dimension ("The Proximity-Image Effect") when large discrepancies exist between the auditory and visual targets (Mershon et al., 1980) and particularly when auditory distance information is impoverished (Gardner, 1968). The capture effects observed here are clearly much more subtle.

On the other hand, there are aspects of our results from the A+V condition that are not entirely consistent with visual capture. Research on multisensory perception emphasizes the optimal integration of multisensory information based on the variances of the two modalities (Ernst and Banks, 2002; Alais and Burr, 2004). According to this optimal integration model, the variance of the combined bimodal information should be lower than either modality alone. Additionally, the model stipulates that the modalities are weighted by the inverse of their variance, so the modality with lower variance is more heavily weighted at the modality integration stage of the perceptual process. For example, vision should be heavily weighted in a spatial task; however, if noise is added to the visual stimulus audition will become more heavily weighted. Therefore, if optimal integration occurred in our study, the A+V condition would be expected to have had lower variance than either the A or V condition alone. This was not observed, which is surprising because even if vision in the A+V condition was weighted 100% by the sensory system, the optimal integration theory still predicts lower variance in the A+V condition. It is possible, however, that this apparent lack of optimal integration may relate to the response method used in our study. Magnitude estimation methods are inherently noisier than the discrimination methods used by previous studies that have demonstrated optimal integration (Ernst and Banks, 2002; Alais and Burr, 2004). It is therefore conceivable that the perceptual noise in the A+V condition was in fact lower than either the A or V condition alone, thus consistent with optimal integration, but the response noise was simply too great to observe this reduction in variance consistent with optimal integration. Nevertheless, the measurement of variability is interesting itself because it has not been studied extensively in distance judgment studies.

Finally, our measurements of distance judgment variability provide additional and important insights into ADP and VDP both within and across individual participants. The inherent variability in distance judgments, particularly in the auditory domain, has not been well quantified prior to this study. In general, distance judgment variability across participants was found to be reduced when visual cues were present, a result that is consistent with past work that used similar response and analysis methods for apparent distance judgments (Zahorik, 2001). This result is inconsistent, however, with recent work by Calcagno et al. (2012), which shows essentially constant judgment variability independent of whether visual target information is provided to the listener. This discrepancy could be due to differences in the type of visual information available. In Calcagno's study the visual information (2–4 LEDs in a dark field) was much more limited than the visual information present in either the present study or the Zahorik (2001) study, which provided multiple depth cues to the target locations. It is also worth noting that there were differences in the number of responses evaluated in summarizing response variability (24 judgments/distance in (Calcagno et al., 2012) vs. 959 judgments/distance in this study), as well as the analysis strategies used to summarize variability (variability of raw judgments in Calcagno et al., 2012 vs. variability of log-transformed judgments in this study and in Zahorik, 2001). We also show that when the judgment variability is expressed as logarithmic deviation from a best-fitting power function for individual subjects, the distributions of this deviation (error) measure are approximately normal. This, in conjunction with the fact that power functions are generally good fits to the data, suggests that the perceived auditory/visual space surrounding the subject has a logarithmically spaced topology. This conclusion is consistent with past work related to ADP (Zahorik, 2002b), as well as visual depth work that demonstrates perceptual foreshortening of faraway objects (Wagner, 1985; Loomis et al., 2002).

CONCLUSIONS

Results from this study indicate that: (1) Distance estimates in all conditions (A, V, A+V) were well-explained by power-function fits; (2) The presence of visual targets increased distance judgment accuracy in the V and A+V conditions compared to the A condition; (3) The A condition had greater unexplained response variance than either the V or A+V condition; (4) The unexplained response variance was approximately normally distributed in logarithmic space for all three conditions. These conclusions are consistent with the notion that visual depth information, when available to the participant, dominates the auditory percept of distance. They are also consistent with the idea that aspects of distance perception in both perceived auditory and perceived visual space appear to be organized logarithmically.

ACKNOWLEDGMENTS

We thank Gina Collecchia, Finesse Moreno-Rivera, and Noah Jacobs for their assistance with data collection. Work supported by AFOSR / KY DEPSCoR (FA9550-08-1-0234) and NIH-NEI (R21 EY023767).

REFERENCES

Alais, D., and Burr, D. (2004). The ventriloquist effect results from near-optimal bimodal integration. *Curr. Biol.* 14, 257–262. doi: 10.1016/j.cub.2004.01.029

Ashmead, D. H., Davis, D. L., and Northington, A. (1995). Contribution of listeners' approaching motion to auditory distance perception. *J. Exp. Psychol. Hum. Percept. Perform.* 21, 239–256. doi: 10.1037/0096-1523.21.2.239

Blauert, J. (1997). *Spatial Hearing: The Psychophysics of Human Sound Localization.* Cambridge, MA: MIT press.

Calcagno, E. R., Abregu, E. L., and Manuel, C. E. (2012). The role of vision in auditory distance perception. *Perception* 41, 175–192. doi: 10.1068/p7153

Coleman, P. D. (1968). Dual role of frequency spectrum in determination of auditory distance. *J. Acoust. Soc. Am.* 44, 631–632. doi: 10.1121/1.1911132

Da Silva, J. A. (1985). Scales for perceived egocentric distance in a large open field: comparison of three psychophysical methods. *Am. J. Psychol.* 98, 119–144. doi: 10.2307/1422771

Ernst, M. O., and Banks, M. S. (2002). Humans integrate visual and haptic information in a statistically optimal fashion. *Nature* 415, 429–433. doi: 10.1038/415429a

Gardner, M. B. (1968). Proximity image effect in sound localization. *J. Acoust. Soc. Am.* 43, 163. doi: 10.1121/1.1910747

Gogel, W. C. (1969). The sensing of retinal size. *Vision Res.* 9, 1079–1094. doi: 10.1016/0042-6989(69)90049-2

ISO-3382. (1997). *3382. Acoustics–Measurement of The Reverberation Time of Rooms With Reference To Other Acoustical Parameters.* Geneva: International Standards Organization.

Jack, C. E., and Thurlow, W. R. (1973). Effects of degree of visual association and angle of displacement on the "ventriloquism" effect. *Percept. Mot. Skills* 37, 967–979. doi: 10.2466/pms.1973.37.3.967

Loomis, J. M., Philbeck, J. W., and Zahorik, P. (2002). Dissociation between location and shape in visual space. *J. Exp. Psychol. Hum. Percept. Perform.* 28, 1202–1212. doi: 10.1037/0096-1523.28.5.1202

Mershon, D. H., Ballenger, W. L., Little, A. D., McMurtry, P. L., and Buchanan, J. L. (1989). Effects of room reflectance and background noise on perceived auditory distance. *Perception* 18, 403–416. doi: 10.1068/p180403

Mershon, D. H., and Bowers, J. N. (1979). Absolute and relative cues for the auditory perception of egocentric distance. *Perception* 8, 311–322. doi: 10.1068/p080311

Mershon, D. H., Desaulniers, D. H., Amerson, T. L., and Kiefer, S. A. (1980). Visual capture in auditory distance perception: proximity image effect reconsidered. *J. Aud. Res.* 20, 129–136.

Mershon, D. H., and King, L. E. (1975). Intensity and reverberation as factors in the auditory perception of egocentric distance. *Percept. Psychophys.* 18, 409–415. doi: 10.3758/BF03204113

Middlebrooks, J. C., and Green, D. M. (1991). Sound localization by human listeners. *Annu. Rev. Psychol.* 42, 135–159. doi: 10.1146/annurev.ps.42.020191.001031

Mills, A. W. (1958). On the minimum audible angle. *J. Acoust. Soc. Am.* 30, 237–246. doi: 10.1121/1.1909553

Rife, D. D., and Vanderkooy, J. (1989). Transfer-function measurement with maximum-length sequences. *J. Audio Eng. Soc.* 37, 419–444.

Sedgwick, H. A. (1986). "Space perception," in *Handbook of Perception and Human Performance*, Vol. 1, eds K. R. Boff, L. Kaufman, and J. P. Thomas (New York, NY: Wiley), 21-1–21-57.

Thurlow, W. R., and Jack, C. E. (1973). Certain determinants of the "ventriloquism effect." *Percept. Mot. Skills* 36, 1171–1184. doi: 10.2466/pms.1973.36.3c.1171

Vroomen, J., and de Gelder, B. (2004). Temporal ventriloquism: sound modulates the flash-lag effect. *J. Exp. Psychol. Hum. Percept. Perform.* 30, 513–518. doi: 10.1037/0096-1523.30.3.513

Wagner, M. (1985). The metric of visual space. *Percept. Psychophys.* 38, 483–495. doi: 10.3758/BF03207058

Wightman, F. L., and Kistler, D. J. (1989). Headphone simulation of freefield listening. I: stimulus synthesis. *J. Acoust. Soc. Am.* 85, 858–867. doi: 10.1121/1.397557

Zahorik, P. (2001). Estimating sound source distance with and without vision. *Optom. Vis. Sci.* 78, 270–275. doi: 10.1097/00006324-200105000-00009

Zahorik, P. (2002a). Assessing auditory distance perception using virtual acoustics. *J. Acoust. Soc. Am.* 111, 1832–1846. doi: 10.1121/1.1458027

Zahorik, P. (2002b). Direct-to-reverberant energy ratio sensitivity. *J. Acoust. Soc. Am.* 112, 2110–2117. doi: 10.1121/1.1506692

Zahorik, P., Brungart, D. S., and Bronkhorst, A. W. (2005). Auditory distance perception in humans: a summary of past and present research. *Acta Acust. United Acust.* 91, 409–420.

3

The moving minimum audible angle is smaller during self-motion than during source motion

W. Owen Brimijoin* and Michael A. Akeroyd

Scottish Section, Institute of Hearing Research, Medical Research Council/Chief Scientist Office, Glasgow, UK

***Correspondence:**
W. Owen Brimijoin, Scottish Section, Institute of Hearing Research, Medical Research Council/Chief Scientist Office, New Lister Building, Glasgow Royal Infirmary, 10-16 Alexandra Parade, Glasgow G31 2ER, UK
e-mail: owen@ihr.gla.ac.uk

We are rarely perfectly still: our heads rotate in three axes and move in three dimensions, constantly varying the spectral and binaural cues at the ear drums. In spite of this motion, static sound sources in the world are typically perceived as stable objects. This argues that the auditory system—in a manner not unlike the vestibulo-ocular reflex—works to compensate for self motion and stabilize our sensory representation of the world. We tested a prediction arising from this postulate: that self motion should be processed more accurately than source motion. We used an infrared motion tracking system to measure head angle, and real-time interpolation of head related impulse responses to create "head-stabilized" signals that appeared to remain fixed in space as the head turned. After being presented with pairs of simultaneous signals consisting of a man and a woman speaking a snippet of speech, normal and hearing impaired listeners were asked to report whether the female voice was to the left or the right of the male voice. In this way we measured the moving minimum audible angle (MMAA). This measurement was made while listeners were asked to turn their heads back and forth between ± 15° and the signals were stabilized in space. After this "self-motion" condition we measured MMAA in a second "source-motion" condition when listeners remained still and the virtual locations of the signals were moved using the trajectories from the first condition. For both normal and hearing impaired listeners, we found that the MMAA for signals moving relative to the head was ~1–2° smaller when the movement was the result of self motion than when it was the result of source motion, even though the motion with respect to the head was identical. These results as well as the results of past experiments suggest that spatial processing involves an ongoing and highly accurate comparison of spatial acoustic cues with self-motion cues.

Keywords: spatial hearing, head movements, auditory motion, sound localization, motion tracking, self-motion compensation

INTRODUCTION

Listeners make continual head movements, be they intentional head turns, reflexive orienting responses, or small involuntary movements. Because the ears are attached to the head and the head is never perfectly still, this means that the acoustic world must also be in constant motion. We nonetheless perceive the auditory world to be relatively stable. The underlying mechanisms that permit this percept are unknown. The visual system incorporates a low-level mechanism that counteracts the motion of the head, the "vestibulo-ocular reflex" (VOR). Using input from the vestibular and proprioceptive systems, the VOR works to physically move the eyes in direct opposition to one's own head motion, more or less stabilizing the projection of images on the surface of the retina (Lorente De No, 1933). Such a mechanical solution is not possible in the auditory system due to the simple fact that the ears are fixed to the sides of the head. Thus each time the head turns, the acoustic world at the ears turns in the opposite direction. We refer to this as "self motion" and contrast it with "source motion": that which is due to the source of sound itself moving.

While both head motions and physically moving sound sources in the world result in acoustic movement at the ears, self motion is not perceived as a moving sound: simple introspection will demonstrate that the acoustic world appears to remain relatively stable as the head turns. By analogy with the VOR, it is sensible to suggest that there exists a fundamental mechanism by which the moving auditory world is perceptually stabilized (Lewald and Karnath, 2000; Lewald et al., 2000). Evidence directly supporting such a mechanism, however, remains somewhat circumstantial, despite there being a wealth of studies showing a tight integration between motion and auditory spatial perception in general. Heads are essentially in continual motion (König and Sussman, 1955) and movements have been shown to increase the accuracy of sound localization judgments (Thurlow and Runge, 1967; Perrett and Noble, 1997); in particular they have been shown to play a critical role in resolving the front/back position of a sound source (Wightman and Kistler, 1999; Brimijoin and Akeroyd, 2012; Kim et al., 2013). Head motions have also been linked to the degree to which sound sources are externalized (Brimijoin et al., 2013). Vestibular stimulation has been shown to shift a listener's subjective auditory midline (Lewald and Karnath, 2000); and, in a complementary fashion, rotating auditory stimuli can induce an illusion of rotational self motion (Lackner, 1977). A number of related studies are discussed at the end of this manuscript, but here it should be noted that together they suggest that vestibular information is thoroughly integrated with auditory spatial information. To our knowledge, however, no study has directly tested whether self motion is processed differently from source motion, nor has any examined the impact of compensation for self-generated motion.

If there is an auditory stabilization mechanism that works to at least partially cancel out self-generated movements, it is reasonable to expect that it would provide a more stable background against which a listener could judge the position and/or motion of auditory sources. Such a scenario leads to the following prediction: listeners' performance on moving spatial auditory tasks should be better when the acoustic movement in question is generated by their own motion than when it is generated by the source itself. We tested this prediction using a measurement of the *moving* minimum audible angle (MMAA), which we define to be the smallest angular separation between two simultaneous, moving sound sources that is needed for a listener to be able to tell that the two sources are in separate directions. The MMAA is a generalization of the classical minimum audible angle (MAA), which uses sounds that are static (Mills, 1958). Also, the MMAA should not be confused with the minimum audible movement angle (MAMA), which is the smallest detectable motion of a sound (Perrott and Tucker, 1988). We measured the MMAA using two simultaneous signals, separated in space rather than sequential signals, marking a slight departure from traditional methods of measuring the MAA (though note that the MAA for concurrent sounds has been measured previously; Perrott, 1984).

The use of high speed infrared motion tracking (see Brimijoin and Akeroyd, 2012) allowed us to tightly control the movement of virtual signals. In this way we were able to measure the performance of listeners when presented with self motion vs. source motion while ensuring that the actual movement itself was identical in the two conditions. We found an advantage for spatial processing during movement when the movement in question was self motion rather than source motion. This advantage was similar in size across a wide range of ages and levels of hearing impairment.

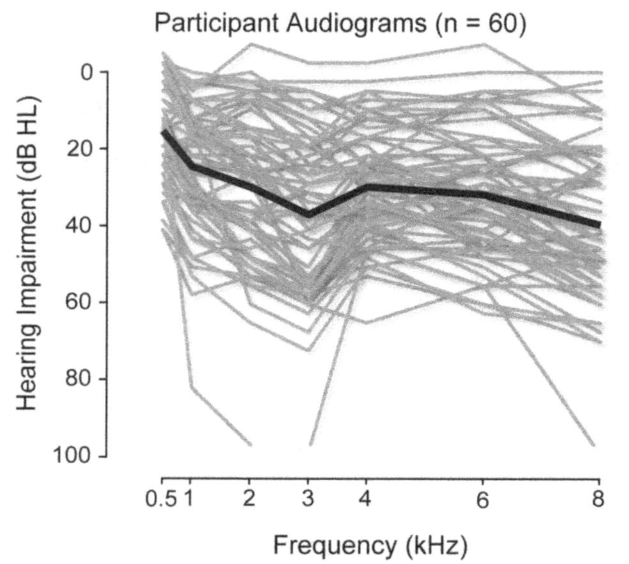

FIGURE 1 | Audiograms for the participants. The individual audiograms, measured at 500, 1000, 2000, 3000, 4000, 6000, and 8000 Hz, of all listeners are plotted in gray. The mean audiograms are plotted as solid black lines.

METHODS

LISTENERS

We recorded complete data sets (i.e., had successful motion tracking throughout all conditions) and made MAA and MMAA measurements for 60 listeners. Audiograms for the complete subject pool are shown in **Figure 1**. The individual audiogram in decibels Hearing Level (dB HL) of each listener is plotted in gray and the mean for all listeners is plotted as a solid black line. Hearing thresholds were measured at 250, 500, 1000, 2000, 3000, 4000, 6000, and 8000 Hz for both left and right ears. For the purposes of analysis, mean thresholds were computed for each ear by averaging the hearing threshold at 500, 1000, 2000, and 4000 Hz. All listeners had less than 15 dB of difference in their mean hearing thresholds between the two ears.

Each listener was seated in a quiet, sound-treated room and presented with pairs of simultaneous signals over headphones consisting of a man and a woman speaking 1-s duration snippets of speech. The sentence fragments were drawn from the Adaptive Sentence List corpus (Macleod and Summerfield, 1987); these sentences were sampled at 44.1 kHz, but low pass filtered at 10 kHz, and presented at a comfortable listening level (typically between 65 and 80 dB sound pressure level). The signals were processed using virtual acoustics to appear to come from different directions. For each of the four conditions (see below) the male and female voices differed in direction by any of 10 values (±1°, 2°, 4°, 8°, and 16°, chosen pseudo-randomly on each trial) and the mean presentation angle of the two signals was randomly varied across five angles (−16°, −8°, 0°, 8°, and 16°, where 0° corresponds to directly in front, negative to the left, and positive to the right). The listeners were asked to determine whether the female voice was to the left or the right of the male voice, regardless of the pair's absolute position in space. The order of male-female separation angle within the conditions was randomized, but within blocks listeners always performed the head-moving condition first, as the trajectories measured here were used in the source-motion condition.

MOTION TRACKING

Motion tracking was performed in a sound-treated room using a commercial infrared camera system (Vicon MX3+) using methods described previously (Brimijoin et al., 2010). Six cameras were placed above the listener, behind and ahead, and were pointed toward the listener. The system tracked 9-mm diameter reflective spheres; these "markers" were placed on a head-mounted "crown" worn by the listeners. The motion-tracking system was queried from Matlab and returned three-dimensional

Cartesian coordinates of the crown markers at a sample rate of 100 Hz. Arctangent transforms converted these coordinates to the three Euler angles of yaw, pitch, and roll. These angles were accurate to within approximately 0.1°.

VIRTUAL SOUND FIELD REPRODUCTION

We used linearly-interpolated manikin (KEMAR, Burkhard and Sachs, 1975) binaural room impulse responses (BRIR), measured at 1.0 m, to create virtual sound locations in the horizontal plane (Wierstorf et al., 2011). When a signal is filtered using BRIRs and played back over headphones, the result is audio that seems to be emanating from a particular direction relative to the head. The use of BRIRs instead of free-field loudspeakers allowed us to create two directly comparable experimental conditions. To measure self- vs. source-motion acuity using loudspeakers would require a comparison between statically presented signals while the head was moving, and dynamically panned signals while the head was kept still. As the signal processing in these two cases is different, we opted to use virtual acoustics to create acoustically identical conditions that differed only in whether the presented motion was specified relative to the head or relative to the world. It should be noted that the use of generic BRIRs recorded solely in the horizontal plane does carry with it two drawbacks: (1) the realism of the simulation was partly dependent on the similarity of the participant's head to that of the KEMAR manikin; and (2) neither head rotations in the vertical plane nor head translations were accounted for, potentially decreasing the realism of the acoustic simulation, and/or the perceived source elevation (although listeners were given feedback on the ideal head movements during a trial period). The use of this database, however, allowed us to create two experimental conditions that were acoustically identical to one another without the complexity and time requirements associated with measuring hundreds of individualized BRIRs.

Every 10 ms, the listener's head direction was measured by the motion tracking system and the two closest BRIRs from the database were selected and then linearly interpolated with one another to give a BRIR corresponding to the actual direction. The interpolation was performed as a weighted sum in the time domain. This technique was computationally efficient enough to allow us to do real time processing, but could in principle result in interpolated BRIRs with doubled attenuated peaks. We largely avoided this problem by using a BRIR library that was measured in 1° intervals (Wierstorf et al., 2011), meaning that the time difference between angle-adjacent BRIRs was smaller than the sample period (1/44100)[1]. The interpolated 512-sample long BRIR was then convolved with a 512-sample long chunk of audio and the last 441 samples (corresponding to 10 ms) were sent to an audio buffer. The time position in the acoustic signal was then incremented by 441 samples and the process was repeated. Transitions between buffer segments were smoothed using a 32-sample linear crossfade. The audio buffering was handled using playrec (www.playrec.co.uk), a custom Matlab audio protocol built on the PortAudio API. All together, these methods could change the virtual location of two audio signals every 10 ms with a total movement-to-change latency of between 22 and 33 ms. Our experience was that the method was smooth, and none of the sounds had perceptible jumps, transitions, or clicks.

STATISTICAL ANALYSIS

The data across the 10 values of male-female separation angles for each condition defined a psychometric function for percent-correct vs. separation angle. The absolute values of the separation of the male and female voice (i.e., positive vs. negative subtended angles) were averaged to yield five points on each psychometric function. These were fitted with a logistic function using "nlinfit" from the Statistics Toolbox for Matlab release 2012a (The Mathworks, Natick MA). Values of MMAA, defined as the separation angle needed to give a performance of 75%, were calculated from the logistic fits. We used SPSS v21 (IBM, Armonk NY) to perform an ANOVA on the MMAA values as a function of listening condition. We made two *post-hoc* comparisons to determine whether there were significant differences between the two static-signal conditions and between the two moving-signal conditions. Alpha was set to 0.05 for the ANOVA and the Bonferroni correction was used for all *post-hoc* tests.

PROCEDURE

We ran four sets of conditions (**Figure 2**). In all conditions the listeners were asked to report the relative position of the female voice with respect to the male voice. In two of the conditions, we asked listeners to remain still in the ring of loudspeakers, in the other two, the listener was asked to turn his/her head back and forth continually between two visual markers at ±15° while we used motion tracking to determine the orientation of the listener's head every 10 ms. The listeners were given feedback until their rotations were within a few degrees of this target motion and their peak velocities were roughly 45°/s.

In one of the four conditions, the self-motion condition, the pair of signals were dynamically filtered so that they appeared to remain fixed at particular absolute directions with respect to the world as the listeners turned (see Brimijoin et al., 2013 for a more complete methods description). In the source-movement condition, listeners were asked to remain still and were played signals that moved according to randomly chosen motion trajectories recorded in the self-motion condition. It should be noted that although listeners were asked to remain still, our experience is that they still made continual micromotions. These $< 0.5°$ head motions aside, the signals in the self-motion and source-motion conditions shared the identical acoustic movements, but the movement was in the first instance perfectly correlated with the listener's own head motion (self motion) whereas in the second it was entirely uncorrelated (source motion). We also ran two control conditions, in which the signals did not use dynamically interpolated BRIRs but instead were fixed with respect to the head, whether the listener was static or moving. Note that only in the head static/signal static condition does our measurement correspond to a classic simultaneous MAA.

Thus the experiment was conducted using a 2 × 2 design in which listeners were asked to either remain static or to move their heads and presented with pairs of signals that were either static or

[1] It should be noted that linear interpolation of BRIRs can never result in a BRIR that is identical to one actually measured at the interpolated location, but the fine-grained nature of the database we used minimized this problem.

moving with respect to the head (see **Figure 2**). The four conditions were: (1) head static/source static, (2) head moving/source static, (both 1 and 2 being standard headphone presentation), (3) head static/source dynamic (source motion), and (4) head moving/source dynamic (self motion).

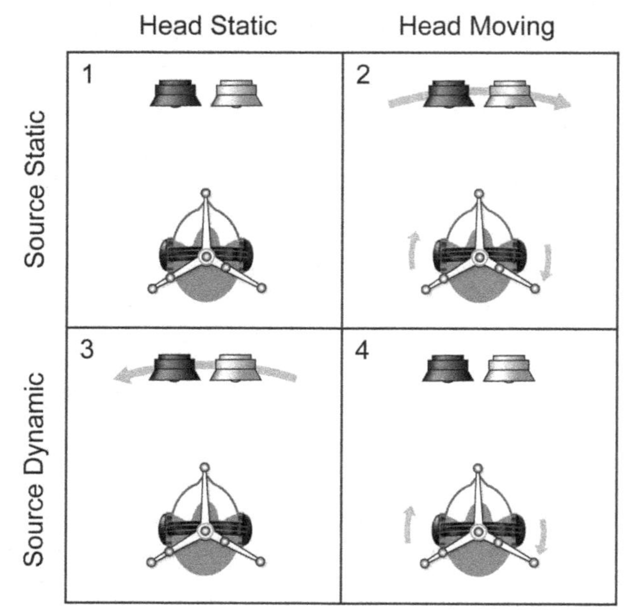

FIGURE 2 | The 2 × 2 experiment design. Tests of the minimum audible angle were conducted in four conditions: **(1)** listeners were asked to remain static and the signal was not moved, **(2)** listeners were asked to turn their heads and the signal moved with them, **(3)** listeners were asked to remain static and the signals were moved, and **(4)** listeners were asked to turn their heads and the signal was adjusted so as to appear to remain still with respect to the world.

RESULTS

PSYCHOMETRIC FUNCTIONS

The across-listener mean psychometric functions of proportion correct relative localization are shown in **Figure 3A**. For all conditions, the mean proportion correct increased as a function of the separation of the male and female voices. While the 75% threshold differences are reported below, it may be observed that the difference in performance between the two signal static conditions (top two curves) suggests that listeners were most easily able to discriminate the left/right positions of separated signals when both the listener and the signals did not move (solid diamonds). When the listeners were required to turn their heads back and forth and the signal moved with them (open diamonds), their mean performance appeared to drop. The offset in the two "source dynamic" curves suggests that listeners were better able to discriminate the position of signals that moved in realistic opposition to their head movements (open circles) than those that appeared to move arbitrarily in space (solid circles).

MINIMUM AUDIBLE ANGLE MEASUREMENTS

Figure 3B plots the mean MMAAs calculated from the logistic fits to each listener's psychometric functions. A Two-Way repeated measures ANOVA confirmed a significant main effect of signal type (static vs. dynamic) [$F_{(3,236)} = 195.7, p < 0.001$]. This result is due to the large difference between the MAA measurements and the MMAA measurements, arguing that the dynamically moving signals were associated with an increased difficulty in discriminating the two target signal positions. The ANOVA revealed no effect of head movement [$F_{(3,236)} = 4.4$, $p = 0.40$] but a significant interaction between movement and signal type [$F_{(1,236)} = 52.9$, $p < 0.005$]. The lack of a main effect of head movement is due to an opposite influence of head movement seen in the two signal conditions.

In the "signal static" conditions, the MAAs were between 3 and 4°, but in the self-motion condition they averaged 5.4°, and in the

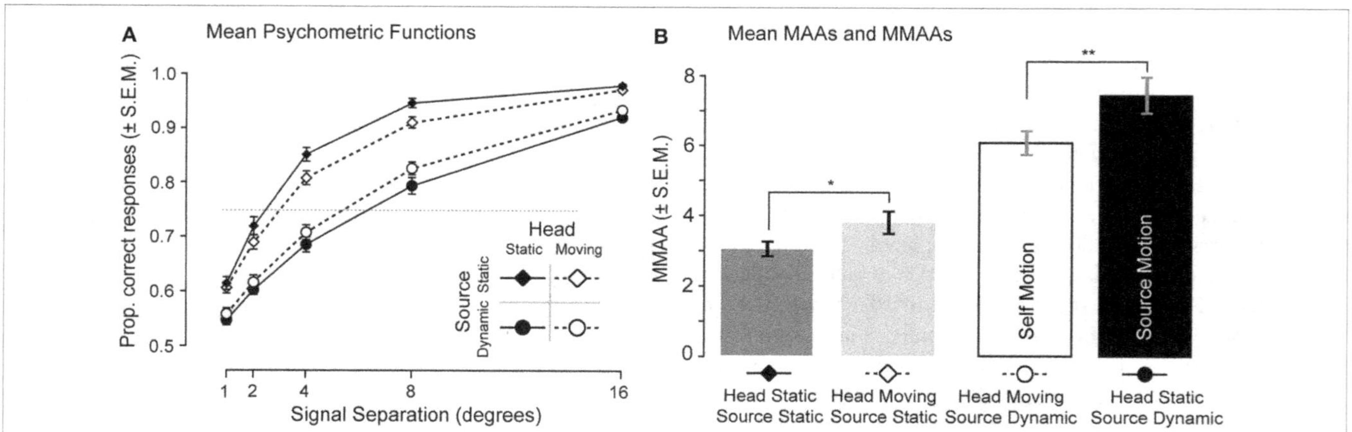

FIGURE 3 | Psychometric functions and measurements of the minimum audible angle. (A) The mean psychometric functions for all listeners are plotted for all four conditions including: (1) head static/source static (solid diamonds), (2) head moving/source static (open diamonds), (3) head static/source dynamic (solid circles), and (4) head moving/source dynamic (open circles). Error bars show ±1 standard error. **(B)** The results of logistic fits to individual psychometric functions show that the MMAA was larger for source motion (black bar) than for self motion (white bar), and that both of these were larger than for the source static conditions (gray bars). A single asterisk represents differences in means significant at an alpha of 0.05, and a double asterisk an alpha of 0.01.

source-motion condition they averaged 6.6°. *Post-hoc* contrasts using a Bonferonni correction revealed a significant difference in MMAAs between the two dynamic signal conditions (a mean difference of 1.2°, $p < 0.01$). A *post-hoc* test also showed that there was a significant difference between the two signal-static conditions (mean difference in MMAA of 0.7°, $p < 0.05$), arguing that signals fixed relative to the head were less easily discriminated in position when the listener was moving than they were when the listener was static.

The classical, static-signal MAA has been previously shown to increase as a function of hearing impairment (Häusler et al., 1983). **Figure 4A** shows the results of an attempt to replicate this finding, plotting MAA for static signals as a function of hearing impairment. While the variance in MAA measurements appears to increase as a function of hearing impairment, an R^2 value of 0.03 for static heads and an R^2 of 0.07 for moving heads suggests that the mean MAA for statically presented signals did not increase with level of hearing impairment. The discrepancy between these results and those of Häusler et al. (1983) may be due to the fact that our measurements of the MAA were all made in front of the listener, rather than off to the sides where Häusler et al. observed the greatest effect of hearing impairment. **Figure 4B** plots the mean MAA values as a function of age and also showed no significant correlations (R^2 of 0.04 and 0.01 for head static and head moving, respectively).

For the dynamic signal stimuli (whether self- or source motion), the MMAA for dynamic sounds also did not increase with hearing impairment (**Figure 5A**). There was an apparent increase in variance as a function of hearing impairment, but the correlations were low for both conditions [R^2 of 0.02 and 0.06 for self motion (head moving) and source motion (head static), respectively]. Apart from a similar increase in variance, no effect of age was found for the MMAA either (**Figure 5B**) (R^2 of 0.02 and 0.01 for self motion and source motion, respectively).

CONDITION-DEPENDENT DIFFERENCES IN THE MINIMUM AUDIBLE ANGLE

Figure 6A plots the difference in MMAA between the source-motion and self-motion conditions (the "self-motion advantage") as a function of hearing impairment plotted as open circles with a histogram in 0.5° bins on the right y-axis. The majority of the points fall above the zero line (also shown by the distribution

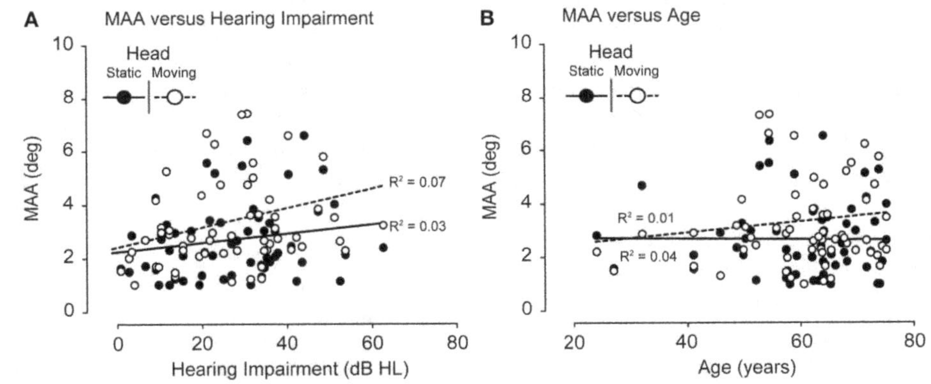

FIGURE 4 | (A) Static MAA as a function of hearing impairment. No increase in MAA was observed as a function of hearing impairment for either the head moving (open circles, dotted line) or the head static conditions (filled circles, solid line). **(B)** MAA as a function of age. No increase in MAA was observed as a function of age for either the head moving (open circles, dotted line) or the head static conditions (filled circles, solid line).

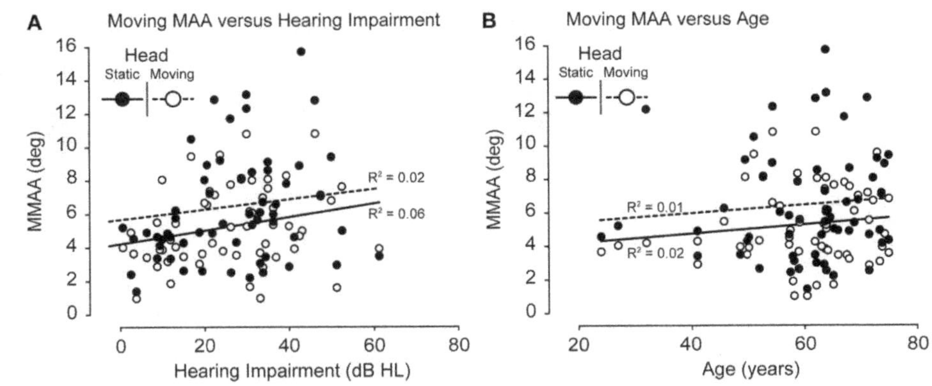

FIGURE 5 | (A) MMAA as a function of hearing impairment. No increase in MMAA was observed as a function of hearing impairment for either the head-moving (open circles, dotted line) or head-static (filled circles, solid line) conditions. **(B)** MMAA as a function of age. No increase in MMAA was observed as a function of age for either the head-moving (open circles, dotted line) or the head-static conditions (filled circles, solid line).

of the histogram), confirming the slight advantage for processing self motion, although there was no consistent effect of level of hearing impairment on the self-motion advantage. A similar analysis may be found in **Figure 6B**, but in this case these data are the difference between the MAAs found in the two signal static conditions. The consistent pattern is that there was a slight disadvantage in MAA performance when listeners were required to turn their heads and the acoustic world moved with them (a histogram of these data points is found on the right y-axis). No effect of level of hearing impairment on this difference was found.

DISCUSSION

Listeners had lower MMAAs when the signals moved in a way that was correlated with the listener's own movement (self motion) compared to when they were uncorrelated (source motion). These results demonstrate that there is a relative advantage in spatial processing when listeners are tested using self motion as compared to source motion. This advantage is maintained even in the older, impaired auditory system, as is evidenced by the consistent difference in the self- vs. source-motion conditions across listeners of all levels of hearing impairment and age. These data are consistent with the hypothesis that the percept of sound source location is at least partially corrected for self-generated motion, providing a more stable background against which a listener can judge the position of auditory sources.

Despite the evidence for a self-motion processing advantage, there appeared to be a consistent *disadvantage* associated with head movement for the signal static conditions (see **Figure 6B**). There are two possible explanations for this phenomenon, the first is that requiring listeners to move makes them less able to process spatial cues, the second is that the disadvantage is the result of the signals not moving in a behaviorally relevant manner (i.e., moving with the head). The first would imply that the advantage observed in MMAA processing is an underestimation of the true self-motion advantage, since listeners in the self-motion condition were required to turn their heads, incurring an obligatory movement penalty[2]. The second explanation is that the synchronous movement of the auditory world with the head in the signal static conditions causes a mismatch between the expected and actual movement of the signal. We have previously demonstrated that auditory externalization drops significantly when sound fields are artificially moved with the head (Brimijoin et al., 2013), a finding that was interpreted to be due to the mismatch between the movement of the head and the movement of the signal. Such a mismatch could also be responsible for the apparent MMAA movement disadvantage observed in the current study. Given the evidence of the impact of unrealistic sound field movement on auditory externalization, we feel that the second explanation for the motion disadvantage is more likely.

It should be noted that listeners were better able to determine the relative position of two sound sources when they were statically presented as compared to when they were dynamically moved. This impact on performance was consistent whether listeners moved their heads or not. The difference could be attributable to two factors: first that our method of dynamically adjusting the location of signals in virtual acoustic space resulted in a more diffuse, or "smeared" location percept, and second, that it is more difficult to judge the relative position of two simultaneously moving signals. Given our current data set, we are unable to assess the relative validity of these two explanations.

More generally speaking, however, to compare the movement of the head with the movement of the acoustic world would require both accurate auditory spatial processing and accurate processing of self motion. There is extensive interconnection between the central vestibular and auditory systems (Abraham et al., 1977), starting as low as the cochlear nucleus

[2]Another factor that could contribute to an underestimation of the actual self-motion advantage is that of an order effect. By necessity of the study design the self-motion condition had to be run before the world-motion condition in each block. If listeners performed better over time, then the source-motion condition could be easier on average for the subject.

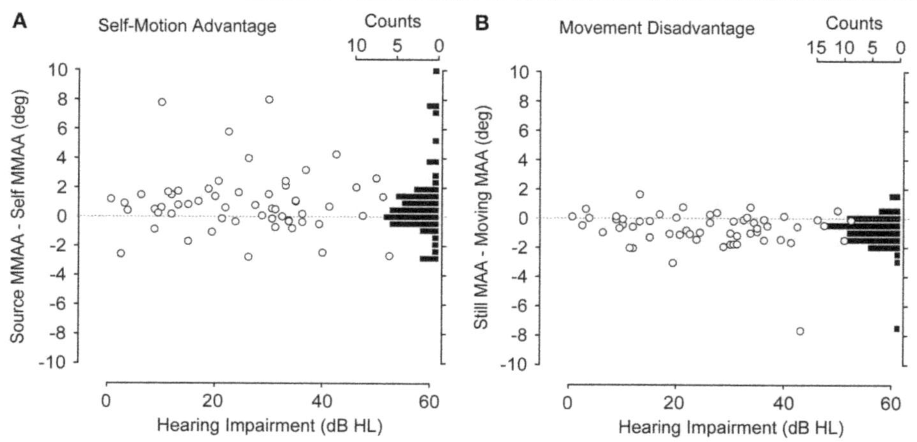

FIGURE 6 | (A) Self-motion advantage. The open circles are the MMAAs measured during self motion subtracted from the MMAAs measured during source motion. The histograms to the right are binned data. The majority of points fall above the zero difference line (dotted line). **(B)** Movement disadvantage. The open circles are MAAs measured during head movements subtracted from the MAAs measured while listeners kept their heads still. The histograms to the right are binned data. The majority of points fall below the zero difference line (dotted line).

(Burian and Gstoettner, 1988), so making it likely that the auditory system incorporates vestibular input at multiple stages of processing. Indeed one could argue that the lack of a clearly defined vestibular cortex responding exclusively to vestibular signals (Guldin and Grüsser, 1998; Chen et al., 2010) would suggest that vestibular information is heavily integrated into the other senses prior to or in conjunction with the arrival of sensory input to the cortex. There are documented interactions between vestibular input and auditory spatial perception, such as the "audiogyral illusion" (Clark and Graybiel, 1949; Lester and Morant, 1970): when listeners are seated in a rotating room, their spatial auditory localization is shifted in the opposite direction from the rotation of the room. A related phenomenon, known as the "audiogravic illusion" (Graybiel and Niven, 1951), demonstrates that linear acceleration affects sound localization by shifting the perceived location of signals opposite to the acceleration of the listener. These studies provide evidence that physical motion can cause spatial auditory displacement. It has also been shown that moving sounds can induce the percept of self motion (for a review see Väljamäe, 2009). Taken together with the common observation that the world does not seem to spin in the opposite direction as one's head turns, the present evidence, allied to the previous data, becomes compelling: vestibular input is on some level deeply linked to auditory input.

Whether, however, the vestibular system works to simply subtract one's own motion from the movement of the acoustic world is a more difficult hypothesis to test. The eye movement driven by the vestibular-ocular reflex that largely subtracts self motion from the visual world can be easily observed, whereas any self-motion subtraction that might exist in the auditory system must be accomplished computationally, rendering it more problematic to observe experimentally. The evidence for a self-motion advantage presented in the current study is *suggestive* of a subtraction, but cannot be considered prima facie evidence for such a mechanism. Eye movements, for example, likely play a role in spatial auditory coordinate transformation. Strict geometric rules govern how the position of real world acoustic signals change with respect to the position and angle of the head (Wallach, 1940), none of which are in any way affected by the position of the eyes, but eye position has been shown to affect spatial localization (Lewald and Ehrenstein, 1996; Lewald, 1997, 1998). Furthermore, eye position influences audiovestibular interaction as well (Van Barneveld and Van Opstal, 2010), arguing that on some level that the primary driver of self-motion subtraction may be the eye movement itself. Certainly the best understood auditory spatial coordinate transformation is that which is driven by eye position. Psychophysically this transformation was described in the 1990s (Lewald and Ehrenstein, 1996; Lewald, 1997, 1998) and there is a growing body of physiological work that compliments this behavioral work. For example, the responses of neurons in the inferior colliculus have been shown to be modulated by eye position (Groh et al., 2001; Zwiers et al., 2004). Auditory receptive fields of neurons in the superior colliculus have also been shown to shift with eye position in both cats (Jay and Sparks, 1984, 1987) and primates (Hartline et al., 1995). An interaction between eye movements and head movements surely plays a role in spatial auditory processing, but we did not track the eye position of our participants. We asked listeners to fixate at a point directly ahead of their bodies as they turned their heads. Since we did not use an eye tracker, how reliably they maintained fixation is unknown, so this remains an issue. Furthermore in terms of general visual input, the use of virtual acoustics in isolation carries with it an inevitable mismatch between audition and vision. The impact of such a mismatch was mitigated somewhat in our experiment because the listeners were seated at the center of a ring of 24 loudspeakers, meaning that there was always a loudspeaker within 15° of the simulated acoustic angle. That said, future work will have to examine the important role of vision and eye movements in this phenomenon.

Another potential factor is that of proprioception: when the head turns, the flexing of muscles and the changing angle of the neck produces somatosensory stimulation that may also be integrated into both the percept of motion and of sound source location. Indeed it has been shown that straining the head against the rotation of a chair can abolish the audiogyral illusion (Lester and Morant, 1970). On the other hand, it has been demonstrated that proprioception plays a lesser role than that of the vestibular system in the discrimination of front/back location (Kim et al., 2013). Regardless of whether such input may be integrated into spatial auditory perception, since we were not able to replicate the natural movements of our listeners using a programmable motion-controlled chair, proprioception remains out of the scope of the current study. It should be noted that the movements in our study consisted of roughly sinusoidal back and forth rotations, necessarily involving angular acceleration. It is unknown whether the effects observed in our study would be the same for a listener turning at a constant rotational velocity and thereby reducing both proprioceptive and vestibular cues, so this too remains an open question. However, despite the fact that our study could not take into account eye movements, constant rotation, or proprioceptive input, we argue that our results are nevertheless attributable to a basic difference in the processing of self motion and world motion.

CONCLUSIONS

We found that for all age groups and levels of hearing impairment, the MMAA during self motion was smaller than during source motion. Thus listeners are more accurate at processing self-generated acoustic motion than source generated-motion. These results suggest that auditory spatial perception is at the very least continually informed by self motion; that is, listeners are engaged in constant and ongoing comparison between their own movement and the apparent movement of the auditory world. Furthermore, we find that the data are consistent with the hypothesis that self motion is at least partially compensated for, providing a more stable backdrop against which spatial location and "real" movement may be better discriminated.

ACKNOWLEDGMENTS

The work was supported by the Medical Research Council (grant number U135097131) and by the Chief Scientist Office of the Scottish Government. The PortAudio API bridge between Matlab and the MOTU soundcard was written by Robert Humphrey (www.playrec.co.uk). The authors would like to thank William Whitmer for reading drafts of this manuscript.

REFERENCES

Abraham, L., Copack, P. B., and Gilman, S. (1977). Brain stem pathways for vestibular projections to cerebral cortex in the cat. *Exp. Neurol.* 55, 436–448. doi: 10.1016/0014-4886(77)90012-7

Brimijoin, W. O., and Akeroyd, M. A. (2012). The role of head movements and signal spectrum in an auditory front/back illusion. *Iperception* 3, 179–182. doi: 10.1068/i7173sas

Brimijoin, W. O., Boyd, A. W., and Akeroyd, M. A. (2013). The contribution of head movement to the externalization and internalization of sounds. *PLoS ONE* 8:e83068. doi: 10.1371/journal.pone.0083068

Brimijoin, W. O., Mcshefferty, D., and Akeroyd, M. A. (2010). Auditory and visual orienting responses in listeners with and without hearing-impairment. *J. Acoust. Soc. Am.* 127, 3678–3688. doi: 10.1121/1.3409488

Burian, M., and Gstoettner, W. (1988). Projection of primary vestibular afferent fibres to the cochlear nucleus in the guinea pig. *Neurosci. Lett.* 84, 13–17. doi: 10.1016/0304-3940(88)90329-1

Burkhard, M., and Sachs, R. (1975). Anthropometric manikin for acoustic research. *J. Acoust. Soc. Am.* 58, 214–222. doi: 10.1121/1.380648

Chen, A., Deangelis, G. C., and Angelaki, D. E. (2010). Macaque parieto-insular vestibular cortex: responses to self-motion and optic flow. *J. Neurosci.* 30, 3022–3042. doi: 10.1523/JNEUROSCI.4029-09.2010

Clark, B., and Graybiel, A. (1949). The effect of angular acceleration on sound localization: the audiogyral illusion. *J. Psychol.* 28, 235–244. doi: 10.1080/00223980.1949.9916005

Graybiel, A., and Niven, J. (1951). The effect of a change in direction of resultant force on sound localization: the audiogravic illusion. *J. Exp. Psychol.* 42, 227. doi: 10.1037/h0059186

Groh, J. M., Trause, A. S., Underhill, A. M., Clark, K. R., and Inati, S. (2001). Eye position influences auditory responses in primate inferior colliculus. *Neuron* 29, 509–518. doi: 10.1016/S0896-6273(01)00222-7

Guldin, W., and Grüsser, O. (1998). Is there a vestibular cortex? *Trends Neurosci.* 21, 254–259. doi: 10.1016/S0166-2236(97)01211-3

Hartline, P., Vimal, R. P., King, A., Kurylo, D., and Northmore, D. (1995). Effects of eye position on auditory localization and neural representation of space in superior colliculus of cats. *Exp. Brain Res.* 104, 402–408. doi: 10.1007/BF00231975

Häusler, R., Colburn, S., and Marr, E. (1983). Sound localization in subjects with impaired hearing: spatial-discrimination and interaural-discrimination tests. *Acta Otolaryngol.* 96, 1–62. doi: 10.3109/00016488309105590

Jay, M. F., and Sparks, D. L. (1984). Auditory receptive fields in primate superior colliculus shift with changes in eye position. *Nature* 309, 345–347. doi: 10.1038/309345a0

Jay, M. F., and Sparks, D. L. (1987). Sensorimotor intergration in the primate superior colliculus. II. coordinates of auditory signals. *J. Neurophysiol.* 57, 35–55.

Kim, J., Barnett-Cowan, M., and Macpherson, E. A. (2013). Integration of auditory input with vestibular and neck proprioceptive information in the interpretation of dynamic sound localization cues. *Proc. Meet. Acoust.* 19:050142. doi: 10.1121/1.4799748

König, G., and Sussman, W. (1955). Zum Richtungshören in der Median-Sagittal-Ebene [On directional hearing in the medial-saggital planes]. *Arch. Ohren-Nasen-Kehlkopfheilk* 167, 303–307. doi: 10.1007/BF02107754

Lackner, J. R. (1977). Induction of illusory self-rotation and nystagmus by a rotating sound-field. *Aviat. Space Environ. Med.* 48, 129–131.

Lester, G., and Morant, R. B. (1970). Apparent sound displacement during vestibular stimulation. *Am. J. Psychol.* 83, 554–566. doi: 10.2307/1420689

Lewald, J. (1997). Eye-position effects in directional hearing. *Behav. Brain. Res.* 87, 35–48. doi: 10.1016/S0166-4328(96)02254-1

Lewald, J. (1998). The effect of gaze eccentricity on perceived sound direction and its relation to visual localization. *Hear. Res.* 115, 206–216. doi: 10.1016/S0378-5955(97)00190-1

Lewald, J., Dorrscheidt, G. J., and Ehrenstein, W. H. (2000). Sound localization with eccentric head position. *Behav. Brain. Res.* 108, 105–125. doi: 10.1016/S0166-4328(99)00141-2

Lewald, J., and Ehrenstein, W. H. (1996). The effect of eye position on auditory lateralization. *Exp. Brain. Res.* 108, 473–485. doi: 10.1007/BF00227270

Lewald, J., and Karnath, H.-O. (2000). Vestibular influence on human auditory space perception. *J. Neurophysiol.* 84, 1107–1952.

Lorente De No, R. (1933). The vestibulo-ocular reflex arc. *Arch. Neurol. Psychiat.* 30, 245–291. doi: 10.1001/archneurpsyc.1933.02240140009001

Macleod, A., and Summerfield, Q. (1987). Quantifying the contribution of vision to speech perception in noise. *Br. J. Audiol.* 21, 131–141. doi: 10.3109/03005368709077786

Mills, A. W. (1958). On the minimum audible angle. *J. Acoust. Soc. Am.* 30, 237–246. doi: 10.1121/1.1909553

Perrett, S., and Noble, W. (1997). The contribution of head motion cues to localization of low-pass noise. *Percept. Psychophys.* 59, 1018–1026. doi: 10.3758/BF03205517

Perrott, D. R. (1984). Concurrent minimum audible angle: a re-examination of the concept of auditory spatial acuity. *J. Acoust. Soc. Am.* 75, 1201–1206. doi: 10.1121/1.390771

Perrott, D. R., and Tucker, J. (1988). Minimum audible movement angle as a function of signal frequency and the velocity of the source. *J. Acoust. Soc. Am.* 83, 1522. doi: 10.1121/1.395908

Thurlow, W. R., and Runge, P. S. (1967). Effect of induced head movements on localization of direction of sounds. *J. Acoust. Soc. Am.* 42, 480–488. doi: 10.1121/1.1910604

Väljamäe, A. (2009). Auditorily-induced illusory self-motion: a review. *Brain Res. Rev.* 61, 240–255. doi: 10.1016/j.brainresrev.2009.07.001

Van Barneveld, D., and Van Opstal, A. (2010). Eye position determines audiovestibular integration during whole-body rotation. *Eur. J. Neurosci.* 31, 920–930. doi: 10.1111/j.1460-9568.2010.07113.x

Wallach, H. (1940). The role of head movements and vestibular and visual cues in sound localization. *J. Exp. Psychol.* 27, 339–367. doi: 10.1037/h0054629

Wierstorf, H., Geier, M., Raake, A., and Spors, S. (2011). "A free database of head related impulse response measurements in the horizontal plane with multiple distances," in *130th AES Convention* (London, UK).

Wightman, F. L., and Kistler, D. J. (1999). Resolution of front-back ambiguity in spatial heading by listener and source movement. *J. Acoust. Soc. Am.* 105, 2841–2853. doi: 10.1121/1.426899

Zwiers, M. P., Versnel, H., and Van Opstal, A. J. (2004). Involvement of monkey inferior colliculus in spatial hearing. *J. Neurosci.* 24, 4145–4156. doi: 10.1523/JNEUROSCI.0199-04.2004

4

Perceptual factors contribute more than acoustical factors to sound localization abilities with virtual sources

Guillaume Andéol[1]*, Sophie Savel[2] and Anne Guillaume[3]

[1] Département Action et Cognition en Situation Opérationnelle, Institut de Recherche Biomédicale des Armées, Brétigny sur Orge, France
[2] Laboratoire de Mécanique et d'Acoustique, Centre National de la Recherche Scientifique, UPR 7051, Equipe Sons, Aix-Marseille Université, Centrale Marseille, Marseille, France
[3] Laboratoire d'Accidentologie, de Biomécanique et d'Étude du Comportement Humain, Nanterre, France

***Correspondence:**
Guillaume Andéol, Département Action et Cognition en Situation Opérationnelle, Institut de Recherche Biomédicale des Armées, BP 73, 91223 Brétigny sur Orge, France
e-mail: guillaume.andeol@irba.fr

Human sound localization abilities rely on binaural and spectral cues. Spectral cues arise from interactions between the sound wave and the listener's body (head-related transfer function, HRTF). Large individual differences were reported in localization abilities, even in young normal-hearing adults. Several studies have attempted to determine whether localization abilities depend mostly on acoustical cues or on perceptual processes involved in the analysis of these cues. These studies have yielded inconsistent findings, which could result from methodological issues. In this study, we measured sound localization performance with normal and modified acoustical cues (i.e., with individual and non-individual HRTFs, respectively) in 20 naïve listeners. Test conditions were chosen to address most methodological issues from past studies. Procedural training was provided prior to sound localization tests. The results showed no direct relationship between behavioral results and an acoustical metrics (spectral-shape prominence of individual HRTFs). Despite uncertainties due to technical issues with the normalization of the HRTFs, large acoustical differences between individual and non-individual HRTFs appeared to be needed to produce behavioral effects. A subset of 15 listeners then trained in the sound localization task with individual HRTFs. Training included either visual correct-answer feedback (for the test group) or no feedback (for the control group), and was assumed to elicit perceptual learning for the test group only. Few listeners from the control group, but most listeners from the test group, showed significant training-induced learning. For the test group, learning was related to pre-training performance (i.e., the poorer the pre-training performance, the greater the learning amount) and was retained after 1 month. The results are interpreted as being in favor of a larger contribution of perceptual factors than of acoustical factors to sound localization abilities with virtual sources.

Keywords: sound localization, perceptual learning, procedural learning, head-related transfer function, individual differences

INTRODUCTION

Individuals receive information about their environment mainly via the visual and auditory sensory modalities. The auditory system has lower spatial resolution than the visual system, but allows perception beyond the visual field and in darkness. However, there is no direct encoding of space in the auditory system. Auditory space perception relies on the processing of binaural cues (i.e., interaural differences in the level and time of arrival of the incoming sound wave) for the left/right dimension, and spectral cues (i.e., filtering of the incoming sound wave by the listener's upper body, which corresponds to the head-related transfer function, HRTF) for the up/down and front/back dimensions. These direction-dependent cues are transformed into a complex audio-spatial map, which depends on anatomical characteristics and develops through experience with sensory—mainly visual (King, 2009)—feedback. Audio-spatial maps have been found to be highly plastic throughout life (Clifton et al., 1988; Hofman et al., 1998; Otte et al., 2013). Experience-dependent plasticity provides a potential neural basis for training-induced perceptual improvements in performance.

Large individual differences in localization ability have been reported, even in young normal-hearing adults (Wightman and Kistler, 1989; Makous and Middlebrooks, 1990; Wenzel et al., 1993; Populin, 2008; Savel, 2009). These individual differences were mainly observed under experimental conditions that are assumed to involve spectral cues: localization in the up/down and front/back dimensions (Wightman and Kistler, 1989; Wenzel et al., 1993) and in noise (Best et al., 2005). Two main contributing factors to localization abilities have therefore been proposed: spectral cues, and perceptual processes involved in the analysis of these cues. Several studies have assessed the contributions of these two factors separately.

It has been proposed that localization abilities depend mainly on the physical saliency of the acoustical cues carried by HRTFs.

According to this hypothesis, the performance of listeners with poorer abilities would be hampered by insufficiently salient spectral cues. This hypothesis was initially supported by the finding that listeners with poor localization performance substantially improved when these listeners used the HRTFs of other listeners who had better performance (Butler and Belendiuk, 1977; Wenzel et al., 1988; Asano et al., 1990). However, the physical saliency of spectral cues was not quantified, and more recent studies, involving more listeners, did not confirm this finding (Møller et al., 1996; Middlebrooks, 1999b). A recent study assessed the spectral shape prominence of 15 individual HRTFs, and found no relationship between this acoustical metrics and localization performance in noise (Andéol et al., 2013).

Alternatively, it has been proposed that providing listeners with other-than-their-own HRTFs should affect their localization performance regardless of the saliency of spectral cues (Wenzel et al., 1993; Møller et al., 1996; Middlebrooks, 1999b). Four studies compared the localization performance obtained using the individual's own HRTFs (normal cues) to the performance obtained using non-individual HRTFs (modified cues) in the same listeners. The two studies involving listeners with previous experience in localization tests reported a difference in performance between HRTFs (Møller et al., 1996; Middlebrooks, 1999b). Conversely, the two studies involving naïve listeners reported no difference (Bronkhorst, 1995; Begault et al., 2001). The latter negative findings may have been due to the involvement of naïve listeners, who usually have more variable performance—perhaps due to differences in the speed of procedural learning (e.g., handling of the response device, Djelani et al., 2000; Majdak et al., 2010). There were multiple other methodological differences between the four studies[1]. Reports of a lack of difference in performance could also result from insufficiently large "interspectral distance" (ISD) between individual and non-individual HRTFs (as defined by Middlebrooks, 1999a). On the other hand, the reports of large differences might be explained merely by the fact that the listeners did not learn to use the cues provided by the non-individual HRTFs. Perceptual learning produces a recalibration of the audio-spatial map (Hofman et al., 1998; Carlile and Blackman, 2013). By simulating complete recalibration, Majdak et al. (2014) showed that using non-individual HRTFs should have a moderate impact on sound localization performance. However, they found that non-acoustical factors (attention, perceptual abilities) would be highly relevant for predicting sound localization performance.

Non-acoustical factors, such as perceptual processes, have been proposed to explain the large individual differences reported in studies about discrimination between front and rear sources (Wightman and Kistler, 1999) and about sound localization in noise (Andéol et al., 2011, 2013). The perceptual processes involved in the analysis of spectral cues (Drennan and Watson, 2001; Sabin et al., 2012) and sound localization accuracy with individual HRTFs (Majdak et al., 2010) were both found to improve with training in the auditory task. In the latter study, acoustical cues were kept constant but sensory (visual) feedback was provided during training. The resulting improvement in localization performance was assumed to reflect perceptual learning. However, increased exposure to the experimental environment (e.g., apparatus) and/or procedural learning (i.e., learning of the task contingencies) could have also contributed to the observed improvement.

In the present study, we assessed the contributions of acoustical and perceptual factors to sound localization abilities with virtual sources under experimental conditions that were chosen specifically to address the confounds present in previous studies—i.e., factors that could interfere with, or mask, the actual contribution of the factor investigated. Twenty naïve listeners were given procedural training prior to sound localization tests in "classical" conditions (anechoic environment, constant target/head distance, large range of azimuths and elevations). Acoustical and perceptual factors were separately manipulated, and the resulting effects on localization performance were assessed.

To investigate the role of acoustical cues, sound localization performance was measured with individual and non-individual HRTFs (normal and modified cues). We quantified the "spectral strength," which is assumed to quantify the amount of spectral detail, of each HRTF (Andéol et al., 2013), and the ISD between individual and non-individual HRTFs. The following observations would be in favor of a substantial contribution of acoustical factors to sound localization abilities with virtual sources: a relationship between performance and spectral strength with individual HRTFs, a difference in performance between individual and non-individual HRTFs, and a relationship between this behavioral difference and the ISD between HRTFs.

The role of perceptual processes was investigated as follows. A subset of 15 listeners performed training to the sound localization task with individual HRTFs. Seven listeners received visual correct-answer feedback during training (test group) and eight received no feedback (control group). The amount of training-induced learning was assessed by comparing pre- and post-test performance. The persistence of learning was assessed by a follow-up post-test. In studies of perceptual training, it is often assumed that the training regimen elicits more efficient perceptual learning if correct-answer feedback is provided (Amitay et al., 2010), particularly for complex tasks (Garcia et al., 2013). For sound localization, it has even been suggested that no perceptual learning can occur if no feedback is provided (Recanzone et al., 1998; Irving and Moore, 2011). We therefore assumed that the training regimen in the present study elicited perceptual learning for the test group only. For this group, significant training-induced improvements in localization performance would indicate that perceptual learning occurred. The finding of a relationship between the amount of learning and the performance as measured prior to training for the test group would therefore reflect the contribution of a common—perceptual in this case—factor to the two behavioral metrics. Taken together, these results would indicate a large contribution of perceptual factors to sound localization abilities with virtual sources.

[1] Middlebrooks (1999b) used a "classical" protocol with an absolute localization task, a virtual sound source simulated in an anechoic environment, a large range of source elevations and azimuths, and constant target/listener distance. Møller et al. (1996) used a non-anechoic environment and variable target distances. Bronkhorst (1995) used a forced-choice localization task. Begault et al. (2001) restrained the target positions to the horizontal plane.

MATERIALS AND METHODS

OVERVIEW OF THE STUDY

To test the hypotheses presented in the Introduction, two consecutive experiments were conducted. In the first experiment, the role of acoustical factors was assessed by comparing the localization performance obtained using individual HRTFs (normal acoustical cues) to that obtained using non-individual HRTFs (modified cues). The spectral strength of each HRTF, and the ISD between individual and non-individual HRTFs, were evaluated. Prior to the sound localization tests, each listener performed procedural training with visual targets to reduce the contribution of procedural factors to the results. The second experiment assessed the role of perceptual factors by comparing localization performance prior to and following a 5-day training regimen. A first group received visual feedback (test group) and a second group (control group) received no feedback. An improvement of performance for the first group would be in favor of a contribution of perceptual factors to sound localization abilities with virtual sources, because acoustical factors were constant during training. The control group allowed to assess the potential contribution of other factors (familiarization, procedural learning,...) to the observed training-induced improvements.

LISTENERS

Twenty-five naïve listeners participated (11 females, mean age 27 ± 5 years; right-handed according to the Edinburgh Handedness Inventory, see Oldfield, 1971). All had normal hearing (thresholds of 15 dB HL or less at octave frequencies from 0.125 to 8 kHz) and normal otoscopy. None had history of auditory pathology. Written informed consent was obtained, in agreement with the guidelines of the Declaration of Helsinki and the Huriet law on biomedical research in humans. Listeners were paid 10 €/h for their participation. After completion of the study, the data from five listeners were excluded due to errors in the processing of their HRTFs (see below).

EXPERIMENTAL APPARATUS

The localization experiment was conducted inside a sphere, which was located in a 30-m^2, light and sound-attenuating (<0.02 Lux and 35 dBA) room. The setup was a black sphere with a radius of 1.4 m that was truncated at its base (1.2 m below center, elevation = −60°). This sphere represented the perceptual space of the listener during testing (see **Figure 1**). Three lines of optical fibers were used to visually indicate the medial vertical, medial horizontal, and medial frontal planes on the interior surface of the sphere. A network of 619 optical fibers, each connected to one LED, was distributed on the sphere. The LEDs (color = red, size = 1° of visual angle, luminance = 10 cd/m^2), when turned on, were used either as visual targets or as feedback signals.

The listener was seated on a stool that was adjusted so as to match the center of the listener's head with that of the sphere. During testing, the matching was verified using an electromagnetic sensor (Polhemus Fastrack) mounted on the headphones (Beyer DT990Pro). Listeners used a "God Eye Localization Pointing" system (GELP, Gilkey et al., 1995) to provide their localization responses. The GELP was composed of a plastic globe (radius = 15 cm) that represented a reduced version of the listener's perceptual space and a stylus. Listeners had to point the stylus on the globe so that the vector "center of the globe to stylus tip" had the same direction as the vector "center of the listener's head to perceived target direction on the sphere." The position of the stylus tip was recorded using an electromagnetic sensor (Polhemus Fastrack), whose transmitter was mounted on the bar supporting the globe. To help the transfer of representation from perceptual to response spaces, the globe contained a figurine's head that represented the listener's head at the center of the sphere, and white circles that represented the three main planes (medial horizontal, medial vertical, and medial frontal). The position of the LEDs relative to the listener's head varied in azimuth from 0 to 360° and in elevation from −60 to 90°. The angular separation between LEDs was 15 or 20°.

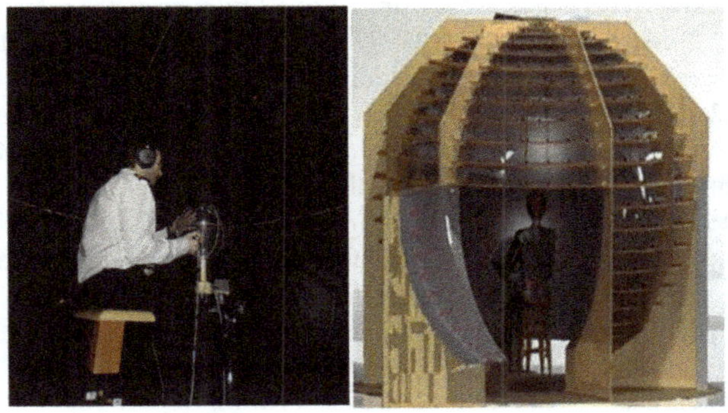

FIGURE 1 | Interior view (left) and exterior schematic view (right) of the experimental apparatus.

MEASUREMENT AND SPECTRAL CHARACTERIZATION OF HRTFs

One non-individual (Neumann KU-100 dummy head) and 25 individual (listeners) HRTFs were measured in a semi-anechoic room (Illsonic Sonex Audio) using the procedure described in Andéol et al. (2013). Directional transfer functions (DTFs) were then derived from each HRTF using the method proposed by Middlebrooks (1999a). DTFs only contain the directional components of the HRTF, and are independent of the characteristics of the microphone or of its positioning into the ear canal. To compute DTFs, each HRTF has to be divided by the square root of the weighted sum of squared HRTFs that have been measured for each sound source direction. The weights are adjusted to take into account the non-uniform distribution of sound directions. The spectral strength, which corresponds to the ISD between a flat spectrum and the magnitude spectrum of the DTF, was computed for each HRTF using the procedure described in Andéol et al. (2013). The ISD between individual and non-individual HRTFs was quantified as the difference in DTF.

As a result of an error in DTFs computation (i.e., use of the HRTF measured for the 90° elevation instead of the weighted sum of squared HRTFs), which was detected after collection of the behavioral data, five listeners were excluded from the study. They had ISDs between correctly and incorrectly assessed DTFs greater than the smallest ISD between individual and non-individual HRTFs in the 25-listener cohort (9.5 dB^2). ISDs between correct and incorrect DTFs ranged from 1.1 to 6.6 dB^2 across the remaining 20 listeners (see **Table 1**). These values are below the ISDs between individual and non-individual HRTFs (range = 9.5 to 17.2 dB^2). However, to verify that the error in DTFs was unlikely to affect the behavioral results reported below, five of the 20 listeners performed an additional localization test with individual HRTFs, using their correct and incorrect DTFs. The results showed little or no effect of the difference in DTF (see Appendix). We therefore refer below to "individual HRTFs" in spite of the small error in DTF presentation.

STIMULI

Stimuli for sound localization tests were digitally generated at a 48.8-kHz sampling rate, 24-bit resolution using a real-time processor (RX6 Tucker-Davis Technologies), and were converted to the analog domain, routed to a headphone buffer (HB7 Tucker-Davis Technologies) and presented through headphones (Beyer DT990Pro). The stimulus was a 150-ms (including 10-ms on/off cosine-squared ramps) burst of pink noise that was filtered between 0.05 and 14 kHz using sixth-order and seventh-order Butterworth filters, respectively. The overall stimulus level was 60 dB SPL.

PROCEDURES

Listeners ($N = 20$ after removal of five listeners) performed procedural training with the GELP using visual targets (3 consecutive days) and then completed sound localization pre-tests with individual and non-individual HRTFs in counterbalanced order (2 days). A subset of 15 listeners then performed training to the sound localization task with individual HRTFs (5 days) followed by sound localization "immediate" post-tests with individual and non-individual HRTFs in fixed order (2 days). All except one trained listeners performed a "long-term" post-test with individual HRTFs (1 month after the immediate post-tests).

The directions of the visual or auditory targets were chosen as follows. For sound localization tests, virtual auditory targets were created by interpolating the directions used for the HRTF measurement. The target directions were determined using 119-point meshes mapped onto the surface of the perceptual space (shortened at −60° of elevation) using the Hypermesh (Altair, MI, USA) software. Three different meshes were used for the pre-test, immediate post-test, and long-term post-test. A 7° azimuth translation was applied so that the directions tested using individual HRTFs were different from those tested using non-individual HRTFs. For the procedural and auditory trainings, the target directions corresponded to the positions of the optical fibers on the surface of the sphere. The surface of the sphere was divided into eight areas defined by the intersection of the median horizontal, vertical and frontal planes. For a given session of procedural or auditory training, the target directions were randomly but equally chosen among the eight areas. The target directions varied between sessions. Thus, the sets of 119 (sound localization tests) or 120 (auditory training) target directions varied between training sessions, between pre- and post-tests, and between individual and non-individual HRTFs.

Table 1 | Individual value of the ISD between correct and incorrect DTFs (in dB^2).

Listener	ISD (dB^2)
L8	3.6
L9	4.4
L11	1.6
L12	1.4
L13	1.8
L14	2.5
L15	3.5
L17	3.9
L18	3.3
L21	2.2
L22	6.6
L23	1.3
L24	2.2
L26	4.9
L27	1.2
L28	2.7
L30	3.8
L31	4.1
L33	1.1
L34	1.3

Procedural training

The setup and response device were the same as those used for auditory tests. The procedural training stage had two goals: (1) familiarize the listener with the experimental environment and (2) reduce experimental noise related to the use of the response device (i.e., pointing errors in the transfer of representation from egocentric perceptual space to allocentric response space). Visual targets were used to prevent auditory learning.

Once the listener was installed in the sphere, a visual cross was turned on to indicate the "straight ahead" direction (azimuth and elevation = 0°). The listener oriented to the straight ahead direction and pressed the stylus button. The cross was turned off and a red visual target was then presented on the sphere by turning on one LED. For trials with no feedback, listeners had to indicate the perceived direction of the visual target using the GELP, and to validate their response by pressing the stylus button. For trials with feedback, listeners pointed to the perceived direction without pressing the stylus button. If the spherical angular error between actual and pointed directions was below the "permissible" error (=8° for day 1; = error measured for the last no-feedback block of the preceding day—2° for days 2 and 3), a "hit" sound was emitted. Otherwise, the listener had to modify the pointed direction until they reached permissible error. The trial ended either by the emission of the hit sound or after 30 s. The position of the target changed from trial to trial. The listeners performed three training sessions (duration = 1 h 30 each). For each session, two blocks of 40 trials with correct-answer feedback (15–20 min) alternated with three blocks of 32 trials with no feedback (12–15 min) in fixed order (no/with/no/with/no feedback).

The spherical angular error averaged across the 20 listeners decreased from 9.2° (±1.6) for the first to 6.6° (±1.3) for the last no-feedback blocks. Individual errors were stable across, at least, the last three no-feedback blocks (repeated measure ANOVA, error at no-feedback blocks as the within-listener factor, post-hoc Tukey-HSD: $p > 0.50$).

Sound localization tests

Before each presentation of the auditory target, the listener's position relative to the straight ahead direction was verified using the electromagnetic sensor. In case of a deviation above 5°, a message required the listener to rectify their position. Once the listener was correctly positioned, the auditory target was presented over headphones at one of 119 possible virtual directions on the sphere. The listener was free to move after the offset of the auditory target. The listener had to indicate the perceived direction using the GELP. There was no time restriction but listeners were encouraged to respond quickly. No correct-answer feedback was provided. The set of 119 directions was repeated six times (total number of trials = 714). The responses collected at the first repetition were excluded from the analyses. Each pre- and post-test had an overall duration of 1.5–2 h, and was divided into three series of four 60-trial blocks (54 for the last one). Listeners had to stay inside the sphere during between-block breaks (1.5 min) but were allowed to leave the setup during between-series breaks (10 min).

Auditory training

The auditory stimuli used during training had the same characteristics as those used in the sound localization pre- and post-tests except that only individual HRTFs were used. Each of the five training sessions included three 20-min blocks of 40 trials, with 8-min breaks between blocks. For the test group ($N = 7$), training consisted in providing the listener with trial-by-trial visual feedback (red LED turned on during 250 ms after the listener's response) as to the correct auditory target direction. Listeners were instructed to search for the red light, face it, and come back to the straight-ahead position. The auditory target + visual feedback sequence was replayed at least once. Listeners were then allowed to replay the sequence as many times as they wished. Training for the test group was similar to that used in the study by Majdak et al. (2010), except that their listeners were allowed only one sequence replay. For the control group ($N = 8$), training sessions were identical to pre- and post-tests sessions, except for the number of trials (660 trials instead of 714) that allowed the training duration to be similar for the two groups. The events and listener's actions during testing are listed in **Table 2**.

Table 2 | Order of events and listener's actions during auditory training.

Events	Listener's actions
Straight ahead indicator turned on	Face the straight ahead indicator
Auditory target presentation	Indicate the target direction using GELP
Visual feedback (red light) turned on	Face the red light and come back
Straight ahead indictor turned on	Face the straight ahead indicator
Visual feedback turned off	
Auditory target re-presentation	
Visual feedback turned on	Choose to replay the auditory target + visual feedback sequence or to move to the next trial

DATA ANALYSIS

Localization responses were computed using a three-pole coordinate system (Kistler and Wightman, 1992). In this system, the position of a point is coded by the three following angles: the left/right angle in the medial vertical plane (direction in the left/right dimension), the front/back angle in the medial frontal plane (direction in the front/back dimension), and the up/down angle in the medial horizontal plane (direction in the up/down dimension). This coordinate system has the advantage that a given angular distance corresponds to a constant distance on the sphere for all spatial regions. Conversely, in two-pole—lateral/polar (Middlebrooks, 1999b) and azimuth/elevation (Oldfield and Parker, 1984)—coordinate systems, a compression of space occurs when points are close to the poles. Another advantage of the three-pole system is the distinction between spatial dimensions that depend on different localization cues or processes: binaural cues for localization in the left/right dimension (Strutt, 1907), spectral-shape analysis (Wightman and Kistler, 1993) or determination of the main spectral-notch position (Butler and Belendiuk, 1977) for localization in the up/down dimension, and comparison of the levels of different bandwidths (Wightman and Kistler, 1997) or more complex cues (Bronkhorst, 1995; Zhang and Hartmann, 2010) for localization in the front/back dimension.

Scatterplots of raw data (i.e., target against response directions) are provided in **Figures 2–4** for the up/down, front/back, and left/right dimensions, respectively. Because left/right judgments remain generally accurate with non-individual HRTFs (Wightman and Kistler, 1997), and individual differences in localization abilities were mainly observed for up/down and front/back dimensions, statistical analyzes were performed for the latter two dimensions only.

Numerous studies have reported frequent front/back (response pointing to the frontal hemifield for a target presented in the rear or vice versa) and up/down reversals (response pointing to above 0° elevation for a target presented at below 0° elevation or vice versa) in localization responses. Such reversals drastically increase angular errors, unless they are excluded or corrected (e.g., a response at −50° elevation is transformed into 50°). We therefore assessed the following localization scores: up/down angular error after correction of up/down reversals (in °), and down → up, up → down, and front/back reversal rates (in %). Up/down errors were separately assessed for "high," "middle," and "low" target elevations (elevation = 25 to 75°, −15 to 15°, −60 to −25°, respectively). Responses at ±15° front/back angles and those at ±20° up/down angles were not considered as front/back and up/down reversals, respectively.

The within- and across-listener paired comparisons listed below were statistically assessed using Wilcoxon tests. Relationships between two metrics were assessed using Spearman correlation coefficients. Two-tailed p-values are reported below.

To examine the role of acoustical factors, we assessed:

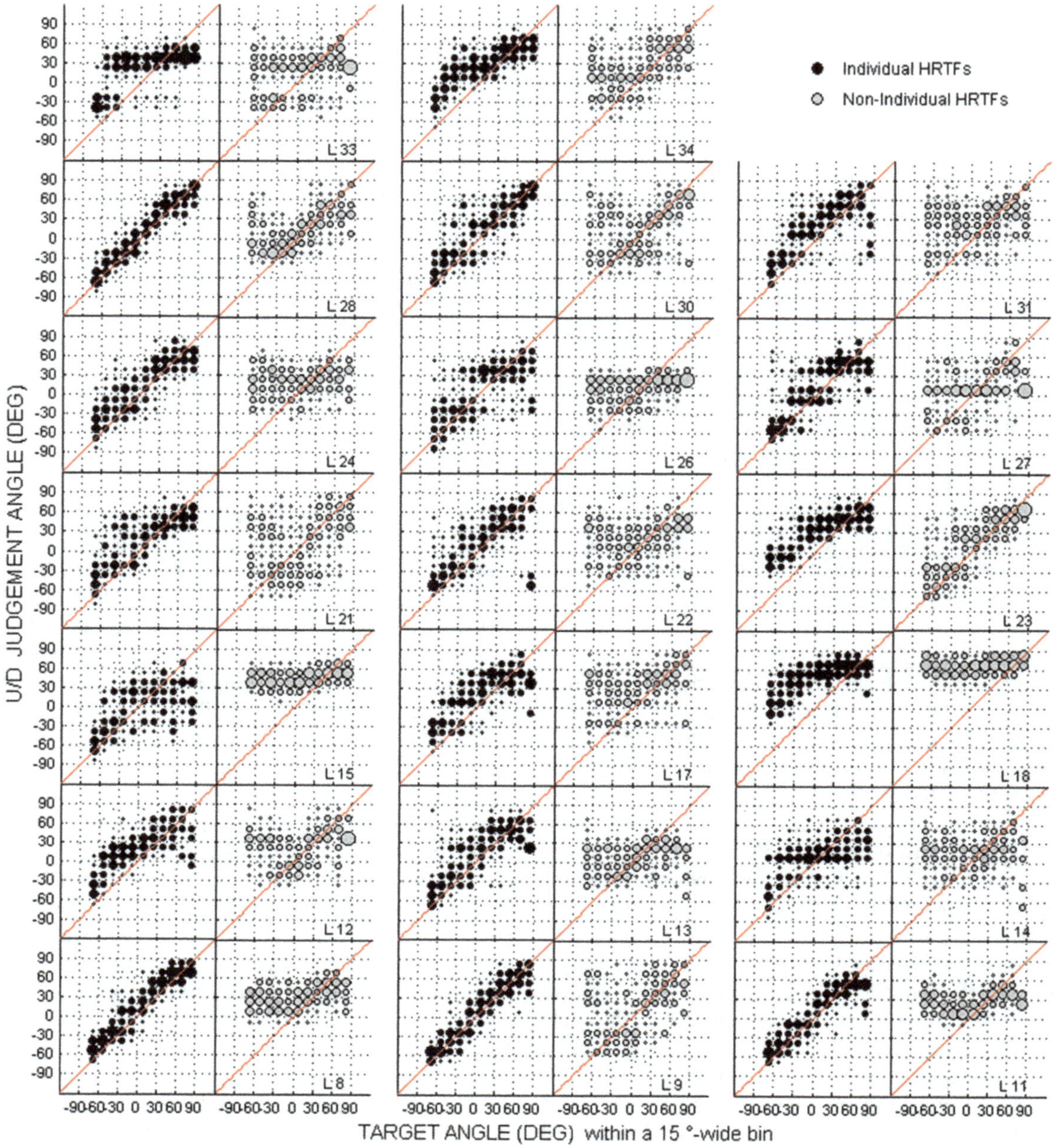

FIGURE 2 | Individual judgment position against target position with individual and non-individual HRTFs (black and gray dots, respectively) at the pre-test in the up/down dimension. Each panel couple is for a different listener ($N = 20$).

(1) The relationship between spectral strength and pre-test performance with individual HRTFs for the 20-listener cohort.
(2) The individual and cohort differences between individual and non-individual HRTFs in pre-test performance.
(3) The relationship between this behavioral difference and the ISD between individual and non-individual HRTFs for the cohort.

To examine the role of perceptual factors, we first computed individual amounts of training-induced improvement (i.e., pre-test – post-test difference in score, referred to below as "learning amount") with individual HRTFs. Then, we determined for each listener whether learning was significant using a Wilcoxon test (pre-test against post-test scores). Finally, we assessed within each trained group:

(1) The relationship between learning amount at the immediate post-test and pre-test score.
(2) Whether the listeners with significant learning at the immediate post-test had similar immediate and long-term post-test scores.

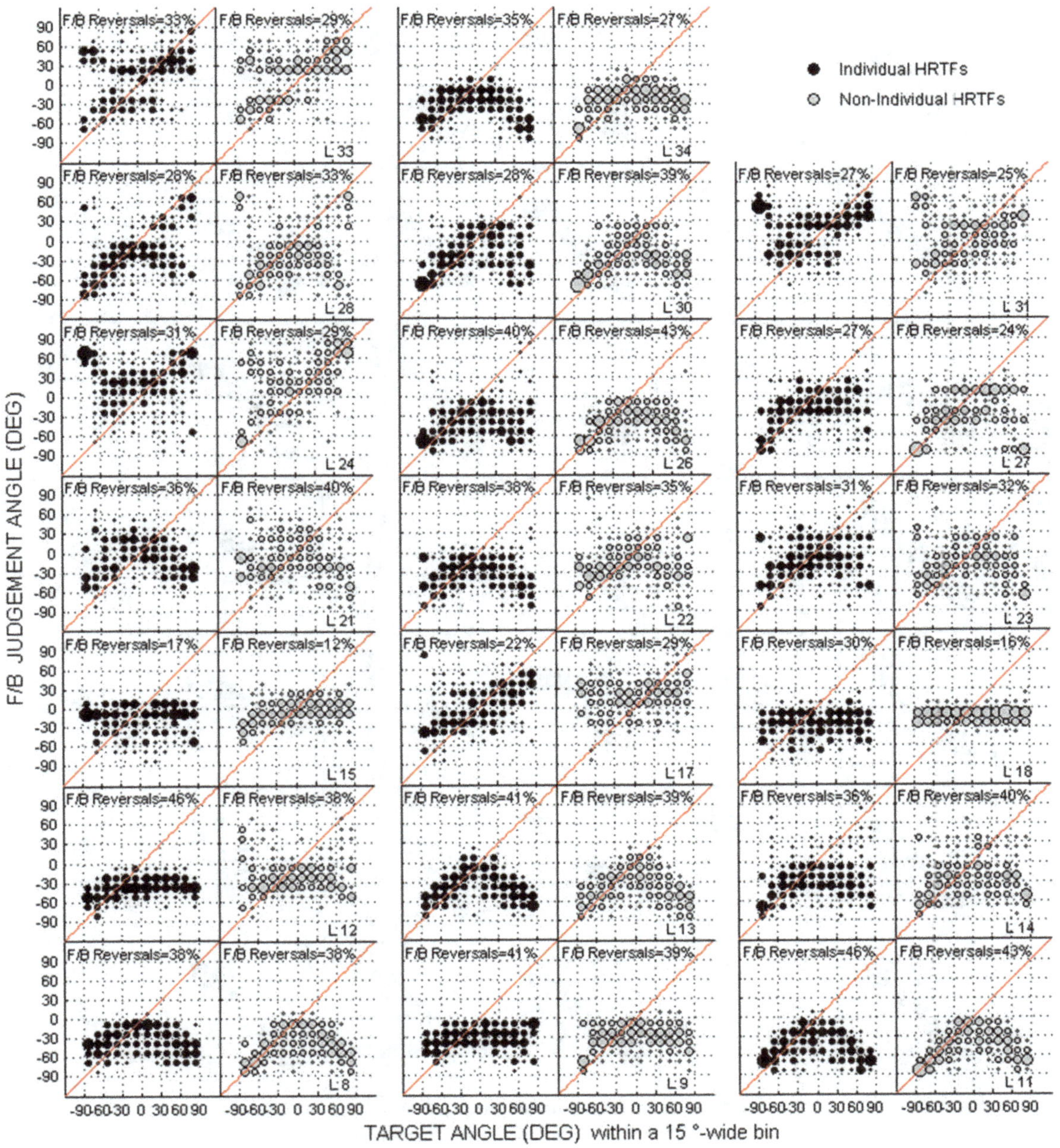

FIGURE 3 | Same as Figure 2 but for the front/back dimension. The front/back reversal rate for individual and non-individual HRTFs are indicated in each panel couple.

RESULTS

RELATIONSHIP BETWEEN SPECTRAL STRENGTH AND PRE-TEST PERFORMANCE WITH INDIVIDUAL HRTFs

With individual HRTFs, no relationship was found between spectral strength and performance at the pre-test (see **Figure 5**), regardless of whether performance was expressed in terms of up/down angular errors (high elevations: $R = -0.21$, $p = 0.37$; middle elevations: $R = 0.32$, $p = 0.16$; low elevations: $R = 0.14$, $p = 0.56$), up/down reversals (up → down: $R = -0.11$, $p = 0.64$; down → up: $R = -0.01$, $p = 0.95$), or front/back reversals ($R = -0.01$, $p = 0.99$). However, the spectral strength of the non-individual HRTFs was weaker than that of all individual HRTFs (12.8 dB^2 vs. 17.6 to 45.0 dB^2) for the low elevation region, where (down → up) reversals were significantly more frequent with non-individual than with individual HRTFs.

DIFFERENCE BETWEEN INDIVIDUAL AND NON-INDIVIDUAL HRTFs AT THE PRE-TEST

For up/down errors (see **Figures 2, 6A–C**), only a few listeners (1, 6, and 6 for high, middle, and low target elevations, respectively) individually showed significant differences between HRTFs. The lack of difference was observed regardless of whether listeners

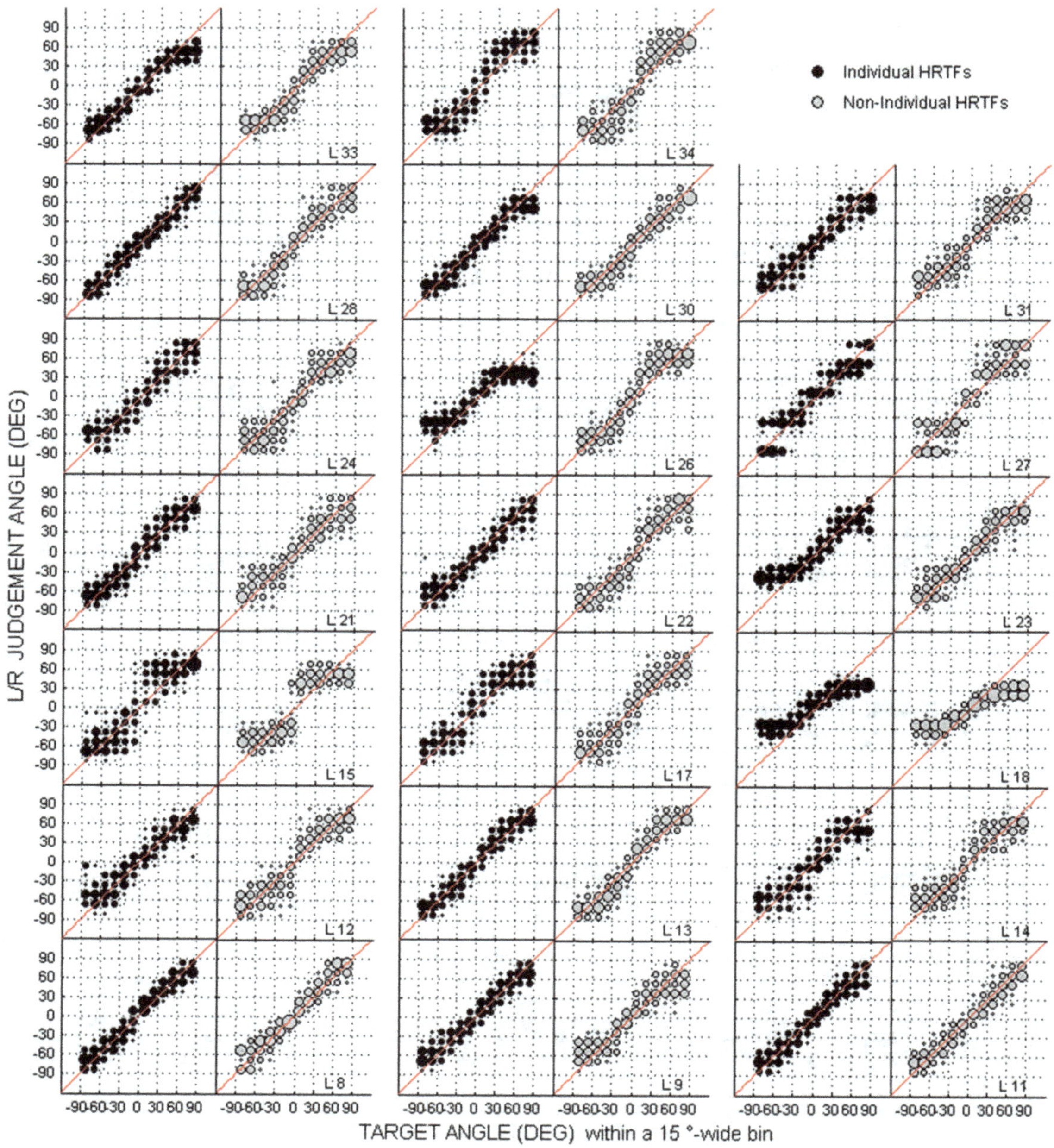

FIGURE 4 | Same as Figure 2 but for the left/right dimension.

had large or small errors, and is therefore unlikely to have been due to a floor effect. The difference between HRTFs as assessed for the cohort was significant for high target elevations (median up/down error ± 1 inter-quartile range = 18 ± 3° with individual HRTFs < 19 ± 5° with non-individual HRTFs, $p = 0.004$) but was not significant for middle (24 ± 8° vs. 23 ± 8°, $p = 0.52$) and low target elevations (23 ± 6° vs. 21 ± 8°, $p = 0.99$). Up → down reversals were infrequent with individual HRTFs (see **Figure 6D**). The difference between HRTFs was small but significant for six listeners and for the cohort (median = 3 ± 5% with individual HRTFs vs. 5 ± 7% with non-individual HRTFs, $p = 0.03$). Down → up reversals were more frequent than up → down reversals, and increased with non-individual HRTFs (see **Figure 6E**). The difference between HRTFs was significant for 17 listeners and for the cohort (median = 20 ± 14% < 51 ± 26%, $p < 0.001$). For front/back reversals (see **Figures 3, 6F**), only two listeners individually showed significant difference between HRTFs. The difference for the cohort was not significant (median = 35 ± 10% ≈ 35 ± 11%, $p = 0.37$). Visual inspection of raw data in the left/right dimension indicates no difference between HRTFs (see **Figure 4**).

RELATIONSHIP BETWEEN BEHAVIORAL DIFFERENCE AND ISD BETWEEN INDIVIDUAL AND NON-INDIVIDUAL HRTFs

The ISD values varied across target regions and listeners (**Figure 7**), but were essentially—except for high

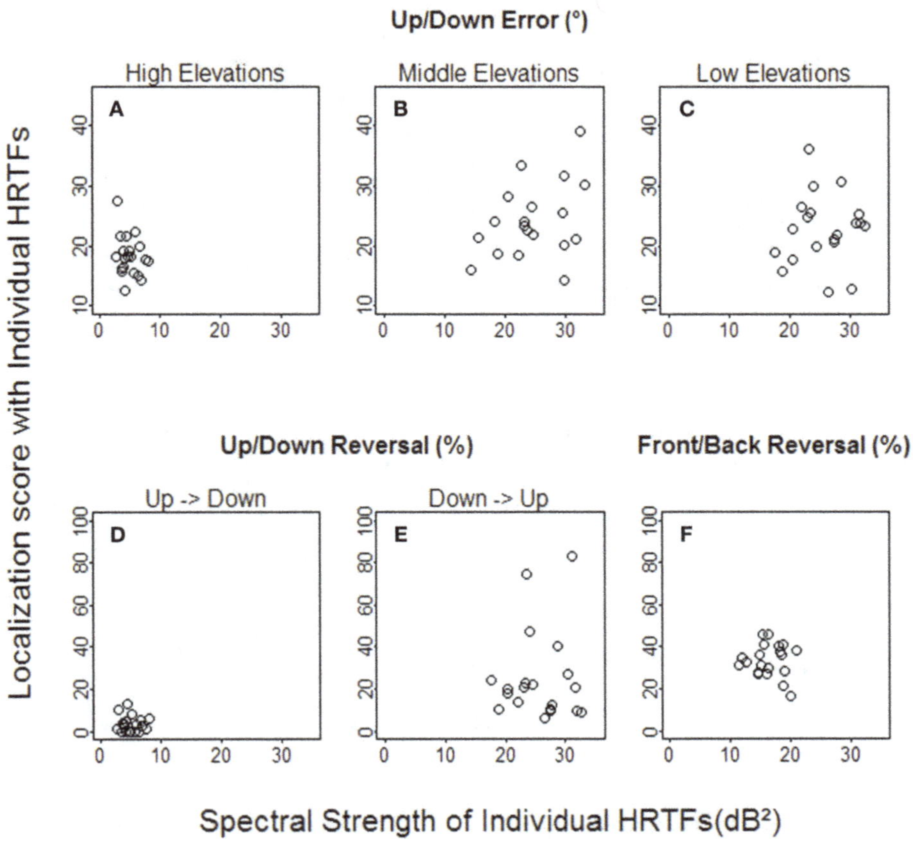

FIGURE 5 | Individual localization scores at the pre-test against spectral strength with individual HRTFs. (A–C) Up/down errors (in °) for high, middle, and low target elevations. **(D–F)** Up → down, down → up, and front/back reversal rates (in %).

elevations—well-above 10 dB^2, which should be large enough to produce behavioral effects according to the results from a past study (Middlebrooks, 1999b). However, we found no *positive* correlation between the signed difference in localization score and the ISD between non-individual and individual HRTFs (up/down errors: $R = -0.03$, $p = 0.90$ for high elevations, $R = -0.07$, $p = 0.77$ for middle elevations, $R = -0.42$, $p = 0.037$ for low elevations; up → down reversals: $R = 0.32$, $p = 0.16$; down → up reversals: $R = 0.37$, $p = 0.11$; front/back reversals: $R = -0.02$, $p = 0.93$). Note that if the listeners who had *lower* scores with non-individual HRTFs than with individual HRTFs were excluded from analyses, no correlation was significant.

SIGNIFICANCE OF LEARNING WITH INDIVIDUAL HRTFs

Individual raw data collected at the pre-test and the post-test for the two groups are provided for the up/down and front/back dimensions in **Figures 8**, **9**, respectively. In the up/down dimension, the listeners from the test group mostly showed substantial training-induced improvement in performance (i.e., post-test responses closer to perfect performance than pre-test responses, see left panels in **Figure 8**), but those from the control group showed little or no improvement (see right panels in **Figure 8**). For up/down errors, many listeners from the test group (2, 4, and 4/7 for high, middle, and low target elevations, respectively) but only a few listeners from the control group (2, 1, and 2/8, respectively) showed significant learning (see filled symbols above the dashed lines in **Figures 10A–C**). Up → down reversals were infrequent prior to training but nonetheless significantly decreased with training for one listener from the test group and for two listeners from the control group (see **Figure 10D**). Down → up reversals were frequent prior to training and significantly decreased with training for four listeners from the test group but for no listener from the control group (see filled symbols above the dashed line in **Figure 10E**). In the front/back dimension, post-test responses were similar to pre-test responses for all except one listener (L27) from the control group (see right panels in **Figure 9**), but frequently came closer to perfect performance with training for the test group, particularly for targets presented in front (see left panels in **Figure 9**). Learning as assessed on front/back reversal rates was significant for three listeners from the test group but for no listener from the control group (see filled symbols above the dashed line in **Figure 10F**).

At the pre-test, no significant difference was observed between the test and control groups (up/down errors: 16 ± 4° vs. 18 ± 2°, $p = 0.28$ for high elevations, 24 ± 6° vs. 25 ± 10°, $p = 0.87$ for middle elevations, 24 ± 7° vs. 22 ± 7°, $p = 0.61$ for low elevations; up → down reversals: 2 ± 4% vs. 3 ± 3%, $p = 0.44$; down → up reversals: 20 ± 22% vs. 19 ± 12%, $p = 0.69$;

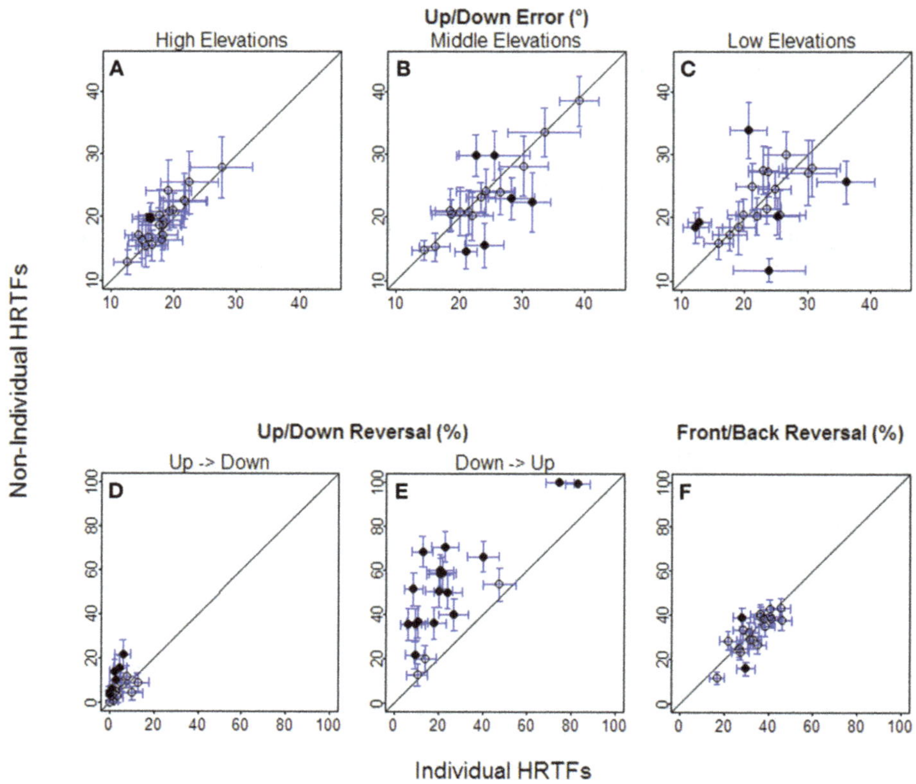

FIGURE 6 | Individual localization scores with non-individual against with individual HRTFs at the pre-test. (A–C) Up/down errors (in °) for high, middle, and low target elevations. **(D–F)** Up → down, down → up, and front/back reversal rates (in %). Each symbol is for a different listener. Circles and bars represent the means and 95% confidence intervals averaged across about 30 (up/down error) to 96 (front/back reversals) target positions. Filled circles indicate the listeners with significant difference between individual and non-individual HRTFs according to Wilcoxon tests.

front/back reversals: 38 ± 8% vs. 32 ± 6%, $p = 0.19$). At the post-test, the test group had significantly smaller up/down errors for middle and low target elevations, and smaller down → up reversal rates, than the control group (22 ± 6° vs. 27 ± 7°, $p = 0.004$, 15 ± 3° vs. 21 ± 15°, $p = 0.02$, and 12 ± 9% vs. 23 ± 20%, $p = 0.01$, respectively). However, no significant between-group difference was observed in up/down errors for high target elevations and in up → down reversals (15 ± 3° vs. 15 ± 2°, $p = 0.54$ and 2 ± 2% vs. 0.3 ± 2%, $p = 0.17$, respectively).

RELATIONSHIP BETWEEN LEARNING AMOUNT AND PRE-TEST RESULTS WITH INDIVIDUAL HRTFs

The correlations between learning amount and pre-test score were assessed for each variable and group. For up/down errors, learning significantly increased with the pre-test score for the test group ($R = 0.96$, $p = 0.003$ for all target elevations), whereas no correlation was found for the control group ($R = 0.14$, $p = 0.75$; $R = 0.31$, $p = 0.46$; $R = 0.50$, $p = 0.22$ for high, middle, and low elevations, respectively). For up/down reversals, the correlations were significant for the test group (up → down: $R = 0.93$, $p = 0.003$; down → up: $R = 0.98$, $p < 0.001$) but were not for the control group (up → down: $R = 0.55$, $p = 0.17$; down → up: $R = 0.49$, $p = 0.22$). For front/back reversals, no correlation was significant (test group: $R = 0.75$, $p = 0.07$; control group: $R = -0.02$, $p = 0.98$).

Furthermore, to check whether the improvement in performance reflected or not an adaptation to errors in DTF computation (see Section Measurement and Spectral Characterization of HRTFs), the correlations between learning amount and ISD between correct and incorrect DTFs were assessed. No *positive* correlation was found for any variable and group (test group: $R = 0.07$, $p = 0.91$; $R = -0.07$, $p = 0.91$; $R = -0.79$, $p = 0.048$ for high, middle, and low elevations, respectively. $R = 0.68$, $p = 0.11$; $R = -0.29$, $p = 0.56$; $R = -0.07$, $p = 0.91$ for up → down, down → up, and front/back reversals, respectively. Control group: $R = -0.16$, $p = 0.71$; $R = 0.30$, $p = 0.47$; $R = 0.01$, $p = 0.98$ for high, middle, and low elevations, respectively. $R = 0.20$, $p = 0.63$; $R = 0.61$, $p = 0.11$; $R = -0.08$, $p = 0.84$ for up → down, down → up, and front/back reversals, respectively).

RETENTION OF LEARNING WITH INDIVIDUAL HRTFs

All listeners with significant learning at the immediate post-test showed no significant difference in score between immediate and long-term post-tests (3/3 in the test group for down → up reversals and 2/2 in the control group for up → down reversals; 1/1, 3/3, and 3/3 in the test group and 2/2, 1/1, and 2/2 in the control group for up/down angular errors for high, middle and low elevations, respectively; 2/2 in the test group for front/back reversals).

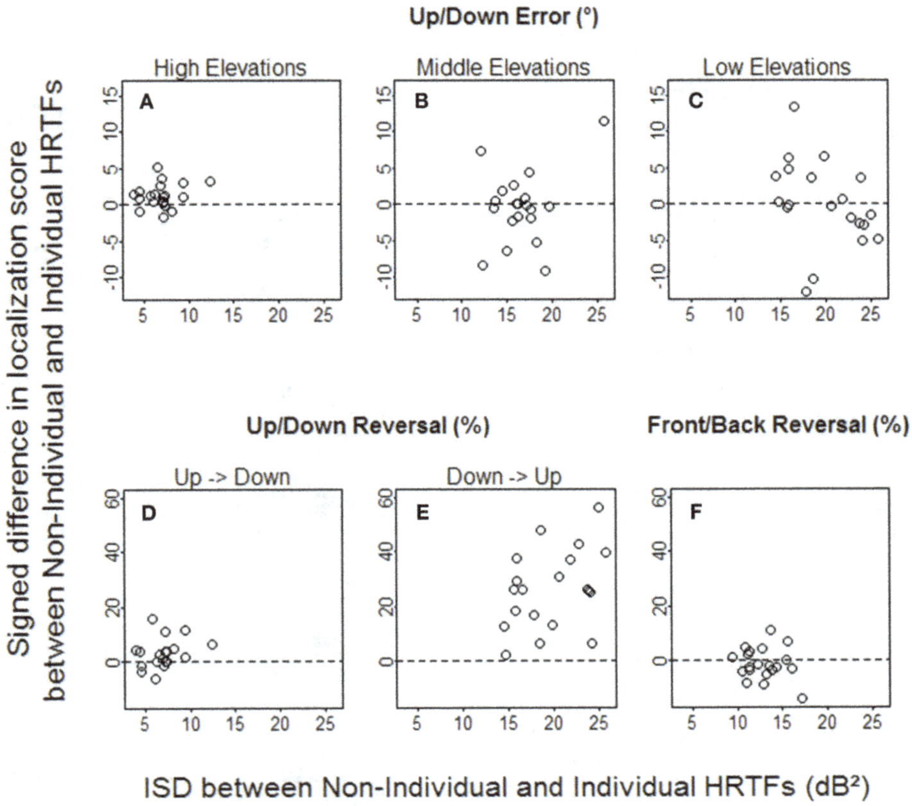

FIGURE 7 | Individual signed differences in localization score against ISD between non-individual and individual HRTFs. (A–C) Up/down errors (in °) for high, middle, and low target elevations. **(D–F)** Up → down, down → up, and front/back reversal rates (in %).

DISCUSSION

ROLE OF ACOUSTICAL FACTORS

To examine the contribution of acoustical factors to sound localization abilities with virtual sources, we assessed for 20 naïve listeners the relationship between the spectral strength and the localization performance with individual HRTFs, the difference in performance between individual and non-individual HRTFs (normal and modified cues), and its relationship with the ISD between HRTFs. Localization performance was measured in terms of up/down angular errors following correction of reversals for three target elevations (high, middle, low), up → down reversals, down → up reversals, and front/back reversals rates. We found no relationship between spectral strength and performance with individual HRTFs nor between behavioral difference and ISD between HRTFs. The only sizeable difference in performance between HRTFs appeared in the low elevation region. In that region, where the acoustical differences between HRTFs (in terms of spectral strength and ISD) were the largest, we noted that the target was perceived in the lower (i.e., correct) hemisphere with individual HRTFs but in the upper (i.e., incorrect) hemisphere with non-individual HRTFs. Past studies involving trained listeners found sizeable differences in localization performance between individual and non-individual HRTFs in both front/back and up/down dimensions (Møller et al., 1996; Middlebrooks, 1999b). Those involving naïve listeners reported little or no difference in the front/back dimension (Bronkhorst, 1995; Begault et al., 2001), as for the present study, but they also reported no difference in the up/down dimension, contrary to the present study.

Concerning the front/back dimension, the present findings indicate that the lack of difference in past studies was unlikely due to a floor effect in the (poor) performance of listeners with no prior experience in the task (Bronkhorst, 1995), or to an insufficient ISD between individual and non-individual HRTFs (Middlebrooks, 1999b). First, our listeners performed procedural training prior to auditory tests, which prevented exposure to the experimental environment and response device from affecting the results. Second, the lack of behavioral difference between HRTFs in the auditory task was observed regardless of whether the listener had good or poor performance. Third, most values of ISD between individual and non-individual HRTFs were assumed to be sufficiently large to affect behavioral results according to the results from a past study (Middlebrooks, 1999b).

Front/back reversal rates were substantially higher in the present study using individual HRTFs than in free-field past studies (Wightman and Kistler, 1989; Carlile et al., 1997; Martin et al., 2001). Higher front/back reversal rates for virtual sources presented with individual cues than for real sources have previously been reported (Wightman and Kistler, 1989; Middlebrooks, 1999b). These difference could possibly result from headphone

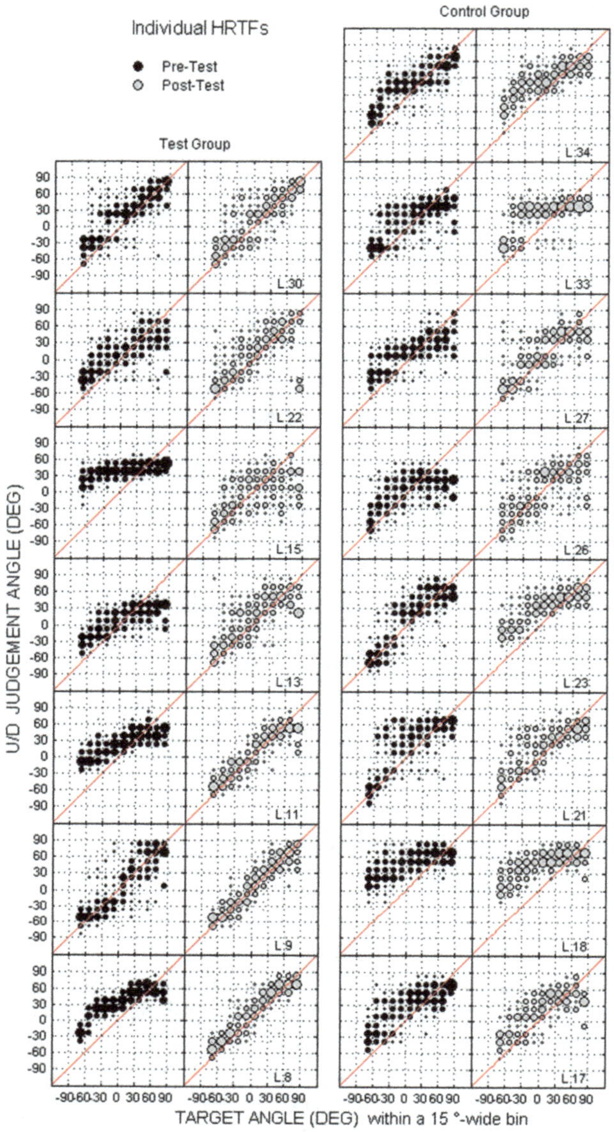

FIGURE 8 | Individual judgment position against target position with individual HRTFs at the pre- and post-tests (black and gray dots, respectively) for the test and control listeners (left and right columns, respectively) in the up/down dimension. Each panel couple is for a different listener.

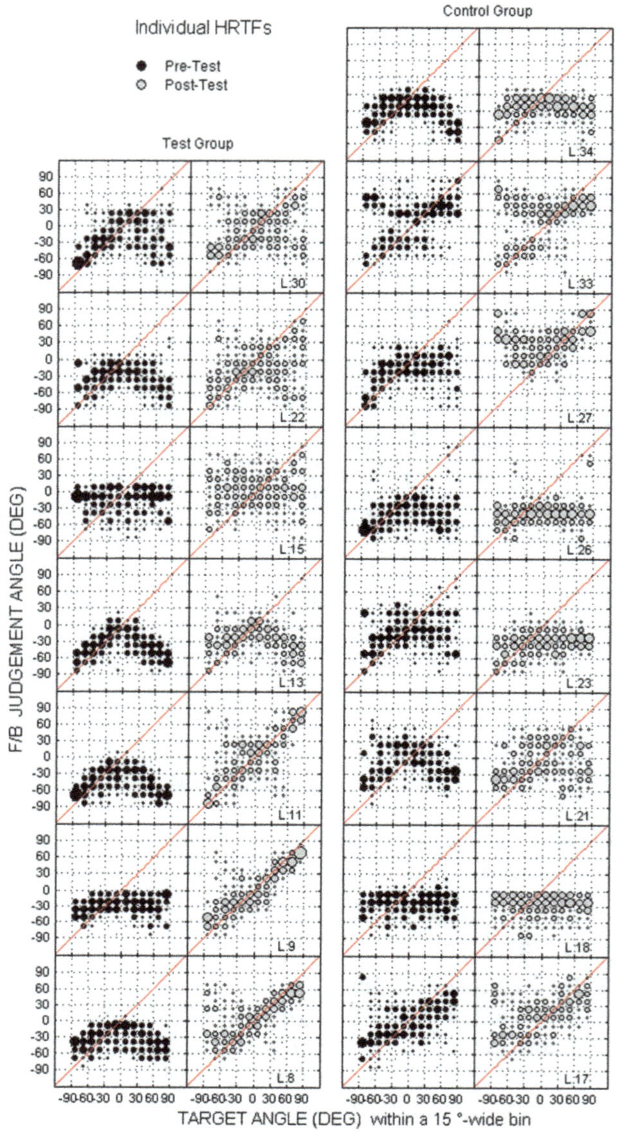

FIGURE 9 | Same as in Figure 8 but for front/back dimension.

transfer function issues (Wightman and Kistler, 2005), degree of spatial resolution during the HRTF measurement, and/or errors in DTF computation (present study, see Section Measurement and Spectral Characterization of HRTFs). In the present study, the error in DTF computation was present in both individual and non-individual HRTFs, and could therefore have reduced the behavioral differences between HRTFs.

Concerning the up/down dimension, the discrepancy between the present study and Bronkhorst (1995) and Begault et al. (2001) studies could arise from methodological issues. Bronkhorst used other listeners' HRTFs as non-individual HRTFs. Given our observations, this has probably reduced the differences in spectral strength—and therefore the behavioral differences—between individual and non-individual HRTFs. In the Begault et al. (2001) study, the auditory target positions were limited to the horizontal plane, excluding the low elevation region where we observed the strongest difference between individual and non-individual HRTFs.

We also suggested that the discrepancy between the four past studies (Bronkhorst, 1995; Møller et al., 1996; Middlebrooks, 1999b; Begault et al., 2001) could arise from differences in experimental protocol (see Footnote 1). In the present study, we used a "classical" protocol, which resembles the protocol used in a past study that reported a difference between HRTFs (Middlebrooks, 1999b). Beyond differences in the listener's characteristics (naïve in the present study but trained in the past study), we explain the discrepancy between the present and Middlebrooks's studies in

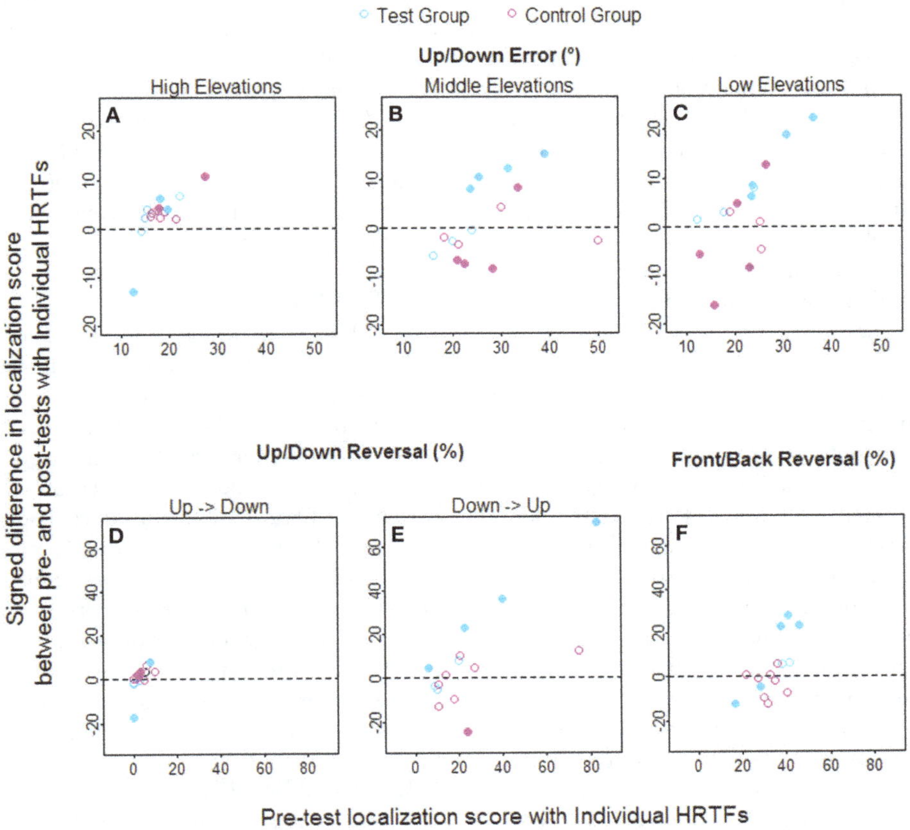

FIGURE 10 | Individual learning amounts (pre-test minus post-test localization score) against pre-test scores for the test and control listeners (blue and pink symbols, respectively) with individual HRTFs. (A–C) Up/down errors (in °) for high, middle, and low target elevations. **(D–F)** Up → down, down → up, and front/back reversal rates (in %). Filled symbols indicate the listeners with significant difference between pre- and post-tests according to Wilcoxon tests.

terms of data analysis. Middlebrooks assessed reversals without distinction between the up/down and front/back dimensions, and angular (polar) errors following correction of reversals using a more conservative criterion than ours.

To sum-up, the lack of correlation between spectral strength and performance with individual HRTFs showed that this acoustical factor is not a good predictor of performance. Another acoustical factor is the degree of matching between the listener's individual localization cues and those provided by the signal to localize. Our results suggest that large mismatch is needed to produce behavioral effects. However, the validity of this statement is limited by the remaining uncertainty in the quality of the HRTFs.

ROLE OF PERCEPTUAL FACTORS

To examine the contribution of perceptual factors to sound localization abilities with virtual sources, a subset of 15 listeners performed training to the sound localization task with fixed acoustical cues (individual HRTFs). The listeners were provided with either sensory (visual) or no correct-answer feedback. We expected the training regimen to elicit perceptual learning, that is, an improvement in the perceptual processes involved in the analysis of acoustical cues, for the "test" group who received feedback. Beyond the use of feedback, the perceptual and procedural contributions to training-induced improvements in performance are rarely separated (Robinson and Summerfield, 1996; Wright and Fitzgerald, 2001). In the present study, the improvement observed following auditory training was unlikely to be triggered by procedural learning for several reasons. First, the listeners performed procedural training with non-auditory stimuli over 3 days prior to sound localization tests, which resulted in optimal and steady ability to handle the response device. Second, further exposure to the procedural aspects of the task during auditory training resulted in significant improvements for only a few listeners from the control group. Third, individual differences in learning amount were larger in the present study (see **Figure 10**) than those reported for procedural learning in a past study (training to interaural time and level differences, Wright and Fitzgerald, 2001). In addition, we observed that the training-induced improvements were retained after 1 month. This suggests that the improvement was not due to modification of the listening strategy, or to a temporary increase in the listener's attentional resources (Goldstone, 1998).

It could seem counter-intuitive that an improvement in sound localization performance is still possible despite a lifetime of localization learning. However, training-induced improvements with normal cues and correct-answer feedback have been reported in previous studies, including for the "most robust" localization ability (i.e., localization of real sources in the left/right dimension, see Savel, 2009; Irving and Moore, 2011). Moreover, improvements in the front/back dimension could result from increased weighting of spectral cues but decreased weighting of dynamic cues—available in everyday life conditions but unavailable in the present experiment (Wightman and Kistler, 1999)—to front/back discrimination following training. Part of the training-induced improvement observed with individual HRTFs could result from exposure to abnormal cues (i.e., incorrect DTFs). In agreement, there are multiple reports of learning of—adaptation to—abnormal spectral cues with exposure (Hofman et al., 1998; Van Wanrooij and Van Opstal, 2005; Carlile and Blackman, 2013). However, the ISD between normal and abnormal spectral cues (i.e., between correct and incorrect DTFs, see **Table 1** and Appendix) in the present study was probably too small to produce significant improvement (Van Wanrooij and Van Opstal, 2005). Moreover, no positive correlation was found between the amount of improvement and the ISD between correct and incorrect DTFs.

Our findings confirm the results of a previous study that reported substantial improvement in sound localization with individual HRTFs after a similar training protocol (Majdak et al., 2010). Our results indicate furthermore that this improvement might not be explained by procedural learning.

As perceptual learning is often stimulus-specific, findings of a generalization of learning to untrained stimuli or conditions are mostly believed to reflect task or procedural learning (Wright and Zhang, 2009). However, it has been suggested that generalization could also reflect perceptual learning (Ahissar, 2001). In this case, the learning involves—often high level—sensory processes that are not specific to the task. In the present study, we assessed whether the listeners from the test and control groups who showed significant learning following auditory training in the trained condition (individual HRTFs) also showed significant learning in an untrained condition (non-individual HRTFs). No learning generalization was observed for the localization responses in the front/back dimension, but most listeners from the test group showed generalization for up/down reversals and up/down errors. Because these listeners had received procedural training, we assume that the generalization was perceptual. The generalization observed could mean that the training improved sensory processes that are not specific to sound localization with individual HRTFs. One of these processes could be, for example, the analysis of the spectral shape of the stimulus (Andéol et al., 2013), a process that is involved regardless of the HRTFs set. Overall, the results indicate that training-induced modifications of perceptual processes had substantial effects on localization performance with virtual sources.

Moreover, we found that the training-induced learning amount was related to the pre-training performance (i.e., poorer initial performance led to larger learning amount), a result also observed in several previous studies (Wright and Fitzgerald, 2001; Amitay et al., 2005; Astle et al., 2013). This correlation is in favor of a contribution of common—here perceptual—factors to the two metrics. In other words, our results suggest that perceptual processes account for individual differences in sound localization abilities with virtual sources in naïve listeners.

Taken together, these results are consistent with a large contribution of perceptual processes to sound localization abilities with virtual sources. Majdak et al. (2014) recently reached a similar conclusion using a sound localization model. By modifying model parameters relative to acoustical or non-acoustical factors, they found that non-acoustical factors (such as for example perceptual abilities to process localization cues) were better predictors of performance than acoustical factors (quality of the directional cues in the HRTFs).

CONCLUSION

The study assessed the contributions of acoustical and perceptual factors to the ability to localize virtual sound sources presented in quiet for naïve normal-hearing young adults. The spectral strength of the HRTFs did not seem to be a relevant acoustical factor to account for localization performance. Only large modifications of acoustical localization cues seemed to produce behavioral effects, although technical issues with the normalization of the HRTFs might have blurred part of the results. Auditory training with visual correct-answer feedback and constant acoustical cues substantially improved performance. These findings are consistent with a greater role of perceptual factors than of acoustical factors in sound localization abilities with virtual sources. Further research is needed to assess whether the present results generalize to the case of localization in free field.

ACKNOWLEDGMENTS

This work was supported in part by the French Procurement Agency (Direction Générale de l'Armement, DGA). The authors thank Jean Christophe Bouy for software development, Lionel Pellieux for HRTFs measurements and signal processing manipulations, and the two reviewers for many helpful comments.

REFERENCES

Ahissar, M. (2001). Perceptual training: a tool for both modifying the brain and exploring it. *Proc. Natl. Acad. Sci. U.S.A.* 98, 11842–11843. doi: 10.1073/pnas.221461598

Amitay, S., Halliday, L., Taylor, J., Sohoglu, E., and Moore, D. R. (2010). Motivation and intelligence drive auditory perceptual learning. *PLoS ONE* 5:e9816. doi: 10.1371/journal.pone.0009816

Amitay, S., Hawkey, D. J. C., and Moore, D. R. (2005). Auditory frequency discrimination learning is affected by stimulus variability. *Percept. Psychophys.* 67, 691–698. doi: 10.3758/BF03193525

Andéol, G., Guillaume, A., Micheyl, C., Savel, S., Pellieux, L., and Moulin, A. (2011). Auditory efferents facilitate sound localization in noise in humans. *J. Neurosci.* 31, 6759–6763. doi: 10.1523/JNEUROSCI.0248-11.2011

Andéol, G., Macpherson, E. A., and Sabin, A. T. (2013). Sound localization in noise and sensitivity to spectral shape. *Hear. Res.* 304, 20–27. doi: 10.1016/j.heares.2013.06.001

Asano, F., Suzuki, Y., and Sone, T. (1990). Role of spectral cues in median plane localization. *J. Acoust. Soc. Am.* 88, 159–168. doi: 10.1038/srep01158

Astle, A. T., Li, R. W., Webb, B. S., Levi, D. M., and McGraw, P. V. (2013). A Weber-like law for perceptual learning. *Sci. Rep.* 3:1158. doi: 10.1038/srep01158

Begault, D. R., Wenzel, E. M., and Anderson, M. R. (2001). Direct comparison of the impact of head tracking, reverberation, and individualized head-related transfer functions on the spatial perception of a virtual speech source. *J. Audio Eng. Soc.* 49, 904–916.

Best, V., van Schaik, A., Jin, C., and Carlile, S. (2005). Auditory spatial perception with sources overlapping in frequency and time. *Acta Acust. United Acust.* 91, 421–428.

Bronkhorst, A. W. (1995). Localization of real and virtual sound sources. *J. Acoust. Soc. Am.* 98, 2542–2553. doi: 10.1121/1.413219

Butler, R. A., and Belendiuk, K. (1977). Spectral cues utilized in the localization of sound in the median sagittal plane. *J. Acoust. Soc. Am.* 61, 1264–1269. doi: 10.1121/1.381427

Carlile, S., and Blackman, T. (2013). Relearning auditory spectral cues for locations inside and outside the visual field. *J. Assoc. Res. Otolaryngol.* 15, 249–263. doi: 10.1007/s10162-013-0429-5

Carlile, S., Leong, P., and Hyams, S. (1997). The nature and distribution of errors in sound localization by human listeners. *Hear. Res.* 114, 179–196. doi: 10.1016/S0378-5955(97)00161-5

Clifton, R. K., Gwiazda, J., Bauer, J. A., Clarkson, M. G., and Held, R. M. (1988). Growth in head size during infancy: implications for sound localization. *Dev. Psychol.* 24, 477–483. doi: 10.1037/0012-1649.24.4.477

Djelani, T., Porschmann, C., Sahrhage, J., and Blauert, J. (2000). An interactive virtual-environment generator for psychoacoustic research II: collection of head-related impulse responses and evaluation of auditory localization. *Acta Acust. United Acust.* 86, 1046–1053.

Drennan, W. R., and Watson, C. S. (2001). Sources of variation in profile analysis. I. Individual differences and extended training. *J. Acoust. Soc. Am.* 110, 2491–2497. doi: 10.1121/1.1408310

Garcia, A., Kuai, S.-G., and Kourtzi, Z. (2013). Differences in the time course of learning for hard compared to easy training. *Front. Psychol.* 4:110. doi: 10.3389/fpsyg.2013.00110

Gilkey, R. H., Good, M. D., Ericson, M. A., Brinkman, J., and Stewart, J. M. (1995). A pointing technique for rapidly collecting localization responses in auditory research. *Behav. Res. Methods Instrum. Comput.* 27, 1–11. doi: 10.3758/BF03203614

Goldstone, R. L. (1998). Perceptual learning. *Annu. Rev. Psychol.* 49, 585–612. doi: 10.1146/annurev.psych.49.1.585

Hofman, P. M., Van Riswick, J. G., and Van Opstal, A. J. (1998). Relearning sound localization with new ears. *Nat. Neurosci.* 1, 417–421. doi: 10.1038/1633

Irving, S., and Moore, D. R. (2011). Training sound localization in normal hearing listeners with and without a unilateral ear plug. *Hear. Res.* 280, 100–108. doi: 10.1016/j.heares.2011.04.020

King, A. J. (2009). Visual influences on auditory spatial learning. *Philos. Trans. R. Soc. Lond. B Biol. Sci.* 364, 331–339. doi: 10.1098/rstb.2008.0230

Kistler, D. J., and Wightman, F. L. (1992). A model of head-related transfer functions based on principal components analysis and minimum-phase reconstruction. *J. Acoust. Soc. Am.* 91, 1637–1647. doi: 10.1121/1.402444

Majdak, P., Baumgartner, R., and Laback, B. (2014). Acoustic and non-acoustic factors in modeling listener-specific performance of sagittal-plane sound localization. *Front. Psychol.* 5:319. doi: 10.3389/fpsyg.2014.00319

Majdak, P., Goupell, M. J., and Laback, B. (2010). 3-D localization of virtual sound sources: effects of visual environment, pointing method, and training. *Atten. Percept. Psychophys.* 72, 454–469. doi: 10.3758/APP.72.2.454

Makous, J. C., and Middlebrooks, J. C. (1990). Two-dimensional sound localization by human listeners. *J. Acoust. Soc. Am.* 87, 2188–2200. doi: 10.1121/1.399186

Martin, R. L., McAnally, K. I., and Senova, M. A. (2001). Free-field equivalent localization of virtual audio. *J. Audio Eng. Soc.* 49, 14–22.

Middlebrooks, J. C. (1999a). Individual differences in external-ear transfer functions reduced by scaling in frequency. *J. Acoust. Soc. Am.* 106, 1480–1492. doi: 10.1121/1.427176

Middlebrooks, J. C. (1999b). Virtual localization improved by scaling nonindividualized external-ear transfer functions in frequency. *J. Acoust. Soc. Am.* 106, 1493–1510. doi: 10.1121/1.427147

Møller, H., Sørensen, M. F., Jensen, C. B., and Hammershøi, D. (1996). Binaural technique: do we need individual recordings? *J. Audio Eng. Soc.* 44, 451–469.

Oldfield, R. C. (1971). The assessment and analysis of handedness: the Edinburgh inventory. *Neuropsychologia* 9, 97–113. doi: 10.1016/0028-3932(71)90067-4

Oldfield, S. R., and Parker, S. P. (1984). Acuity of sound localisation: a topography of auditory space. I. Normal hearing conditions. *Perception* 13, 581–600. doi: 10.1068/p130581

Otte, R. J., Agterberg, M. J. H., Van Wanrooij, M. M., Snik, A. F. M., and Van Opstal, A. J. (2013). Age-related hearing loss and ear morphology affect vertical but not horizontal sound-localization performance. *J. Assoc. Res. Otolaryngol.* 14, 261–273. doi: 10.1007/s10162-012-0367-7

Populin, L. C. (2008). Human sound localization: measurements in untrained, head-unrestrained subjects using gaze as a pointer. *Exp. Brain Res.* 190, 11–30. doi: 10.1007/s00221-008-1445-2

Recanzone, G. H., Makhamra, S. D. D. R., and Guard, D. C. (1998). Comparison of relative and absolute sound localization ability in humans. *J. Acoust. Soc. Am.* 103, 1085–1097. doi: 10.1121/1.421222

Robinson, K., and Summerfield, A. Q. (1996). Adult auditory learning and training. *Ear Hear.* 17, 51S–65S. doi: 10.1097/00003446-199617031-00006

Sabin, A. T., Eddins, D. A., and Wright, B. A. (2012). Perceptual learning of auditory spectral modulation detection. *Exp. Brain Res.* 218, 567–577. doi: 10.1007/s00221-012-3049-0

Savel, S. (2009). Individual differences and left/right asymmetries in auditory space perception. I. Localization of low-frequency sounds in free field. *Hear. Res.* 255, 142–154. doi: 10.1016/j.heares.2009.06.013

Strutt, J. W. (1907). On our perception of sound direction. *Philos. Mag.* 13, 214–232. doi: 10.1080/14786440709463595

Van Wanrooij, M. M., and Van Opstal, A. J. (2005). Relearning sound localization with a new ear. *Nat. Neurosci.* 25, 5413–5424. doi: 10.1523/JNEUROSCI.0850-05.2005

Wenzel, E. M., Arruda, M., Kistler, D. J., and Wightman, F. L. (1993). Localization using nonindividualized head-related transfer functions. *J. Acoust. Soc. Am.* 94, 111–123. doi: 10.1121/1.407089

Wenzel, E. M., Wightman, F. L., Kistler, D. J., and Foster, S. H. (1988). Acoustic origins of individual differences in sound localization behavior. *J. Acoust. Soc. Am.* 84, S79. doi: 10.1121/1.2026486

Wightman, F., and Kistler, D. (2005). Measurement and validation of human HRTFs for use in hearing research. *Acta Acust. United Acust.* 91, 429–439.

Wightman, F. L., and Kistler, D. J. (1989). Headphone simulation of free-field listening. II: psychophysical validation. *J. Acoust. Soc. Am.* 85, 868–878. doi: 10.1121/1.397558

Wightman, F. L., and Kistler, D. J. (1993). "Sound localization," in *Human Psychophysics Springer Handbook of Auditory Research*, eds W. A. Yost, A. N. Popper, and R. R. Fay (New York, NY: Springer), 155–192.

Wightman, F. L., and Kistler, D. J. (1997). "Factors affecting the relative salience of sound localization cues," in *Binaural and Spatial Hearing in Real and Virtual Environments,* eds R. H. Gilkey and T. H. Anderson (Mahwah, NJ: Lawrence Erlbaum Associates), 1–23.

Wightman, F. L., and Kistler, D. J. (1999). Resolution of front-back ambiguity in spatial hearing by listener and source movement. *J. Acoust. Soc. Am.* 105, 2841–2853. doi: 10.1121/1.426899

Wright, B. A., and Fitzgerald, M. B. (2001). Different patterns of human discrimination learning for two interaural cues to sound-source location. *Proc. Natl. Acad. Sci. U.S.A.* 98, 12307–12312. doi: 10.1073/pnas.211220498

Wright, B. A., and Zhang, Y. (2009). A review of the generalization of auditory learning. *Philos. Trans. R. Soc. Lond. B Biol. Sci.* 364, 301–311. doi: 10.1098/rstb.2008.0262

Zhang, P. X., and Hartmann, W. M. (2010). On the ability of human listeners to distinguish between front and back. *Hear. Res.* 260, 30–46. doi: 10.1016/j.heares.2009.11.001

APPENDIX

An error in DTFs computation was detected following collection of behavioral data. To assess whether this error influenced behavioral results, we compared the performance with individual HRTFs obtained using correct DTFs to that obtained using incorrect DTFs in five listeners. The methods were similar to those used to compare individual and non-individual HRTFs (set of 119 target positions, six repetitions) except that the type of DTFs (correct or incorrect) randomly changed from trial to trial. Each listener performed 1428 trials over 2 days. The first 119 trials of each day, which contained approximately the same number of trials with correct and with incorrect DTFs, were excluded from the analyses. Visual inspection of the raw data in the left/right, front/back, and up/down dimensions showed similar results for correct and incorrect DTFs for each listener (**Figure A1**), including listener L22 who had the highest ISD between DTFs (6.6 dB^2). Wilcoxon tests showed better performance with correct than with incorrect DTFs for only one of 30 comparisons (5 listeners × 6 variables, see **Table A1**): listener (L22) for up/down errors for high elevations (17° *vs.* 13°, $p = 0.005$). The differences between DTFs for the 5-listener group were not significant (up/down error: 17 ± 2° *vs.* 15 ± 3°, $p = 0.06$; 26 ± 7° *vs.* 26 ± 4°, $p = 0.19$; 19° ± 4 *vs.* 19 ± 6°, $p = 0.63$ for high, middle, and low target elevations, respectively; up → down reversals: 2 ± 01% *vs.* 2 ± 3%, $p = 0.99$; down → up reversals: 13 ± 9% *vs.* 19 ± 14%, $p = 0.58$; Front/back reversals: 38 ± 8% *vs.* 32 ± 6%, $p = 0.19$).

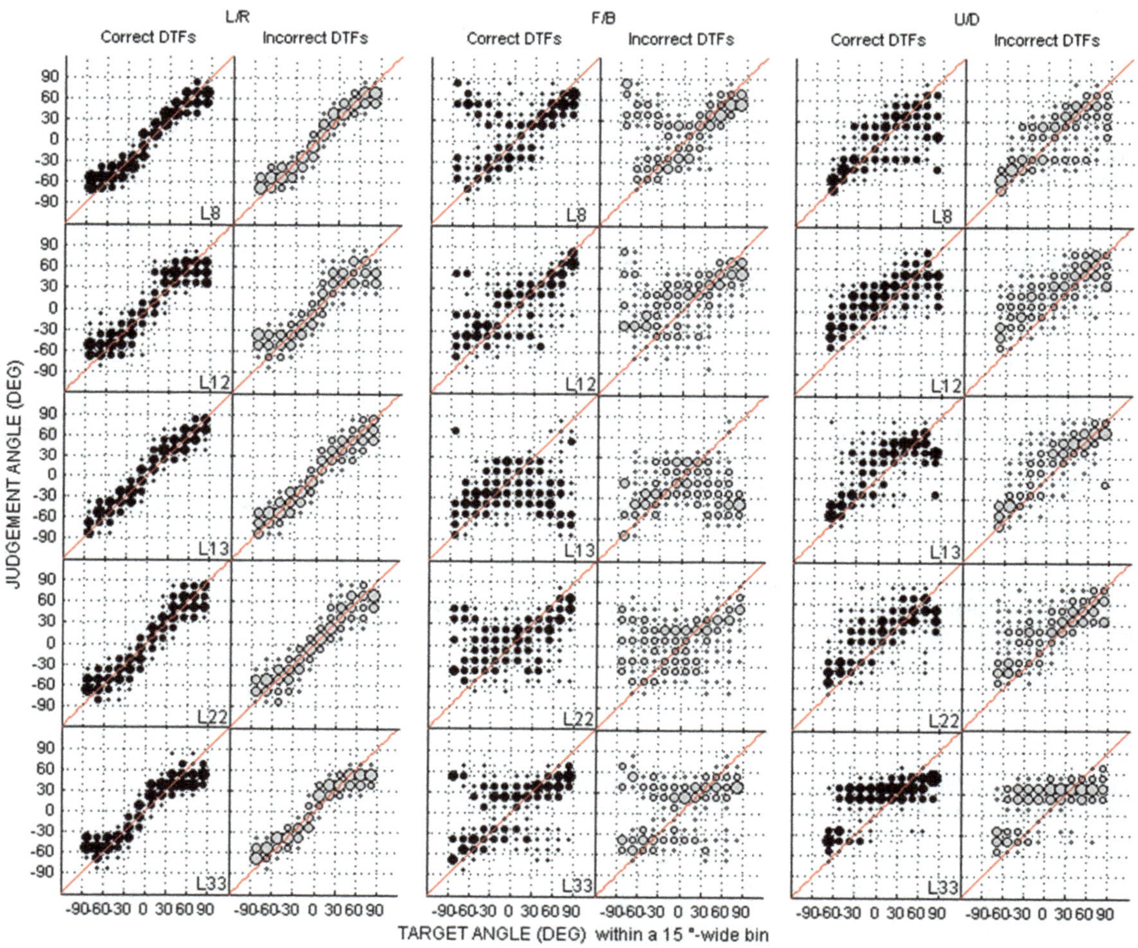

FIGURE A1 | Individual judgment position against target position using correct and incorrect DTFs (black and gray dots, respectively) with individual HRTFs in the left/right, up/down, and front/back dimensions. Each panel couple is for a different listener ($N = 5$).

Table A1 | Comparison between correct and incorrect DTFs for each variable and each listener.

			L22	L8	L13	L12	L33
Spectral strength of the individual HRTFs (dB^2)		Incorrect DTFs	21.0	18.3	15.6	15.4	12.8
		Correct DTFs	15.6	15.2	13.3	14.0	11.9
Inter-DTF (Incorrect – Correct) ISD (dB^2)			6.6	3.6	1.8	1.4	1.1
Up/down error (°)	High elevations	Incorrect DTFs	17	22	15	18	16
		Correct DTFs	13	19	14	18	15
		Difference	P = 0.005	*ns*	*ns*	*ns*	*ns*
	Middle elevations	Incorrect DTFs	26	22	29	21	29
		Correct DTFs	26	22	29	25	29
		Difference	*ns*	*ns*	*ns*	*ns*	*ns*
	Low elevations	Incorrect DTFs	20	16	15	29	19
		Correct DTFs	22	15	15	29	19
		Difference	*ns*	*ns*	*ns*	*ns*	*ns*
Up → down reversals (%)		Incorrect DTFs	3	9	2	1	2
		Correct DTFs	1	12	2	0	4
		Difference	*ns*	*ns*	*ns*	*ns*	*ns*
Down → up reversals (%)		Incorrect DTFs	19	3	13	11	35
		Correct DTFs	24	3	10	19	35
		Difference	*ns*	*ns*	*ns*	P = 0.030	*ns*
Front/back reversals (%)		Incorrect DTFs	26	24	30	19	32
		Correct DTFs	30	21	32	24	32
		Difference	*ns*	*ns*	*ns*	*ns*	*ns*

5

Reaching nearby sources: Comparison between real and virtual sound and visual targets

Gaëtan Parseihian[1*†], Christophe Jouffrais[2] and Brian F. G. Katz[1*]

[1] *Laboratoire de Mécanique et d'Informatique pour les Sciences de l'Ingénieur, LIMSI - CNRS, Universite Paris Sud, Orsay, France*
[2] *IRIT, CNRS, Université de Toulouse, Toulouse, France*

***Correspondence:**
Gaëtan Parseihian, Laboratoire de Mécanique et d'Acoustique, CNRS - UPR 7051, 31 Chemin Joseph Aiguier, 13402 Marseille Cedex 20, Marseille, France
e-mail: parseihian@lma.cnrs-mrs.fr;
Brian F. G. Katz, Audio Acoustics Group, LIMSI-CNRS, BP 133, 91403 Orsay, France
e-mail: brian.katz@limsi.fr

†Present address:
Gaëtan Parseihian, CNRS, Aix-Marseille Université, Centrale Marseille, LMA UPR 7051, 13402 Marseille, France

Sound localization studies over the past century have predominantly been concerned with directional accuracy for far-field sources. Few studies have examined the condition of near-field sources and distance perception. The current study concerns localization and pointing accuracy by examining source positions in the peripersonal space, specifically those associated with a typical tabletop surface. Accuracy is studied with respect to the reporting hand (dominant or secondary) for auditory sources. Results show no effect on the reporting hand with azimuthal errors increasing equally for the most extreme source positions. Distance errors show a consistent compression toward the center of the reporting area. A second evaluation is carried out comparing auditory and visual stimuli to examine any bias in reporting protocol or biomechanical difficulties. No common bias error was observed between auditory and visual stimuli indicating that reporting errors were not due to biomechanical limitations in the pointing task. A final evaluation compares real auditory sources and anechoic condition virtual sources created using binaural rendering. Results showed increased azimuthal errors, with virtual source positions being consistently overestimated to more lateral positions, while no significant distance perception was observed, indicating a deficiency in the binaural rendering condition relative to the real stimuli situation. Various potential reasons for this discrepancy are discussed with several proposals for improving distance perception in peripersonal virtual environments.

Keywords: auditory localization, near-field pointing, nearby sound sources, virtual auditory display, spatial hearing, sound target, visual target

INTRODUCTION

The basic mechanisms of sound localization have been well studied in the last century (see Blauert, 1997). These studies have primarily examined azimuth and elevation localization accuracy using a variety of reporting techniques. Several studies have examined distance perception under a variety of acoustic conditions, though typically for frontally positioned sources in the far-field. Few studies have examined spatial hearing in the near-field and even fewer for positions significantly low in elevation.

For sources located in the near field, several studies (see Brungart and Rabinowitz, 1999; Shinn-Cunningham et al., 2000) have shown through analysis of proximal-region Head-Related Transfer Function (HRTF) measurements a dramatic increase in Interaural Level Difference (ILD) cues for sources within 1 m of a listener's head for positions away from the median plane. This increase is the consequence of two factors. First, due to head shadowing, the more proximate is the source from the head, the more high frequency attenuation is observed on the contralateral acoustic trajectory. Second, as acoustic waves follow an attenuation inverse-square law relationship between distance and intensity, the differences in path length between the two acoustic trajectories reaching each ear for near sources is proportionally bigger than for far sources. This leads to greater and more easily noticeable ILD. In contrast, the Interaural Time Delay (ITD) cue is roughly independent of distance in the proximal region. Although there is a slight increase of ITD for nearest distances, it occurs only near the lateral positions where the ITD is large and where listeners are relatively insensitive to ITD changes (see Hershkowitz and Durlach, 1969). Considering the spectral cues' variation in near field, Brungart and Rabinowitz (1999) have shown that the features of the HRTF that significantly change with elevation are not strongly dependent on the distance. However, as the source approaches the head, the angle of the source relative to the ear can differ from the angle of the source relative to the center of the head. This creates an acoustic parallax effect that laterally shifts some of the high-frequency features of the HRTF (see Brungart, 1999).

Only few studies have aimed to evaluate sound source localization performances in the near-field. Ashmead et al. (1990) evaluated the perception of the relative distances of frontal sources near one and two meters with only intensity cues in an anechoic room. They found a smallest noticeable change in distance of 5% (e.g., a distance of 5 cm at 1 m) whereas Strybel and Perrott (1984) found a change of 10% and Simpson and Stanton (1973) of 20%. Concerning the response methods for the localization of nearby object, Brungart et al. (2000) compared four response methods with visual targets and found a superiority of the direct pointing method over the other methods. With this method, the authors highlight an overall error of 7.6% in distance and of 5° in azimuth when subjects pointed toward visual targets. In an experiment performed to evaluate proximal-region localization performances, Brungart et al. (1999) found an increase in azimuth error as the sound approached the head, a distance independency of elevation performance, and a strong azimuth dependency of distance localization performances. This study was performed without amplitude-based distance cues using sources distributed from −40° to 60° in elevation, 15 to 100 cm in distance, and situated in the right hemisphere of the subject.

In Shinn-Cunningham et al. (2005), the authors analyzed the distortions of the spatial acoustic cues induced by the presence of reverberant energy. They measured Binaural Room Impulse Responses (BRIRs) on a KEMAR manikin for several nearby sound sources positions in a classroom. Their results highlighted a reduction of the ILD depending on acoustic properties of the environment as well as on the location of the listener in the environment. Furthermore, monaural spectral cues are less reliable in the ear farther from the sound source whereas ITD can still be recovered from the BRIRs. These systematics distortions are mostly prominent when the listener is oriented with one ear toward a wall. With a perceptual study on the effect of near field sound source spectrum on lateral localization in virtual reverberant simulation, Ihlefeld and Shinn-Cunningham (2011) showed a compression of the perceived angle toward the center for lateral sources (more than 45° from the median plane). This effect grows with increasing distance (as Direct/Reverberant ratio decreases) and it is greater for low-frequency sounds than for high-frequency sounds. Exploring the effect of simulated reverberant space on near field distance perception, Kopčo and Shinn-Cunningham (2011) showed lower performances for the evaluation of frontal sources than for lateral sources. They highlighted a high influence of sound spectrum on distance perception and explain it by assuming that near distances are evaluated using a fixed Direct/Reverberant mapping with distance that vary with frequencies.

Exploitation of the human capacities for spatial auditory perception often involves the creation of virtual auditory environments. The basis of this technique has been described in detail by Begault (1994) and Xie (2013). Such virtual reality simulations have been used in numerous studies, for example in the study of spatial cognition by Afonso et al. (2010), the treatment of phobias by Viaud-Delmon et al. (2008), the perception of architectural spaces by acoustic information by the blind by Picinali et al. (2014), interactive multidimensional data sonification and exploration by Férey et al. (2009), training systems to improve localization ability by Honda et al. (2007) and Parseihian and Katz (2012b), as well as in navigation systems for the blind by Wilson et al. (2007); Walker and Lindsay (2006). However, the vast majority of virtual auditory applications have focused on either far-field virtual sources, or virtual sources in the near horizontal plane and higher elevations. Very few studies have addressed very low elevations and proximal source positions.

In the context of the development of a specific integrated near- and far-field navigation and guidance system using spatial audio rendering (see Katz et al., 2012) this study concerns not only the accuracy in pointing to the direction of an auditory source (azimuth and elevation), but the accuracy in indicating the exact position of an anechoic auditory source. One situation of specific interest is the ability to locate an auditory source when positioned on a table-top type surface, which would be the position for which the user would be guided. This context considers both near and low elevation source positions.

The current study proposes an evaluation of basic auditory localization and pointing accuracy for sources low elevation in the peripersonal space. This condition examines an area rarely studied in previous literature. While not carried in anechoic conditions, the current study is performed in an acoustically damped room with very low reverberation. As such, the results can be compared to previous anechoic and non-anechoic condition studies, with the understanding that some minor room effect is present. Accuracy is evaluated as a function of pointing hand used, in an attempt to examine if there is any bias relative to hand dominance in the reporting task. This experiment explores localization and pointing accuracy for source positions spanning azimuths of ±120°.

A subsequent evaluation examines the potential of errors in position reporting due to biomechanical related effects rather than auditory perception limitations. A visual condition using the same test protocol serves as a control condition, with results showing that pointing accuracy is good and similar anywhere around the subject. To address the contextual situation, the subsequent study also includes a secondary preliminary investigation exploring how the peripersonal pointing accuracy depends on a virtual implementation of distance cues using an anechoic binaural simulation. This subsequent experiment explores localization and pointing accuracy over a reduced angular range, with source positions spanning azimuths of ±60°.

The following section provides an overview of the experimental design with each individual experiment being detailed in subsequent sections.

REACHING TO SOUND SOURCES

In order to investigate sound localization and pointing accuracy in the peripersonal space, two exploratory experiments have been designed and carried out. The first experiment evaluates general localization accuracy and specifically examines the effect of the pointing hand, dominant vs. secondary, for the pointing task. The second experiment compares the localization and pointing accuracy in peripersonal space for two additional stimulus types relative to the first experiment. Firstly, comparisons are made to visual stimuli, in an attempt to identify any common reporting errors due to difficulties relating to the pointing task. Secondly, the experimental platform is reproduced using a virtual audio display employing binaural synthesis, in an attempt to provide a benchmark for localization and pointing accuracy in the peripersonal space in a virtual environment.

All experiments were carried out in the same conditions, using the common protocol and experimental platform, in order to facilitate comparisons. Details of the protocol and platform are provided in the following section. Specific details associated with a given experiment are described in the subsequent sections along with the results of the two experiments.

STIMULI

A brief sound stimulus was used for the two experiments in order to prevent active localization related to dynamic cues during head movement. It consisted of a train of three, 40 ms Gaussian broadband noise bursts (50–20000 Hz) with 2 ms Hamming ramps at onset and offset and 30 ms of silence between each burst. This stimulus was chosen following (Macé et al., 2012), where the effect of repetition and duration of the burst on localization accuracy was analyzed for blind and sighted individuals. Their results showed an improvement in accuracy between three repeated 40 ms bursts and a single 200 ms burst. The overall level of the train was approximately 60 dBA, measured at the ear position.

SETUP

The experimental setup used for both experiments consists of a semicircle platform of 1 m radius. It contained 35 sound sources distributed on five semi-circular rows spaced by 13 cm (radii at: 33, 46, 59, 72, and 85 cm); each row contained seven sources spaced by 30° (**Figure 1**). For the real sound condition, the sources comprised 35 small loudspeakers (ref: CB990, 8 Ohms, 3 Watt) placed under an acoustically transparent grid. Acoustically absorbing foam covered the mounting board between loudspeakers. Subjects were seated on a swivel chair with their head placed over the center of the semi-circle and at a height of 65 cm. Each loudspeaker was oriented to the subject's head in order to avoid loudspeaker directivity variations. All sources were equalized to present the same spectral response (speakers responses were flattened with twelve cascaded biquad filters) and level calibrated at the center of the listening head position (± 1 dB SPL). The spectral equalization suppressed potential supplementary localization cues and learning effects for a given loudspeaker. The loudness equalization suppressed the distance attenuation intensity cue so as to avoid potential relative judgments and to place the listener in an unfamiliar condition (the subject doesn't know the source and its "natural" level) as in Brungart et al. (1999).

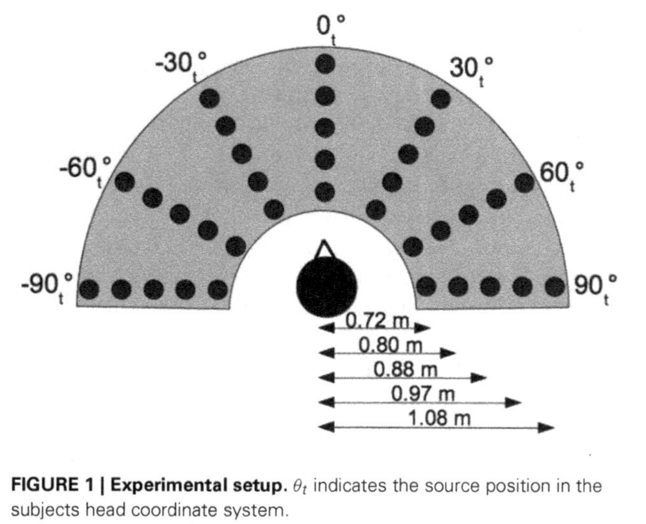

FIGURE 1 | Experimental setup. θ_t indicates the source position in the subjects head coordinate system.

For the first experiment the subject's head was tracked with a 6-DoF position/orientation sensor (Optitrack motion capture system—precision: 0.2° in azimuth, 5 mm in distance) positioned on the top of the head, and hand position was tracked with a sensor positioned over the extremity of the hand (on the tip of the three middle fingers). The position of the hand was calculated relative to the 6-DoF head tracker shifted to the center of the head. For the second experiment, hand positions were measured with the Optitrack motion capture system and head orientation was monitored with a magnetic sensor [Flock of Bird, Ascension Technology—angular precision (yaw, pitch, roll): 0.5°].

The experimental setup was located in a dark and acoustically damped low reverberant space (reverberation time ≈ 300 ms in the mid frequency region) in order to avoid any visual or auditory cues from the experimental platform and surrounding environment.

EXPERIMENT 1: POINTING HAND EFFECT

The aim of experiment 1 was to measure pointing/reaching accuracy toward real sound sources. This accuracy was then evaluated as a function of the pointing hand and source location. In addition to source position, the effect of the reporting method, specifically dominant vs. non-dominant hand, was evaluated.

MATERIALS AND METHODS

Subjects

A total of 15 adult subjects (3 women and 12 men, mean age = 28 years, $SD = 6$) served as paid volunteers; all were healthy. An audiogram was performed on each subject before the experiment to ensure that his or her audition was normal (defined as thresholds no greater than 15 dB hearing level in the range of 125–8000 Hz). All were naive regarding the purpose of the experiment and the sets of spatial locations selected for the experiment. All were self-reported right handed; no handedness measure was performed to establish their dominant hand. This study was performed in accordance with the ethical standards of the Declaration of Helsinki (revised Edinburgh 2000) and written informed consent was obtained from all subjects prior to the experiment (after receiving instructions about the experiment).

Experimental procedure

The localization task consisted in reporting the perceived position of a brief static sound sample using a hand placing technique. Each subject was instructed to orient him- or her-self straight ahead and keep his/her head fixed, in a reference position at the center of the system, 0.65 m over the table, during the brief sound stimulus presentation. Before each trial, the subject's head position was automatically compared to the reference position and the subject was asked to correct the position if there was no concordance (±5 cm for position and ±3° for orientation). After presentation of the stimulus, the subject was instructed to place the tip of his/her hand on the table at the location of the perceived sound source and to validate the response with a MIDI button in front of the subject, placed near the center of the inner arc, using their other hand. In this manner, the subject was stationary during stimulus presentation, avoiding dynamic cues. The reported position was calculated between the initial head center position/orientation when the stimulus was played and the final extremity of the hand position when the listener validated the target. No feedback was provided regarding the actual target location.

Preliminary experiments using the semi-circle table showed that sources at the extreme azimuths posed problems as they were too close to the edge of the table which unintentionally provided subjects a tactile reference point. As such, the experimental protocol was modified to use only 25 sources (from $-60_t°$ to $60_t°$ in **Figure 1**) with two subject orientations in order to cover a larger range of tested relative azimuths. For each hand, a total of 35 sources were tested with 7 different azimuths ($-60_r°$, $-30_r°$, $0_r°$, $30_r°$, $60_r°$, $90_r°$, and $120_r°$), where θ_r represents the source azimuth relative to the subject's head orientation and θ_t represents the source azimuth in the table reference frame. The experiment was realized in four phases:

(a) Subject faced the -60°_t line and reported 25 source locations (0°_r, 30°_r, 60°_r, 90°_r, and 120°_r) using the 1st (dominant, right) hand.
(b) Subject faced the -60°_t line and reported 15 source locations (-60°_r, -30°_r, and 0°_r) using the 2nd (non-dominant, left) hand.
(c) Subject faced the $+60^\circ_t$ line and reported 25 source locations (0°_r, 30°_r, 60°_r, 90°_r, and 120°_r) using the 2nd (non-dominant, left) hand.
(d) Subject faced the $+60^\circ_t$ line and reported 15 source locations (-60°_r, -30°_r, and 0°_r) using the 1st (dominant, right) hand.

All locations were repeated 5 times and randomly presented for each phase in five blocks of 25 locations (phases *a* and *c*) or 15 locations (phases *b* and *d*). A total of 400 locations were presented during the experiment and the total duration was around 90 min.

Data analysis

Because of technical validation problems with several participants (some subjects had a tendency to validate the reported position before the end of their hand placement movement), all trials with reported positions significantly above the table's surface (>10 cm) have been removed from further analysis (0.68% of all the trials).

Accuracy was calculated by measuring the bias and dispersion between the sound source and reported position in head spherical coordinates (azimuth, elevation, and distance). Due to the platform's configuration, distance and elevation of the source relative to the head are interdependent. As such, results were analyzed across two components: azimuth and distance relative to the subject.

As source locations were calculated in head coordinates, initial distances of 0.33, 0.46, 0.59, 0.72, and 0.85 m from the center of the platform corresponded to actual distances of $d_1 = 0.729$, $d_2 = 0.796$, $d_3 = 0.885$, $d_4 = 0.970$, and $d_5 = 1.078$ m from the center of the head (located 0.65 m above the platform).

Some front/back confusion errors were observed for rendered sources at lateral positions. These were identified according to the conventional definition of front/back confusion (proposed by Wightman and Kistler, 1989): if the angle between the target and the judged position is bigger than the angle between the target and the mirror of the judgment about the interaural axis, the judgment is considered as a confusion; combined with exclusion zone of Martin et al. (2001) (both the target and the judged position of the sound source do not fall within a narrow exclusion zone of ±7.5° around 90° axis). Due to the occurrence of such confusions (8.3% of all the trials), the analysis were performed both on the azimuth with front/back confusions present and on the azimuth after correcting front/back confusions by mirroring the judgment across the interaural axis ("corrected azimuth").

Statistical analyses were performed with repeated measurement analysis of variance (ANOVA) after verifying the datas distribution normality of unsigned azimuth error and signed distance error with Shapiro-Wilk tests on each hand, azimuth and distance conditions (only two conditions over fourteen were slightly skewed for the azimuth error). A Tukey *post-hoc* was used to assess differences between conditions.

RESULTS

Figure 2A presents the mean pointed position (with corrected azimuth) for the 1st and 2nd hand condition with the precision estimated by the 50% confidence ellipse linked to each position. For each target, 50% confidence ellipses were computed across all the subjects and all the conditions according to the method proposed by Murdoch and Chow (1996). The angle of the ellipse is determined by the covariance of the data and the magnitudes of the ellipse axes depend on the variance of the data. These plots highlight a compression of the reported distance dependent on the stimuli angle and a shift of the reported azimuth dependent on the stimuli angle and distance. For example, the azimuth error at 90° is larger for nearer sources and distance perception appears better at lateral angles. Azimuth and distance errors have been analyzed as a function of reporting hand, stimuli azimuth, and stimuli distance.

Azimuth error

Figure 2B represents the reported azimuth (without front/back confusion correction) as a function of stimuli azimuth. Unsigned azimuth error and front/back confusion rates as a function of azimuth are presented in **Table 1**. These results highlight good pointing accuracy with low variability in the frontal direction ($-30° \leq \theta_r \leq 30°$) with a mean unsigned error of 6.7°, and lower accuracy with greater variability toward the sides with a mean error of 17.8°. Lateral locations were underestimated. Front/back confusion analysis (**Table 1**) shows high levels of confusions from back to front at 120° and some confusions from front to back at −60° and 60°. The azimuth error at 120° when correcting front/back confusions is 15.9° against 39.2° without corrections. Surprisingly, one can observe some front/back confusions at 0° and 30° although the subjects were aware of the platform geometry. The standard deviation of azimuth error (around 15°) shows the high inter-subject variability. The mean of the standard deviation of azimuth error over subjects (7.9 ± 3.2°) shows a lower intra-subject variability.

Overall performance shows similar errors in the median plan and greater differences on the side, but with a slight difference

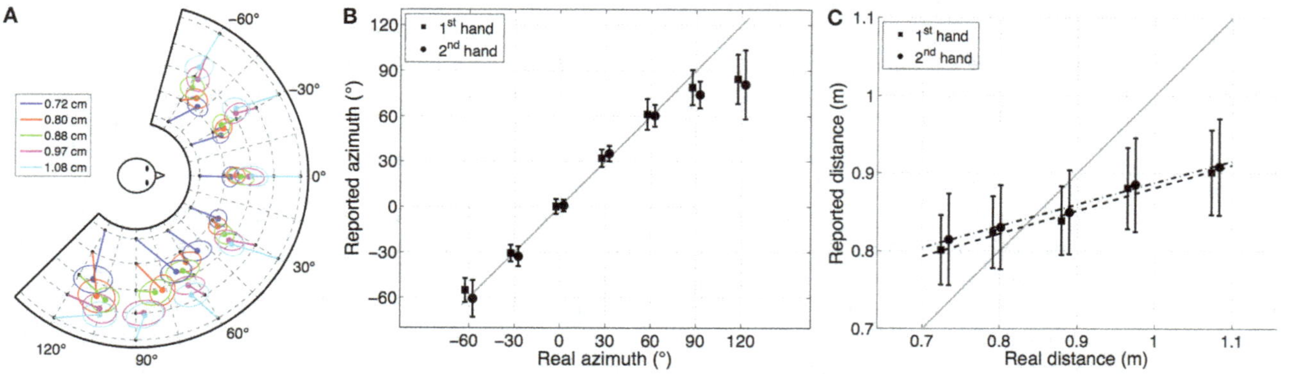

FIGURE 2 | (A) (Color on-line) Mean of all subjects' reported location with 50% confidence ellipse linked to source location for the dominant hand condition. Front/back confusion corrected. Good directional pointing accuracy in the median plane, larger compression of reported distances in front than in side. **(B)** Mean of all subjects' reported azimuth as a function of the target azimuth for both hand conditions. Error bars show one standard deviation across the subjects. Gray line shows unity. For the sake of readability, results corresponding to the different hand conditions have been slightly horizontally shifted. This plot shows a good pointing accuracy on the frontal hemisphere and lower accuracy on the side. **(C)** Mean of all subjects' reported distance as a function of target distance with mean of linear regression slope for 1st and 2nd hand across all azimuths. Gray line shows unity. Error bars show one standard deviation across the subjects. Reported distance is linear but compressed.

Table 1 | Mean of absolute azimuth and corrected azimuth error in degree (standard deviations in parenthesis) and front/back confusion rate as a function of stimuli azimuth.

	Azimuth	−60°	−30°	0°	30°	60°	90°	120°	Total
Azimuth	1st hand	9.3 (7.8)	6.7 (5.4)	6.5 (7.8)	7.1 (5.8)	11.1 (8.9)	15.2 (12.4)	36.1 (12.4)	12.3 (14.6)
Error	2nd hand	11.9 (9.7)	6.9 (5.9)	6.1 (7.4)	8.2 (7.3)	9.2 (8.0)	17.7 (12.0)	42.0 (23.5)	13.6 (16.2)
Corrected	1st hand	9.3 (7.8)	6.7 (5.4)	6.4 (5.9)	7.1 (5.8)	10.7 (8.1)	15.2 (12.4)	15.9 (11.8)	9.7 (9.1)
azim. error	2nd hand	11.3 (8.7)	6.9 (5.9)	6.0 (5.4)	8.1 (7.2)	9.2 (7.9)	17.7 (12.0)	11.8 (8.8)	9.6 (8.7)
F/B	1st hand	0.0	0.0	0.1	0.0	3.5	0.0	56.5	7.5
Conf. (%)	2nd hand	4.3	0.0	0.1	0.3	0.8	0.0	66.3	9.1

when using the dominant (1st) or non-dominant (2nd) hand. A repeated measure ANOVA performed on front/back confusion rate with pointing hand as a factor shows no significant differences between the two conditions [$F_{(1,\,14)} = 2.53, p = 0.13$]. A repeated measure 3-factor ANOVA (Hand∗Azimuth∗Distance) performed on the absolute corrected azimuth error highlights a significant effect of azimuth [$F_{(6,\,84)} = 19.14, p < 10^{-5}$] and distance [$F_{(4,\,56)} = 6.63, p < 0.001$] but no effect of hand reporting condition [$F_{(1,\,14)} = 0.01, p = 0.91$]. The *post-hoc* analysis performed on the azimuth indicates significant differences in performance between central positions (−30°, 0°, and 30°), lateral positions (−60° and 60°), and extreme positions (90° and 120°). The *post-hoc* analysis performed on distance highlights significantly poorer azimuth estimation for the nearest positions ($d = 0.33$ m). Interaction analysis shows an effect of Hand∗Azimuth [$F_{(6,\,84)} = 4.59, p < 0.001$] with significant differences in azimuth performances for the 1st and 2nd hand condition at 120°; no interaction effect of Hand∗Distance [$F_{(4,\,56)} = 0.35, p = 0.84$]; and an interaction effect of Azimuth∗Distance [$F_{(24,\,336)} = 7.43, p < 10^{-5}$].

Distance error

Figure 2C shows the average mean reported source distance as a function of sound source distance. This figure highlights a compressed but still linear perception of distance in the range of the tested region. The mean distance error across subjects, and the slope of the regression line and goodness-of-fit criteria r^2 calculated over the five trials for each azimuth and hand condition are shown in **Table 2**.

These results highlight difficulty regarding distance perception and a tendency to overestimate sound distance for the two nearest distances and to underestimate it for the others. Global error is ≈ 10 cm which equated to 11% relative error. This error is lower at the sides (9.2 cm) than toward the front (10.4 cm). Although distance perception was compressed (with a mean regression slope of 0.30 ± 0.11), **Figure 2C** shows a quasi linear perception of distance in the range of the tested region (36 cm). The comparison of regression slope across stimuli angles (**Table 2**) highlights better distance perception to the side (at −60°, 60°, and 90°) than toward the front. Standard deviation of the distance error (around 8 cm) indicates high inter-subject variability. The mean of the standard deviation of the distance error across subjects (7.6 ± 1.0 cm) also indicates intra-subject variability. Regarding the mean of the regression slope across subjects ($m = 0.29 \pm 0.11$), inter-subject variability is quite large (the subject with lowest distance perception obtaining a mean slope of 0.12 ± 0.18 and the subject with highest distance perception a mean slope of 0.52 ± 0.11).

followed the axis of a motorized turntable (B&K 9640), which allowed variation of its orientation within the horizontal plane. The interaural axis of the KEMAR dummy head was centered (at 1.9 m from the loudspeaker) using a set of three coincident laser beams. The axis of the turntable coincided with a line extending through the center of the dummy head, therefore minimizing displacements during rotations of the turntable. The measurement set was obtained using the sweep-sine excitation technique at a sample rate of 44.1 kHz (RME Fireface 800 audio interface). The free-field HRTF was obtained through normalization (direct deconvolution through division in the complex frequency domain) by the free-field system response without the KEMAR present. The resulting HRIR was windowed (rectangular) to a length of 256 samples. The window was positioned to include 20 samples before the first peak as evaluated over all positions. In order to render all the sound source positions, it was necessary to measure the HRTF over the entire sphere. The set used contained measurement from −90° to 90° in elevation in steps of 5°, and from −180° to 180° in azimuth in steps of 5°.

The HRTF was decomposed into spectral component (representing spectral cues) and pure delay (representing ITD cues). A spatial interpolation of the spectral component was realized (see Aussal et al., 2013). The spatialization engine used a hybrid HRTF, where the modeled individual interaural time difference (ITD) based on head and shoulder circumference (see Aussal et al., 2012) was combined with the KEMAR spectral component. Binaural sound sources were rendered using a real-time spatialization engine based on full-phase HRIR convolution. ILD cues were modified to account for contralateral level difference for near distances using a spherical head model and a parallax effect correction was implemented for distances inferior to 1 m (HRIR were selected taking into account the angle of the source relative to the ear rather than the angle relative to the head center) (see Katz et al., 2011, 2012).

Thus, in the *virtual sound* condition, the available distance cues consisted of ILD variations as well as localization spectral cues associated with the corrected HRTF angles position. No near field correction was made for ITD variations with distance. Furthermore, an additional distance cue consisted in the spectral variations corresponding to the elevation changes linked to the distance due to the configuration of the table top setup. No additional propagation paths or reflections were simulated.

In order to improve reporting performance of the binaural rendering using non-individual HRTF, three preliminary adaptation sessions of 12 min were conducted according to the method proposed by Parseihian and Katz (2012b). Briefly, this method consists of a training game allowing the subject to perform a rapid exploration of the spatial map of the virtual rendering by an auditory-kinesthetic closed-loop. These training sessions were performed 3 days in a row, 12 min per day, the last session being immediately prior to the main experiment.

Data analysis

Analysis of results was performed following the same parameters as the first experiment: azimuth and distance relative to the subject. With subject's head located 0.60 m over the table, the sources were at distances of 0.685, 0.756, 0.842, 0.937, and 1.040 m from the subject's head center.

No front/back confusions (observed as pointing to the back) were observed. However, during the debriefing, some subjects reported having heard sources behind them or inside their head and pointed toward the table edge. As it is difficult to detect these pointing instances as front/back confusions, we looked for outliers in the dataset. First, a total of 48 trials with reported positions lying outside the table were preliminarily removed from the data (0.80% of all the trials; 0.00% of *real sound* condition trials, 1.55% of *virtual sound* condition trials, and 0.85% of *visual* condition trials.) Second, trials with signed azimuth error or signed distance error exceeding a fixed limit were removed. The upper limit was defined as $Q_3 + 1.5 \times (Q_3 - Q_1)$ and the lower limit as $Q_1 - 1.5 \times (Q_3 - Q_1)$ with Q_1 and Q_3 respectively the first and the third data quartile. Outside these limits the reported locations were tagged as outliers. A total of 244 trials were removed from the data (4.11% of all the trials; 6.45% of *real sound* condition trials, 2.14% of *virtual sound* condition trials, and 4.45% of *visual* condition trials.)

Statistical analyses were performed with repeated measurement analysis of variance (ANOVA) after verifying the datas distribution normality of unsigned azimuth error and signed distance error with Shapiro-Wilk tests on each hand, azimuth and distance conditions. A Tukey *post-hoc* was used to assess differences between conditions.

RESULTS

The mean reported positions linked to target locations for each rendering condition are presented in **Figure 3** with 50% confidence ellipse. These plots allow one to evaluate the error bias across the three conditions. For *visual* sources, lateral localization accuracy is quite good while the nearest distances are overestimated. For *real sound* sources, the reported distance is compressed and a lateral shift appears mostly at −60° and 60°. For *virtual sound* sources, all lateral sources are shifted toward the sides and there is no apparent distance perception. In the following sections these results are analyzed in terms of azimuth and distance bias and dispersion.

Azimuth error

Figure 4A presents the mean and standard deviation of reported azimuth as a function of stimuli azimuth. The mean and standard deviation of the unsigned azimuth error are presented in **Table 3**. First, the *visual* condition shows good estimation of azimuth, with a low variability (mean error of 2.79° ± 4.51°). For frontal locations, the mean unsigned error is 1.61° ± 1.27°. This error increases with azimuth to 2° for ±30° locations and to 4° for ±60° locations, as does the dispersion. It can be noticed that the lateral error corresponds to a slight underestimation of the azimuth. Second, results for *real sound* condition are similar to the first experiment's results. They highlight good accuracy at 0° with a mean error of 5.7°, and lower accuracy at the sides. Third, *virtual sound* condition showed lower performance results in terms of azimuth estimation. The mean absolute error at 0° is 10.79° ± 10.03°. The ±30° and ±60° locations are shifted by

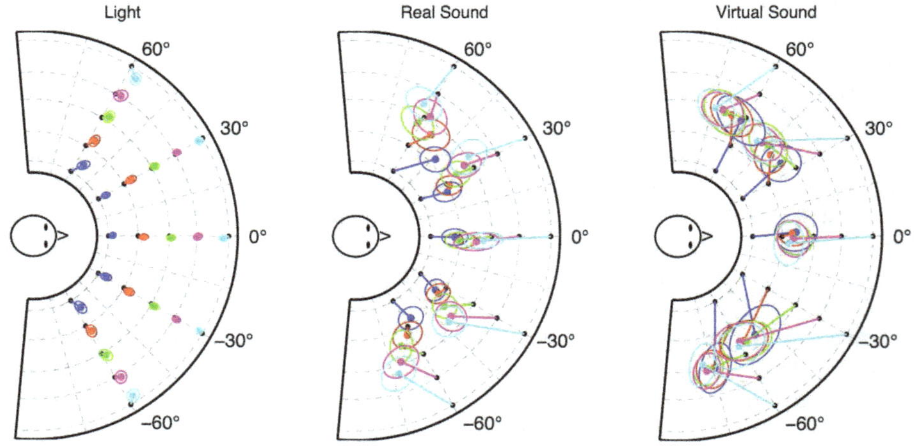

FIGURE 3 | Mean of all subjects' reported location with 50% confidence ellipse linked to source location for each rendering condition: *visual* (left), *real sound* (center), and *virtual sound* (right).

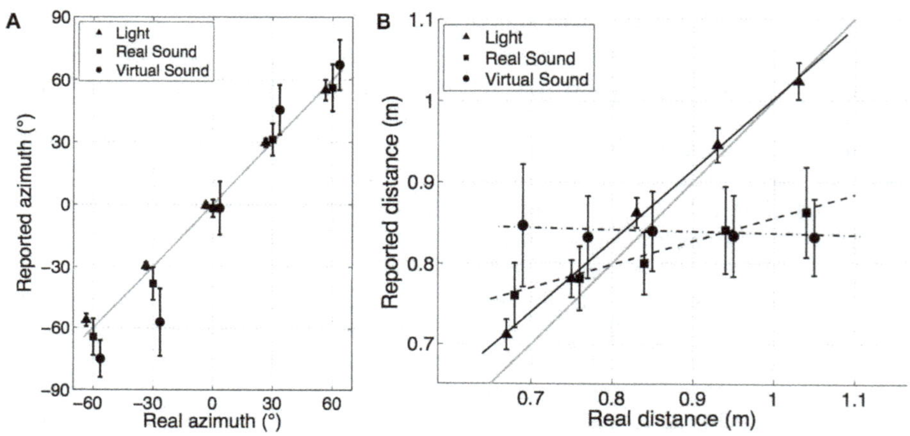

FIGURE 4 | (A) Mean of all subjects' reported azimuth as a function of stimuli azimuth for each rendering condition: *visual* (▲), *real sound* (■), and *virtual sound* (•). Error bars show one standard deviation across the subjects. Gray line shows unity. **(B)** Mean of all subjects' reported distance as a function of stimuli distance for each rendering condition: *visual* (▲), *real sound* (■), and *virtual sound* (•). Error bars show one standard deviation across the subjects for each condition. Solid gray lines show linear regression curves for each modality. Gray line shows unity.

Table 3 | Mean absolute azimuth error in degree (standard deviations in parenthesis) for each rendering condition as a function of stimuli azimuth.

Condition	–60°	–30°	0°	30°	60°	Total
Visual	3.85 (5.84)	1.94 (2.97)	1.61 (1.27)	1.99 (2.56)	4.51 (6.56)	2.79 (4.51)
Real sound	11.08 (8.15)	10.66 (8.22)	5.70 (4.61)	7.08 (5.81)	11.30 (8.27)	9.18 (7.54)
Virtual sound	16.75 (9.04)	28.17 (17.43)	10.79 (10.03)	16.83 (13.78)	14.44 (9.97)	17.48 (13.76)

approximately 15° to the side (except −30° locations which are reported at −60°).

A repeated measures 3-factor ANOVA (Condition∗Azimuth∗Distance) was performed on the mean absolute azimuth error of each subject, highlighting a significant effect of condition [$F_{(2,38)} = 61.75$; $p < 10^{-5}$]. The *post-hoc* test revealed a significant difference between each condition. Azimuth errors are significantly lower for the *visual* condition compared to the sound conditions and are significantly greater for *virtual sound* condition compared to the two others. The interaction analysis showed a significant effect of Condition∗Azimuth [$F_{(8,152)} = 15.62$; $p < 10^{-5}$] and of Condition∗Distance [$F_{(8,152)} = 9.71$; $p < 10^{-5}$]. The *post-hoc* test on Condition∗Azimuth highlights no effect of the azimuth on the *visual* condition, but it shows a significant difference of performance between 0° and lateral positions (−60° and 60°) for stationary during stimulus presentation, avoiding dynamic cues. The reported position was calculated between the initial head center position/orientation when the stimulus was played and the final extremity of the hand position when the listener validated the target. No feedback was provided regarding the actual target location.

Preliminary experiments using the semi-circle table showed that sources at the extreme azimuths posed problems as they were too close to the edge of the table which unintentionally provided subjects a tactile reference point. As such, the experimental protocol was modified to use only 25 sources (from $-60_t°$ to $60_t°$ in **Figure 1**) with two subject orientations in order to cover a larger range of tested relative azimuths. For each hand, a total of 35 sources were tested with 7 different azimuths ($-60_r°$, $-30_r°$, $0_r°$, $30_r°$, $60_r°$, $90_r°$, and $120_r°$), where θ_r represents the source azimuth relative to the subject's head orientation and θ_t represents the source azimuth in the table reference frame. The experiment was realized in four phases:

(a) Subject faced the -60°_t line and reported 25 source locations (0°_r, 30°_r, 60°_r, 90°_r, and 120°_r) using the 1st (dominant, right) hand.
(b) Subject faced the -60°_t line and reported 15 source locations (-60°_r, -30°_r, and 0°_r) using the 2nd (non-dominant, left) hand.
(c) Subject faced the $+60^\circ_t$ line and reported 25 source locations (0°_r, 30°_r, 60°_r, 90°_r, and 120°_r) using the 2nd (non-dominant, left) hand.
(d) Subject faced the $+60^\circ_t$ line and reported 15 source locations (-60°_r, -30°_r, and 0°_r) using the 1st (dominant, right) hand.

All locations were repeated 5 times and randomly presented for each phase in five blocks of 25 locations (phases *a* and *c*) or 15 locations (phases *b* and *d*). A total of 400 locations were presented during the experiment and the total duration was around 90 min.

Data analysis

Because of technical validation problems with several participants (some subjects had a tendency to validate the reported position before the end of their hand placement movement), all trials with reported positions significantly above the table's surface (>10 cm) have been removed from further analysis (0.68% of all the trials).

Accuracy was calculated by measuring the bias and dispersion between the sound source and reported position in head spherical coordinates (azimuth, elevation, and distance). Due to the platform's configuration, distance and elevation of the source relative to the head are interdependent. As such, results were analyzed across two components: azimuth and distance relative to the subject.

As source locations were calculated in head coordinates, initial distances of 0.33, 0.46, 0.59, 0.72, and 0.85 m from the center of the platform corresponded to actual distances of $d_1 = 0.729$, $d_2 = 0.796$, $d_3 = 0.885$, $d_4 = 0.970$, and $d_5 = 1.078$ m from the center of the head (located 0.65 m above the platform).

Some front/back confusion errors were observed for rendered sources at lateral positions. These were identified according to the conventional definition of front/back confusion (proposed by Wightman and Kistler, 1989): if the angle between the target and the judged position is bigger than the angle between the target and the mirror of the judgment about the interaural axis, the judgment is considered as a confusion; combined with exclusion zone of Martin et al. (2001) (both the target and the judged position of the sound source do not fall within a narrow exclusion zone of ±7.5° around 90° axis). Due to the occurrence of such confusions (8.3% of all the trials), the analysis were performed both on the azimuth with front/back confusions present and on the azimuth after correcting front/back confusions by mirroring the judgment across the interaural axis ("corrected azimuth").

Statistical analyses were performed with repeated measurement analysis of variance (ANOVA) after verifying the datas distribution normality of unsigned azimuth error and signed distance error with Shapiro-Wilk tests on each hand, azimuth and distance conditions (only two conditions over fourteen were slightly skewed for the azimuth error). A Tukey *post-hoc* was used to assess differences between conditions.

RESULTS

Figure 2A presents the mean pointed position (with corrected azimuth) for the 1st and 2nd hand condition with the precision estimated by the 50% confidence ellipse linked to each position. For each target, 50% confidence ellipses were computed across all the subjects and all the conditions according to the method proposed by Murdoch and Chow (1996). The angle of the ellipse is determined by the covariance of the data and the magnitudes of the ellipse axes depend on the variance of the data. These plots highlight a compression of the reported distance dependent on the stimuli angle and a shift of the reported azimuth dependent on the stimuli angle and distance. For example, the azimuth error at 90° is larger for nearer sources and distance perception appears better at lateral angles. Azimuth and distance errors have been analyzed as a function of reporting hand, stimuli azimuth, and stimuli distance.

Azimuth error

Figure 2B represents the reported azimuth (without front/back confusion correction) as a function of stimuli azimuth. Unsigned azimuth error and front/back confusion rates as a function of azimuth are presented in **Table 1**. These results highlight good pointing accuracy with low variability in the frontal direction ($-30° \le \theta_r \le 30°$) with a mean unsigned error of 6.7°, and lower accuracy with greater variability toward the sides with a mean error of 17.8°. Lateral locations were underestimated. Front/back confusion analysis (**Table 1**) shows high levels of confusions from back to front at 120° and some confusions from front to back at −60° and 60°. The azimuth error at 120° when correcting front/back confusions is 15.9° against 39.2° without corrections. Surprisingly, one can observe some front/back confusions at 0° and 30° although the subjects were aware of the platform geometry. The standard deviation of azimuth error (around 15°) shows the high inter-subject variability. The mean of the standard deviation of azimuth error over subjects (7.9 ± 3.2°) shows a lower intra-subject variability.

Overall performance shows similar errors in the median plan and greater differences on the side, but with a slight difference

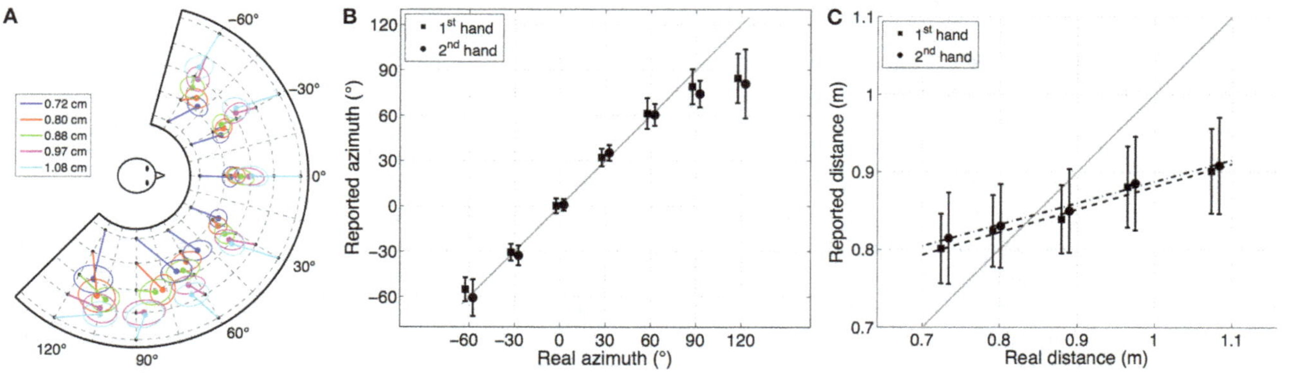

FIGURE 2 | (A) (Color on-line) Mean of all subjects' reported location with 50% confidence ellipse linked to source location for the dominant hand condition. Front/back confusion corrected. Good directional pointing accuracy in the median plane, larger compression of reported distances in front than in side. **(B)** Mean of all subjects' reported azimuth as a function of the target azimuth for both hand conditions. Error bars show one standard deviation across the subjects. Gray line shows unity. For the sake of readability, results corresponding to the different hand conditions have been slightly horizontally shifted. This plot shows a good pointing accuracy on the frontal hemisphere and lower accuracy on the side. **(C)** Mean of all subjects' reported distance as a function of target distance with mean of linear regression slope for 1st and 2nd hand across all azimuths. Gray line shows unity. Error bars show one standard deviation across the subjects. Reported distance is linear but compressed.

Table 1 | Mean of absolute azimuth and corrected azimuth error in degree (standard deviations in parenthesis) and front/back confusion rate as a function of stimuli azimuth.

	Azimuth	−60°	−30°	0°	30°	60°	90°	120°	Total
Azimuth	1st hand	9.3 (7.8)	6.7 (5.4)	6.5 (7.8)	7.1 (5.8)	11.1 (8.9)	15.2 (12.4)	36.1 (12.4)	12.3 (14.6)
Error	2nd hand	11.9 (9.7)	6.9 (5.9)	6.1 (7.4)	8.2 (7.3)	9.2 (8.0)	17.7 (12.0)	42.0 (23.5)	13.6 (16.2)
Corrected	1st hand	9.3 (7.8)	6.7 (5.4)	6.4 (5.9)	7.1 (5.8)	10.7 (8.1)	15.2 (12.4)	15.9 (11.8)	9.7 (9.1)
azim. error	2nd hand	11.3 (8.7)	6.9 (5.9)	6.0 (5.4)	8.1 (7.2)	9.2 (7.9)	17.7 (12.0)	11.8 (8.8)	9.6 (8.7)
F/B	1st hand	0.0	0.0	0.1	0.0	3.5	0.0	56.5	7.5
Conf. (%)	2nd hand	4.3	0.0	0.1	0.3	0.8	0.0	66.3	9.1

when using the dominant (1st) or non-dominant (2nd) hand. A repeated measure ANOVA performed on front/back confusion rate with pointing hand as a factor shows no significant differences between the two conditions [$F_{(1,\ 14)} = 2.53, p = 0.13$]. A repeated measure 3-factor ANOVA (Hand∗Azimuth∗Distance) performed on the absolute corrected azimuth error highlights a significant effect of azimuth [$F_{(6,\ 84)} = 19.14, p < 10^{-5}$] and distance [$F_{(4,\ 56)} = 6.63, p < 0.001$] but no effect of hand reporting condition [$F_{(1,\ 14)} = 0.01, p = 0.91$]. The *post-hoc* analysis performed on the azimuth indicates significant differences in performance between central positions (−30°, 0°, and 30°), lateral positions (−60° and 60°), and extreme positions (90° and 120°). The *post-hoc* analysis performed on distance highlights significantly poorer azimuth estimation for the nearest positions ($d = 0.33$ m). Interaction analysis shows an effect of Hand∗Azimuth [$F_{(6,\ 84)} = 4.59$, $p < 0.001$] with significant differences in azimuth performances for the 1st and 2nd hand condition at 120°; no interaction effect of Hand∗Distance [$F_{(4,\ 56)} = 0.35, p = 0.84$]; and an interaction effect of Azimuth∗Distance [$F_{(24,\ 336)} = 7.43$, $p < 10^{-5}$].

Distance error

Figure 2C shows the average mean reported source distance as a function of sound source distance. This figure highlights a compressed but still linear perception of distance in the range of the tested region. The mean distance error across subjects, and the slope of the regression line and goodness-of-fit criteria r^2 calculated over the five trials for each azimuth and hand condition are shown in **Table 2**.

These results highlight difficulty regarding distance perception and a tendency to overestimate sound distance for the two nearest distances and to underestimate it for the others. Global error is ≈ 10 cm which equated to 11% relative error. This error is lower at the sides (9.2 cm) than toward the front (10.4 cm). Although distance perception was compressed (with a mean regression slope of 0.30 ± 0.11), **Figure 2C** shows a quasi linear perception of distance in the range of the tested region (36 cm). The comparison of regression slope across stimuli angles (**Table 2**) highlights better distance perception to the side (at −60°, 60°, and 90°) than toward the front. Standard deviation of the distance error (around 8 cm) indicates high inter-subject variability. The mean of the standard deviation of the distance error across subjects (7.6 ± 1.0 cm) also indicates intra-subject variability. Regarding the mean of the regression slope across subjects ($m = 0.29 \pm 0.11$), inter-subject variability is quite large (the subject with lowest distance perception obtaining a mean slope of 0.12 ± 0.18 and the subject with highest distance perception a mean slope of 0.52 ± 0.11).

Table 2 | Mean of absolute distance error (standard deviations in parenthesis), slope of the regression line and goodness-of-fit criteria r^2 for each azimuth and hand condition.

	Azimuth	−60°	−30°	0°	30°	60°	90°	120°	Total
Absolute distance error (cm)	1st hand	9.5 (7.6)	9.9 (7.7)	10.7 (8.9)	10.5 (8.4)	8.7 (6.3)	8.6 (6.4)	10.0 (7.4)	9.8 (7.8)
	2nd hand	9.8 (7.8)	10.6 (8.5)	10.5 (8.5)	10.1 (8.1)	9.0 (7.1)	9.4 (7.2)	12.1 (9.2)	10.3 (8.2)
Regression slope	1st hand	0.31 (0.17)	0.29 (0.14)	0.21 (0.16)	0.25 (0.12)	0.38 (0.12)	0.40 (0.17)	0.30 (0.19)	0.31 (0.15)
	2nd hand	0.34 (0.14)	0.24 (0.12)	0.24 (0.15)	0.26 (0.15)	0.35 (0.14)	0.34 (0.14)	0.22 (0.21)	0.28 (0.15)
Goodness-of-fit r^2	1st hand	0.53	0.46	0.22	0.38	0.60	0.51	0.32	0.43
	hand	0.55	0.40	0.31	0.41	0.52	0.48	0.23	0.41

Performance analysis as a function of reporting hand condition showed few differences between 1st and 2nd hand. In both cases, distance perception was virtually the same, however, with higher variability in the 2nd hand condition. A repeated measure 3-factor ANOVA (Hand∗Azimuth∗Distance) performed on signed distance error highlights a significant effect of azimuth [$F_{(6, 84)} = 70.09$, $p < 10^{-5}$], a significant effect of distance [$F_{(4, 56)} = 572.78$, $p < 10^{-5}$] and no effect of hand [$F_{(1, 14)} = 0.88$, $p = 0.36$]. The *post-hoc* analysis performed on the azimuth shows significant differences in distance evaluation between 60° and 90° positions (which lead to the best distance evaluation) and the others positions. The *post-hoc* analysis performed on distance highlights significant differences between all distances positions, with over estimation of the distance for nearest positions (d_1 and d_2) and under estimation for the others (d_3, d_4, and d_5). Interaction analysis shows an effect of Azimuth∗Distance [$F_{(24, 336)} = 4.47$, $p < 10^{-5}$]; no effect of Hand∗Azimuth [$F_{(6, 84)} = 1.62$, $p = 0.15$] and no effect of Hand∗Distance [$F_{(4, 56)} = 1.82$, $p = 0.14$].

Regression slopes are virtually equal in the two conditions (0.30 ± 0.11 for 1st hand and 0.28 ± 0.11 for 2nd hand) as well as the goodness of fit. A 2-factor ANOVA (Hand∗Azimuth) performed on the regression slope showed no effect of the reporting hand [$F_{(1, 14)} = 3.36$, $p = 0.09$] and an effect of the azimuth [$F_{(6, 84)} = 4.47$, $p < 0.001$]. The *post-hoc* test revealed a significant difference between regression slopes calculated for 0° azimuths and those calculated for 60° and 90° azimuths. No Hand∗Azimuth interaction was observed.

Distance accuracy in the studied zone was poorer than azimuth accuracy. Although distance error clearly depends on the distance of the stimuli (linear regression), it is compressed toward the center of the reporting area.

DISCUSSION

The results of this experiment show a large variability between subjects. Despite this disparity, the results highlight the capacity of listeners to perceive and report a sound target within a general error of ≈ 13°, and an error of ≈ 6–7° in the frontal zone. In this zone, distance perception is poorer and compressed to the middle of the platform. Although distance perception was almost linear in the range of the tested region, the low value of the regression slope (around 0.3) highlights the difficulty in perceiving and reporting target stimuli using the sound cues provided.

The poor performance for distance perception can be explained in several ways. First, the small range variation of distances (from 0.72 to 1.08 m, total variation 0.36 m) is an important limitation factor. Second, the normalization of the stimulus amplitude to eliminate global distance attenuation cues and relative level differences makes distance judgments more difficult. Third, the suppression of the reverberant field with absorbent material reduces potential distance cues due to binaural variations and spatially coherent reflection information.

Since the setup of this experiment differs from previous studies, precise comparison is difficult. It is however possible to make comparisons with Brungart et al. (1999) (carried out in an anechoic room), considering their results for frontal and lateral zones with elevations below −20° and distances between 0.5 and 1.0 m. For azimuth perception, Brungart et al. (1999) reported a lateral error of 13.4° (between 60° and 120°) and a frontal error of 16.1° (between −60° and 60°). Results of our study, with errors of 18° for lateral angle and 7° for the frontal zone, show an opposite trend to their results. First, this difference can be explained by the front/back confusion suppression applied by Brungart et al. (1999). Results are more similar with suppression of front/back confusions in our results (lateral error ≈ 13°). Despite this, the difference in azimuth error in the frontal zone is surprising. In our study, subjects were more precise in the frontal zone, which is coherent with classical localization results summarized by Blauert (1997) for greater distances. One explanation could be the difference in reporting technique; reported locations were calculated relative to a position sensor mounted on the end of a 20 cm wooden wand in Brungart's experiment and directly to the hand in the present experiment. For distance perception, studies from Brungart et al. (1999) and Kopčo and Shinn-Cunningham (2011) reported more accurate results than the current work, with regression slopes around 0.90 in the lateral zone and around 0.70 in the frontal zone (compared to 0.34 and 0.25 respectively in the current study). Although the three studies show the same tendency of improved distance perception for lateral positions, the distance perception in the current study is significantly worse. One can note the different range of distances value used in these studies (from 0.7 to 1.1 m in our study, from 0.1 to 1.0 m in Brungart's study, and from 0.15 to 1.7 m in Kopčo and Shinn-Cunningham, 2011). One major difference in test conditions was that elevation angles varied from approximately −65° to −37° in the current study while they varied from approximately −40°

to −20° in Brungart et al. (1999) and were equal to zero in Kopčo and Shinn-Cunningham (2011). Where as Brungart's experiment took place in anechoic condition (with ILD as the main distance cue), and Kopčo and Shinn-Cunningham (2011)'s experiment in low reverberant conditions (TR ≈ 600 ms, with ILD and D/R as the main distance cues), the present experiment took place in an acoustically damped low reverberant space (TR ≈ 300 ms), where it can be assumed that listeners used both ILD and few near-ear D/R changes with distance, but also HRTF changes correlated to elevation's variations. Thus, the low distance perception in this study might be principally due to the small range of distances rather than the lack of distance cues. Future experiments in anechoic field are necessary to evaluate the influence of elevation cues in this type of situation.

Some bias for the nearest positions to the side may be linked to biomechanical limitations. Effectively, it is difficult to correctly place the hand near the body for lateral positions (especially at azimuth from 60° to 120°) and this may influence results by shifting the pointed position toward the center. However, similar compression and shift effects can be found in the results obtained by Soechting and Flanders (1989) with a pointing bias toward the remembered position of a short visual stimulus. In their experiment, results highlighted a slight compression of perceived distances when the platform was 40 cm below the head, and a slight shift toward the center for lateral targets (at −45° and −45°). Instead of arguing for biomechanical limitations, they showed that errors in pointing to remembered targets were due to approximations in sensorimotor transformations between extrinsic (target location in space) and intrinsic (limb orientation) reference frames (see Soechting and Flanders, 1989). This question is further addressed in experiment 2 which considers stimuli of different modalities, in order to identify common pointing task errors separate from the perceptual nature of the stimuli.

In summary, results highlight similar accuracy for pointing task toward sound sources in the frontal space with dominant and non-dominant hand. Common results as a function of hand choice allow for the elimination of reporting hand consideration in future experiments, offering greater flexibility in task design and reporting protocol for the participants.

EXPERIMENT 2: REAL SOUND, VIRTUAL SOUND, AND VISUAL TARGETS

The aim of experiment 2 was two-fold. In order to address questions concerning observed localization and pointing errors in certain regions as their cause being attributed to either perceptual or biomechanical limitations a visual stimulus was included, as a contrast to the auditory stimulus of the previous experiment. Any observed bias errors in both the auditory and visual conditions could indicate a common origin, such as biomechanical limitations in reporting accuracy to certain positions.

In order to address the applied context of using virtual or augmented audio reality for creating sound objects in the peripersonal space, and to identify possible limitations of current implementations of binaural rendering technology, a virtual audio stimulus was also included.

Due to the additional number of stimulus conditions, the range of stimulus positions was reduced to ±60°.

MATERIAL AND METHODS

Subjects

A total of 20 adult subjects (3 women and 17 men, mean age = 26 years, *SD* = 4), different from the first study, served as paid volunteers. An audiogram was performed on each subject before the experiment to ensure that their audition was normal (defined as thresholds no greater than 15 dB hearing level in the range of 125–8000 Hz). All were naive regarding the purpose of the experiment and the sets of spatial positions selected for the experiment. This study was performed in accordance with the ethical standards of the Declaration of Helsinki (revised Edinburgh 2000) and written informed consent was obtained from all subjects prior to the experiment (after receiving instructions about the experiment).

Experimental procedure

As with the first experiment, the task consisted in reporting the perceived location of a static remembered target using a hand placement technique validated by a MIDI button. The experimental procedure was the identical to the first experiment (see Section 3.1.2) except that the reference position was 0.60 m above the table surface (0.05 m lower than the first experiment due to tracking instabilities). This experiment was divided into three blocks of 100 trials, each block lasting approximately 15 min and corresponding to a different condition (real sound, virtual sound, and visual target). For each condition, 25 locations were tested with 5 different azimuths (−60°, −30°, 0°, 30°, and 60°) and 5 different distances (33, 46, 59, 72, and 85 cm). All locations were repeated 4 times. Each condition was divided in 4 blocks (for the four repetitions) with a pseudo-random order for the locations. The stimuli used for the three conditions were:

- *Visual*: single 200 ms flash of a white disc (same total duration as the two sound conditions) having a 1 cm diameter, projected on the table covered by a black cloth using an overhead video projector;
- *Real sound*: three repeated 40 ms bursts rendered over loudspeaker's table as in experiment 1;
- *Virtual sound*: three repeated 40 ms bursts rendered over stereo open ear headphone (model Sennheiser HD570) spatialized using a non-individual HRTF set measured on a KEMAR mannequin (described in Section 4.1.3).

All stimuli were presented in the peripersonal space and were off before the beginning of the reporting movement.

The order of the two sound conditions was counterbalanced in order to suppress any potential learning effect. The visual condition was always at the end of the experiment so as to not influence the subject with the location of the sound sources.

KEMAR HRTF

The HRTF of a KEMAR mannequin was measured for the purpose of this experiment. The measurement was performed in an anechoic room (see LISTEN, 2004 for room details). The mannequin was equipped with a pair of omnidirectional in-ear microphones (DPA 4060) according to a blocked meatus protocol. The mannequin was fixed to a metal support that followed the axis of a motorized turntable (B&K 9640), which allowed variation of its orientation within the horizontal plane. The interaural axis of the KEMAR dummy head was centered (at 1.9 m from the loudspeaker) using a set of three coincident laser beams. The axis of the turntable coincided with a line extending through the center of the dummy head, therefore minimizing displacements during rotations of the turntable. The measurement set was obtained using the sweep-sine excitation technique at a sample rate of 44.1 kHz (RME Fireface 800 audio interface). The free-field HRTF was obtained through normalization (direct deconvolution through division in the complex frequency domain) by the free-field system response without the KEMAR present. The resulting HRIR was windowed (rectangular) to a length of 256 samples. The window was positioned to include 20 samples before the first peak as evaluated over all positions. In order to render all the sound source positions, it was necessary to measure the HRTF over the entire sphere. The set used contained measurement from −90° to 90° in elevation in steps of 5°, and from −180° to 180° in azimuth in steps of 5°.

The HRTF was decomposed into spectral component (representing spectral cues) and pure delay (representing ITD cues). A spatial interpolation of the spectral component was realized (see Aussal et al., 2013). The spatialization engine used a hybrid HRTF, where the modeled individual interaural time difference (ITD) based on head and shoulder circumference (see Aussal et al., 2012) was combined with the KEMAR spectral component. Binaural sound sources were rendered using a real-time spatialization engine based on full-phase HRIR convolution. ILD cues were modified to account for contralateral level difference for near distances using a spherical head model and a parallax effect correction was implemented for distances inferior to 1 m (HRIR were selected taking into account the angle of the source relative to the ear rather than the angle relative to the head center) (see Katz et al., 2011, 2012).

Thus, in the *virtual sound* condition, the available distance cues consisted of ILD variations as well as localization spectral cues associated with the corrected HRTF angles position. No near field correction was made for ITD variations with distance. Furthermore, an additional distance cue consisted in the spectral variations corresponding to the elevation changes linked to the distance due to the configuration of the table top setup. No additional propagation paths or reflections were simulated.

In order to improve reporting performance of the binaural rendering using non-individual HRTF, three preliminary adaptation sessions of 12 min were conducted according to the method proposed by Parseihian and Katz (2012b). Briefly, this method consists of a training game allowing the subject to perform a rapid exploration of the spatial map of the virtual rendering by an auditory-kinesthetic closed-loop. These training sessions were performed 3 days in a row, 12 min per day, the last session being immediately prior to the main experiment.

Data analysis

Analysis of results was performed following the same parameters as the first experiment: azimuth and distance relative to the subject. With subject's head located 0.60 m over the table, the sources were at distances of 0.685, 0.756, 0.842, 0.937, and 1.040 m from the subject's head center.

No front/back confusions (observed as pointing to the back) were observed. However, during the debriefing, some subjects reported having heard sources behind them or inside their head and pointed toward the table edge. As it is difficult to detect these pointing instances as front/back confusions, we looked for outliers in the dataset. First, a total of 48 trials with reported positions lying outside the table were preliminarily removed from the data (0.80% of all the trials; 0.00% of *real sound* condition trials, 1.55% of *virtual sound* condition trials, and 0.85% of *visual* condition trials.) Second, trials with signed azimuth error or signed distance error exceeding a fixed limit were removed. The upper limit was defined as $Q_3 + 1.5 \times (Q_3 - Q_1)$ and the lower limit as $Q_1 - 1.5 \times (Q_3 - Q_1)$ with Q_1 and Q_3 respectively the first and the third data quartile. Outside these limits the reported locations were tagged as outliers. A total of 244 trials were removed from the data (4.11% of all the trials; 6.45% of *real sound* condition trials, 2.14% of *virtual sound* condition trials, and 4.45% of *visual* condition trials.)

Statistical analyses were performed with repeated measurement analysis of variance (ANOVA) after verifying the datas distribution normality of unsigned azimuth error and signed distance error with Shapiro-Wilk tests on each hand, azimuth and distance conditions. A Tukey *post-hoc* was used to assess differences between conditions.

RESULTS

The mean reported positions linked to target locations for each rendering condition are presented in **Figure 3** with 50% confidence ellipse. These plots allow one to evaluate the error bias across the three conditions. For *visual* sources, lateral localization accuracy is quite good while the nearest distances are overestimated. For *real sound* sources, the reported distance is compressed and a lateral shift appears mostly at −60° and 60°. For *virtual sound* sources, all lateral sources are shifted toward the sides and there is no apparent distance perception. In the following sections these results are analyzed in terms of azimuth and distance bias and dispersion.

Azimuth error

Figure 4A presents the mean and standard deviation of reported azimuth as a function of stimuli azimuth. The mean and standard deviation of the unsigned azimuth error are presented in **Table 3**. First, the *visual* condition shows good estimation of azimuth, with a low variability (mean error of 2.79° ± 4.51°). For frontal locations, the mean unsigned error is 1.61° ± 1.27°. This error increases with azimuth to 2° for ±30° locations and to 4° for ±60° locations, as does the dispersion. It can be noticed that the lateral error corresponds to a slight underestimation of the azimuth. Second, results for *real sound* condition are similar to the first experiment's results. They highlight good accuracy at 0° with a mean error of 5.7°, and lower accuracy at the sides. Third, *virtual sound* condition showed lower performance results in terms of azimuth estimation. The mean absolute error at 0° is 10.79° ± 10.03°. The ±30° and ±60° locations are shifted by

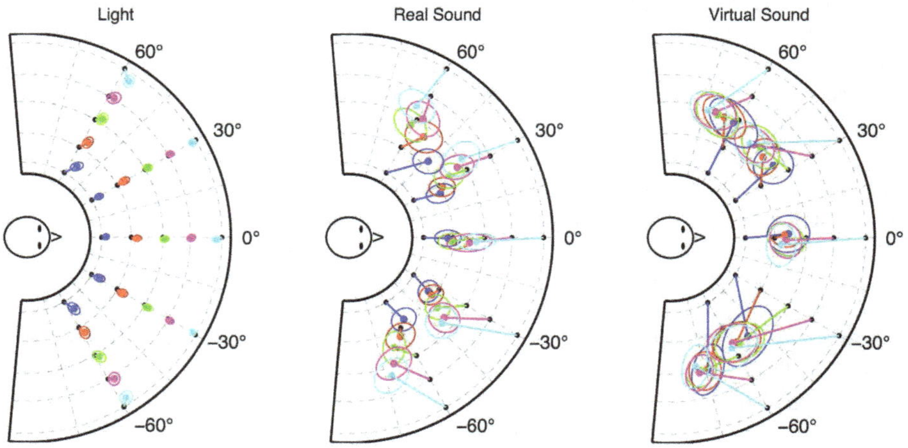

FIGURE 3 | Mean of all subjects' reported location with 50% confidence ellipse linked to source location for each rendering condition: *visual* (left), *real sound* (center), and *virtual sound* (right).

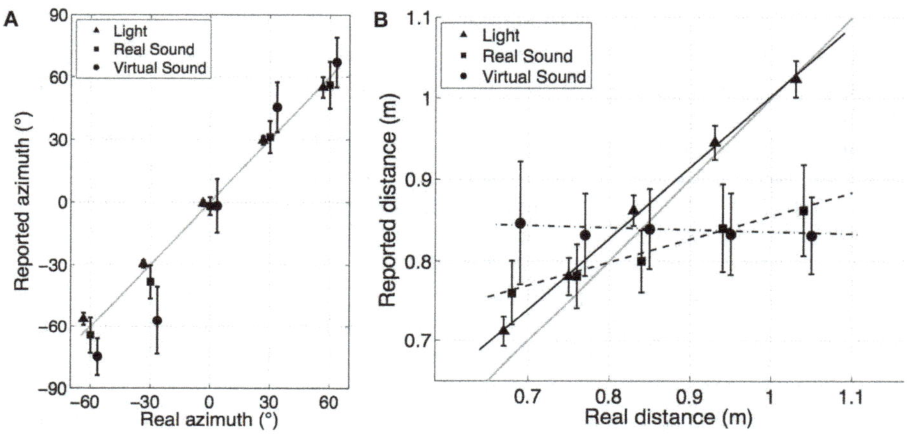

FIGURE 4 | (A) Mean of all subjects' reported azimuth as a function of stimuli azimuth for each rendering condition: *visual* (▲), *real sound* (■), and *virtual sound* (•). Error bars show one standard deviation across the subjects. Gray line shows unity. **(B)** Mean of all subjects' reported distance as a function of stimuli distance for each rendering condition: *visual* (▲), *real sound* (■), and *virtual sound* (•). Error bars show one standard deviation across the subjects for each condition. Solid gray lines show linear regression curves for each modality. Gray line shows unity.

Table 3 | Mean absolute azimuth error in degree (standard deviations in parenthesis) for each rendering condition as a function of stimuli azimuth.

Condition	−60°	−30°	0°	30°	60°	Total
Visual	3.85 (5.84)	1.94 (2.97)	1.61 (1.27)	1.99 (2.56)	4.51 (6.56)	2.79 (4.51)
Real sound	11.08 (8.15)	10.66 (8.22)	5.70 (4.61)	7.08 (5.81)	11.30 (8.27)	9.18 (7.54)
Virtual sound	16.75 (9.04)	28.17 (17.43)	10.79 (10.03)	16.83 (13.78)	14.44 (9.97)	17.48 (13.76)

approximately 15° to the side (except −30° locations which are reported at −60°).

A repeated measures 3-factor ANOVA (Condition∗Azimuth∗Distance) was performed on the mean absolute azimuth error of each subject, highlighting a significant effect of condition [$F_{(2, 38)} = 61.75$; $p < 10^{-5}$]. The *post-hoc* test revealed a significant difference between each condition. Azimuth errors are significantly lower for the *visual* condition compared to the sound conditions and are significantly greater for *virtual sound* condition compared to the two others. The interaction analysis showed a significant effect of Condition∗Azimuth [$F_{(8, 152)} = 15.62$; $p < 10^{-5}$] and of Condition∗Distance [$F_{(8, 152)} = 9.71$; $p < 10^{-5}$]. The *post-hoc* test on Condition∗Azimuth highlights no effect of the azimuth on the *visual* condition, but it shows a significant difference of performance between 0° and lateral positions (−60° and 60°) for *real sound* condition and significant differences between 0° and (−60°, −30°, 30°) and between −30° and other angles for the *virtual sound* condition. For these two conditions the azimuth errors are significantly greater for lateral positions as compared to frontal positions. The *post-hoc* test on Condition∗Distance highlights a significant difference on azimuth estimations between the nearest distance (d_1 and d_2) and the other distances (d_3, d_4, and d_5). In this condition, the azimuth is better estimated for nearer distances.

Distance error

Figure 4B shows the average mean response of reported distance as a function of stimuli distance for the three conditions. This figure highlights the large differences between the rendering conditions: the *visual* condition shows good and linear perception of distance, the *real sound* condition shows similar results as in the first experiment (e.g., compressed but linear perception of the distance in the range of the tested region), and finally there is no apparent distance perception in the *virtual sound* condition. A linear regression analysis was performed on these results. The mean of the linear regression line across the subjects for each rendering condition is shown in **Figure 4B**. The mean distance error across subjects, slope of the regression line, and goodness-of-fit criteria r^2 calculated over the four trials for each azimuth and rendering condition are shown in **Table 4**. The overall mean results represent the mean of results for each subject when considering the entire data set (mean of subject's regression slopes calculated with all the data from one condition, without considering target azimuth).

First, the *real sound* condition results are similar to the first experiment with a mean absolute distance error of 9.6 ± 7.5 cm, and a mean regression slope of 0.30 ± 0.18. The evolution of the distance error as a function of stimuli angle is also as in the first experiment: distance perception was better for lateral angles than in the frontal space. Second, in the *virtual sound* condition, distance perception seems non-existent. The mean distance error is 12.80 cm and the variability covers a large part of the table with a standard deviation of 9.16 cm. The regression slope is practically zero (−0.02 ± 0.27) and the goodness-of-fit of 0.11 ± 0.11 shows that *virtual sound* distance perception cannot be considered as linear for each subject. Analyzing the regression slope as a function of subject shows that 11 subjects (out of 20) obtained a positive regression slope and only two subjects obtained a regression slope superior to 0.1. Third, *visual* condition shows good perception of distance with an absolute error of 2.5 ± 2.5 cm, a regression slope of 0.89 ± 0.06 and a goodness-of-fit of 0.98. Distance error analysis as a function of the target angle highlights a better distance perception in the frontal zone (mean distance error at 0° was 1.88 ± 1.185 cm) than in lateral zones (mean distance error at ±60° was 3.01 ± 3.02 cm).

A repeated measures 3-factor ANOVA (Condition∗Azimuth∗Distance) performed on the mean signed distance error shows a significant effect of the rendering condition [$F_{(2, 38)} = 16.6$; $p < 10^{-5}$]. The *post-hoc* test revealed a significant difference between each condition with better performances obtained with *visual* condition and worst performances obtained with *virtual sound* condition. The analysis of Condition∗Azimuth interaction [$F_{(8, 152)} = 8.95$; $p = 0.005$] shows a significant effect of the azimuth on the distance error in *real sound* condition between 0° and −60° and 60° and in *virtual sound* condition between 0° and the others angles positions. The analysis of Condition∗Distance interaction [$F_{(8, 152)} = 178.72$; $p < 10^{-5}$] highlights significant differences in distance error between furthest distance location (d_4 and d_5) and middle distance locations (d_2, and d_3) for the *real sound* condition and between middle distance location (d_3) and extreme distance locations (d_1, d_4, and d_5) for the *virtual sound* condition. A 2-factor ANOVA (Condition∗Azimuth) performed on the regression slopes calculated for each subject shows a significant effect of the rendering condition [$F_{(2, 38)} = 286.43$; $p < 10^{-5}$] (with each condition significantly different from the others) and no observed effect of azimuth and no interaction effect of Condition∗Azimuth.

DISCUSSION

The results of experiment 2 show a large inter-subject variability, as was observed in experiment 1, which is condition dependent (the highest inter-subject variability was observed for *virtual sound* condition whereas the lowest was observed for the *visual* condition). The results also highlight large differences

Table 4 | Mean absolute distance error (standard deviations in parenthesis), slope of the regression line, and goodness-of-fit criteria r^2 for each azimuth and rendering conditions.

	Azimuth	−60°	−30°	0°	30°	60°	Total
Absolute distance error (cm)	Visual	2.91(2.99)	2.17 (2.14)	1.88 (1.85)	2.22 (2.12)	3.12 (3.06)	2.47 (2.53)
	Real sound	8.68 (6.63)	9.88 (8.15)	10.82 (8.38)	9.50 (7.76)	9.05 (6.27)	9.58 (7.50)
	Virtual sound	12.86 (9.53)	12.89 (9.39)	13.20 (9.46)	12.33 (8.82)	12.75 (8.64)	12.80 (9.16)
Regression slope	Visual	0.88 (0.09)	0.91 (0.06)	0.93 (0.06)	0.91 (0.05)	0.85 (0.08)	0.89 (0.06)
	Real sound	0.34 (0.18)	0.28 (0.16)	0.25 (0.21)	0.31 (0.19)	0.30 (0.16)	0.30 (0.18)
	Virtual sound	−0.05 (0.19)	−0.02 (0.22)	−0.03 (0.16)	0.00 (0.10)	−0.02 (0.24)	−0.02 (0.18)
Goodness-of-fit r^2	Visual	0.98	0.99	0.99	0.99	0.97	0.98
	Real sound	0.52	0.46	0.31	0.46	0.44	0.44
	Virtual sound	0.10	0.10	0.09	0.05	0.18	0.11

in localization/pointing accuracy toward *light*, *real sound*, and *virtual sound* targets both in azimuth and distance.

Results for *real sound* condition show the same performances in azimuth and distance as for experiment 1 in the studied area. Distance perception is almost linear in the range of the tested region but largely compressed to the middle of the platform (regression slope of 0.3). Azimuth perception is better in the frontal zone ($|azimuth| \leq 30°$) than toward the sides ($|azimuth| = 60°$). As seen in experiment 1, some localization biases are observed on the sides. For example, at 60° the azimuth of nearest source positions are underestimated whereas at −60° the azimuth of the farthest source positions is overestimated.

Results of the *virtual sound* condition are significantly poorer than those of the *real sound* condition. Directional pointing is shifted to the side for positions outside the median plane and there is no apparent distance perception (regression slope of 0). This could be attributed to the use non-individual HRTFs, despite the training period. Azimuth distortion errors could be attributed to the ITD individualization model employed and associated errors in the tested region, which exceeds the initial bounds of the developed method. This shift in azimuth perception is common with virtual auditory display and is smaller than the shift observed for example by Boyer et al. (2013) citing an overall azimuth error of 25°, as compared to 17.5° in the present study. However, these results show an opposite trend to the results of Ihlefeld and Shinn-Cunningham (2011), who observed a bias toward the median plane for perceived lateral angle sources more than 45° from the median plane. This difference might be explained by the presence of a reverberant field in the non-individualized BRIR used in their study (since this shift toward the center seems to be linked to the D/R ratio). In addition, the binaural rendering algorithm attempts to compensate for the difference in the distances between the measured HRTF (1.9 m) and the virtual source position. This correction may not be able to correctly reproduce all cues for the evaluated range. Finally, the virtual environment was entirely anechoic, in contrast to the *real sound* condition where, despite acoustic treatment, some acoustic reflections would still exist and could be interpreted by the auditory system.

GENERAL DISCUSSION

This study presents the results of two experiments concerning localization and pointing accuracy in the peripersonal space. In contrast to numerous previous studies which have investigated auditory localization in the far-field by examining azimuth and elevation accuracy, the current studies considers near-field auditory localization associated with typical object positions, specifically for positions located in the region of a tabletop surface.

Evaluation of localization and pointing accuracy to real acoustic sources and consideration of dominant or secondary hand for the reporting task were carried out. Results showed no difference reported azimuth or distance as a function of reporting hand. Mean azimuth errors were 6.7° for frontal source positions, increasing to 17.8° for lateral positions, which were consistently underestimated (reported positions of lateral sources were shifted toward the front of the platform). These results are in contrast to a previous study by Brungart et al. (1999) which considered a similar task. However, several major differences exist between these two studies, including the reporting method (finger vs. stick pointing), source elevations, which spanned from −65° to −37° in the current study compared to −40° to 60° in Brungart et al. (1999), and acoustic conditions (the present study was conducted in a low reverberant space and not an anechoic chamber which may had influence localization in azimuth (Ihlefeld and Shinn-Cunningham, 2011).

Reported distances showed a consistent compression of reported distance toward the center of the experimental platform. Similar trends of response compression have been frequently observed in perceptual scaling paradigms that depend on the range of the presented stimuli (Parducci, 1963) as well as the setup used to collect subjects responses. For example, Zahorik (2002) observed a general overestimation of the nearest distances and an underestimation of farther distances, with distances spanning from 0.3 to 13.79 m.

Comparison of localization and pointing accuracy to real acoustic sources and visual sources of comparable duration using the same reporting technique and experimental platform showed only minor errors in the visual condition. The lack of a common bias in results between stimulus modalities indicates that the observed errors in performance are due to other factors than biomechanical difficulties in the reporting task. Mean reported azimuth errors were comparable between these two conditions. Some distance compression was observed for visual stimuli with compression being directed toward the farthest distance, while a greater degree of compression was observed for auditory stimuli where compression was directed toward the center of the middle of the platform.

A final comparison between real acoustic sources and binaurally rendered acoustic virtual sources highlighted several limitations of the binaural rendering. Reported source azimuths exhibited increased errors with azimuths being consistently overestimated toward more lateral positions. In addition, no differences were observed in reported distances relative to the rendered distance, meaning that there was no perceived distance variation between virtual sources. Numerous factors can be considered in trying to determine the cause of such lack of perception, such as the purely anechoic synthesis conditions vs. the present, while minimal, room effect of the experimental room and the use of non-individual HRTF's (despite efforts to individualize the measured dataset and the inclusion of a learning phase). In the context of an auditory guidance system in the peripersonal space, considering the observed limitations, additional cues would be necessary to aid the user in estimating the distance to the auditory target object. First, the use of a continuous sound allowing the user to move their head during localization, thus taking advantages of dynamic changes of the acoustic cues, is well known to improve directional localization (see Middlebrooks and Green, 1991). Second, Boyer et al. (2013) have highlighted the role of the auditory-motor loop in pointing to an auditory source by displaying the source position in a hand centered coordinate system. With such a shift of coordinates, the localization cue differences are largely increased when the user moves his or her hand toward the target, thus increasing movement accuracy. Finally, localization performances can be enhanced by simulating a reverberant environment (see Shinn-Cunningham et al., 2005; Kopčo and Shinn-Cunningham, 2011), by increasing the cue variations in a specific range (see Shinn-Cunningham et al., 1998), by adding continuous modification of the stimuli using a variety of sonification metaphors (see Parseihian et al., 2012), or with static and coded cues according to distance intervals using a hierarchical auditory icon system (see Parseihian and Katz, 2012a).

FUNDING

This work was supported in part by the French National Research Agency (ANR) through the TecSan program (project NAVIG ANR-08TECS-011) and the Midi-Pyrénées region through the APRRTT program. Additional funding was provided by an internal research grant by the LIMSI-CNRS and the French Inter-ministerial R&D fund (project FUI-AAP14 BiLi, www.bili-project.org) concerning binaural listening with support from "Cap Digital—Paris Region."

REFERENCES

Afonso, A., Blum, A., Katz, B., Tarroux, P., Borst, G., and Denis, M. (2010). Structural properties of spatial representations in blind people : scanning images constructed from haptic exploration or from locomotion in a 3-D audio virtual environment. *Mem. Cogn.* 38, 591–604. doi: 10.3758/MC.38.5.591

Ashmead, D. A., Leroy, D., and Odom, R. D. (1990). Perception of relative distances of nearby sound sources. *Percept. Psychophys.* 47, 326–331. doi: 10.3758/BF03210871

Aussal, M., Alouges, F., and Katz, B. (2012). "Itd interpolation and personalization for binaural synthesis using spherical harmonics," in *Audio Engineering Society UK Conference* (York).

Aussal, M., Alouges, F., and Katz, B. (2013). "A study of spherical harmonics interpolation for hrtf exchange," in *Proceedings of Meetings on Acoustics* (Montreal, QC).

Begault, D. (1994). *3-D Sound for Virtual Reality and Multimedia.* Cambridge: Academic Press.

Blauert, J. (1997). *Spatial Hearing, The Psychophysics of Human Sound Localization.* Cambridge: MIT Press.

Boyer, E. O., Babayan, B. M., Bevilacqua, F., Noisternig, M., Warusfel, O., Roby-Brami, A., et al. (2013). From ear to hand: the role of the auditory-motor loop in pointing to an auditory source. *Front. Comput. Neurosci.* 7:26. doi: 10.3389/fncom.2013.00026

Brungart, D., Durlach, N., and Rabinowitz, W. (1999). Auditory localization of nearby sources. II. localization of a broadband source. *J. Acoust. Soc. Am.* 106, 1956–1968. doi: 10.1121/1.427943

Brungart, D., and Rabinowitz, W. (1999). Auditory localization of nearby sources. Head-related transfer functions. *J. Acoust. Soc. Am.* 106, 1465–1479. doi: 10.1121/1.427180

Brungart, D., Rabinowitz, W., and Durlach, N. (2000). Evaluation of response methods for the localization of nearby objects. *Attent. Percept. Psychophys.* 62, 48–65. doi: 10.3758/BF03212060

Brungart, D. S. (1999). "Auditory parallax effects in the hrtf for nearby sources," in *Proceedings of 1999 IEEE Workshop on Applications of Signal Processing to Audio and Acoustics* (New York, NY).

Férey, N., Nelson, J., Martin, C., Picinali, L., Bouyer, G., Tek, A., et al. (2009). Multisensory VR interaction for protein-docking in the CoRSAIRe project. *Vir. Real.* 13, 273–293. doi: 10.1007/s10055-009-0136-z

Hershkowitz, R., and Durlach, N. (1969). Interaural time and amplitude jnds for a 500-hz tone. *J. Acoust. Soc. Am.* 46, 1464–1467. doi: 10.1121/1.1911887

Honda, A., Shibata, H., Gyoba, J., Saitou, K., Iwaya, Y., and Suzuki, Y. (2007). Transfer effects on sound localization performances from playing a virtual three-dimensional auditory game. *Appl. Acoust.* 68, 885–896. doi: 10.1016/j.apacoust.2006.08.007

Ihlefeld, A., and Shinn-Cunningham, B. (2011). Effect of source spectrum on sound localization in an everyday reverberant room. *J. Acoust. Soc. Am.* 130, 324–333. doi: 10.1121/1.3596476

Katz, B., Dramas, F., Parseihian, G., Gutierrez, O., Kammoun, S., Brilhault, A., et al. (2012). NAVIG: guidance system for the visually impaired using virtual augmented reality. *J. Technol. Disabil.* 24, 163–178. doi: 10.3233/TAD-2012-0344

Katz, B., Rio, E., and Piccinali, L. (2011). *LIMSI Spatialization Engine.* Inter Deposit Digital Number: F.001.340014.000.S.P.2010.000.31235.

Kopčo, N., and Shinn-Cunningham, B. (2011). Effect of stimulus spectrum on distance perception for nearby sources. *J. Acoust. Soc. Am.* 130, 1530–1541. doi: 10.1121/1.3613705

LISTEN (2004). *HRTF Database.* Available online at: http://recherche.ircam.fr/equipes/salles/listen/

Macé, M. J. M., Dramas, F., and Jouffrais, C. (2012). "Reaching to sound accuracy in the peri-personal space of blind and sighted humans," in *Computers Helping People with Special Needs: 13th International Conference, ICCHP 2012*, eds K. Miesenberger, A. Karshmer, P. Penaz, and W. Zagler (Linz: Springer-Verlag), 636–643.

Martin, R. L., McAnally, K. I., and Senova, M. A. (2001). Free-field equivalent localization of virtual audio. *J. Audio Eng. Soc.* 49, 14–22.

Middlebrooks, J. C., and Green, D. M. (1991). Sound localization by human listeners. *Ann. Rev. Psychol.* 42, 135–159. doi: 10.1146/annurev.ps.42.020191.001031

Murdoch, D. J., and Chow, E. D. (1996). A graphical display of large correlation matrices. *Am. Stat.* 50, 178–180.

Parducci, A. (1963). Range-frequency compromise in judgment. *Psychol. Monogr. Gen. Appl.* 77, 1–50. doi: 10.1037/h0093829

Parseihian, G., Conan, S., and Katz, B. (2012). "Sound effect metaphors for near field distance sonification," in *Proceedings of the 18th International Conference on Auditory Display (ICAD 2012)* (Atlanta).

Parseihian, G., and Katz, B. (2012a). Morphocons: a new sonification concept based on morphological earcons. *J. Audio Eng. Soc.* 60, 409–418.

Parseihian, G., and Katz, B. (2012b). Rapid head-related transfer function adaptation using a virtual auditory environment. *J. Acoust. Soc. Am.* 131, 2948–2957. doi: 10.1121/1.3687448

Picinali, L., Afonso, A., Denis, M., and Katz, B. F. (2014). Exploration of architectural spaces by the blind using virtual auditory reality for the construction of spatial knowledge. *Int. J. Hum. Comput. Stud.* 72, 393–407. doi: 10.1016/j.ijhcs.2013.12.008

Shinn-Cunningham, B. G., Durlach, N. I., and Held, R. M. (1998). Adapting to supernormal auditory localization cues. I. Bias and resolution. *J. Acoust. Soc. Am.* 103, 3656–3666. doi: 10.1121/1.423088

Shinn-Cunningham, B. G., Kopčo, N., and Martin, T. J. (2005). Localizing nearby sound sources in a classroom: Binaural room impulse responses. *J. Acoust. Soc. Am.* 117, 3100–3115. doi: 10.1121/1.1872572

Shinn-Cunningham, B. G., Santarelli, S., and Kopčo, N. (2000). Tori of confusion: binaural localization cues for sources within reach of a listener. *J. Acoust. Soc. Am.* 107, 1627–1636. doi: 10.1121/1.428447

Simpson, W., and Stanton, L. (1973). Head movement does not facilitate perception of the distance of a source of sound. *Am. J. Psychol.* 86, 151–159. doi: 10.2307/1421856

Soechting, J., and Flanders, M. (1989). Sensorimotor representations for pointing to targets in three-dimensional space. *J. Neurophysiol.* 62, 582–594.

Strybel, T., and Perrott, D. (1984). Discrimination of relative distance in the auditory modality: the success and failure of the loudness discrimination hypothesis. *J. Acoust. Soc. Am.* 76, 318. doi: 10.1121/1.391064

Viaud-Delmon, I., Znaïdi, F., Bonneel, N., Suied, C., Warusfel, O., N'Guyen, K.-V., et al. (2008). "Auditory-visual virtual environments to treat dog phobia," in *Proceedings 7th ICDVRAT with ArtAbilitation* (Maia).

Walker, B., and Lindsay, J. (2006). Navigation performance with a virtual auditory display: effects of beacon sound, capture radius, and practice. *Hum. Factors* 48, 265–278. doi: 10.1518/001872006777724507

Wightman, F. L., and Kistler, D. J. (1989). Headphone simulation of free-field listening. II: psychophysical validation. *J. Acoust. Soc. Am.* 85, 868–878. doi: 10.1121/1.397558

Wilson, J., Walker, B., Lindsay, J., Cambias, C., and Dellaert, F. (2007). "Swan: system for wearable audio navigation," in *Proceedings of the 2007 11th IEEE International Symposium on Wearable Computers* (Washington, DC: IEEE Computer Society), 1–8. doi: 10.1109/ISWC.2007.4373786

Xie, B. (2013). *Head-Related Transfer Function and Virtual Auditory Display, 2nd Edn.* Plantation, FL: J. Ross Publishing Incorporated.

Zahorik, P. (2002). Assessing auditory distance perception using virtual acoustics. *J. Acoust. Soc. Am.* 111, 1832–1846. doi: 10.1121/1.1458027

6

The influence of vision on sound localization abilities in both the horizontal and vertical planes

Vanessa Tabry[1,2], Robert J. Zatorre[1,2] and Patrice Voss[1,2]*

[1] Department of Neurology and Neurosurgery, Montreal Neurological Institute, McGill University, Montreal, QC, Canada
[2] International Laboratory for Brain, Music and Sound Research (BRAMS), Montreal, QC, Canada

***Correspondence:**
Patrice Voss, Department of Neurology and Neurosurgery, Montreal Neurological Institute, McGill University, 3801 rue University, Montréal, QC H3A 2B4, Canada
e-mail: patrice.voss@mcgill.ca

Numerous recent reports have suggested that individuals deprived of vision are able to develop heightened auditory spatial abilities. However, most such studies have compared the blind to blindfolded sighted individuals, a procedure that might introduce a strong performance bias. Indeed, while blind individuals have had their whole lives to adapt to this condition, sighted individuals might be put at a severe disadvantage when having to localize sounds without visual input. To address this unknown, we compared the sound localization ability of eight sighted individuals with and without a blindfold in a hemi-anechoic chamber. Sound stimuli were broadband noise delivered via two speaker arrays: a horizontal array with 25 loudspeakers (ranging from −90° to +90°; 7.5°) and a vertical array with 16 loudspeakers (ranging from −45° to +67.5°). A factorial design was used, where we compared two vision conditions (blindfold vs. non-blindfold), two sound planes (horizontal vs. vertical) and two pointing methods (hand vs. head). Results show that all three factors significantly interact with one another with regards to the average absolute deviation error. Although blindfolding significantly affected all conditions, it did more so for head-pointing in the horizontal plane. Moreover, blindfolding was found to increase the tendency to undershoot more eccentric spatial positions for head-pointing, but not hand-pointing. Overall, these findings suggest that while proprioceptive cues appear to be sufficient for accurate hand pointing in the absence of visual feedback, head pointing relies more heavily on visual cues in order to provide a precise response. It also strongly argues against the use of head pointing methodologies with blindfolded sighted individuals, particularly in the horizontal plane, as it likely introduces a bias when comparing them to blind individuals.

Keywords: sound localization, vision, pointing methods, spatial hearing, blindness

INTRODUCTION

It has been proposed that the blind compensate for their lack of vision by sharpening their auditory abilities (Niemeyer and Starlinger, 1981; Muchnick et al., 1991; Gougoux et al., 2004). In particular, auditory spatial processing has been a topic of particular interest due to its high relevance for spatial navigation. There have been multiple reports of enhanced sound localization abilities in early blind humans (Ashmead et al., 1998; Lessard et al., 1998; Doucet et al., 2005; Gougoux et al., 2005) as well as enhanced auditory spatial discrimination abilities (Röder et al., 1999; Voss et al., 2004) in the horizontal (azimuthal) plane. Other findings, however, point to degraded auditory spatial abilities when having to localize sounds in the vertical plane (Zwiers et al., 2001; Lewald, 2002). Aside from the obvious difference in auditory spatial planes studied, another important potential source for this discrepancy relates to the use of different pointing methods. While the studies reporting enhancements typically used hand pointing procedures to measure subjects, the latter used either head pointing (Zwiers et al., 2001) or a swivel pointer that was fixed in front of the subjects (Lewald, 2002). Overall, these findings raise interesting questions on how the visual status of an individual interacts with other factors such as the auditory spatial plane and the pointing method used when having to localize sounds in the environment.

The selection of an appropriate pointing method in sound localization studies comparing the sighted to the blind should therefore be given careful attention, because the two subpopulations may differ in their proficiency in using the same pointing method (e.g., hand pointing or head pointing). This is an issue of particular importance because in most studies comparing the sighted and the blind, the sighted are transiently visually deprived, which may hamper their ability to use a pointing method to localize a target. On the other hand, the early blind may be more proficient with the pointing method, having developed non-visual compensatory mechanisms to orient body parts toward specific directions. As such, potential differences in pointing ability may partially account for previously shown differences in sound localization performance between the two groups. Further, vision is more heavily weighted comparatively to proprioception in judgments requiring multisensory integration, and so exerts a strong bias on proprioception (Hay et al., 1965; Pick and Warren,

1969; Rossetti et al., 1995). Indeed, while sighted children show a decrease in the relative importance of proprioception in multisensory integration with age, blind children do not, likely because in their case, vision does not become the dominant localizing modality, as it does in the sighted (Pick and Warren, 1969). Additionally, the directive control of vision over proprioception has been shown to increase with long-term visual experience (Birch and Lefford, 1963). Consequently, both populations may differentially rely on proprioceptive cues when having to explicitly localize sound sources; not to mention that the reliance on such cues could differ depending on the pointing method (head vs. hand).

To better ascertain the relative sound localization abilities of the sighted and blind, it is vital to identify pointing methods whose accuracy are as little affected as possible by transient or developmental visual deprivation, in order to isolate and reduce potential biases in the responses that are unrelated to spatial sound perception. In the current study, we addressed the issue of whether transient visual deprivation of sighted individuals (i.e., removal of visual feedback cues) would differentially affect different pointing methods. We also assessed whether the lack of visual feedback would have a differential effect on localization in orthogonal sound planes (vertical vs. horizontal). To address these questions we used a 2 × 2 × 2 factorial design, where we compared two visual conditions (blindfold vs. non-blindfold), two pointing methods (hand pointing vs. head pointing) and two auditory spatial planes (horizontal vs. vertical). We predicted main effects of visual condition where performance would be best without the blindfold, and of auditory spatial plane given the higher auditory spatial resolution of the human auditory system in the horizontal plane (see Makous and Middlebrooks, 1990). While we did not necessarily expect a main effect of pointing method (see Haber et al., 1993), we were particularly interested in determining if possible interaction effects could exist between the visual condition and pointing method given the different proprioceptive cues that underlie head and hand pointing. Similarly, we predicted an interaction between visual condition and auditory spatial plane, where blindfolding would have a greater effect on performance in the vertical plane given the poorer performance of blind individuals in the vertical plane (Zwiers et al., 2001; Lewald, 2002).

MATERIALS AND METHODS

PARTICIPANTS

The participants were eight right-handed sighted volunteers (four male, mean age: 22 ± 2.98 years), with no history of neurological disease. They gave their written informed consent in accordance with guidelines approved by the Montreal Neurological Institute (MNI) and the *Centre de Recherche Interdisciplinaire en Réadaptation* (CRIR), and received monetary compensation for participating. Each participant was tested in two separate 1-h long sessions that were approximately 1 week apart. The participants have self-reported normal or corrected-to-normal vision. Standard audiometric assessments were performed for all participants and indicated normal and comparable hearing in both ears.

CONDITIONS

Three variables were manipulated for each subject when having to localize sounds: visual condition (blindfold vs. no blindfold), pointing method (head pointing vs. hand pointing), and auditory spatial plane (horizontal vs. vertical). As a result of this 2 × 2 × 2 factorial design, each subject performed the task under eight conditions, which were counterbalanced across all subjects. Trial runs were completed over two separate testing sessions that were held approximately 1 week apart.

MATERIALS AND STIMULI

Sound localization tests were controlled by a custom-designed Matlab script (r.2009a; MathWorks) and stimuli were generated using TDT System 3 (Tucker-Davis-Technology). The stimuli consisted of 100 ms pink noise bursts (10 ms rise/fall times) presented at 60 dB SPL as measured at the center of the array.

The experiment was carried out in a hemi-anechoic chamber (2.5 × 5.5 × 2.5 m). The acoustic apparatus used to test sound localization consisted of 25 loudspeakers on the horizontal plane and 16 on the vertical plane, mounted on two semicircular railings with a radius of 90 cm (see **Figure 1**). Each location was sampled four times in each of the eight experimental conditions. The positions of the loudspeakers ranged from −90 to +90° on the horizontal plane, and from −37.5 to +67.5° on the vertical plane; thus providing a spatial resolution of 7.5° on both planes. Subjects were seated such that the speakers in the horizontal plane were positioned at ear level and those in the vertical plane were aligned with the subjects' mid-sagittal plane. The loudspeaker located at the crossing of both railings was therefore located at 0° azimuth, 0° elevation. The loudspeakers were hidden by a thin black cotton sleeve in such a way that the distance to the speakers could be seen, but not their spacing, size, or exact location. In addition, two fabric rulers were put in place along the semicircular railings; this was done so that an experimenter present could note laser-pointed locations (see procedure).

PROCEDURE

Subjects were seated in a fixed chair in front of the two semicircular railings and were required to indicate the location of short noise bursts delivered through a randomly selected loudspeaker. Subjects were also instructed to maintain a head position pointing straight ahead until the end of the stimulus presentation, and were required to return to that position prior to starting the next trial (failure to do so would result in the inability to start the next trial; see also "*Recording method*" below for more details). Prior to beginning the experimental conditions, subjects performed practice trials until they felt at ease with the recording apparatus (typically 10–15 trials). They were also given short breaks when needed between trial blocks. Subjects were allowed to turn their shoulders if necessary when indicating peripheral sources. No headrest was mounted on the chair, in order to reduce the probability of obstructing head movements to extreme spatial locations. Trials were run in blocks of either horizontal or vertical trials. In each block the error was only computed in one dimension (either horizontal or vertical) in accordance with the auditory plane being tested, and the subjects always knew in advance which plane was being tested prior to starting each block.

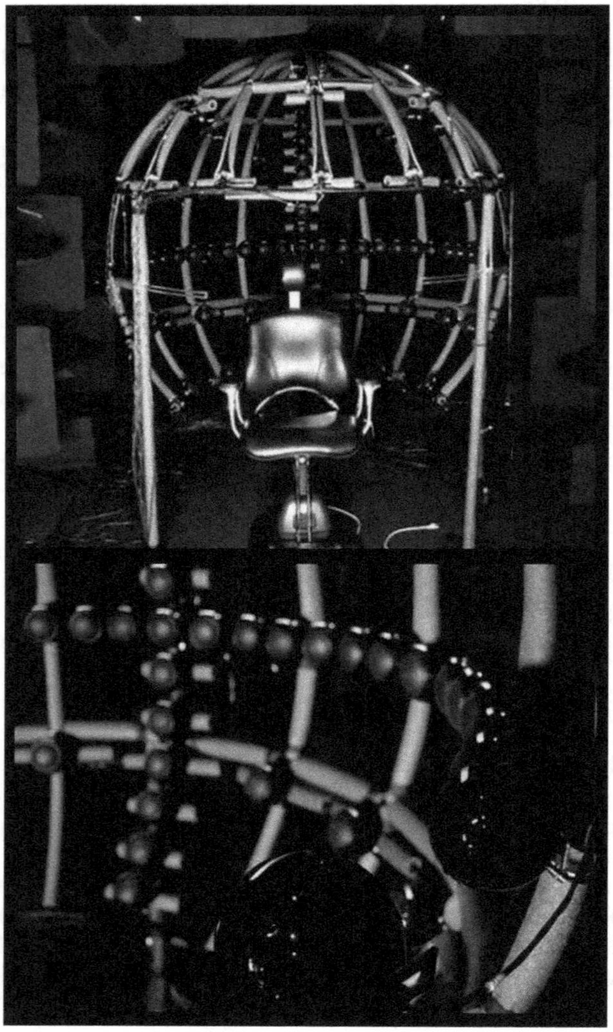

FIGURE 1 | Sound localization setup. Illustrated here is the hemi-anechoic chamber and the acoustic apparatus used to test sound localization. The bottom panel provides a close-up of the arrays of loudspeakers along the horizontal and vertical midlines. The additional speakers were not used in the current experiment.

RECORDING METHOD

Head-tracking apparatus

Subjects wore an elastic cap with a magnetic receiver of a 3D digitizer system (ISOTRAK II, Polhemus) that recorded the head position, and that was mounted with a laser pointer directing its beam straight ahead. Prior to each trial subjects were instructed to face the crossing point of both axes (0° azimuth, 0° elevation) and to record their head position with a button-press on a remote once they were satisfied with the position of the head. Following a trial, subjects were required to return to their initial position (centered on 0° azimuth, 0° elevation) and press the button on the remote. When the head was properly positioned, a brief high-frequency tone was played via the speaker directly above the head to indicate a correct head position, and was followed by the sound burst to be localized. In the event of an improper head positioning, a lower-frequency tone would be played and the subject was required to reposition their head appropriately.

Head pointing

As mentioned above, a laser pointer was mounted onto the subjects' heads along with the magnetic receiver of the digitizer system. When localizing a sound burst, subjects were instructed to orient their heads so that their noses pointed toward the perceived location of the sound source, and to hold still for a moment until an experimenter in the room could note the pointed location.

Hand pointing

Following the sound bursts, subjects were asked to point to its location with a hand held laser-pointer (in their dominant hand; all right-handed). The location was again marked down by an experimenter present in the room.

ANALYSIS

Three different dependant variables were entered into separate 2 (visual condition: blindfold vs. no blindfold) × 2 (pointing method: head pointing vs. hand pointing) × 2 (auditory spatial plane: horizontal vs. vertical) repeated measures ANOVAs: average overall unsigned error, average signed error and slope of the regression curve of the signed error as a function of the target location in space. The *unsigned error* consisted of the average absolute deviation (in degrees) of the response from the target location, irrespective of whether responses were undershooting or overshooting the target, and was taken to be a measure of overall accuracy. The *signed error* consisted in the average signed deviation from target, and was taken to indicate potential directional response biases (e.g., tendency to present a leftward or rightward shift in the horizontal plane). Lastly, the *slope* of the regression curve served as indicator of how the signed error varied as a function of target eccentricity.

RESULTS

Single trials with absolute errors that were larger than 3 standard deviations above the mean deviation per target location were considered outliers and removed from our analysis. As such, 0.75% of the total number of trials ($n = 10496$) were excluded. An additional 0.27% of the trials were discarded due to the subjects not holding the laser in position long enough for the experimenter to take note of the position.

ABSOLUTE ERROR

The main effect of visual condition was found to be significant, as subjects localized sounds more accurately without the blindfold [$F_{(1, 7)} = 25.84$, $p < 0.001$]. The main effect of auditory spatial plane was also significant, as horizontal sources were located more accurately then vertical ones [$F_{(1, 7)} = 32.15$, $p < 0.001$]. The main effect of pointing method was however non-significant [$F_{(1, 7)} = 0.60$, $p = 0.465$]. The *auditory plane* × *pointing method* interaction was also found to be significant [$F_{(1, 7)} = 17.69$, $p = 0.004$]. We then broke down the interaction into components by looking at the simple effects of each condition. This revealed that performance on the horizontal plane was better for hand-pointing than for head-pointing ($p = 0.026$), whereas head-pointing was better than hand-pointing on the vertical plane ($p = 0.035$).

Both the *auditory plane* × *visual condition* [$F_{(1, 7)} = 0.26$, $p = 0.625$] and the *pointing method* × *visual condition* [$F_{(1, 7)} = 1.80$, $p = 0.222$] interactions were found to be non-significant. However, a significant triple interaction was found between the effects of the pointing method, the visual condition and the auditory spatial plane on sound localization performance ($F_{(1, 7)} = 6.45$; $p = 0.039$). When examining the simple effects (illustrated in **Figure 2**), it was found that this interaction is primarily driven by the fact that the pointing methods do not differ from one another in most conditions (all $p > 0.3$), with the exception of the *blindfold-horizontal* conditions where head pointing was significantly less accurate than hand pointing ($p = 0.029$). The effect of blindfolding was however significant for all conditions [*hand-horizontal* ($p = 0.019$), *head-horizontal* ($p = 0.009$), *hand-vertical* ($p = 0.047$), *head-vertical* ($p = 0.025$)]. The effect was nonetheless greater for head pointing in the horizontal plane, where the average absolute error increased by 6.9°; all other blindfold-related increases were of 4.0° or less (see **Figure 2**).

SIGNED ERROR

Figure 3 shows the mean signed error in all conditions. A repeated measures 2 × 2 × 2 was performed on the signed error in the same manner as it was for the unsigned error. No main effects or interactions were found to be significant (all $p > 0.146$).

REGRESSION SLOPE

As can be seen in **Figure 3**, signed error tended to increase as a function of target eccentricity and subjects tended to undershoot target locations. To address potential differences across the conditions, first-order regression curves were fitted to the signed error plots as a function of target location (see also **Figure 3**). These slopes can be taken as an index of the tendency to undershoot or overshoot target locations. We performed a similar 2 × 2 × 2 ANOVA to those above, but this time using the regression slope as the dependant measure. There was a significant main effect of visual condition, where the slope was steeper for blindfolded trials [$F_{(1, 7)} = 6.87$, $p = 0.034$], and of auditory spatial plane [$F_{(1, 7)} = 40.25$, $p < 0.001$], where the slope was steeper for the vertical plane. There was also a main effect of pointing [$F_{(1, 7)} = 6.27$, $p = 0.041$], where the slope for head pointing was found to be steeper than for hand pointing. However, a *visual condition* × *pointing method* interaction was also found to be significant [$F_{(1, 7)} = 18.59$, $p = 0.004$]. This effect was due to the fact that while blindfolding had no significant effect on the slope when hand-pointing ($p = 0.341$), it had a significant effect on it when head-pointing ($p = 0.005$). Accordingly, the slope associated with each pointing method did not differ with visual feedback ($p = 0.215$), whereas it was steeper for head pointing when blindfolded ($p = 0.006$). Overall, these results indicate that blindfolding increases the tendency to undershoot target locations for head-pointing only, and not hand-pointing. All other interaction effects failed to reach significance (all $p > 0.314$).

DISCUSSION

The purpose of the present study was primarily to investigate the effects of blindfolding and choice of pointing method on the sound localization performance of sighted individuals. In addition to the oft-studied horizontal plane, we included sound localization tasks presented along the vertical median plane, which generally requires individuals to use a different set of localization cues (Batteau, 1967; Gardner and Gardner, 1973). The addition of the vertical plane was done to ascertain whether blindfolding or the choice of pointing method would have a differential effect on the two auditory planes. Results showed that all three factors significantly interact with one another with regards to the average absolute localization error. Although blindfolding significantly affected all conditions, it did more so

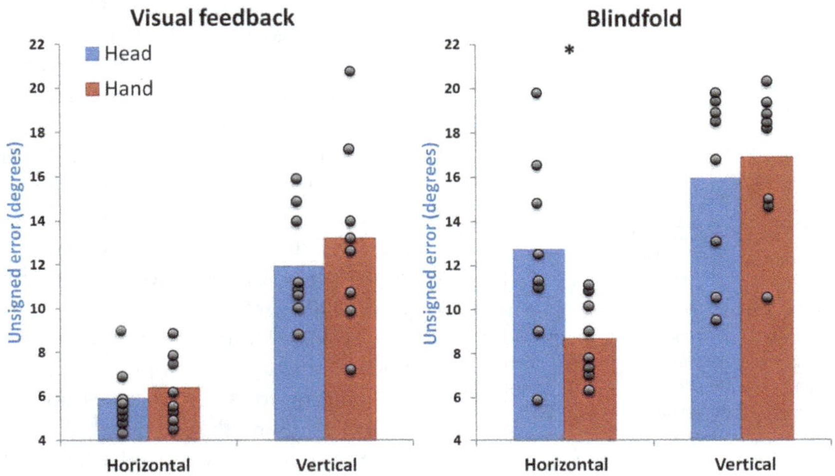

FIGURE 2 | Triple interaction. Shown here is the significant interaction effect on the unsigned error between all three independent variables. Error bars represent the standard error of the mean. The gray dots represent the average localization error for each subject under each condition and illustrate the strong variability between subjects, particularly for the blindfolded conditions. The asterisk (*) indicates a significant difference between pointing methods for a given auditory plane and visual condition ($p < 0.05$).

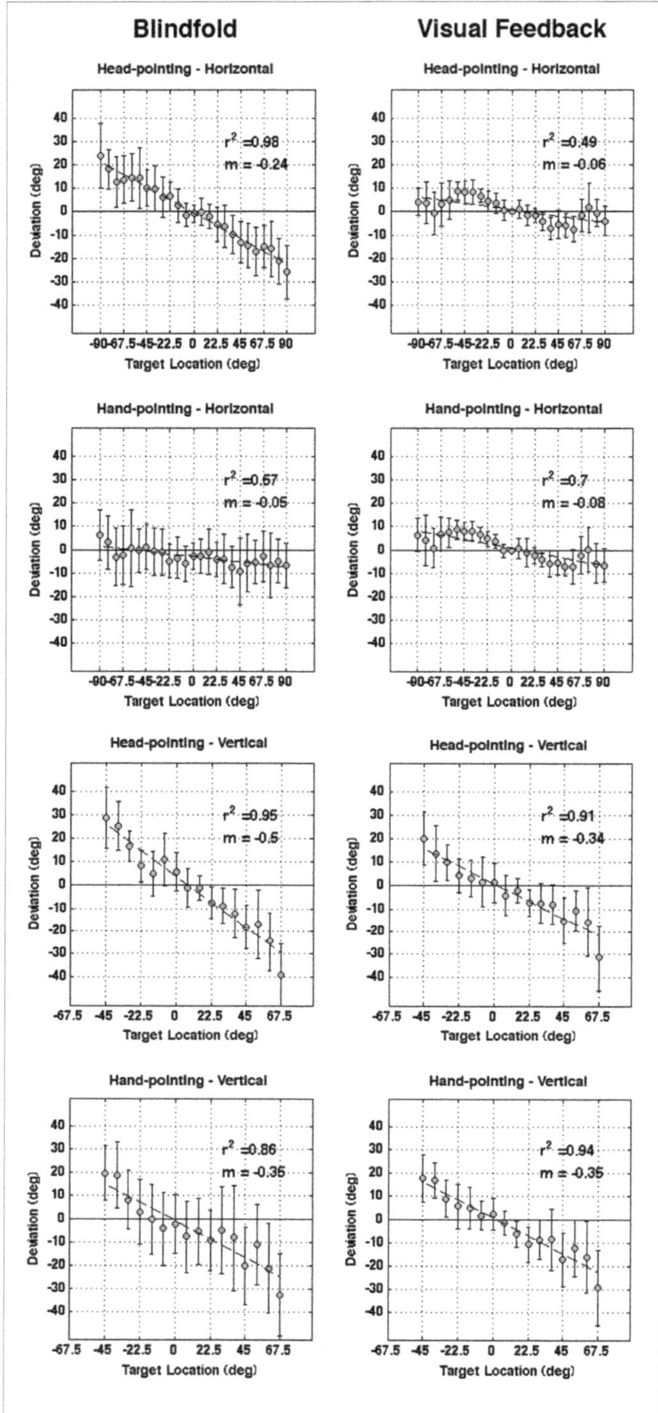

FIGURE 3 | Signed error plots. Illustrated here are the signed error plots for each condition as a function of target location. Overlaid on top of the plots are first-order regression curves that were fitted to the signed error plots, for which the slopes can be taken as an index of the tendency to undershoot or overshoot target locations. In general, signed error tended to increase (undershoot) as a function of target eccentricity, and was further increased by blindfolding. However, this effect was primarily driven by the head pointing trials, as blindfolding did not have a significant effect on hand pointing. There was also a significant effect of auditory spatial plane, where the slope was greater for trials on the vertical plane.

for head-pointing in the horizontal plane. Moreover, blindfolding was found to increase the tendency to undershoot more eccentric spatial positions for head-pointing, but not hand-pointing.

EFFECT OF AUDITORY PLANE AND POINTING METHOD

As expected, sound locations on the horizontal plane were more accurately localized than those on the vertical plane, where there is a strong tendency to undershoot the source locations (see **Figure 3**). This is highly consistent with previous findings demonstrating that auditory spatial resolution is far greater in the horizontal plane than in the vertical one (Oldfield and Parker, 1984; Makous and Middlebrooks, 1990). Although there was no global difference between the pointing methods, they provided different levels of accuracy with respect to the planes in which sounds were presented, as evidenced by the *auditory plane × pointing method* interaction. It was found that head-pointing was more accurate for localizing vertical targets (by approximately 1°), whereas hand pointing was more accurate for localization in the horizontal plane (by approximately 2°). However, a triple interaction revealed that this effect was primarily driven by the blindfolded conditions (discussed further below). In the conditions where visual feedback was available, the two pointing methods were not significantly different from one another (see **Figure 2**). While there is little comparative data for localization in the vertical plane, this result is consistent with previous findings indicating that both methods are comparable to one another for localization in the horizontal plane (Haber et al., 1993; Majdak et al., 2010). Although, there was a significant effect of pointing method on the slope of the regression curve, this was also driven by the effect of blindfolding, as the slope did not differ between pointing methods when visual feedback was available.

EFFECT OF BLINDFOLDING

The presence of visual feedback was found to lead to a significantly lower absolute localization error compared to performance on the same task when blindfolded. Although blindfolding increased this error for both pointing methods and for both auditory planes, this effect was greater for head pointing conditions, and was especially strong for head pointing in the horizontal plane (see **Figure 2**). Blindfolding also significantly increased the amount of undershooting for head-pointing (particularly for eccentric spatial positions), but not for hand pointing (as reflected by the regression curves slope seen in **Figure 3**). Overall, these effects of visual feedback on head pointing in the horizontal plane are highly consistent with the findings of Lewald et al. (2000), who showed that localizing with the head in darkness reduced localization accuracy and increased the tendency to undershoot target locations in the horizontal plane.

Pointing to sound sources in normal visual conditions arguably requires the combined and weighted processing of visual and proprioceptive cues. Indeed, matching a target position with the hand is better performed while having access to both visual and proprioceptive cues than with either modality alone (van Beers et al., 1999). Here we showed that blindfolding significantly increased the absolute localization error for both auditory spatial planes and both pointing methods. However, in the horizontal plane, the effect of blindfolding was shown to be greater for head than for hand pointing. Overall, our results suggest a greater dependence on visual cues for orienting one's head toward a specific location in space than for orienting one's arm. Indeed, blindfolding was shown to significantly affect both the average deviation from the target (in the horizontal plane) and the tendency to undershoot them more so for head-pointing trials.

So why would blindfolding (i.e., the removal of visual input and feedback) affect both pointing methods differently in the horizontal plane but not in the vertical plane? One possible explanation stems from the fact that the most peripheral positions in the vertical condition weren't as eccentric as those used in the horizontal plane; however this is also true for hand pointing conditions and therefore seems like an unlikely cause of the discrepancy. An alternative point of view could be that both pointing methods should be considered more or less equal (as evidenced in three of the four conditions), and that blindfolding for some reason induces a more pronounced effect specifically on head pointing in the horizontal plane. Why this is the case is also unclear. One possibility is the existence of different underlying physical restrictions in rotating the head, shoulders and elbows. This however cannot constitute the primary cause of the difference since the two methods were not statistically different from one another when visual feedback was present. Moreover, the effect of blindfolding for head-pointing was greatest for the horizontal plane, which argues for the existence of an alternative explanation.

The greater undershooting with head pointing in the horizontal plane, compared with the vertical plane, could potentially result from a greater sensitivity to eye movements when making gaze shifts. While it has been clearly documented that small but significant sound localization shifts occur in the opposite direction in response to eccentric gaze (Lewald and Ehrenstein, 1996; Lewald, 1997; Getzmann, 2002), those in the vertical plane are largely dependent on the movement of the head on the neck, whereas horizontal shifts can be augmented with movements from the shoulders, hips and body. One way to address this issue in future work would be to have the subjects perform the sound localization in complete darkness (as opposed to being blindfolded) in order to measure gaze shifts during the localization trials. Alternatively, the increase in undershooting targets when head-pointing in the horizontal plane might also arise due to a shift in the subjective auditory median plane (SAMP) of the head when deprived of visual input. The SAMP might be shifted or biased in the direction of a heard sound while moving toward it, which would lead subjects to undershoot targets due to having the perception of having pointed more eccentrically. This effect has previously been reported (Lewald et al., 2000) where head-pointing to a remembered sound source in darkness produced an undershooting in sound localization responses, that was largely corrected, as in the present study, when laser-pointed feedback of the objective median plane of the head was available. It is thus possible that the visual feedback provided by the laser pointer counteracts the manifestation of such a shift. The lesser impact of blindfolding on hand-pointing on the other hand, could potentially be due to the higher reliability of proprioceptive signals from the arm and hand compared to those provided by the vestibular and head/ neck muscle proprioceptive signals when localizing with the head. Since the present study was not specifically designed to address these issues, further experiments are required in order to fully answer such questions.

A potential caveat of the current experimental design relates to the use of the laser pointer, in that it may have provided a form of super-accurate feedback that is not normally available. This means that the subjects' performance in the non-blindfolded conditions might be better than otherwise expected. While the use of the laser pointing here also served as a means for the experimenter to record the data, future studies may consider alternative recording methods to eliminate this possible bias. Although the average localization error recorded here with the laser pointer when hand-pointing in the horizontal plane (6.36°) does not appear to be markedly better than those previously obtained without the added visual feedback provided by a laser pointer (e.g., Gougoux et al., 2005: 7.61°), future within-experiment control conditions would be best suited to address this issue. Lastly, also unclear at this point is whether it is specifically the localization response that is affected by removal of visual input, or whether the spatial percept itself is also affected. Further experimentation with auditory spatial tasks that do not require an overt motor response (e.g., sound source discrimination tasks) would likely provide valuable insights into this issue.

IMPLICATIONS FOR STUDIES WITH THE BLIND

The present findings demonstrate the effect of performing sound localization tasks while blindfolded and provide compelling evidence that it significantly reduces performance, and does so predominantly under particular circumstances. This observation raises important implications for studies comparing the sound localization abilities of sighted and blind individuals, as the present data argue that specific methodologies should be avoided when doing so. Specifically, in light of the present findings, the use of head-pointing procedures to localize sounds should be avoided, particularly for investigations interested in the horizontal plane. This is particularly important when considering that this discrepancy between pointing methods in the horizontal plane was not found for blind individuals (Haber et al., 1993).

ACKNOWLEDGMENTS

We thank all the individuals that volunteered to participate in this study as well as the Institut Nazareh et Louis-Braille (INLB) for its assistance in recruiting blind participants. We also thank Marc Schönwiesner and Régis Trapeau for their assistance in programming the tasks and setting up the equipment. This research was funded by the Canadian Institutes of Health Research.

REFERENCES

Ashmead, D. H., Wall, R. S., Ebinger, K. A., Eaton, S. B., Snook-Hill, M. M., and Yang, X. (1998). Spatial hearing in children with visual disabilities. *Perception* 27, 105–122. doi: 10.1068/p270105

Batteau, D. W. (1967). The role of the pinna in human localization. *Proc. R. Soc. Lond. B Biol. Sci.* 168, 158–180. doi: 10.1098/rspb.1967.0058

Birch, H. G., and Lefford, A. (1963). Intersensory development in children. *Monogr. Soc. Res. Child Dev.* 28, 1–47. doi: 10.2307/1165681

Doucet, M. E., Gagné, J. P., Leclerc, C., Lassonde, M., Guillemot, J. P., and Lepore, F. (2005). Blind subjects process auditory spectral cues more efficiently than sighted people. *Exp. Brain Res.* 160, 194–202. doi: 10.1007/s00221-004-2000-4

Gardner, M. B., and Gardner, R. S. (1973). Problem of localization in the medial plane: effect of pinnae cavity occlusion. *J. Acoust. Soc. Am.* 53, 400–408. doi: 10.1121/1.1913336

Getzmann, S. (2002). The effect of eye position and background noise on vertical sound localization. *Hear. Res.* 169, 130–139. doi: 10.1016/S0378-5955(02)00387-8

Gougoux, F., Lepore, F., Lassonde, M., Voss, P., Zatorre, R. J., and Belin, P. (2004). Neuropsychology: pitch discrimination in the early blind. *Nature* 430, 309. doi: 10.1038/430309a

Gougoux, F., Zatorre, R. J., Lassonde, M., Voss, P., and Lepore, F. (2005). A functional neuroimaging study of sound loclization: visual cortex activity predicts performance in early-blind individuals. *PLoS Biol.* 3:e27. doi: 10.1371/journal.pbio.0030027

Haber, L., Haber, R. N., Penningroth, S., Novak, K., and Radgowski, H. (1993). Comparison of nine methods of indicating the direction to objects: data from blind adults. *Perception* 22, 35–47. doi: 10.1068/p220035

Hay, J., Pick, H. L. Jr., and Ikeda, K. (1965). Visual capture produced by prism spectacles. *Psychon. Sci.* 2, 215–216

Lessard, N., Paré, M., Lepore, F., and Lassonde, M. (1998). Early-blind human subjects localize sound sources better than sighted subjects. *Nature* 395, 278–280. doi: 10.1038/26228

Lewald, J. (1997). Eye-position effects in directional hearing. *Behav. Brain Res.* 87, 35–48. doi: 10.1016/S0166-4328(96)02254-1

Lewald, J. (2002). Vertical sound localization in blind humans. *Neuropsychologia* 40, 1868–1872. doi: 10.1016/S0028-3932(02)00071-4

Lewald, J., Dörrscheidt, G. J., and Ehrenstein, W. H. (2000). Sound localization with eccentric head position. *Behav. Brain Res.* 108, 105–125. doi: 10.1016/S0166-4328(99)00141-2

Lewald, J., and Ehrenstein, W. H. (1996). The effect of eye position on auditory lateralization. *Exp. Brain Res.* 108, 473–485. doi: 10.1007/BF00227270

Majdak, P., Goupell, M. J., and Laback, B. (2010). 3-D localization of virtual sound sources: effects of visual environment, pointing method, and training. *Atten. Percept. Psychophys.* 72, 454–69. doi: 10.3758/APP.72.2.454

Makous, J. C., and Middlebrooks, J. C. (1990). Two-dimensional sound localization by human listeners. *J. Acoust. Soc. Am.* 87, 2188–200. doi: 10.1121/1.399186

Muchnick, C., Efrati, M., Nemeth, E., Malin, M., and Hildesheimer, M. (1991). Central auditory skills in blind and sighted subjects. *Scand. Audiol.* 20, 19–23. doi: 10.3109/01050399109070785

Niemeyer, W., and Starlinger, I. (1981). Do the blind hear better? II. Investigations of auditory processing in congenital and early acquired blindness. *Audiology* 20, 510–515. doi: 10.3109/00206098109072719

Oldfield, S. R., and Parker, S. P. A. (1984). Acuity of sound localisation: a topography of auditory space. I Normal hearing conditions. *Perception* 3, 581–600. doi: 10.1068/p130581

Pick, H. L. Jr., and Warren, D. H. (1969). Sensory conflict in judgments of spatial direction. *Percept. Psychophys.* 6, 203–205. doi: 10.3758/BF03207017

Röder, B., Teder-Sälejärvi, W., Sterr, A., Rösler, F., Hillyard, S. A., and Neville, H. J. (1999). Improved auditory spatial tuning in blind humans. *Nature* 400, 162–166. doi: 10.1038/22106

Rossetti, Y., Desmurget, M., and Prablanc, C. (1995). Vectorial coding of movement: vision, proprioception, or both? *J. Neurophysiol.* 74, 457–463.

van Beers, R. J., Sittig, A. C., and Denier van der Gon, J. J. (1999). Localization of a seen finger is based exclusively on proprioception and on vision of the finger. *Exp. Brain Res.* 125, 43–49. doi: 10.1007/s002210050656

Voss, P., Gougoux, F., Lassonde, M., Fortin, M., Guillemot, J. P., and Lepore, F. (2004). Early- and late-onset blind individuals show supra-normal auditory abilities in far space. *Curr. Biol.* 14, 1734–1738. doi: 10.1016/j.cub.2004.09.051

Zwiers, M. P., Van Opstal, A. J., and Cruysberg, J. R. M. (2001). A spatial hearing deficit in early blind individuals. *J. Neurosci.* 21, RC142:1–5.

7

Sensitivity to temporal fine structure and hearing-aid outcomes in older adults

Elvira Perez*, Abby McCormack and Barrie A. Edmonds

NIHR Nottingham Hearing Biomedical Research Unit, School of Medicine, University of Nottingham, Nottingham, UK

****Correspondence:***
Elvira Perez, Division of Psychiatry and Applied Psychology, School of Medicine, Institute of Mental Health, University of Nottingham, Triumph Rd., Nottingham, NG7 2TU, UK
e-mail: elvira.perez@nottingham.ac.uk

Objective: To investigate the effect of sensitivity to temporal fine structure (TFS) on subjective measures of hearing aid outcome.

Design: Prior to receiving hearing aids, participants completed a test to assess sensitivity to TFS and two self-assessment questionnaires; the Glasgow Hearing Aid Benefit Profile (GHABP), and the Speech, Spatial and Qualities of hearing (SSQ-A). Follow-up appointments, comprised three self-assessment questionnaires; the GHABP, the SSQ-B, and the International Outcome Inventory for Hearing Aid Outcomes (IOI-HA).

Study sample: 75 adults were recruited from direct referral clinics.

Results: Two thirds of participants were found to have good sensitivity to TFS; listeners with good sensitivity to TFS rated their hearing abilities higher at pre-fitting (SSQ-A) than those with poor sensitivity to TFS. At follow-up, participants with good sensitivity to TFS showed a smaller improvement on SSQ-B over listeners with poor sensitivity to TFS. Among the questionnaires, only the SSQ showed greater sensitivity to measure subjective differences between listeners with good and poor sensitivity to TFS.

Conclusions: The clinical identification of a patient's ability to process TFS information at an early stage in the treatment pathway could prove useful in managing expectations about hearing aid outcomes.

Keywords: lateralization, interaural phase difference, audiology, older adults, hearing aids

INTRODUCTION

Presbycusis is characterized by gently-sloping high-frequency hearing loss. It is often first revealed to the listener through a reduced understanding of conversational speech, particularly when there is a source of background noise. A common treatment for presbycusis is provision of hearing aids. Hearing aids make understanding speech much easier for the vast majority of people in a range of situations. However, listening in complex or noisy environments can remain challenging for some people even after provision of amplification (Moore et al., 1999). As the ability to understand speech is only moderately associated with audiometric threshold (Ching et al., 1998), factors other than reduced audibility may contribute to the communication difficulties experienced by some patients. For example, when competing sound sources are spatially separated, spatial hearing plays an important role for speech intelligibility. It is well established that certain acoustical and perceptual mechanisms can lead to large speech intelligibility improvements (e.g., Zurek, 1993; Freyman et al., 1999). However, listeners have to have access to spatially salient acoustic cues to be able to take advantage of those mechanisms. Previous research showed that spatial hearing is mediated by various types of binaural acoustic cues: interaural time differences (ITDs), which, for on-going tones, translate to interaural phase differences (IPDs), interaural level differences (ILDs), and monaural spectral cues (see Blauert, 1983 for a review). ITDs arise as a result of the physical separation of a listener's ears and provide information about the left-right position of a sound source. ITDs are perceptually most potent below about 1–0.75 kHz and there is evidence regarding neural firing tracking the phase of a signal up to about 1.5 kHz, (Neher et al., 2009 for a review). Registration of IPDs reflect fine structure coding and are presumed to involve the comparison of phase-locked inputs in the two ears, a process that forms the basis of the coincidence detection model of binaural hearing (Jeffress, 1948). Consequently, IPDs provide an accepted metric for neural synchrony and sensitivity to temporal fine structure (TFS).

TFS information is useful (for normal-hearing listeners at least) for frequencies lower than 1000 Hz because TFS information is thought to be important for the perception of F0 information (Moore et al., 1984; Hartmann and Doty, 1996), and for the discrimination of IPDs (Hafter et al., 1979). In this study we have manipulated the IPD of the waveform fine structure for measuring the ITDs of periodic inputs such as pure tones. The TFS test is based on measuring thresholds for detecting an IPD for pure tones, where there is an interaural disparity in the TFS only. Listeners must be sensitive to TFS to detect such a disparity, which is usually heard as a shift in the position of the tone inside the head (Hopkins and Moore, 2010a,b).

It has been suggested that if the amount of TFS information in a speech signal is varied then listeners with sensori-neural hearing loss find the speech less intelligible than normally-hearing listeners (Lorenzi et al., 2006; Hopkins et al., 2008; Hopkins and Moore, 2010a,b). When sensitivity to TFS information is measured with tonal stimuli the relationship with speech intelligibility measures is not so clear. Hopkins and Moore (2011) found that after controlling for hearing loss, sensitivity to monaural TFS was correlated with speech reception thresholds (SRTs), but not sensitivity to binaural TFS cues. Strelcyk and Dau (2009), on the other hand, found that sensitivity to TFS was associated with SRTs against a multi-talker background, but not against an amplitude-modulated noise masker. Nonetheless, it is thought that the ability to exploit TFS information is poorer in adults with sensori-neural loss than normally-hearing listeners (Lacher-Fougere and Demany, 1998; Moore and Skrodzka, 2002; Hopkins et al., 2008; Strelcyk and Dau, 2009; Ardoint et al., 2010; Hopkins and Moore, 2010a,b), and varies among listeners with similar audiometric configurations (Hopkins et al., 2008; Strelcyk and Dau, 2009; Hopkins and Moore, 2010a,b). Consequently, it is thought that sensitivity to TFS information could account for some of the variability observed in the amount of benefit that patients report to receive from hearing aids. However, to our knowledge there is no evidence in the literature describing the effect of reduced sensitivity to TFS information on actual hearing-aid outcomes, as might be determined in the clinic.

The aim of this study was to investigate the effect of sensitivity to TFS information on hearing-aid outcomes. In an earlier report (Perez et al., 2012), a group of presbycusic participants completed tests of sensitivity to TFS information, temporal resolution (gap detection) and frequency resolution (notched-noise). We found that sensitivity to TFS information appeared to contribute to the degree of difficulty these participants reported experiencing on self-report questionnaires prior to the fitting of their hearing aids (portions of this data are also reported here for ease of reading). In the current report, we followed these patients for a period of 6 months after their hearing aid fittings to determine whether listeners with good sensitivity also perform better on hearing-aid outcomes. We hypothesized that those listeners with good sensitivity to TFS information would experience better hearing-aid outcomes than those with impaired TFS processing abilities.

METHODS

PROCEDURE

The recruitment of participants was made via leaflets distributed to patients attending Nottingham Audiological Services for a direct referral assessment. All participants that enrolled in the study met the following selection criteria: (a) followed General Practice (GP) direct-referral route to audiology, (b) 50+ years of age, (c) bilaterally symmetrical sensori-neural hearing loss, (d) had not previously worn a hearing aid, (e) normal or corrected-to-normal vision. Our sample comprised 75 adults (44 men and 31 women) with a mean age of 72.24 ± 0.82 (range age 51–85 years) with mild-to-moderate hearing loss. Ethical approval for this study was obtained from the Derbyshire Research Ethics Committee.

Participants were tested by a member of the research team on three occasions. The first testing session took place prior to the patient being fitted with a hearing aid. During this session, participants completed a short test to determine their sensitivity to TFS and a number of self-report assessment questionnaires. The second and third research appointments took place 3- and 6-month post-hearing-aid fitting, in which participants completed a number of self-report outcome questionnaires.

SELF-REPORT QUESTIONNAIRES

In order to ascertain the degree of difficulty experienced prior to provision of a hearing aid in a range of listening scenarios, all participants were asked to complete the first part of the Glasgow Hearing Aid Benefit Profile (GHABP: Gatehouse, 1999) and the Speech, Spatial and Qualities of Hearing (SSQ-A: Gatehouse and Noble, 2004) questionnaires during the first testing session. Part one of the GHABP asks participants to rate themselves using a 5-point ordinal scale on two dimensions: Initial Disability and Handicap on four pre-specified listening circumstances which may commonly occur in the lives of people with hearing loss, (e.g., "*Listening to the television with other family or friends when the volume is adjusted to suit other people*") and four self-nominated listening scenarios which allows the listener to specify additional listening circumstances of importance and relevance to their everyday communication circumstances (e.g., "*Listening to music in a concert hall.*"). Higher ratings on each of these dimensions indicate greater levels of difficulty or worry. The SSQ-A asks participants to rate their listening abilities using an ordinal scale (0–10) on three sub-scales: Speech, Spatial, and Qualities on 14, 17, and 18 pre-specified listening scenarios respectively (e.g., Speech sub-scale: "you are talking with one other person and there is a TV on in the same room. Without turning the TV down, can you follow what the person you're talking to says?") Higher ratings on the SSQ-A indicate greater levels of perceived ability.

In order to ascertain the degree of benefit experienced after receiving a hearing aid, participants were asked to complete the second part of the GHABP, the SSQ-B (Jensen et al., 2009), and the International Outcome Inventory for Hearing Aids (IOI-HA, Cox and Alexander, 2002). The second part of the GHABP uses four pre-defined subscales for monitoring hearing-aid outcomes: Usage, Benefit, Residual Disability (difficulties still present while using the hearing aid), and Satisfaction. The SSQ-B is very similar to the SSQ-A, but asks participants to compare their hearing abilities now (aided) with their abilities prior to provision of a hearing aid on an ordinal scale ranging from −5 (much worse) to +5 (much better). The IOI-HA questionnaire uses a 5-point nominal scale (e.g., "helped not at all" through to "helped very much") to record self-report scores for seven outcome dimensions: Use, Benefit, Residual Activity Limitation (difficulties still present while using the hearing aid that affect the users day-to-day activities), Satisfaction, Residual Participation Restriction (difficulties still present while using the hearing aid that affect the users social interactions), Impact on Others, and Quality of Life. For example, Residual Activity Limitation is assessed with the following question: "Think again about the situation where you most wanted to hear better. When you use your present hearing aid(s), how much difficulty do you STILL have in that situation?"

These questionnaires can be accessed online at:

http://www.ihr.mrc.ac.uk/products/display/questionnaires

http://www.harlmemphis.org/index.php/clinical-applications/ioi-ha/

HEARING ASSESSMENTS

Hearing thresholds/0.25–8 kHz

Air-conduction audiometry without masking was used to calculate hearing thresholds at 0.25, 0.5, 1, 2, 4, and 8 kHz in accordance with the British Society of Audiology (BSA) guidelines (2011) by a qualified audiologist as part of the routine direct referral assessment process using a Siemens Unity 1 or 2 audiometers with TDH39 headphones. Air-conduction audiometry without masking consists on measuring the quietest percept of a sound (target tone). Participants are asked to press a button as soon as they hear a tone and keep it pressed for as long as they hear the tone, no matter which ear they hear it in. Participants are asked to release the button as soon as they no longer hear the tone. According the BSA guidelines, the professional administrating the audiometry should start presenting the tones at the better-hearing ear (according to the subject's account) and at 1000 Hz. Next, test 2000, 4000, 8000, 500, and 250 Hz in that order. It is also recommended to vary the length of the tone presentation to ensure that the timing of each tone is not predictable.

TFS/0.5 kHz

Sensitivity to TFS was measured using the TFS-LF method (Hopkins and Moore, 2010a,b) over Sennheiser HD-25. The task utilizes a two-interval two-alternative forced choice (2I-2AFC) task. Each interval contained four 0.5 kHz pure tones in either *AAAA* or *ABAB* sequences. In *AAAA* intervals, all the tones were presented diotically. In *ABAB* intervals, the first and third tones were diotic whilst the 2nd and 4th tones were presented with an IPD (ΔØ). Participants were asked to identify which interval contained the tones that appeared to change in location. A two-up, one-down adaptive procedure was used to vary ΔØ. At the beginning of a run ΔØ was set to a maximum value of 180°. Thresholds were calculated by measuring the geometric mean of ΔØ at the last six turn points which corresponded to the 71% correct point. However, the adaptive procedure terminated early if this maximum value was reached twice before the second turn point, or at all after the second turn point. In this situation, the program reverted to a non-adaptive (method of constant measures) procedure in which a further 40 trials were presented with ΔØ fixed at its maximum value and a percentage correct score was calculated. Discriminability index (d′) values for the TFS test were calculated using a table of d′ values for two-alternative forced choice procedures (Hacker and Ratcliff, 1979) which was 0.78. For Thresholds measured using the percent-correct procedure we followed Hopkins and Moore (2010a,b) approach by linearly extrapolating the threshold value of ΔØ needed for 71% correct from the d′ scores, so that results from percent-correct and adaptive procedures could be compared.

$$(\Delta\text{Ø extrapolated} = (0.78 \times 180°)/d' \text{ from percent correct procedure})$$

All participants concluded a practice run to ensure they understood the task. Signals used in the measurement of TFS were presented with a sampling rate of 44.1 kHz, using a PC and an external sound card (ECHO Gina 3D).

All hearing assessments were conducted in a double-walled, sound proof booth

STATISTICAL METHODOLOGY

The statistical methodology employed in this study includes basic descriptive analysis, *post-hoc* paired-sample *t*-tests, One-Way ANOVA and Pearson correlations. Calculation of discriminability index (d′) values for the TFS is described in section Hearing assessments, TFS/0.5 kHz.

RESULTS

PRE-FITTING ASSESSMENTS

Although hearing thresholds were classified to be bilaterally symmetric, the six-frequency pure-tone average hearing thresholds measured at the better ear and the poorer ear (34.5 ± 1.04 dB HL at the better ear) were found to be significantly different [$t_{(1, 74)} = -9.12$, $p < 0.001$]. Audiogram for left and right is shown in **Figure 1**.

In the following sections, we describe how age and hearing loss related to the self-reported assessments of hearing difficulty measured on the GHABP and SSQ-A. Whilst it was anticipated that hearing loss would account for most of the variability observed in hearing difficulties reported, we hypothesized that some of the variability observed in the difficulties experienced by these patients might be explained by their sensitivity to TFS information.

Glasgow hearing aid benefit profile (GHABP): assessment questionnaire

Participants reported experiencing "Great difficulty" (3.06 ± 0.57) on the Initial Disability sub-scale and "Moderate" levels of worry on the Handicap sub-scale (2.9 ± 0.78). Initial Disability and Handicap scores were strongly correlated with one another, but were not correlated with age or audiometric threshold (see **Table 1**). In addition to the four pre-defined listening scenarios described in the GHABP, participants had the option of nominating an additional four listening scenarios. All participants completed the four pre-defined listening

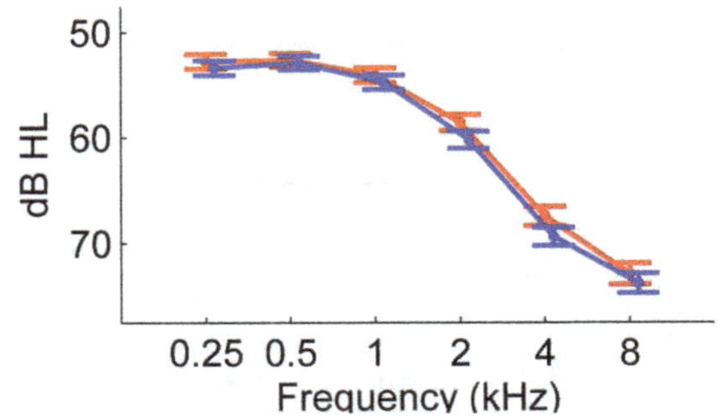

FIGURE 1 | Mean air-conduction PTA thresholds of 75 participants measured for right (red circles) and left (blue circles) ears. Error bars show ±1 standard error of the mean.

scenarios and 26 provided self-nominated scenarios: five participants self-nominated a single additional scenario, six participants provided two self-nominated scenarios, seven participants provided three self-nominated scenarios, and eight participants provided four self-nominated scenarios. For those participants who provided self-nominated scenarios, the four pre-defined listening situations (S1–S4) were scored as significantly less difficult [Initial Disability: $t_{(1,\ 28)} = -7.72$, $p < 0.01$] and less worrying [Handicap: $t_{(1,\ 28)} = -7.95$, $p < 0.01$] than the self-nominated listening situations (See **Figure 2**).

Speech, spatial and qualities of hearing: assessment (SSQ-A)

The majority of participants reported moderate levels of hearing ability on the Speech, Spatial and Qualities sub-scales (see **Figure 3**). Correlations are described in **Table 2**.

SENSITIVITY TO TEMPORAL FINE STRUCTURE (TFS)

Altogether, 49 participants completed the TFS-LF task using the adaptive procedure while 26 participants reverted to the method of constant measures (i.e., discriminating tones with a fixed phase shift of 180°). Sensitivity to TFS information was confirmed by comparing discriminability index (d′) values for the two groups (see **Figure 3A**). The participants that completed the adaptive version of the test were found to have significantly greater sensitivity to TFS information than those listeners who reverted to the constant measures version of the test [$F_{(1,\ 74)} = 31.43, p < 0.01$].

Sensitivity to TFS (d′) was weakly associated with age, and moderately associated with self-report scores of the Spatial and Quality sub-scales of the SSQ-A (see **Table 2**). Participants with good sensitivity to TFS reported significantly greater confidence in their Spatial processing abilities [$F_{(1,\ 73)} = 7.23$, $p < 0.01$] than participants with poorer sensitivity to TFS (see **Figure 3B**).

Table 1 | Results of Pearson correlation for pre-fitting assessment GHABP.

	1	2	3	4
1. Initial disability	–	$r = 0.8^{**}$	$r = 0.2$	$r = 0.1$
2. Handicap	$r = 0.8^{**}$	–	$r = 0.2$	$r = 0.1$
3. Age	$r = 0.2$	$r = 0.2$	–	$r = 0.4^{**}$
4. Audiometry	$r = 0.1$	$r = 0.1$	$r = 0.4^{**}$	–

*Notes: **Correlation is significant at 0.01 (2-tailed).*

HEARING AID OUTCOMES AT THE 3-MONTH FOLLOW-UP

Glasgow hearing aid benefit profile (GHABP): outcome questionnaire

The mean GHABP part two self-report scores for Usage, Benefit, Residual Disability, and Satisfaction are shown in **Figure 2**. For those listeners who provided self-nominated listening scenarios, there were significant differences between pre-defined and self-nominated scenario scores for Benefit [$t_{(1,\ 26)} = 2.89, p = 0.08$], Residual Disability [$t_{(1,\ 26)} = -2.22, p = 0.035$], and Satisfaction [$t_{(1,\ 26)} = 2.99, p = 0.006$].

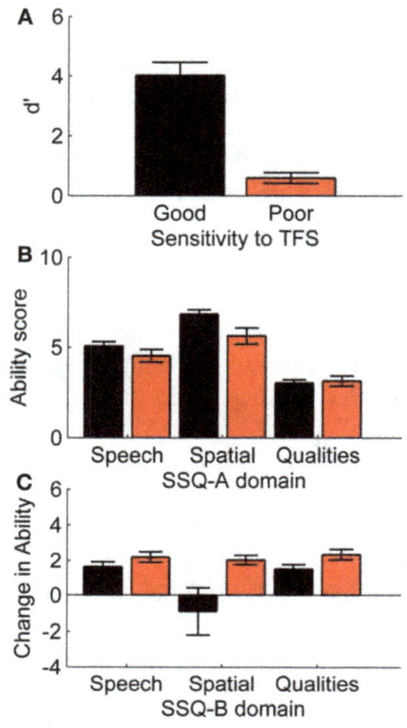

FIGURE 3 | Sensitivity to TFS information and self-reported listening abilities. (A) discriminability index (d′) of participants classified as having good or poor sensitivity on the basis of whether they completed the TFS-LF test adaptively (good sensitivity) or reverted to a method of constant measures (poor sensitivity), **(B)** SSQ-A self-report scores for participants with good sensitivity to TFS information (black bars) or poor sensitivity to TFS information (red bars), **(C)** SSQ-B self-report scores for participants with good sensitivity to TFS information (black bars) or poor sensitivity to TFS information (red bars). Error bars show ±1 standard error of the mean.

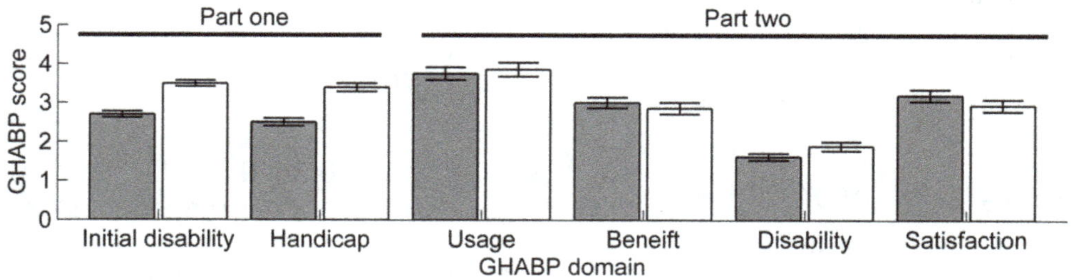

FIGURE 2 | Mean GHABP scores for pre-defined (gray bars) and self-nominated (white bars) scenarios. Error bars show ±1 standard error of the mean.

Table 2 | Results of pearson correlation for pre-fitting assessment SSQ-A and TFS.

		1	2	3	4	5	6	7	8
1.	Speech	–	$r = 0.7^{**}$	$r = 0.7^{**}$	$r = -0.3^{*}$	$r = -0.3^{**}$	$r = -0.3^{**}$	$r = 0.1$	$r = 0.1$
2.	Spatial	$r = 0.7^{**}$	–	$r = 0.7^{**}$	$r = -0.3^{*}$	$r = -0.3^{**}$	$r = -0.3^{**}$	$r = 0.3^{*}$	$r = 0.1$
3.	Qualities	$r = 0.7^{**}$	$r = 0.7^{**}$	–	$r = -0.1$	$r = -0.3^{**}$	$r = -0.3^{**}$	$r = 0.3^{*}$	$r = 0.1$
4.	Audiometry	$r = -0.3^{*}$	$r = -0.3^{*}$	$r = -0.1$	–	$r = 0.1$	$r = 0.1$	$r = -0.1$	$r = 0.4^{**}$
5.	Initial disability	$r = -0.3^{**}$	$r = -0.3^{**}$	$r = -0.3^{**}$	$r = 0.1$	–	$r = 0.8^{**}$	$r = 0.1$	$r = 0.2$
6.	Handicap	$r = -0.3^{**}$	$r = -0.3^{**}$	$r = -0.3^{**}$	$r = 0.1$	$r = 0.8^{**}$	–	$r = 0.1$	$r = 0.2$
7.	TFS (d′)	$r = 0.1$	$r = 0.3^{*}$	$r = 0.3^{*}$	$r = -0.1$	$r = 0.1$	$r = 0.1$	–	$r = -0.27^{*}$
8.	Age	$r = 0.1$	$r = 0.1$	$r = 0.1$	$r = 0.4^{**}$	$r = 0.2$	$r = 0.2$	$r = -0.27^{*}$	–

Notes: **Correlation is significant at 0.05 level (2-tailed);* ***correlation is significant at 0.01 (2-tailed).*

Table 3 | Results of pearson correlation for GHABP 3-month follow-up.

		1	2	3	4	5	6	7
1.	Usage	–	$r = 0.5^{**}$	$r = 0.5^{**}$	$r = 0.1$	$r = 0.3^{*}$	$r = 0.3^{*}$	$r = -0.36^{*}$
2.	Benefit	$r = 0.5^{**}$	–	$r = 0.5^{**}$	$r = -0.4^{**}$	$r = -0.1$	$r = -0.1$	$r = 0.2$
3.	Satisfaction	$r = 0.5^{**}$	$r = 0.5^{**}$	–	$r = -0.4^{**}$	$r = -0.1$	$r = -0.1$	$r = 0.2$
4.	Residual disability	$r = 0.1$	$r = -0.4^{**}$	$r = -0.4^{**}$	–	$r = 0.1$	$r = 0.1$	$r = 0.1$
5.	Handicap	$r = 0.3^{*}$	$r = -0.2$	$r = -0.1$	$r = 0.1$	–	$r = 0.1$	$r = 0.2$
6.	Initial disability	$r = 0.3^{*}$	$r = -0.2$	$r = -0.1$	$r = 0.1$	$r = -0.1$	–	$r = 0.2$
7.	Age	$r = -0.36^{*}$	$r = 0.2$	$r = 0.2$	$r = 0.1$	$r = 0.2$	$r = 0.2$	–

Notes: **Correlation is significant at 0.05 level (2-tailed);* ***correlation is significant at 0.01 (2-tailed).*

Table 4 | Results of pearson correlation for SSQ-B 3-month follow-up.

	Speech-B	Spatial-B	Qualities-B
Speech-B	–	$r = 0.7^{**}$	$r = 0.7^{**}$
Spatial-B	$r = 0.7^{**}$	–	$r = 0.7^{**}$
Qualities-B	$r = 0.7^{**}$	$r = 0.7^{**}$	–
Speech-A	$r = 0.5^{**}$	$r = 0.5^{**}$	$r = 0.5^{**}$
Spatial-A	$r = 0.5^{**}$	$r = 0.5^{**}$	$r = 0.5^{**}$
Qualities-A	$r = 0.5^{**}$	$r = 0.5^{**}$	$r = 0.5^{**}$
Usage	$r = -0.4^{**}$	$r = -0.4^{**}$	$r = -0.4^{**}$
Benefit	$r = -0.4^{**}$	$r = -0.4^{**}$	$r = -0.4^{**}$
Satisfaction	$r = -0.4^{**}$	$r = -0.4^{**}$	$r = -0.4^{**}$
Residual disability	$r = -0.3^{**}$	$r = -0.3^{**}$	$r = -0.3^{**}$
Hearing thresholds (0.25 kHz right ear)	$r = 0.1$	$r = 0.3^{*}$	$r = 0.1$
Age	$r = 0.1$	$r = 0.1$	$r = 0.1$

Notes: **Correlation is significant at 0.05 level (2-tailed);* ***correlation is significant at 0.01 (2-tailed).*

There was no association between GHABP self-reported outcomes and severity of hearing loss, or sensitivity to TFS information. Significant associations are described in **Table 3**.

Speech, spatial and qualities: benefit (SSQ-B)

Participants reported moderate improvements in listening ability on all three sub-scales of the SSQ-B (Speech, 1.9; Spatial 1.3; Qualities 1.9). See **Table 4** for associations between SSQ-B outcomes and other variables.

Participants with poor sensitivity to TFS (constant-measures TFS group) reported experiencing greater levels of improvement on all three of the SSQ-B sub-scales. Ratings of improvement were significant different between the two groups on the Qualities $[F_{(1, 67)} = 4.22, p < 0.05]$ sub-scale. It can be seen from **Figure 3C** that, on average, listeners with good sensitivity to TFS information reported a decrement in their spatial processing abilities following hearing aid provision.

International outcome inventory for hearing aids (IOI-HA)

Self-reported outcomes obtained on the seven questions of the IOI-HA were strongly associated with one another, however, usage did not correlate with Residual Activity Limitations or Residual Participation Restrictions; Satisfaction was not associated with Impact on Others. There were no associations with age, hearing loss (better ear average) or sensitivity to TFS. However, Impact on Others was associated with degree of hearing loss at 4 kHz for the left ear. See **Table 5** for associations between IOI-HA dimensions, GHABP post-fitting sub-scales and SSQ-B outcomes.

HEARING-AID OUTCOMES AT THE 6-MONTH FOLLOW-UP

Of the original sample of 75 people who participated at the 3-month follow-up, only 54 attended the 6-month follow-up appointment (72% retention rate). The association between age and GHABP Residual Disability was preserved at the 6-month follow-up ($r = -0.36$, $p \leq 0.05$) which suggests that this relationship is fairly stable. The association first observed at the 3-month follow-up between low-frequency hearing loss and

Table 5 | Results of pearson correlation for IOI-HA 3-month follow-up.

	Usage	Benefit	RAL	Satisfaction	RPR	IoO	QL
Usage	–	$r = 0.5^{**}$	$r = 0.2$	$r = 0.5^{**}$	$r = 0.2$	$r = 0.4^{**}$	$r = 0.4^{**}$
Benefit	$r = 0.5^{**}$	–	$r = 0.4^{**}$	$r = 0.8^{**}$	$r = 0.3^{*}$	$r = 0.8^{**}$	$r = 0.3^{*}$
RAL	$r = 0.1$	$r = 0.4^{**}$	–	$r = 0.3^{*}$	$r = 0.3^{*}$	$r = 0.3^{*}$	$r = 0.3^{*}$
Satisfaction	$r = 0.5^{**}$	$r = 0.8^{**}$	$r = 0.3^{*}$	–	$r = 0.2^{*}$	$r = 0.1$	$r = 0.2^{*}$
RPR	$r = 0.1$	$r = 0.3^{*}$	$r = 0.3^{*}$	$r = 0.2^{*}$	–	$r = 0.2^{*}$	$r = 0.2^{*}$
IoO	$r = 0.4^{**}$	$r = 0.8^{**}$	$r = 0.3^{*}$	$r = 0.1$	$r = 0.2^{*}$	–	$r = 0.2^{*}$
QL	$r = 0.4^{**}$	$r = 0.3^{*}$	$r = 0.3^{*}$	$r = 0.2^{*}$	$r = 0.2^{*}$	$r = 0.2^{*}$	–
Age	$r = 0.1$	$r = 0.1$	$r = 0.1$	$r = 0.1$	$r = 0.1$	$r = 0.1$	$r = 0.1$
Audiometry	$r = 0.1$	$r = 0.1$	$r = 0.1$	$r = 0.1$	$r = 0.1$	$r = 0.1$	$r = 0.1$
Hearing threshold (4 kHz left ear)	$r = 0.1$	$r = 0.1$	$r = 0.1$	$r = 0.1$	$r = 0.1$	$r = 0.3^{*}$	$r = 0.1$
TFS (d′)	$r = 0.1$	$r = 0.1$	$r = 0.1$	$r = 0.1$	$r = 0.1$	$r = 0.1$	$r = 0.1$
Usage GHABP	$r = 0.6^{**}$	$r = 0.2^{*}$	$r = 0.1$	$r = 0.1$	$r = 0.1$	$r = 0.3^{*}$	$r = 0.3^{*}$
Benefit GHABP	$r = 0.4^{*}$	$r = 0.6^{**}$	$r = 0.4^{*}$	$r = 0.5^{**}$	$r = 0.4^{*}$	$r = 0.4^{*}$	$r = 0.4^{*}$
Satisfaction GHABP	$r = 0.4^{*}$	$r = 0.3^{*}$	$r = 0.4^{*}$	$r = 0.6^{**}$	$r = 0.4^{*}$	$r = 0.5^{*}$	$r = 0.4^{*}$
Residual disability GHABP	$r = 0.1$	$r = 0.3^{*}$	$r = 0.3^{*}$	$r = 0.1$	$r = 0.1$	$r = 0.2^{*}$	$r = 0.2^{*}$
Speech-B	$r = 0.4^{*}$	$r = 0.5^{**}$	$r = 0.4^{*}$	$r = 0.2^{*}$	$r = 0.7^{**}$	$r = 0.2^{*}$	$r = 0.7^{**}$
Spatial-B	$r = 0.5^{**}$	$r = 0.4^{*}$	$r = 0.5^{**}$	$r = 0.1$	$r = 0.2^{*}$	$r = 0.5^{**}$	$r = 0.2^{*}$
Qualities-B	$r = 0.7^{**}$	$r = 0.2^{*}$	$r = 0.2^{*}$	$r = 0.1$	$r = 0.1$	$r = 0.2^{*}$	$r = 0.7^{**}$

*Notes: *Correlation is significant at 0.05 level (2-tailed); **correlation is significant at 0.01 (2-tailed). RAL, Residual Activity Limitation; RPR, Residual Participation Restriction; IoO, Impact on Others; and QL, Quality of Life.*

self-reported outcome was also observed at the 6-month follow-up appointment. Thus although, presbycusis is generally accepted to reflect high-frequency loss, consideration of low-frequency audiometric configurations appears to be important to self-reported outcomes. **Table 6** provides a summary of some of the key findings from this visit.

Differences in outcome reported at the 3- and 6-month follow-up appointments were compared using *post-hoc* paired-sample *t*-tests for each of the self-report sub-scales. There were no significant improvements in outcome as measured on the GHABP or the SSQ-B over the 6-month follow-up period. However, IOI-HA Usage ratings increased at the 6-month follow-up [$t_{(1, 49)} = -2.09$, $p < 0.05$], and IOI-HA Residual Activity Limitations decreased during the same period [$t_{(1, 48)} = -2.27$, $p < 0.05$]. Participants with the poorest sensitivity to TFS continued to experience better outcomes (SSQ-B) at the 6-month follow-up than those with good sensitivity to TFS [Speech: $F_{(1, 48)} = 5.38$, $p < 0.05$; Qualities: $F_{(1, 48)} = 4.36$, $p < 0.05$].

DISCUSSION

In this observational case series, we monitored the auditory rehabilitation of 75 older adults for a period of 6-months following receipt of their first hearing aid. All patients received standard audiological management pathways (initial audiological assessment and provision of hearing aids) for sensori-neural hearing loss. No experimental interventions or treatment groups were used. However, patients did complete a non-standard pre-fitting assessment to determine sensitivity to TFS information, and a range of non-standard pre- and post-fitting self-report questionnaires. The main purpose of this study was to assess how sensitivity to TFS information contributed to the hearing difficulties that the group faced pre- and post-provision of hearing aids.

SENSITIVITY TO TEMPORAL FINE STRUCTURE

It is generally accepted that speech perception deteriorates with increasing age (Plomp and Mimpen, 1979; Duquesnoy, 1983; Dubno et al., 2002) and hearing loss (Houtgast and Festen, 2008). A number of studies have shown that listeners with sensori-neural hearing loss are less able to exploit TFS cues for speech understanding than normally-hearing controls (Lorenzi et al., 2006; Hopkins et al., 2008; Ardoint et al., 2010; Hopkins and Moore, 2010a,b). However, there is no evidence to indicate that sensitivity to TFS information is dependent on the severity of hearing loss. For instance, previous studies have not found any association between sensitivity to TFS information and audiometric configuration (Hopkins and Moore, 2007; Strelcyk and Dau, 2009). This indicates that impairments to the processing of TFS information are relatively independent of hearing loss. Our results corroborate previous results as there was no association between sensitivity to TFS information at 0.5 kHz and audiometric thresholds. Age and sensitivity to TFS were associated with one another, but only weakly. In a recent study, however, Moore et al. (2012), found sensitivity to TFS worsen with age when assessing in a sample of 39 adults with ages ranging from 61 to 83 years (mean 69 years) with age-related hearing loss.

We found a number of self-report outcomes to be moderately associated with sensitivity to TFS information. For instance, prior to the receipt of a hearing aid, participants with good sensitivity to TFS information reported having better Spatial hearing (e.g., *Can you tell right away whether it is the person on your left or your right, without having to look?*) and Qualities of hearing (e.g., *Can you easily ignore other sounds when trying to listen to something?*) than participants with poor sensitivity to TFS on the SSQ-A. However, participants with poor sensitivity to TFS reported experiencing greater improvements on the Spatial and

Table 6 | Results of pearson correlation for 6-month follow-up outcomes with degree if hearing loss.

	Hearing thresholds (0.25 kHz)	Hearing thresholds (0.5 kHz)	Hearing thresholds (1 kHz)	Hearing thresholds (2 kHz)
Usage GHABP	$r = 0.2$	$r = 0.2$	$r = 0.2$	$r = 0.1$
Benefit GHABP	$r = 0.3$*	$r = 0.3$*	$r = 0.2$	$r = 0.1$
Satisfaction GHABP	$r = 0.1$	$r = 0.3$*	$r = 0.1$	$r = 0.1$
Residual disability GHABP	$r = 0.1$	$r = 0.2$	$r = 0.1$	$r = 0.1$
Speech-B	$r = 0.3$*	$r = 0.3$*	$r = 0.1$	$r = 0.1$
Spatial-B	$r = 0.3$*	$r = 0.3$*	$r = 0.1$	$r = 0.1$
Qualities-B	$r = 0.1$	$r = 0.3$*	$r = 0.2$	$r = 0.2$
Usage IOI-HA	$r = 0.1$	$r = 0.1$	$r = 0.2$	$r = 0.2$
Benefit IOI-HA	$r = 0.1$	$r = 0.1$	$r = 0.1$	$r = 0.2$
RAL IOI-HA	$r = 0.1$	$r = 0.1$	$r = 0.2$	$r = 0.2$
Satisfaction IOI-HA	$r = 0.3$*	$r = 0.3$*	$r = 0.2$	$r = 0.2$
RPR IOI-HA	$r = 0.1$	$r = 0.1$	$r = 0.2$	$r = 0.3$*
IoO IOI-HA	$r = 0.1$	$r = 0.1$	$r = 0.3$* (right ear only)	$r = 0.3$*
QL IOI-HA	$r = 0.1$	$r = 0.1$	$r = 0.05$	$r = 0.1$

*Notes: *Correlation is significant at 0.05 level (2-tailed). RAL, Residual Activity Limitation; RPR, Residual Participation Restriction; IoO, Impact on Others; and QL, Quality of Life.*

Qualities of hearing dimensions of the SSQ-B than the participants with good sensitivity to TFS at the 3-month follow-up, and Speech and Qualities of hearing at the 6-month follow-up. These results suggest that listeners with poor sensitivity to TFS may experience poorer spatial and qualities of hearing than listeners with good sensitivity to TFS prior to their hearing aid fitting, and therefore, experience by contrast greater hearing aid benefit as their initial score was lower and consequently had more "opportunities for improvement" than listeners with good sensitivity to TFS information. Given these differences in self-reported listening abilities and the relative independence of TFS sensitivity and audibility, it appears that an assessment of a patient's sensitivity to low-frequency binaural TFS information could prove useful in managing the expectations of patients who are due to receive a hearing aid. Differences in expectations could, at least partly, explain the observed patter of results in which patients with high sensitivity to TFS may have higher expectations, and consequently more difficult to fulfill, while patients with poor sensitivity to TFS may have lower expectations, easier to fulfill. Perhaps with better management options that take sensitivity to TFS information into account this advantage could be increased further. For instance, there is some evidence to suggest that choice of compression algorithm could be informed by knowledge of a patient's ability to process TFS information (Moore, 2008).

SELF-REPORTED HEARING AID OUTCOMES

Good practice guidelines for adult audiology in the UK (Department of Health, 2007) recommend that patients receive a follow up visit sometime after provision of hearing aids (normally 8–12 weeks post-fitting) in which an assessment of patient outcomes should be undertaken. There are a number of methods available to monitor hearing-aid outcomes including subjective (self-report questionnaires) and objective measures of speech intelligibility (e.g., speech reception threshold). However, GHABP (Gatehouse, 1999) is the recommended outcome tool for assessing hearing-aid outcomes. In the current study, we employed three self-report questionnaires to monitor hearing-aid outcome, as previous research has shown that outcomes can vary markedly from one assessment tool to another (Humes, 1999; Lunner, 2003; Walden and Walden, 2004). Our results also revealed marked differences in outcome as measured on different outcome tools, and suggest that a multifaceted appraisal of hearing-aid outcome might be warranted.

We found that, while the GHABP pre-fitting dimensions (i.e., Handicap and Initial Disability) were highly associated with one another, they were not associated with age, severity of hearing loss or GHABP post-fitting outcomes. At the 3-month outcome assessment the four GHABP outcome dimensions (Usage, Benefit, Residual Disability, and Satisfaction) were strongly associated with one another, but again largely independent of age and severity of hearing loss. Moreover, there was a striking dichotomy between self-reports obtained on the pre-defined and self-nominated listening scenarios. The individual needs that may arise when measuring hearing aid benefit across different domains can be better captured when the hearing aid user is giving the opportunity to self-nominate specific scenarios. Those self-nominated scenarios may be very specific and only relevant to a single hearing aid user. While the GHABP is sensitive for capturing those meaningful and idiosyncratic listening difficulties, our results showed that those dimensions are not associated to TFS. These findings limit the efficacy of the GHABP as an outcome tool, at least when comparing group data, but highlight its sensitivity in characterizing patient's needs and therefore treatment improvement (e.g., managing expectations and hearing aid fittings). The SSQ-A and SSQ-B, on the other hand, showed high levels of consistency between pre- and post-fitting assessments, and were moderately correlated with GHABP pre-fitting dimensions; the SSQ questionnaires were also the only ones, in this study, to reveal subjective differences between listeners with good and poor sensitivity to TFS. It has been reported that the severity of hearing loss is associated with the amount of hearing aid benefit and satisfaction (Walden and Walden, 2004) or hearing aid usage (Bertoli et al., 2009) that patients report. We found that, the associations between self-report scores, age and hearing loss (4-frequency PTA at better ear) were generally weak. Outcome scores for Benefit and Satisfaction (GHABP), Speech, Spatial and Qualities (SSQ-B), and Satisfaction (IOI-HA) showed moderate associations with audiometric threshold, but only at low frequencies (0.25 and 0.5 kHz), and that this effect was stronger at the 6-month follow-up than at the 3-month follow-up. Results also showed that the severity of high-frequency loss was inversely associated with the Residual Participation Restrictions and the Impact on Others dimensions of the IOI-HA at the 6-month follow-up, indicating that those patients with the greatest levels of high-frequency hearing loss were least worried about the impact of their hearing loss on their daily lives and the lives of others. We also found that participant reports of hearing aid usage and benefit increased significantly over the 6-month follow-up period. However, neither outcome dimension increased significantly on a single outcome tool (Usage as measured on the IOI-HA increased during this period, but Usage on the GHABP did not; reports of Benefit on the GHABP increased over this period, but Benefit on the IOI-HA did not). Such variability in outcome highlights the differences in test sensitivity of the different methods, and the inherent limitations of restricting the clinical assessment of outcome to a single tool.

CONCLUSION

In the current study, our hypothesis was that those patients with good sensitivity to TFS would have significantly better outcomes than those with poor sensitivity. Our results show that assessing sensitivity to TFS information could prove important to the management of the expectations of first-time hearing aid users. We found that, new hearing aid users with good sensitivity to TFS reported experiencing less debilitating hearing difficulties prior to provision of hearing aids, but also reported experiencing the least amount of improvement following provision of hearing aids compared to listeners with poor sensitivity to TFS. The TFS test employed in this study (TFS-LF: Hopkins and Moore, 2010a,b was designed to be quick, easy and clinically relevant). We have shown that even if a listener does not find the task easy, the test can be used to categorize listeners into two groups (good or poor sensitivity) that differ on subjective and objective measures of hearing aid outcome. These results provide further evidence about the role of TFS processing in understanding the difficulties faced by older listeners, and indicate that an assessment of sensitivity to TFS information could play a role in shaping the management of patients receiving hearing aids.

ACKNOWLEDGMENTS

This report is independent research by the National Institute for Health Research Biomedical Research Unit Funding Scheme. The views expressed in this publication are those of the author(s) and not necessarily those of the NHS, the National Institute for Health Research or the Department of Health. We would like to thank three anonymous reviewers for their insightful and constructive comments, which contributed greatly to the overall quality and clarity of this manuscript.

REFERENCES

Ardoint, M., Sheft, S., Fleuriot, P., and Lorenzi, C. (2010). Perception of temporal fine-structure cues in speech with minimal envelope cues for listeners with mild-to-moderate hearing loss. *Int. J. Audiol.* 49, 823–831. doi: 10.3109/14992027.2010.492402

Bertoli, S., Staehelin, K., Zemp, E., Schindler, C., Bodmer, D., and Probst, R. (2009). Survey on hearing aid use and satisfaction in Switzerland and their determinants. *Int. J. Audiol.* 48, 183–195. doi: 10.1080/14992020802572627

Blauert, J. (1983). *Spatial Hearing: The Psychophysics of Human Sound Localization.* Cambridge, MA: MIT Press.

British Society of Audiology. (2011). *Pure Tone Air and Bone Conduction Threshold Audiometry with and Without Masking.* Reading: British Society of Audiology.

Ching, T. Y. C., Dillon, H., and Byrne, D. (1998). Speech recognition of hearing-impaired listeners: predictions from audibility and the limited role of high-frequency amplification. *J. Acoust. Soc. Am.* 103, 1128–1140. doi: 10.1121/1.421224

Cox, R. M., and Alexander, G. C. (2002). The International Outcome Inventory for Hearing Aids (IOI-HA): psychometric properties of the English version. *Int. J. Audiol.* 41, 30–35. doi: 10.3109/14992020209101309

Department of Health. (2007). *Transforming Adult Hearing Services for Patients with Hearing Difficulty - A Good Practice* Guide.

Dubno, J. R., Horwitz, A. R., and Ahlstrom, J. B. (2002). Benefit of modulated maskers for speech recognition by younger and older adults with normal hearing. *J. Acoust. Soc. Am.* 111, 2897–2907. doi: 10.1121/1.1480421

Duquesnoy, A. J. (1983). The intelligibility of sentences in quiet and in noise in aged listeners. *J. Acoust. Soc. Am.* 74, 1136–1144. doi: 10.1121/1.390037

Freyman, R. L., Helfer, K. S., McCall, D. D., and Clifton, R. K. (1999). The role of perceived spatial separation in the unmasking of speech. *J. Acoust. Soc. Am.* 106, 3578–3588. doi: 10.1121/1.428211

Gatehouse, S. (1999). A self-report outcome measure for the evaluation of hearing aid fittings and services. *Health Bull.* 57, 424–436.

Gatehouse, S., and Noble, W. (2004). The speech, spatial and qualities of hearing scale (SSQ). *Int. J. Audiol.* 43, 85–99. doi: 10.1080/14992020400050014

Hacker, M. J., and Ratcliff, R. (1979). A revised table of d′ for M-alternative forced choice. *Percept Psychophys.* 26, 168–170. doi: 10.3758/BF03208311

Hafter, E. R., Dye, R. H., and Gilkey, R. H. (1979). Lateralization of tonal signals which have neither onsets nor offsets. *J. Acoust. Soc. Am.* 65, 471–477. doi: 10.1121/1.382346

Hartmann, W. M., and Doty, S. L. (1996). On the pitches of the components of a complex tone. *J. Acoust. Soc. Am.* 99, 567–578.

Hopkins, K., and Moore, B. C. (2007). Moderate cochlear hearing loss leads to a reduced ability to use temporal fine structure information. *J. Acoust. Soc. Am.* 122, 1055–1068. doi: 10.1121/1.2749457

Hopkins, K., Moore, B. C., et al. (2008). Effects of moderate cochlear hearing loss on the ability to benefit from temporal fine structure information in speech. *J. Acoust. Soc. Am.* 123, 1140–1153. doi: 10.1121/1.2824018

Hopkins, K., and Moore, B. C. (2010a). The importance of temporal fine structure information in speech at different spectral regions for normal-hearing and hearing-impaired subjects. *J. Acoust. Soc. Am.* 127, 1595–1608. doi: 10.1121/1.3293003

Hopkins, K., and Moore, B. C. J. (2010b). Development of a fast method for measuring sensitivity to temporal fine structure information at low frequencies. *Int. J. Audiol.* 49, 940–946. doi: 10.3109/14992027.2010.512613

Hopkins, K., and Moore, B. C. J. (2011). The effects of age and cochlear hearing loss on temporal fine structure sensitivity, frequency selectivity, and speech reception in noise. *J. Acoust. Soc. Am.* 130, 334–349. doi: 10.1121/1.3585848

Houtgast, T., and Festen, J. M. (2008). On the auditory and cognitive functions that may explain an individual's elevation of the speech reception threshold in noise. *Int. J. Audiol.* 47, 287–295. doi: 10.1080/14992020802127109

Humes, L. E. (1999). Dimensions of hearing aid outcome. *J. Am. Acad. Audiol.* 10, 26–39.

Jeffress, L. A. (1948). A place theory of sound localization. *J. Comp. Physiol. Psychol.* 41, 35–39. doi: 10.1037/h0061495

Jensen, N. S., Akeroyd, M. A., Noble, W., and Naylor, G. (2009). "The Speech, Spatial and Qualities of Hearing scale (SSQ) as a benefit measure," in *NCRAR conference on The Ear-Brain System: Approaches to the Study and Treatment of Hearing Loss* (Portland, OR).

Lacher-Fougere, S., and Demany, L. (1998). Modulation detection by normal and hearing-impaired listeners. *Audiology* 37, 109–121. doi: 10.3109/00206099809072965

Lorenzi, C., Gilbert, G., Carn, C., Garnier, S., and Moore, B. C. J. (2006). Speech perception problems of the hearing impaired reflect inability to use temporal fine structure. *Proc. Natl. Acad. Sci. U.S.A.* 103, 18866–18869. doi: 10.1073/pnas.0607364103

Lunner, T. (2003). Cognitive function in relation to hearing aid use. *Int. J. Audiol.* 42, S49–S58. doi: 10.3109/14992020309074624

Moore, B. C. (2008). The role of temporal fine structure processing in pitch perception, masking, and speech perception for normal-hearing and hearing-impaired people. *J. Assoc. Res. Otolaryngol.* 9, 399–406. doi: 10.1007/s10162-008-0143-x

Moore, B. C., Glasberg, B. R., Stoev, M., Fullgrabe, C., and Hopkins, K. (2012). The influence of age and high-frequency hearing loss on sensitivity to temporal fine structure at low frequencies. *J. Acoust. Soc. Am.* 131, 1003–1006. doi: 10.1121/1.3672808

Moore, B. C. J., Glasberg, B. R., and Shailer, M. J. (1984). Frequency and intensity difference limens for harmonics within complex tones. *J. Acoust. Soc. Am.* 75, 550–561. doi: 10.1121/1.390527

Moore, B. C. J., Peters, R. W., and Stone, M. A. (1999). Benefits of linear amplification and multichannel compression for speech comprehension in backgrounds with spectral and temporal dips. *J. Acoust. Soc. Am.* 105, 400–411. doi: 10.1121/1.424571

Moore, B. C., and Skrodzka, E. (2002). Detection of frequency modulation by hearing-impaired listeners: effects of carrier frequency, modulation rate, and added amplitude modulation. *J. Acoust. Soc. Am.* 111(1 Pt 1), 327–335. doi: 10.1121/1.1424871

Neher, T., Behrens, T., Carlile, S., Jin, C., Kragelund, L., Petersen, A. S., et al. (2009). Benefit from spatial separation of multiple talkers in bilateral hearing-aid users: effects of hearing loss, age, and cognition. *Int. J. Audiol.* 48, 758–774. doi: 10.3109/14992020903079332

Perez, E., McCormack, A., and Edmonds, B. (2012). "Measuring sensitivity to temporal fine structure in older adults with sensori-neural hearing loss," in *Speech Perception and Auditory Disorders*, eds T. Dau, M. L. Jepsen, T. Poulsen, and J. C. Dalsgaard (Denmark: Centertryk A/S), 183–190.

Plomp, R., and Mimpen, A. M. (1979). Speech-reception threshold for sentences as a function of age and noise level. *J. Acoust. Soc. Am.* 66, 1333–1342. doi: 10.1121/1.383554

Strelcyk, O., and Dau, T. (2009). Relations between frequency selectivity, temporal fine-structure processing, and speech reception in impaired hearing. *J. Acoust. Soc. Am.* 125, 3328–3345. doi: 10.1121/1.3097469

Walden, T. C., and Walden, B. E. (2004). Predicting success with hearing aids in everyday living. *J. Am. Acad. Audiol.* 15, 342–352. doi: 10.3766/jaaa.15.5.2

Zurek, P. M. (1993). "Binaural advantages and directional effects in speech intelligibility," in *Acoustical Factors Affecting Hearing Aid Performance II*, eds G. A. Studebaker and I. Hochberg (Boston: Allyn and Bacon).

8

From ear to body: the auditory-motor loop in spatial cognition

Isabelle Viaud-Delmon[1,2,3]* and Olivier Warusfel[1,2,3]

[1] *CNRS, UMR 9912, Sciences et Technologies de la Musique et du Son, Paris, France*
[2] *Institut de Recherche et Coordination Acoustique/Musique, UMR 9912, Sciences et Technologies de la Musique et du Son, Paris, France*
[3] *Sorbonne Universités, Université Pierre et Marie Curie, UMR 9912, Sciences et Technologies de la Musique et du Son, Paris, France*

***Correspondence:**
Isabelle Viaud-Delmon, CNRS, UMR 9912, Institut de Recherche et Coordination Acoustique/Musique, 1 place Igor Stravinsky, 75004 Paris, France
e-mail: isabelle.viauddelmon@gmail.com

Spatial memory is mainly studied through the visual sensory modality: navigation tasks in humans rarely integrate dynamic and spatial auditory information. In order to study how a spatial scene can be memorized on the basis of auditory and idiothetic cues only, we constructed an auditory equivalent of the Morris water maze, a task widely used to assess spatial learning and memory in rodents. Participants were equipped with wireless headphones, which delivered a soundscape updated in real time according to their movements in 3D space. A wireless tracking system (video infrared with passive markers) was used to send the coordinates of the subject's head to the sound rendering system. The rendering system used advanced HRTF-based synthesis of directional cues and room acoustic simulation for the auralization of a realistic acoustic environment. Participants were guided blindfolded in an experimental room. Their task was to explore a delimitated area in order to find a hidden auditory target, i.e., a sound that was only triggered when walking on a precise location of the area. The position of this target could be coded in relationship to auditory landmarks constantly rendered during the exploration of the area. The task was composed of a practice trial, 6 acquisition trials during which they had to memorize the localization of the target, and 4 test trials in which some aspects of the auditory scene were modified. The task ended with a probe trial in which the auditory target was removed. The configuration of searching paths allowed observing how auditory information was coded to memorize the position of the target. They suggested that space can be efficiently coded without visual information in normal sighted subjects. In conclusion, space representation can be based on sensorimotor and auditory cues only, providing another argument in favor of the hypothesis that the brain has access to a modality-invariant representation of external space.

Keywords: spatial audition, Morris water maze, auditory landmarks, virtual reality, navigation, spatial memory, allocentric representation, auditory scene

INTRODUCTION

We perceive the world around us through multiple senses. When we explore an environment, we produce idiothetic information through vestibular receptors, muscle and joint receptors, and efference copy of commands that generate movement. Visual, auditory, and olfactory stimuli caused by movement can also be used to encode our spatial environment. However, spatial cognition has mainly been studied in experimental situations without auditory information: View-based approaches for spatial memory are the most common. For example, with very few exceptions (e.g., Loomis et al., 1998, 2001; Afonso et al., 2010), landmark based navigation has been studied in vision.

The Morris water maze test is a classical paradigm used to evaluate spatial learning in animal models (Morris, 1981, 1984). It requires the animal to locate a hidden platform, using available room cues, which is submerged below the surface of a large circular arena filled with opaque water. The manipulation of available visual information allows for the determination of the types of cues that are used to solve the task. The Morris water maze has been widely used to investigate which brain structures are involved in spatial memory, and has largely contributed to the discovery of "place cells." Place cells fire when an animal is at a specific location in an environment, providing a stable representation, independent of orientation, of the animal's location.

The Morris water task has been adapted to humans in real settings (e.g., Bohbot et al., 2002) and in virtual environments. Virtual reality analogues have been developed and tested in humans for more than 15 years (e.g., Jacobs et al., 1998; Moffat et al., 1998; Sandstrom et al., 1998; Astur et al., 1998; Hamilton and Sutherland, 1999; Chamizo et al., 2003), all of which centered on the visual modality. As in the water maze, participants are required to find a platform (hidden target) surrounded by a set of landmarks. In rodents, few studies have integrated the auditory modalities in their Morris water maze tasks (Rossier et al., 2000; Watanabe and Yoshida, 2007). Likely due to the difficulty in mastering the acoustic parameters of an experimental environment not conceived for auditory experiments, the results of these studies are not convincing.

We created a virtual sound scene composed of landmarks surrounding a hidden target. We asked participants to actively explore this scene in order to learn to locate the target on the basis of cues provided by the auditory-motor loop. It is known that to localize sound requires the integration of multisensory information and the processing of self-generated movements, therefore a stable representation of an auditory source has to be based on acoustic inputs and their relation to motor states (Aytekin et al., 2008). Here we hypothesized that auditory and motor cues would constitute relevant enough information to build a spatial representation of the scene in the absence of any visual cue.

We devised tests to ascertain which aspects of the organization of the landmarks were involved in determining the locus of search and to understand whether the principles of spatial cognition that have been largely developed on the basis of vision hold as general principles independent of the sensory modality or, conversely, are completely dependent on the stimulated sensory modality.

After the acquisition phase, we first investigated whether the most proximal auditory landmark was used to find the target. In a second test, we maintained the adjacency relations of the landmarks but modified their distance with the target. In a third test, we altered the adjacency relationship between landmarks from those that were learned, creating a conflict between landmark location ("where") and landmark type ("what"). Alterations were made such that one landmark location in the testing configuration maintained identical distance relationships as they were in the learning configuration. In a last test, the boundaries of the surface layout were modified.

It has been suggested that geometric cues are processed separately from non-geometric cues (e.g., Wang and Spelke, 2000; Cheng, 2008), and that different brain activations are associated with boundary-related locations and landmark-related locations (Doeller et al., 2008). There is also a segregation between auditory cortical pathways for the identification and localization of objects (e.g., Rauschecker and Tian, 2000; Ahveninen et al., 2013). We thought that altering the identity of a landmark independently of its location might be a way to distinguish object-related patterns (what) from spatial patterns (where). We therefore expected that the difficulties the participants encountered would be different in function of modifications of the geometrical configuration of the landmarks (like in test 1—Removal and test 2—Rotation), the identity of the landmarks (as in test 3—Switch), or the boundary of the surface layout (as in test 4—Perimeter).

MATERIALS AND METHODS

PARTICIPANTS

Eleven participants (6 females and 5 males; 26.7 ± 4.1 years old) took part in the experiment. All were healthy and reported normal hearing. The study was carried out in accordance with the Declaration of Helsinki. After an explanation of the procedure, all participants signed informed consent releases.

EXPERIMENTAL SETUP

The participants were equipped with wireless headphones, which delivered an auditory virtual environment updated in real time in accordance with their movements in 3D space. A wireless tracking system (video infrared with passive markers) was used to send the coordinates of the subject's head to the sound rendering system with a refreshing rate of 60 Hz. We used the Spat∼ sound rendering engine (Jot and Warusfel, 1995; Jot, 1999) and the ListenSpace auditory scene authoring tool (Delerue and Warusfel, 2002), both developed at Ircam. The rendering system used advanced HRTF-based synthesis of directional cues and room acoustic simulation for the auralization of a realistic acoustic environment. Moving in the virtual environment would for instance modify the level and direction of the direct sound and of the first reflections of each source landmark according to its position and orientation relative to the participant's head. Participants were selected among people whose HRTFs had been previously measured to constitute the Listen HRTF database (http://recherche.ircam.fr/equipes/salles/listen/). Hence, the auditory virtual environment could be rendered binaurally using their individual HRTFs.

Exploration area and auditory virtual environment

The experimental room was 25 × 17 m^2 in size. The auditory virtual environment consisted of 3 distinct landmarks, a target location within the triangle formed by the 3 landmarks, and a delimitated exploration area (see **Figure 1**). Because the landmarks were distinct, semantic information about landmark identity was available.

The landmarks were located in the periphery of a zone covering a surface of 22 m^2, the exploration area, centered in the experimental room. The following three familiar and distinct sound samples were used as constantly active auditory landmarks: a melody played on a piano, a text read by a male voice, and a cicada. The choice of these sound samples was guided by the following criteria: they should be easy to discriminate on the basis of acoustic features (spectro-temporal content) as well as high level semantic content. Moreover they should be constantly active i.e., without periods of silence or abrupt changes. They were positioned on a horizontal plane at 1.60 m from the ground, i.e., on average slightly above the participant's sight level. The three landmarks were equalized so that their rms levels were identical (±1 dB) when the listener was located at the center of the exploration area. An auditory border delineated the exploration area. Whenever the participant crossed the limits of the exploration area a non spatialized sound of wind was rendered and the auditory landmarks were muted. In this case, the participant was instructed to come back inside the area whereupon she/he would be again immersed in the virtual environment. The hidden auditory target was located in a 60 × 60 cm zone. When walking on this zone, the participant activated the non spatialized sound of a whistle.

EXPERIMENTAL PROCEDURE

The experiment lasted 2 h and was composed of a practice trial, 6 acquisition trials, and 4 test trials, each respectively immediately followed by an additional acquisition trial. The experiment ended with a probe trial.

The participants were led blindfolded into the experimental room and remained blindfolded until the end of the experiment. In order to avoid the construction of any mental preset

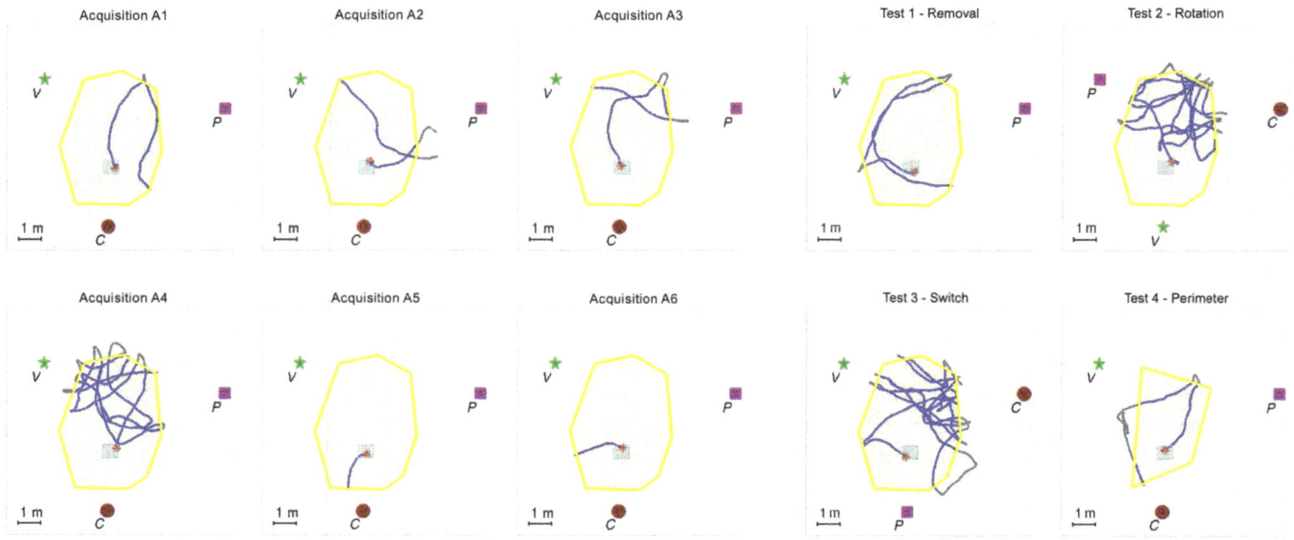

FIGURE 1 | Example of individual data for one participant. The experimental setup is composed of 3 auditory landmarks (red spot, green star and purple square, respectively labeled C for cicada, V for voice, and P for piano) surrounding the exploration zone (area = 22 m^2) delineated by the yellow auditory border (wind heard when outside); "hidden" auditory target (gray squared frame; 40 cm^2) triggering a whistle tone. The same configuration was maintained for the six acquisition trials, labeled from A1 to A6 (left). During the four test trials (right), the auditory landmarks configuration or the shape of the exploration area were modified.

about the space in which they were to perform the task, participants were blindfolded before entering the experimental room. To acclimate the participants with using a locomotor mode without vision, the participants were guided around the room in a preliminary acclimatization phase, after which the experiment started.

Practice (1 trial)

The participant walked in the exploration area to get used to the system and the soundscape. She/he had to search for the hidden auditory target (whistle tone) which was only triggered when entering and standing in a small zone (60 × 60 cm) located within the exploration area. If the participant did not find the target within 2 min, the practice trial terminated and she/he was guided outside of the exploration area, whilst hearing a non-spatialized masking sound (rolling pebbles).

The participants were instructed that their task during the next trials of the experiment was to find a similar target that would be hidden in a different location. Furthermore, they were instructed that the target location would henceforward remain the same for each subsequent trial.

Acquisition phase (6 trials)

The task of the participant was to search for, find, and stand on an initially inaudible target on the arena floor. When the participant found and stood on the target, it became audible, but reverted to being inaudible should the participant moved off it. As soon as the participant had found the target, the trial ended: the target sound and the auditory landmarks were then switched off and replaced with the non-spatialized masking sound (rolling pebbles) that was played until the commencement of the next trial.

Between each trial, the participant was randomly walked around in the experimental room to prevent any knowledge of the surrounding space. For each trial, lasting a maximum of 3 min, the participant started the exploration from a different entry point.

Test phase (4 tests)

For the test phase, the participant was informed that the location of the hidden target was identical to that of the hidden target in the acquisition phase, but that some aspects of the auditory landscape will have been changed from trial to trial.

There were four different conditions for this phase. In the first condition, the most proximal auditory landmark (cicada) was removed, therefore modifying the geometrical configuration of the landmarks (a line rather than a triangle), thus allowing for an evaluation of the participant's reliance on both the triangular configuration and the most proximal landmark (Test 1—Removal). In the second condition, all three auditory landmarks were rotated with respect to the exploration area and the location of the hidden target. As such, the distance relations between the exploration area, the hidden target, and the landmarks were all modified, whereas the geometrical configuration of the landmarks remained the same (Test 2—Rotation). In the third condition, the positions of two of the auditory landmarks (cicada and piano) were switched, while the third one remained unchanged (Test 3—Switch). In the fourth one, the auditory landmarks were unchanged, but the shape of the exploration area perimeter was modified (Test 4—Perimeter). Each of the test trials (capped at 3 min) was immediately followed by the initial configuration used in the acquisition trials in order to reaffirm the participant's familiarity with the original soundscape.

Probe

The final trial was a probe trial that had no more hidden target: the participants were regardless given the same, now impossible, task of finding the hidden target. This trial ended automatically after 2 min.

Debriefing

At the end of the experiment, the participants were guided blindfolded outside of the experimental room. They were then asked to draw a map of the soundscape that they had learnt and to comment on the experience.

DATA ANALYSIS

As the participants explored the environment, the position and orientation of their heads were recorded on average every 60 ms (15 Hz) and subsequently used to calculate their paths taken during the different phases of the experiment (**Figure 1**).

From these recordings, we assessed search time, i.e., the time to reach the hidden target, path length, and boundary crossings for all the trials. In order to study the effect of the tests, the following performance measures were also calculated:

1. Percent quadrant time: Amount of time participants searched in a virtual quadrant (i.e., 25% of total exploration area).
2. Boundary crossing per quadrant: Number of times the participant crossed the boundary of the exploration area per virtual quadrant.

For the tests and probe trial we computed the spatial distribution of the time elapsed in the exploration area, i.e., the percentage of time spent in a given location.

RESULTS

There was a significant reduction of search time in finding the target across the 6 acquisition trials [repeated measures ANOVA, $F_{(5,\ 110)} = 2.86, p = 0.02$], indicating that participants had learnt how to find the hidden target (**Figure 2**). The number of boundary crossings and total length of the path covered followed the same pattern, diminishing with an increase in learning (**Table 1**).

Table 1 | Parameters of level of performance during the different phases of the experiment.

	Path length in m ± *SD*		Boundary crossings ± *SD*	
ACQUISITION PHASE (3 mn max)				
Trial 1	32.6	24.4	7.5	8.5
Trial 2	17	17.7	3.2	5.2
Trial 3	39.6	29.3	7.5	6.5
Trial 4	19.8	12.8	3.6	2.7
Trial 5	15.4	10	1.8	1.3
Trial 6	8.9	9.1	0.9	1.9
TEST PHASE (3 mn max)				
Test 1—Removal	10.2	7.8	1.5	2.1
Test 2—Rotation	55.7	22.2	11.7	4.7
Test 3—Switch	44.7	23.1	7.7	5.8
Test 4—Perimeter	8.3	7.6	1	1.3
Probe (2 mn)	58.7	21.9	8.6	3.8

Boundary crossings represent the number of times participants walked across the limits of the exploration area, triggering the sound of wind.

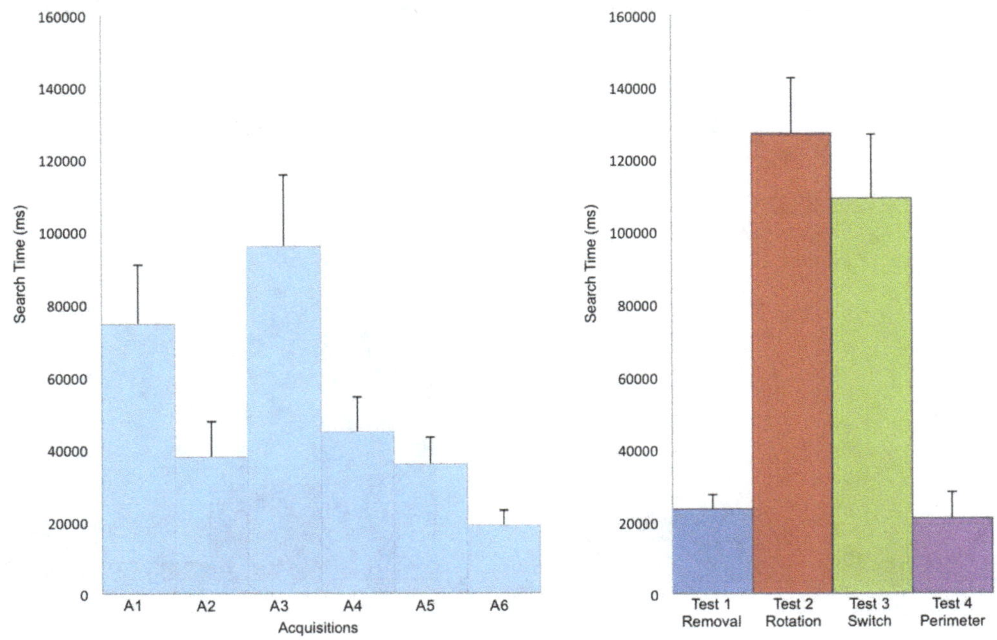

FIGURE 2 | Mean search time in ms to find the target during acquisition (A) and in the tests (B). Search time significantly decreases during the learning phase of the acquisition trials. Performances decreased when the landmarks were rotated (Test 2—Rotation) and when two landmarks were inverted (Test 3—Switch). Error bars represent the standard error of means.

The search time was different according to the modifications tested during the test (see **Figure 2**). The analysis of the virtual quadrants in the tests contrasted bias for the target location with other equivalent locations in the total area (**Figure 3**). Wilcoxon signed rank test indicated that in test 1—Removal (removal of a landmark), participants spent more time in the first quadrant (Q1), in which the target was located, than in the other quadrants (Q2, $z = 2.49$, $p = 0.01$; Q3, $z = 2.8$, $p < 0.01$; Q4, $z = 2.67$, $p < 0.01$). The absence of the closest landmark to the hidden target in Q1 did not seem to have a strong impact on their performance, as indicated by the mean search time. This suggests that the closest landmark to the target was not used as a beacon, but that the two other landmarks were equally used to localize the position of the target.

In test 2—Rotation (rotation of the 3 landmarks in relationship to the exploration area and to the hidden target) and test 3—Switch (inversion of two landmarks), the search time was much higher than in the two other tests. In both tests, both Q2 and Q3 were visited above the chance level: participants spent most of their time in those quadrants looking for the hidden target.

In test 2—Rotation, the manner in which the paths are distributed, clustered in Q2 and Q3, indicates that it is not a singular landmark that serves as a navigational beacon. It is rather the relationship between landmarks, put into evidence by the preserved geometry of the landmarks, and the respective distance between the cicada landmark and the target that seems to serve as the primary strategy (see **Figure 4**).

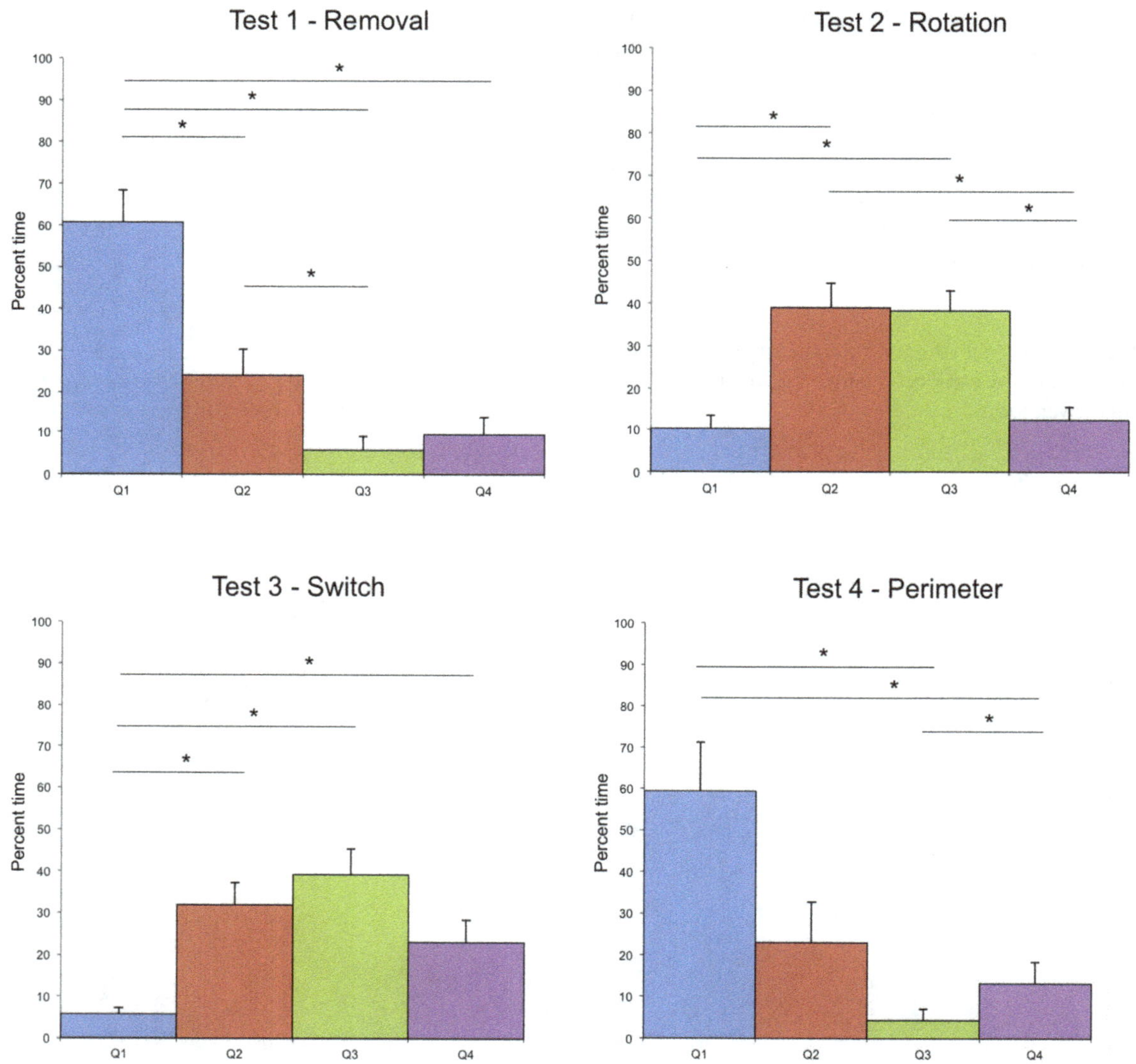

FIGURE 3 | Distribution of mean time spent in each quadrant of the exploration area in the four different tests. Error bars represent the standard error of means, *indicates significant differences. Test 2—Rotation, Wilcoxon signed rank test indicates differences between Q1 and Q2, $z = 2.4$, $p = 0.02$; Q1 and Q3, $z = 2.7$, $p < 0.01$; Q2 and Q4, $z = 2.5$, $p = 0.01$; Q3 and Q4, $z = 2.6$, $p < 0.01$. Test 3—Switch, Wilcoxon signed rank test indicates differences between Q1 and Q2, $z = 2.9$, $p < 0.01$; Q1 and Q3, $z = 2.8$, $p < 0.01$; Q1 and Q4, $z = 2.7$, $p < 0.01$.

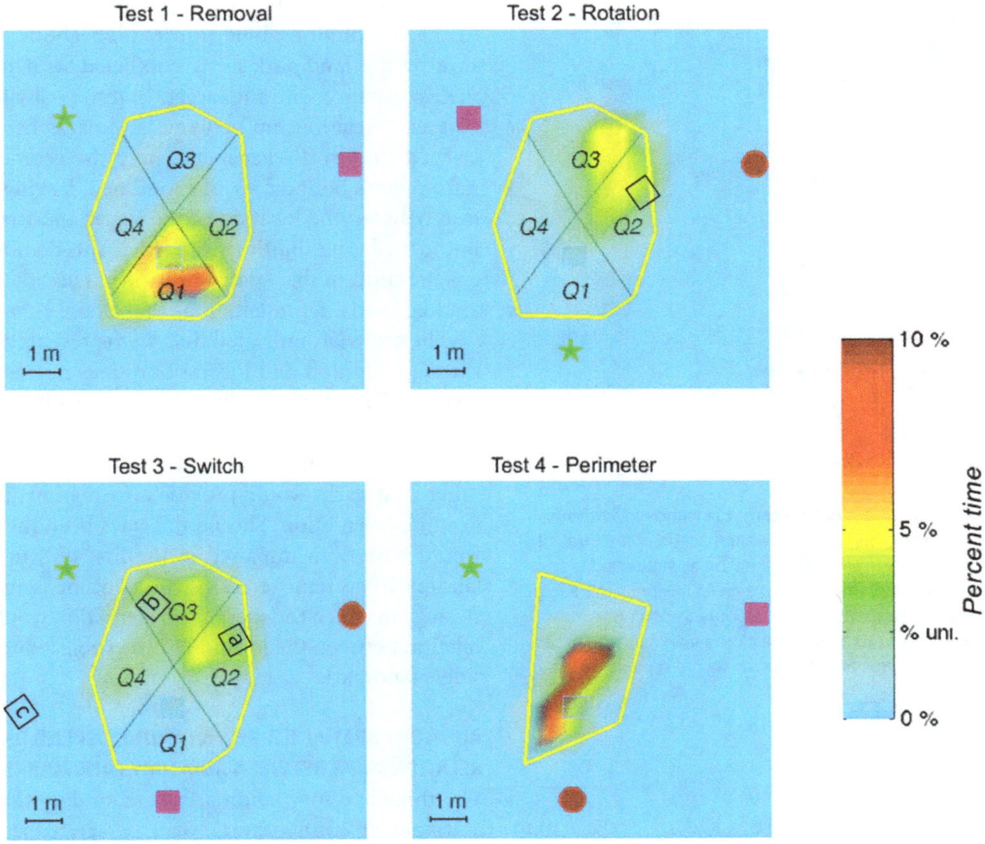

FIGURE 4 | The figure shows the spatial distribution of the time elapsed in the exploration area until the target was found and averaged on all subjects. Color shadings represent percentage of time spent in a given location. The tick label "% uni." on the scale corresponds to the hypothesis of a uniform spatial distribution. The actual position of the target is represented in gray. The red spot represents the cicada landmark, the green star represents the voice landmark, and the purple square represents the piano landmark. In Test 2—Rotation (landmarks rotation) and Test 3—Switch (inversion of 2 landmarks), the black squares represent different hypothetical positions of the target, corresponding to what could be tested by the participants according to their search strategy relative to the initial landmark configuration (angle and distance). Note that in Test 3—Switch, several possibilities could be explored by the participants, according to the characteristics of the auditory environment that was guiding the search (a- preservation of angle between landmarks with distance with cicada as a main cue, b- preservation of angle between landmarks with distance with piano as a main cue, c- preservation of angle between the piano and the voice, ignoring that the cicada is in the back instead of in front). If distance and angle to the voice landmark only were respected, while inversions of cicada and piano ignored, the target would remain located at the same place. The geometrical configuration of the landmarks seems to have been a strong cue in the search, whatever the test situation, as indicated by the heat maps.

In test 3—Switch, only Q1 was significantly different from the 3 other quadrants, which were equally visited, indicating an extension of the area of searching in this test. Indeed, according to the search strategy adopted, several solutions could be investigated by the participant to find the target (**Figure 4**). One of them would lead directly to the target (preservation of distance with the voice landmark together with a preservation of the geometrical organization of the 3 landmarks). This might account for the extension of the search area, and for the shorter search time than in test 2—Rotation.

In test 4—Perimeter (modification of the perimeter of the exploration area), the first quadrant was not significantly more visited than Q2 ($z = 1.5$, $p = 0.1$) and Q2 and Q3 were only marginally significantly different ($z = 1.8$, $p = 0.08$). This might be due to the efficiency of the participants in finding the target in this test, which permitted the participants to maintain the same search pattern across the quadrants. It seems that the modification of the perimeter of the exploration area did not impair the search strategy of the participants (see **Figures 1, 2**).

The analysis of boundary crossing per quadrant led to the same observations than with percent quadrant time, except in test 2—Rotation during which the amount of boundary crossings were slightly higher in Q2 than in Q3 ($z = 1.9$, $p = 0.06$). In this test, the cicada landmark was located in front of Q2, and was more distant to the exploration area than during the acquisition phase. It is possible that participants crossed the boundary several times in this quadrant when attempting to walk toward the cicada, usually the most proximal to the target in the acquisition phase configuration.

For the probe trial (without the hidden target), the heat maps indicate that participants most extensively searched near the target's supposed location (**Figure 5**).

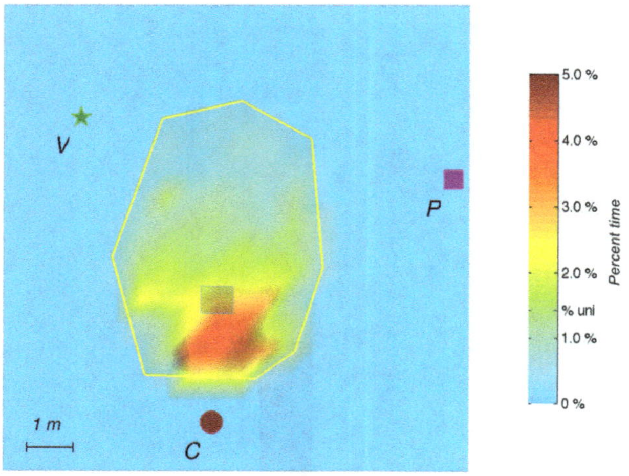

FIGURE 5 | During the Probe, the auditory target is removed without the subject being aware of it. The figure shows the spatial distribution of the time elapsed in the exploration area (2 min) and on all subjects. Color shadings represent percentage of time spent in a given location. The tick label "% uni." on the scale corresponds to the hypothesis of a uniform spatial distribution. The red spot represents the cicada landmark, the green star represents the voice landmark, and the purple square represents the piano landmark.

DEBRIEFING

After the experiment, participants were asked to draw a map of the environment, marking the auditory landmarks and commenting on their strategy. All subjects accurately represented the triangular structure of the landmarks and its relationship to the target, with more or less precision but sometimes with stunning accuracy. Six participants drew instinctively a shape to define the exploration area: circular (4 participants) or rectangular (2 participants). The remaining five participants drew only the auditory sound sources and the target. No participants reported having built a visual mental imagery of the scene. Some participants were able to indicate what the modifications of the auditory landmarks were during the test phase. Only one participant suggested that the shape of the exploration area was different in the last test. One participant reported a path strategy to find the target, following a route along which the target would be found. Six participants described the usage of the angles between the landmarks, half of them also using the distance between the landmarks and the distance with the boundaries of the search area. One participant represented one of the landmarks position without being able to identify it, having forgotten its semantic content.

DISCUSSION

In this experiment, we wanted to explore whether spatial representation in blindfolded, normally sighted participants could be based on sensorimotor and auditory cues only. As indicated by the diminution of search time in the acquisition trials, and by the spatial distribution of the search paths in the probe test, participants had indeed learnt the spatial location of a hidden target without any visual information. The location of the target was surrounded by a set of landmarks. In test 1—Removal, we removed a landmark. In test 2—Rotation, because the geometrical configuration of the landmarks remained the same but was rotated with respect to the exploration zone, information about the target's enclosure by the landmark array conflicted with information about metric distance with the target. In test 3—Switch, we altered the adjacency relationship between landmarks from those that were learned. In test 4—Perimeter, only the geometry of the exploration area's boundaries was modified, leaving the angular relation between the location of the target and the set of landmarks untouched. The abilities that participants demonstrated strengthens the concept that spatial hearing has access to mechanisms for amodal spatial representations (Lakatos, 1993).

The test trials indicated that the representation of space learnt through audition and locomotion does not depend on auditory beacons. The cicada landmark was particularly salient because of its proximity to the boundary: we were thus expecting it to be used as a beacon, marking the nearby hidden target, and that other landmarks would provide information about one's current heading orientation. Should this have been the case, participants would have been impaired in the first test, in which the cicada landmark was removed. This rules out the usage of an egocentric strategy in which the spatial representation would be based on the relation between the location of the subject and the location of a single landmark.

AUDITORY SPATIAL REPRESENTATIONS DEPEND ON GEOMETRIC RELATIONSHIPS BETWEEN AUDITORY LANDMARKS

The three auditory landmarks surrounding the hidden target in a triangular configuration were perceived as one triangle and not as three individual objects, as would be the case with visual objects. The geometry of the exploration array was not coded precisely since there was no coding of a "room," but of individual relationships between walls (acoustically transparent boundary) and landmarks. In audition, there is no enduring representation of environment geometry that serves as a basis for reorientation. In visual environments, the geometric structure surface layout is said to persist much longer than the geometric relationships between distinct objects (Wang and Spelke, 2000). This might be an essential distinction in the contribution of these two sensory modalities to spatial knowledge. Whereas with vision, humans reorient themselves in accordance with the shape of the environment, they cannot do so with audition.

If the general shape of the room did not play a role in the representation of the auditory space, the boundary was a crucial cue (as suggested by the amount of boundary crossings in the different tests), just like in experiments with vision (Hartley et al., 2004). Subjects had to use distal landmark information as well as distance to the exploration area boundary to locate the hidden target. In the water maze tested with rodents, the maze walls are powerful cues used to locate the hidden platform even when they are transparent (Maurer and Derivaz, 2000). Boundaries of the environment play an important role in determining the place cells representation, and do so to an extent depending on their proximity (O'Keefe and Burgess, 1996).

DIRECT ACCESS TO AN ALLOCENTRIC REPRESENTATION THROUGH AUDITION

A major distinction has always been made between spatial representations linked to the observer (egocentric representations) and those that are independent from the observer (allocentric representations). Does this dichotomy exist for auditory perception? Because we can perceive the world only from our own position, it has been proposed that we create allocentric representations only through transformations of egocentric representations (e.g., Nadel and Hardt, 2004). However, this might not be true for auditory information, which might constitute a powerful input to the building of allocentric representations in real-world conditions.

Here we show that under the present experimental conditions, representations that underline place recognition were not purely egocentric: respective distances and directions of all features in the environment seemed to be the features that were looked for by the participants. Patterns of travel did not provide evidence that participants learnt to turn in specific directions at particular places. Only one participant reported at debriefing that his turning decisions depended on local representations of landmarks rather than on a global representation of the scene. However, this participant was perfectly able to draw an allocentric representation of the surface layout. Our results therefore favor the proposition of Holmes and Sholl (2005), stating that spatial information are stored in an allocentric reference system on which is superimposed an egocentric reference system depending on the position that is physically taken by the subject.

Humans may develop distinct types of environmental knowledge on the basis of different sensory cues (Yamamoto and Shelton, 2005). Because visual information is intimately linked to an eye-centered frame of reference, which is forward facing, it may provide an essential basis for landmark coding. Because auditory information allows for the perception of objects outside of reach and vision, they may provide not only egocentric (craniocentric) space representations, but also a direct access to allocentric coding of landmarks in space. Audition gives access to landmarks that are stable: they provide sensory inputs even when the subject turns his/her head from them. It is a crucial difference, which might be the key to the allocentric coding of an auditory scene. We therefore propose that auditory dynamic information allows for a direct coding of space in an allocentric manner.

MOVEMENT TO CALIBRATE SPACE

In the current experiment we could not test any specific hypothesis regarding sensorimotor information and auditory information and how they relate to each other. An additional condition would be to ask the participant to move passively in the auditory scene, e.g., by controlling his/her navigation through a joystick. We have started to test this condition, and preliminary results suggest that learning of the spatial location of the hidden target is impaired when there is an absence of any visual and sensorimotor information linked to self-movement. Further experiments are needed to understand how acoustic inputs are related to motor states and which parameters of the auditory-motor loop are relevant for the building of spatial representations.

Because spatial audition is mainly studied in humans with a fixed position in space, the possibilities of human spatial audition to encode space are often underestimated. There is a gap in the literature on spatial cognition in humans and in animals. In rodents, major categories of spatial cells have been discovered (place cells, head direction cells, grid cells and boundary cells), each of which having a characteristic firing pattern that encodes spatial parameters relating to the animal's current position and orientation (see Hartley et al., 2013 for a recent review). For these experiments, the animals move freely in an arena, integrating sensorimotor cues together with other sensory cues. In humans, it is very seldom that sensorimotor integration is taken into account when studying spatial cognition. This is also the case when studying spatial auditory cognition, which is mainly studied in deprivation of other senses. In spite of the rarity of studies in audition taking movement into account, it has already been suggested that auditory localization processes combine the acoustic input with head position information to encode targets in a body-centered frame rather than an external visual frame of reference (Goossens and van Opstal, 1999), and that dynamically varying acoustic cues are adequately processed to build a representation in world coordinate (Vliegen et al., 2004).

The role of visual information to calibrate auditory spatial cognition has been underlined by many (e.g., Hofman et al., 1998; Zwiers et al., 2003; Sarlat et al., 2006; King, 2009). More recently, the role of sensorimotor calibration of audition emerges as very significant (Aytekin et al., 2008; Boyer et al., 2013; Carlile and Blackman, 2013; Carlile et al., 2014). Here we provide data attesting that when humans can use sensorimotor information, their spatial map of an auditory space is very accurate. When perceived in movement, auditory information is probably of paramount importance to sense space, even in normal sighted humans. The motor calibration of auditory space connects the ear to the body and to the space around us.

ACKNOWLEDGMENT

This work was supported by the French program DEFISENS from the CNRS MI, project Supplé-Sens.

REFERENCES

Afonso, A., Blum, A., Katz, B. F., Tarroux, P., Borst, G., and Denis, M. (2010). Structural properties of spatial representations in blind people: Scanning images constructed from haptic exploration or from locomotion in a 3-D audio virtual environment. *Mem. Cogn.* 38, 591–604. doi: 10.3758/MC.38.5.591

Ahveninen, J., Huang, S., Nummenmaa, A., Belliveau, J. W., Hung, A. Y., Jääskeläinen, I. P., et al. (2013). Evidence for distinct human auditory cortex regions for sound location versus identity processing. *Nat. Comm.* 4:2585. doi: 10.1038/ncomms3585

Astur, R. S., Ortiz, M. L., and Sutherland, R. J. (1998). A characterization of performance by men and women in a virtual morris water task: a large and reliable sex difference. *Behav. Brain Res.* 93, 185–190. doi: 10.1016/S0166-4328(98)00019-9

Aytekin, M., Moss, C. E., and Simon, J. Z. (2008). A sensorimotor approach to sound localization. *Neural Comput.* 20, 603–635. doi: 10.1162/neco.2007.12-05-094

Bohbot, V. D., Jech, R., Růzicka, E., Nadel, L., Kalina, M., Stepánková, K., et al. (2002). Rat spatial memory tasks adapted for humans: characterization in subjects with intact brain and subjects with medial temporal lobe lesions. *Physiol. Res.* 51, S49–S64.

Boyer, E. O., Babayan, B. M., Bevilacqua, F., Noisternig, M., Warusfel, O., Roby-Brami, A., et al. (2013). From ear to hand: the role of the auditory-motor loop in pointing to an auditory source. *Front. Comput. Neurosci.* 7:26. doi: 10.3389/fncom.2013.00026

Carlile, S., Balachandar, K., and Kelly, H. (2014). Accommodating to new ears: the effects of sensory and sensory-motor feedback. *J. Acoust. Soc. Am.* 135, 2002–2011. doi: 10.1121/1.4868369

Carlile, S., and Blackman, T. (2013). Relearning auditory spectral cues for locations inside and outside the visual field. *J. Assoc. Res. Otolaryngol.* 15, 249–263. doi: 10.1007/s10162-013-0429-5

Chamizo, V. D., Aznar-Casanova, J. A., and Artigas, A. A. (2003). Human overshadowing in a virtual pool: simple guidance is a good competitor against locale learning. *Learn. Motiv.* 34, 262–281. doi: 10.1016/S0023-9690(03)00020-1

Cheng, K. (2008). Whither geometry?: troubles of the geometric module. *Trends Cogn. Sci.* 12, 355–361. doi: 10.1016/j.tics.2008.06.004

Delerue, O., and Warusfel, O. (2002). "Authoring of virtual sound scenes in the context of the LISTEN project," in *Proceedings of the 22nd AES Conference* (Espoo), 39–47.

Doeller, C., King, J., and Burgess, N. (2008). Parallel striatal and hippocampal systems for landmarks and boundaries in spatial memory. *Proc. Natl. Acad. Sci. U.S.A.* 105, 5915–5920. doi: 10.1073/pnas.0801489105

Goossens, H. H., and van Opstal, A. J. (1999). Influence of head position on the spatial representation of acoustic targets. *J. Neurophysiol.* 81, 2720–2736.

Hamilton, D. A., and Sutherland, R. J. (1999). Blocking in human place learning: evidence from virtual navigation. *Psychobiology* 27, 453–461.

Hartley, T., Lever, C., Burgess, N., and O'Keefe, J. (2013). Space in the brain: how the hippocampal formation supports spatial cognition. *Philos. Trans. R. Soc. Lond. B Biol. Sci.* 369:20120510. doi: 10.1098/rstb.2012.0510

Hartley, T., Trinkler, I., and Burgess, N. (2004). Geometric determinants of human spatial memory. *Cognition* 94, 39–75. doi: 10.1016/j.cognition.2003.12.001

Hofman, P. M., Riswick, J. G. A. V., and Opstal, A. J. V. (1998). Relearning sound localization with new ears. *Nat. Neurosci.* 1, 417–421. doi: 10.1038/1633

Holmes, M. C., and Sholl, M. J. (2005). Allocentric coding of object-to-object relations in overlearned and novel environments. *J. Exp. Psychol. Learn. Mem. Cogn.* 31, 1069–1078. doi: 10.1037/0278-7393.31.5.1069

Jacobs, W. J., Thomas, K. G. F., Laurance, H. E., and Nadel, L. (1998). Place learning in virtual space II. Topographical relations as one dimension of stimulus control. *Learn. Motiv.* 29, 288–308. doi: 10.1006/lmot.1998.1008

Jot, J. M. (1999). Real-time spatial processing of sounds for music, multimedia and interactive human-computer interfaces. *Multimedia Syst.* 7, 55–69. doi: 10.1007/s005300050111

Jot, J. M., and Warusfel, O. (1995). "A real-time spatial sound processor for music and virtual reality applications," in *Proceedings of ICMC'95* (Banff, AB), 294–295.

King, A. J. (2009). Visual influences on auditory spatial learning. *Philos. Trans. R. Soc. B Biol. Sci.* 364, 331–339. doi: 10.1098/rstb.2008.0230

Lakatos, S. (1993). Recognition of complex auditory-spatial patterns. *Perception* 22, 363–374. doi: 10.1068/p220363

Loomis, J. M., Klatzky, R. L., and Golledge, R. G. (2001). Navigating without vision: basic and applied research. *Optom. Vis. Sci.* 78, 282–289. doi: 10.1097/00006324-200105000-00011

Loomis, J. M., Klatzky, R. L., Philbeck, J. W., and Golledge, R. G. (1998). Assessing auditory distance perception using perceptually directed action. *Percept. Psychophys.* 60, 966–980. doi: 10.3758/BF03211932

Maurer, R., and Derivaz, V. (2000). Rats in a transparent morris watermaze use elemental and configural geometry of landmarks as well as distance to the pool wall. *Spat. Cogn. Comput.* 2, 135–156. doi: 10.1023/A:1011477931753

Moffat, S. D., Hampson, E., and Hatzipantelis, M. (1998). Navigation in a "virtual" maze: sex differences and correlation with psychometric measures of spatial ability in humans. *Evol. Hum. Behav.* 19, 73–87. doi: 10.1016/S1090-5138(97)00104-9

Morris, R. G. M. (1981). Spatial localization does not require the presence of local cues. *Learn. Motiv.* 12, 239–260. doi: 10.1016/0023-9690(81)90020-5

Morris, R. G. M. (1984). Developments of a water-maze procedure for studying spatial learning in the rat. *J. Neurosci. Methods* 11, 47–60. doi: 10.1016/0165-0270(84)90007-4

Nadel, L., and Hardt, O. (2004). The spatial brain. *Neuropsychology* 18, 473–476. doi: 10.1037/0894-4105.18.3.473

O'Keefe, J., and Burgess, N. (1996). Geometric determinants of the place fields of hippocampal neurons. *Nature* 381, 425–428.

Rauschecker, J. P., and Tian, B. (2000). Mechanisms and streams for processing of "what" and "where" in auditory cortex. *Proc. Natl. Acad. Sci. U.S.A.* 97, 11800–11806. doi: 10.1073/pnas.97.22.11800

Rossier, J., Haeberli, C., and Schenk, F. (2000). Auditory cues support place navigation in rats when associated with a visual cue. *Behav. Brain Res.* 117, 209–214. doi: 10.1016/S0166-4328(00)00293-X

Sandstrom, N. J., Kaufman, J., and Huettel, S. A. (1998). Males and females use different distal cues in a virtual environment navigation task. *Cogn. Brain Res.* 6, 351–360. doi: 10.1016/S0926-6410(98)00002-0

Sarlat, L., Warusfel, O., and Viaud-Delmon, I. (2006). Ventriloquism aftereffects occur in the rear hemisphere. *Neurosci. Lett.* 404, 324–329. doi: 10.1016/j.neulet.2006.06.007

Vliegen, J., Van Grootel, T. J., and Van Opstal, A. J. (2004). Dynamic sound localization during rapid eye-head gaze shifts. *J. Neurosci.* 24, 9291–9302. doi: 10.1523/JNEUROSCI.2671-04.2004

Wang, R. F., and Spelke, E. S. (2000). Updating egocentric representations in human navigation. *Cognition* 77, 215–250. doi: 10.1016/S0010-0277(00)00105-0

Watanabe, S., and Yoshida, M. (2007). Auditory cued spatial learning in mice. *Physiol. Behav.* 92, 906–910. doi: 10.1016/j.physbeh.2007.06.019

Yamamoto, N., and Shelton, A. L. (2005). Visual and proprioceptive representations in spatial memory. *Mem. Cogn.* 33, 140–150. doi: 10.3758/BF03195304

Zwiers, M. P., Van Opstal, A. J., and Paige, G. D. (2003). Plasticity in human sound localization induced by compressed spatial vision. *Nat. Neurosci.* 6, 175–181. doi: 10.1038/nn999

9

Factors that account for inter-individual variability of lateralization performance revealed by correlations of performance among multiple psychoacoustical tasks

Atsushi Ochi*[1,2]*, Tatsuya Yamasoba*[2] *and Shigeto Furukawa*[1]

[1] *Human Information Science Laboratory, NTT Communication Science Laboratories, NTT Corporation, Atsugi, Japan*
[2] *Department of Otolaryngology, Faculty of Medicine, University of Tokyo, Tokyo, Japan*

***Correspondence:**
Shigeto Furukawa, Human Information Science Laboratory, NTT Communication Science Laboratories, NTT Corporation, 3-1 Morinosato-wakamiya, Atsugi, Kanagawa 243-0198, Japan
e-mail: furukawa.shigeto@lab.ntt.co.jp

This study explored the source of inter-listener variability in the performance of lateralization tasks based on interaural time or level differences (ITDs or ILDs) by examining correlation of performance between pairs of multiple psychoacoustical tasks. The *ITD*, *ILD*, *Time*, and *Level* tasks were intended to measure sensitivities to ITD; ILD; temporal fine structure or envelope of the stimulus encoded by the neural phase locking; and stimulus level, respectively. Stimuli in low- and high-frequency regions were tested. The low-frequency stimulus was a harmonic complex ($F_0 = 100$ Hz) that was spectrally shaped for the frequency region around the 11th harmonic. The high frequency stimulus was a "transposed stimulus," which was a 4-kHz tone amplitude-modulated with a half-wave rectified 125-Hz sinusoid. The task procedures were essentially the same between the low- and high-frequency stimuli. Generally, the thresholds for pairs of ITD and ILD tasks, across cues or frequencies, exhibited significant positive correlations, suggesting a common mechanism across cues and frequencies underlying the lateralization tasks. For the high frequency stimulus, there was a significant positive correlation of performance between the ITD and Time tasks. A significant positive correlation was found also in the pair of ILD and Level tasks for the low- frequency stimulus. These results indicate that the inter-listener variability of ITD and ILD sensitivities could be accounted for partially by the variability of monaural efficiency of neural phase locking and intensity coding, respectively, depending of frequency.

Keywords: interaural time difference, interaural level difference, level discrimination, correlation, temporal fine structure, phase locking

INTRODUCTION

Performance in lateralization tasks based on interaural time and level differences (ITDs or ILDs), the major cues for horizontal sound localization, often varies markedly among listeners. Lateralization behavior is a product of multiple stages of auditory processing, and thus the listener's performance should reflect the efficiencies of the individual processes by varying degrees. We consider that the processing of the ITD or the ILD in the auditory system consist of two or more stages. The earliest is the peripheral stage, in which the auditory information is processed individually for different ears. At this stage, the temporal structure and intensity of sounds at each ear are encoded to neural signals in the form of the timing and number of auditory nerve firings. The outputs of this stage of processing are fed to processes at the binaural interaction stage, where the relative timing and number of neural firings for the two ears are compared. This binaural interaction stage is followed by the subsequent higher-order processes.

The present study aimed to evaluate the relative contributions of these processing stages to the inter-listener variabilities in lateralization performance. We measured listeners' monaural sensitivities to the temporal structure and intensity of a sound stimulus, as well as their ITD and ILD sensitivities. The hypothesis was that the lateralization performance based on ITD is predominantly determined by the efficiency of temporal structure coding by neural phase-locking at the peripheral processing stage. If this is true, we would expect that the ITD-based lateralization performance correlates with the performance of a non-lateralization task, which reflects sensitivity to the temporal structure of the stimulus that is presumed to be represented by phase locking. A similar hypothesis and prediction are possible in terms of the relationship between ILD-based lateralization and peripheral intensity coding.

The authors are not aware of a study examining the extent to which monaural intensity (or level) encoding efficiency could account for individual differences in ILD sensitivity. On the other hand, the above hypothesis on the relationship between temporal structure coding and ITD sensitivity is supported by studies on the effects of aging and/or hearing-impairment. Groups of aged listeners (Strouse et al., 1998; Hopkins and Moore, 2011) with sensorineural hearing impairment (Strelcyk and Dau, 2009; Hopkins and Moore, 2011) and those with auditory neuropathy (Zeng et al., 2005) exhibited degraded performance more or less specific to the ITD-based lateralization task and to tasks that measure monaural sensitivity to temporal structure, in comparison to control groups. Within-listener correlation between the two types of tasks has also been reported. Strelcyk and Dau

(2009) found a positive correlation between the FM detection threshold (considered to be indicative of sensitivity to the temporal fine structure, TFS) and ITD-based lateralization threshold for hearing-impaired listeners (there was no report for normal-hearing listeners). A similar relationship between the monaural sensitivity to the TFS and the binaural sensitivity to interaural phase differences was also reported for a pooled population of young and aged listeners with and without hearing impairment (Hopkins and Moore, 2011). Nevertheless, it is uncertain whether the positive correlation could be applicable also to the population of normal-hearing listeners. A possibility is that a long-term impairment of a single mechanism (i.e., peripheral TFS coding) affects the efficiency of another independent mechanism (i.e., central binaural processing), leading to an apparent correlation of performance. Strouse et al. (1998) found a strong positive correlation between the monaural temporal-gap detection threshold and ITD discrimination threshold for a group of normal-hearing young listeners, although such a positive correlation was not found for aged listeners. It should be noted, however, that the gap detection task is considered to focus on the sensitivity to the temporal envelope, rather than on that to the cycle-by-cycle TFS of the stimulus.

A secondary aim of the present study was to examine whether mechanisms for processing the ITD (and ILD) are essentially the same across operating frequency regions. It has been argued that essentially the same binaural mechanism is involved in processing ITDs at low and high frequencies, and apparent differences in ITD sensitivities between the frequency regions reflect differences in input to the system (Van De Par and Kohlrausch, 1997; Bernstein, 2001): When high-frequency "transposed stimulus" (see Material and Methods) is used so that the pattern of neural phase locking to the envelope of the stimulus resembles that to TFS of a low-frequency stimulus, listeners' performance for ITD-related tasks should be comparable. Furukawa (2008), however, found that the degree of ITD and ILD cue interaction in lateralization tasks was smaller for low- than for high-frequency regions, even when the inputs to the binaural system were made comparable by using low-frequency tones and high-frequency transposed stimuli. This implies that a more-or-less independent ITD processor exists in the low frequency region, whereas in the high-frequency region, ITD is processed by a mechanism that is common for ILD processing. In this study, we used low- and high-frequency stimuli and examined the relationship between the lateralization tasks and the monaural temporal/intensity-related tasks for each type of the stimuli. Qualitatively different results between the stimulus types would imply the involvement of separate binaural mechanisms in lateralization depending on stimulus frequency.

MATERIALS AND METHODS

LISTENERS AND APPARATUS

Twenty-two adults (10 males and 12 females; 19–43 years old, mean 32.0) participated in the experiment as listeners. All gave written informed consent, which was approved by the Ethics Committee of NTT Communication Science Laboratories. The listeners showed normal audiometric thresholds (<25 dB HL) at frequencies of 250, 500, 1000, 2000, 4000, and 8000 Hz. They had no symptoms of hearing loss and had never been diagnosed as having hearing loss by medical examination. All testing took place in a double-walled sound booth. The listener was seated in front of a computer monitor, which displayed indicators for observation intervals of the forced-choice task and buttons for responses (described later).

Stimuli were digitally synthesized by a personal computer (sampling frequency: 44.1 kHz) and generated by using a digital-to-analog converter with a resolution of 24 bits (M-AUDIO, Transit USB). The signals were amplified and presented to the listener through Sennheiser HDA200 headphones.

MATLAB (Mathworks, Inc.) software was used for stimulus synthesis, experimental control, and data analyses.

STIMULI

The low- and high-frequency stimuli were designed to assess the listener's ability to use information based on neural phase-locking to the stimulus TFS and envelope, respectively, in the ITD and Time tasks. Essentially the same stimuli were used also in the ILD and Level tasks (See section Procedures for the descriptions of the four tasks).

The low-frequency stimulus was a spectrally shaped multi-component complex (SSMC), which was a harmonic complex with a fundamental frequency (F_0) of 100 Hz, consisting of the 7th to 14th harmonics. The components were added in the sine phase. We adopted stimulus parameters as in Moore and Moore (2003) to prevent the listener from using spectral cues (or the excitation-pattern cues) when conducting the tasks: The spectral envelope had a flat passband and sloping edges ($5 \times F_0$ centered at 1100 Hz).The overall level of the complex was 54 dB SPL. Threshold equalizing noise (TEN, Moore et al., 2000), extending from 125 to 15000 Hz, was added to mask combination tones and help ensure that the audible parts of the excitation patterns evoked by the harmonic and frequency-shifted tones were the same in the Time task (described later). The TEN level at 1 kHz was set at 30 dB/ERBN, which was 15 dB below the level of the 1100-Hz component.

The high-frequency stimulus was a "transposed stimulus," which was a 4-kHz tone carrier amplitude-modulated with a half-wave rectified 125-Hz sinusoid. It is considered that the auditory-nerve firing is phase locked to the modulator waveform, which provides the cue for judging the ITD and modulation rate of the stimulus (Van De Par and Kohlrausch, 1997; Bernstein, 2001). For the present stimulus, the modulation frequency of 125 Hz was chosen because that was the frequency with which human listeners exhibited the highest ITD sensitivity in the study by Bernstein and Trahiotis (2002).The overall level of the transposed stimulus was set to 65 dB SPL. A continuous, low-pass filtered Gaussian noise (cutoff frequency 1300 Hz; spectrum level 20 dB SPL) was added to prevent the listener from using any information at low spectral frequencies (e.g., combination tones).

PROCEDURES

General procedure

A two-interval two-alternative forced-choice (2I-2AFC) method was used to measure the listener's sensitivities to stimulus parameters. The listener was instructed to choose the "signal" interval by mouse-clicking one of two buttons displayed on a computer monitor or by pressing a corresponding key on a keyboard. Feedback was given to indicate the correct answer after each response. The two-down/one-up adaptive tracking method was used to estimate discrimination thresholds, corresponding to 70.7% correct (Levitt, 1970). One session of adaptive tracking lasted until twelve turnpoints were obtained. The first two sessions of each task and stimulus type were performed as practice sessions. When the tracking results appeared unstable for a listener with a task, two or three additional practice sessions were added for the listener/task/stimulus. A total of 8–10 sessions besides the practice sessions were conducted for each listener/task/stimulus. The thresholds were computed as the average of all the non-practice sessions. One session set consisted of two consecutive sessions for one task/stimulus. The order of session sets for tasks and stimuli were randomized for each subject in order to reduce the influence of the training and/or order effect.

Task specific procedures

ITD task. In a 2I-2AFC trial, stimuli in the two intervals had ITDs of $+\Delta$ITD/2 and $-\Delta$ITD/2 μs, respectively (positive and negative ITDs indicate right and left advances in time, respectively). Each stimulus was 400-ms long, including 100-ms raised-cosine onset and offset ramps. The raised cosine ramps at the onset and offset of the stimulus were synchronized between the two ears. Signal and non-signal intervals were separated by a 200-ms silent gap. The listeners were required to indicate the direction of the ITD change between the two intervals on the basis of the laterality of sound images. In each tracking session, ΔITD started from 100 to 400 μs, for low- or high-frequency stimuli, respectively. For the first four turnpoints, ΔITD was increased or decreased by a factor of $10^{0.2}$ after one incorrect response or two consecutive incorrect responses, and for the following eight turnpoints, the factor was reduced to $10^{0.05}$. The threshold for the session was computed as the geometric mean of the ΔITD at the last eight turnpoints.

ILD task. In a 2I-2AFC trial, stimuli in the two intervals had ILDs of $+\Delta$ILD/2 and $-\Delta$ILD/2 dB, respectively (positive and negative ILDs indicate higher and lower levels in the right ear, respectively). Each stimulus was 400-ms long, including 20-ms raised-cosine onset and offset ramps. The listeners were required to indicate the direction of the ILD change between the two intervals on the basis of the laterality of sound images. In each tracking session, ΔILD started from 2.5 dB. For the first four turnpoints, ΔILD was increased or decreased by 0.5 dB after one incorrect response or two consecutive incorrect responses, and for the following eight turnpoints, the step size was reduced to 0.25 dB. The threshold for the session was computed as the mean of the ΔILD at the last eight turnpoints. Other details were the same as in the ITD task.

Time task. For the low-frequency stimulus, the listeners were required to detect a common upward frequency shift (Δf Hz) imposed on the individual components of the SSMC with the spectral envelope remaining unchanged. The stimulus parameters and measurement methods for a detection threshold for the frequency shift was in accordance with the "TFS1" test developed by Moore and Sek (2009). It has been reported that such a shift in component frequencies is accompanied with shift in pitch (De Boer, 1956; Schouten et al., 1962; Moore and Moore, 2003). This pitch change was considered to be largely the result of changes in the TFS, since individual frequency components were only intermediately resolved in the auditory periphery (Moore and Moore, 2003) and frequency spacing (corresponding to the periodicity of the envelope) was unchanged. In addition, frequency shifts around a typical threshold value are expected to alter the peripheral excitation pattern by a negligible amount (Moore and Sek, 2009). Therefore, we adopted this task for evaluating the efficiency of neural phase locking to TFS. It should be noted that the pitch of the frequency-shifted SSMC is often ambiguous and listeners could base their judgments not on pitch shifts but on inharmonicity when conducting the tasks (De Boer, 1956; Schouten et al., 1962), and that it was not our intention to use this task for evaluating the pitch mechanism. The "signal" and "non-signal" intervals in the 2I-2AFC method contained RSRS and RRRR sequences, respectively, where R indicates a harmonic complex (i.e., original SSMC) as the reference and S indicates a frequency-shifted SSMC. The listener was required to indicate the signal interval (RSRS).

To assess the peripheral efficiencies of nerural phase locking to stimulus envelope at a high frequency, we adopted a task to measure discriminability of the transposed stimuli with modulation frequencies of 125 Hz and $125 + \Delta f_m$ Hz, referred to as R and S, respectively. Similarly to the low-frequency stimulus, the listener was required to indicate the signal interval (RSRS) as opposed to the non-signal interval (RRRR). When preforming this task, the listeners could base their judgments on changes in pitch associated with the modulation frequency, although the pitch sensation of the transposed stimulus is generally weak and ambiguous (Oxenham et al., 2004).

Commonly for the low- and high-frequency stimuli, an R or S tone had a duration of 100 ms, including 20-ms raised-cosine ramps. There were 100-ms silent intervals between the tones within a sequence in one interval, and there was a 300-ms silent gap between the intervals. In one session of adaptive tracking, Δf or Δf_m was increased or decreased by a factor of $2^{0.5}$ after one incorrect response and after two consecutive correct responses, respectively, for the first four turnpoints. The factor was reduced to $2^{0.25}$ for the following eight turnpoints. The geometric mean of Δf or Δf_m was computed across the last eight turnpoints, which represented the threshold for the session.

The maximum frequency shift, Δf, was limited to 50 Hz (i.e., $0.5 \times F_0$ Hz) in the adaptive tracking for the low-frequency stimulus. For three listeners, the adaptive tracking failed to converge within the maximum Δf limit (50 Hz) for at least one session. For those listeners, their performance was evaluated by the method of constant stimuli, instead of the adaptive method. Subjects were given the same instructions as for the adaptive procedure. A session consisted of 20 trials, and subjects completed five sessions. The Δf was fixed at the maximum value, 50 Hz. The proportion of correct responses was derived from the pooled responses across 10–12 sessions, and converted to d' (Hacker and Ratcliff, 1979). To make the results comparable to the measures obtained by the adaptive method, the threshold was derived on the assumption that d' is proportional to the frequency shift (Hopkins and Moore, 2007) and that the adaptive procedure tracked the 70.7% correct point on the psychometric function, which corresponds to a d' of 0.77 with a 2AFC task. This method sometimes yielded values of the threshold greater than the maximum Δf limit of 50 Hz. Although such large values of thresholds could not be measured empirically, they could be taken as indicators of the listeners' performance.

Level task. In a 2I-2AFC trial, the listeners were required to indicate an interval containing a 400-ms-long SSMC or a transposed stimulus whose central 200-ms portion (including 20-ms raised-cosine ramps) was incremented in level by ΔL dB, while the other non-signal interval contained an original SSMC or a transposed stimulus. In one session of adaptive tracking, ΔL started with 6 dB and was increased or decreased by a factor of 2.68 after one incorrect response and after two consecutive correct responses, respectively, for the first four turnpoints. The factor was reduced to 1.67 for the following eight turnpoints. The geometric mean of ΔL was computed across the last eight turnpoints, which represented the threshold for the session.

RESULTS

Threshold data for individual tasks and listeners are summarized in **Figure 1**. Each symbol and error bar represents the mean and standard error of thresholds of one listener obtained from multiple sessions. Within each task, the listeners are sorted according to the mean threshold. It should be noted that for the ITD and Time tasks, the means and standard errors are represented on a logarithmic scale. Note also that the thresholds for the low- and high-frequency Time tasks are expressed as fractions to F_0 (100 Hz) and modulation rate (125 Hz), respectively. The number in each panel indicates the average across the listeners. One listener (listener number: 10) exhibited an extremely large threshold in the high-frequency Level task (see the rightmost data in the corresponding panel). In the following sections, we report the results of correlation and multiple-regression analyses with and without this listener when they are related to the high-frequency Level task.

Figures 2–4 show scatter plots comparing individual listeners' thresholds between pairs of tasks. Each panel in the figures shows the data for one combination of tasks, representing 22 listeners with data points. For the Time and ITD tasks, we converted the thresholds to a logarithmic scale when plotting the data and computing the Pearson correlation coefficients.

LOW-FREQUENCY STIMULUS

Focusing on the results for the low-frequency stimulus (**Figure 2**), one can see statistically significant positive correlations for pairs of ITD and ILD tasks ($r = 0.55$; $p = 0.008$) and of ILD and Level tasks ($r = 0.67$; $p = 0.001$). The pair of Time and ITD tasks showed a weak negative correlation ($r = -0.26$), which was, however, not statistically significant ($p = 0.252$).

We used a multiple linear regression analysis to further explore the factors that might account for inter-individual variability in the lateralization tasks, which might not be revealed by the single correlation analysis. For a given lateralization task of interest ("target task"; i.e., ITD or ILD task), we regarded the threshold for that task as the dependent variable and the thresholds for the remaining three tasks as the explanatory variables. A significant partial correlation of an explanatory task would suggest that the performance of that explanatory task is a good predictor of the performance of the target task. The size of partial correlation coefficient for each explanatory variable could be interpreted as indicating the size of the effect of the variable (or of mechanisms behind the variable) on the performance of the target task, given the values of the other variables are fixed.

The regression analyses were conducted on the threshold data which had been transformed to z scores (i.e., having a mean of 0 and a standard deviation of 1), for individual tasks. Estimated values of partial correlation coefficients are summarized in **Table 1**, along with p values indicating whether the coefficient was significantly different from zero. For the ITD task as the target, the partial correlation coefficient was significant for the ILD task ($p = 0.015$). As for the ILD task as the target, the coefficients for the ITD and Level tasks were significant ($p = 0.015$ and 0.008, respectively).

HIGH-FREQUENCY STIMULUS

Comparisons between the thresholds of the task types for the high-frequency stimulus are represented in **Figure 3**. Significant correlation were found for pairs of the ITD and ILD tasks ($r = 0.66$, $p = 0.001$), and of the ITD and Time tasks ($r = 0.43$, $p = 0.045$). The correlation of the ILD and Level tasks was not significant ($r = 0.41$, $p = 0.056$; $r = 0.24$, $p = 0.295$, when listener 10 was excluded).

The results of the multiple linear regression analysis are shown in **Table 1**. Consistent with the results of the single correlation analysis, the partial correlation coefficients of the ILD and Time tasks were significant when the ITD task was the target ($p = 0.001$ and 0.026, respectively). The coefficint of the ITD task was significant when the ILD was the target task ($p = 0.001$). Exclusion of listener 10 did not affect the general conclusions of the analysis.

ACROSS-FREQUENCY COMPARISONS

The correlation of task performance across frequencies can be examined in **Figure 3**. When comparing the thresholds for the same task type, one can see that the correlations were significant for all the tasks except the Time task ($r = 0.56, p = 0.007$ for ITD; $r = 0.57, p = 0.005$ for ILD; $r = 0.08, p = 0.721$ for Time; $r = 0.57, p = 0.006$ for Level). The correlation for the Level tasks, however, became non-significant when listener 10 was excluded ($r = 0.31$, $p = 0.165$). A significant correlation for different task types was found in the combination of low-frequency ITD and high-frequency ILD tasks ($r = 0.67$, $p = 0.001$). Significant correlations across frequency regions imply an across-frequency factor that determined the performance of a given task for a frequency region.

Here again, we conducted a multiple linear regression analysis using thresholds (in z scores) of all the combinations of task and stimulus as independent variables. In this analysis, we were specifically interested in the extent to which the performance of one lateralization task could be accounted for by the performances of other tasks, whether the stimuli were in the same or remote

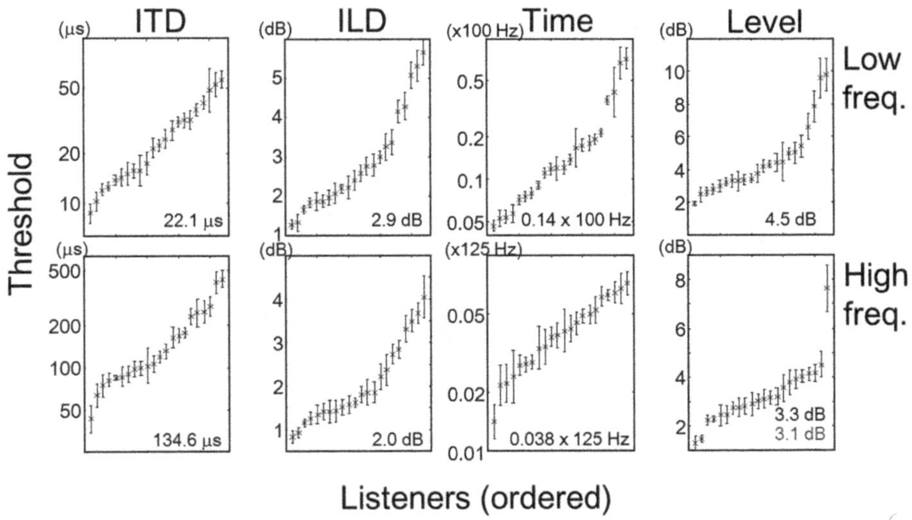

FIGURE 1 | Means and standard errors of individual listeners' thresholds, expressed by the crosses and error bars, respectively. Each panel represents one task, and each set of cross and error bar represents one listener. Within each panel, listeners are sorted according to the mean threshold. Note that for the ITD and Time tasks, the thresholds have been log-transformed. Numbers in the panel indicate the mean across the listeners. In the panel for the high frequency Level task, the number in gray indicates the mean calculated excluding listener 10 (rightmost data).

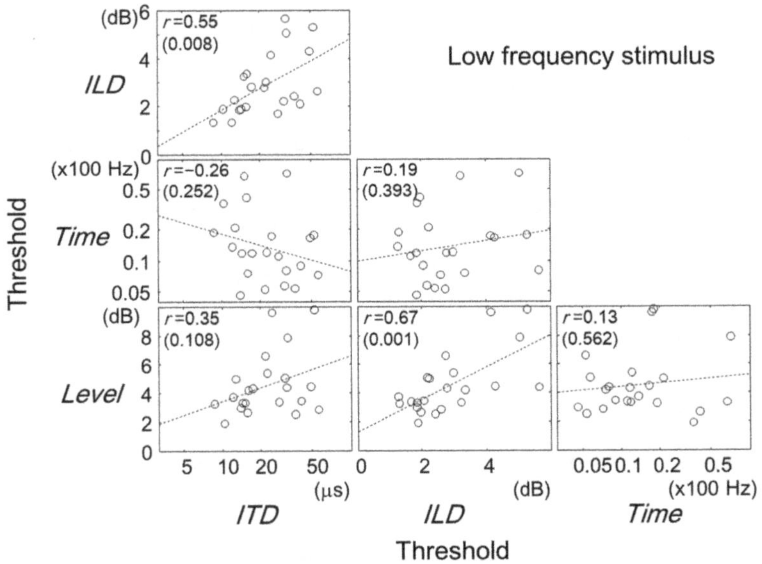

FIGURE 2 | Comparisons of thresholds between tasks for the low-frequency stimulus. Each panel represents one combination of tasks as labeled. Each symbol represents one listener. The broken lines are best-fit straight lines to the data. The Pearson correlation coefficients are shown with their *p*-values in parentheses. Note that for the ITD and Time tasks, the thresholds have been log-transformed. A similar figure has appeared elsewhere (Furukawa et al., 2013).

frequency regions, and in identifying tasks where the performance could predict the performance of the target. We used Akaike's information criterion (AIC) as a basis for selecting most effective combination of variables for the regression while avoiding overfitting (Burnham and Anderson, 2002, p. 63). The AIC values were obtained individually for models with all possible combinations of explanatory variables using the LinearModel.fit function of MATLAB. The combination of variables exhibiting the lowest AIC was employed for constructing the linear model. The results of the analysis are summarized in **Table 2**.

The linear model could account for a relatively large fraction of the variance of the threshold in a target task (R^2 ranged between 0.525 and 0.632). In addition, the results of the variable selection were generally in accordance with the findings described earlier: For a given target task and stimulus frequency, the other lateralization task at the same frequency was selected as an

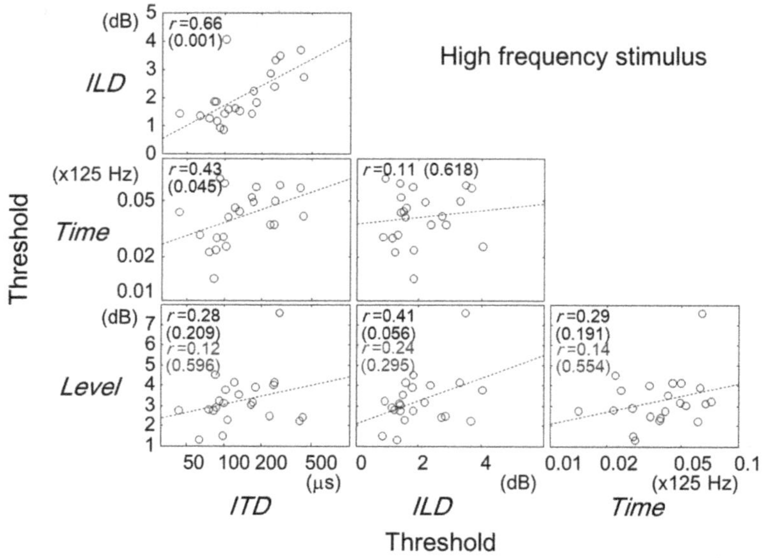

FIGURE 3 | Same as Figure 2 but for the high-frequency stimulus. The correlation coefficients and *p*-values in gray indicates values when listener 10 was excluded.

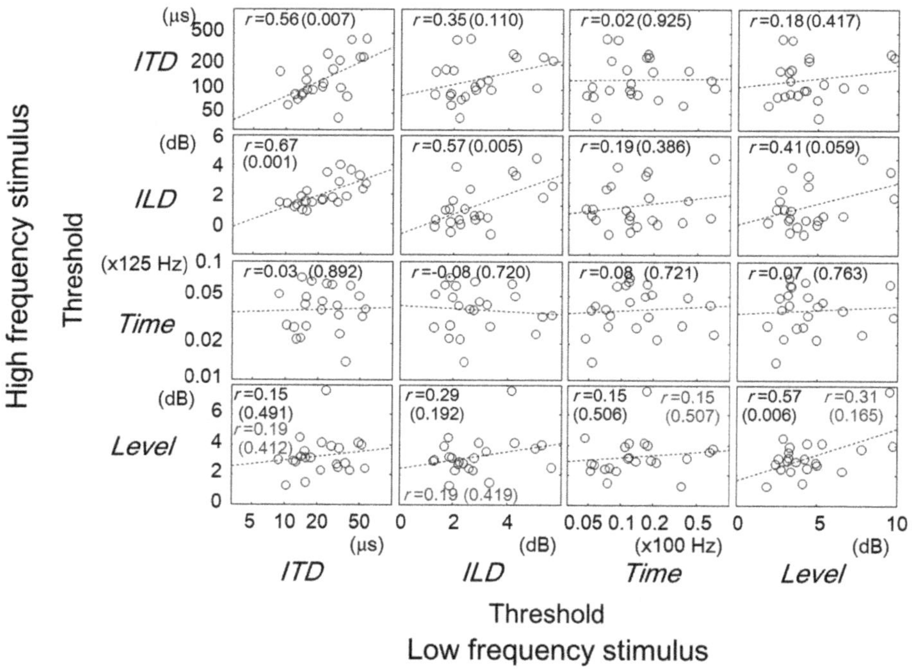

FIGURE 4 | Comparisons of thresholds between tasks for different frequency regions. The panels are arranged so that the horizontal and vertical axes represent the data for the low- and high- frequency stimuli, respectively. Other conventions are the same as in **Figures 2, 3**.

explanatory variable (e.g., for the target of the low-frequency ITD task, the low-frequency ILD task was selected), although the coefficients were not always significantly different from zero. It was also confirmed that for target tasks of ITD and ILD tasks, selected explanatory variables included the Time and Level tasks, respectively. The partial correlation coefficient for the low-frequency ITD task was significant and negative for the target task of low-frequency Time (-0.425; $p = 0.007$). Exclusion of listener 10 affected the result for the target task of high-frequency ILD: the high-frequency Level task was no more selected, and the partial correlation coefficient for the low-frequency Time task became significant (0.346; $p = 0.030$).

Table 1 | Summary of multiple regression analyses for low- and high-frequency stimuli.

Freq.	Target task	Explanatory tasks (p-value) ITD	ILD	Time	Level	Corrected R^2 (p-value)
Low	ITD	–	**0.644**	−0.374	−0.030	0.347
			(0.015)	(0.052)	(0.901)	(0.013)
	ILD	**0.444**	–	0.242	**0.482**	0.550
		(0.015)		(0.139)	(0.008)	(0.001)
High	ITD	–	**0.665**	**0.389**	−0.109	0.509
			(0.001)	(0.026)	(0.541)	(0.001)
			0.645	**0.387**	−0.085	0.477
			(0.001)	(0.031)	(0.623)	(0.003)
	ILD	**0.700**	–	−0.276	0.298	0.483
		(0.001)		(0.137)	(0.090)	(0.002)
		0.720	–	−0.286	0.190	0.495
		(0.001)		(0.147)	(0.290)	(0.008)

Partial correlation coefficients and the p-values are shown for individual explanatory tasks. Note that the analyses were conducted on the z scores of the threshold data. The bold characters indicate statistically significant correlation ($p < 0.05$). The rightmost column shows the multiple coefficients of determination (adjusted for degrees of freedom) and their p-values. For the high frequency stimulus, the results obtained when listener 10 was excluded are also shown in gray.

Table 2 | Summary of multiple regression analyses on all tasks.

Derived formula (p-value for corresponding partial coefficient)	Corrected R^2 (p-value)
$ITD_L = 0.304 \cdot ILD_L - 0.425 \cdot \mathbf{Time_L} + 0.575 \cdot \mathbf{ILD_H}$	0.603
(0.089) (0.007) (0.003)	(<0.001)
$ILD_L = 0.444 \cdot \mathbf{ITD_L} + 0.242 \cdot Time_L + 0.482 \cdot \mathbf{Level_L}$	0.550
(0.015) (0.139) (0.008)	(0.001)
$ITD_H = 0.623 \cdot \mathbf{ILD_H} + 0.362 \cdot \mathbf{Time_H}$	0.525
(0.001) (0.027)	(<0.001)
$ILD_H = 0.545 \cdot \mathbf{ITD_L} + 0.297 \cdot Time_L + 0.298 \cdot ITD_H + 0.201 \cdot Level_H$	0.632
(0.005) (0.051) (0.091) (0.168)	(<0.001)
$ILD_H = 0.632 \cdot \mathbf{ITD_L} + 0.346 \cdot \mathbf{Time_L} + 0.272 \cdot ITD_H$	0.619
(0.002) (0.030) (0.129)	(<0.001)

For each target task, explanatory variables (or tasks) were selected based on the AIC (see text). Each symbol (e.g., ITD_L) represents the threshold (in z score) of the corresponding task and stimulus (subscripts of L and H represent low- and high-frequency stimuli, respectively). Partial correlation coefficients and p-values are shown for individual explanatory tasks. The bold characters indicate statistically significant coefficients ($p < 0.05$). The rightmost column shows the multiple coefficients of determination (adjusted for degrees of freedom) and their p-values. For the high frequency ILD task (ILD_H), a different result of variable selection was obtained when listener 10 was excluded (indicated in gray).

PRINCIPAL COMPONENT ANALYSIS

So far, we have examined associations across tasks through single correlation and the multiple linear regression analyses. Interpretations of the coefficients, however, are often difficult when there are marked correlations among the explanatory variables, which was often the case in the present study. It was possible that the performance of the tasks evaluated in the present study could be explained by one or more common underlying factors. To examine this, we conducted a principal component analysis (PCA) on vectors of the eight tasks obtained from the 22 listeners. Before running the analysis, the threshold data were transformed to a logarithmic scale (for the Time and ITD tasks only) and then to z-scores (all the measures). The results indicated that the data could be accounted for well by the first three principal components (PCs; from PC1 to PC3), which had eigenvalues of 3.33, 1.34, and 1.30, respectively. These three PCs accounted for 74.6% of total variance. The factor loadings (FLs) of the three PCs (indicated by gray-scaled bars) and their squared values (FL^2s) are shown in **Figures 5A,B**, respectively. The FL^2 for a given task by a given PC indicates the proportion to the total variance for the task accounted for by that component.

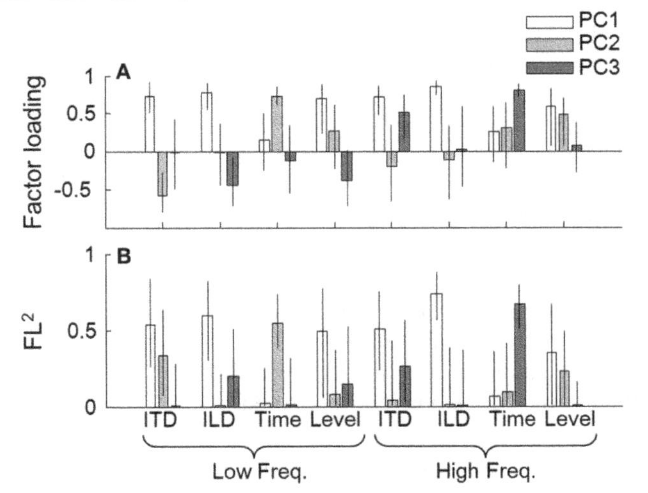

FIGURE 5 | (A) Factor loadings on the individual tasks, derived by the principal component analysis. The loads for the three components (i.e., PC1, PC2, and PC3) are represented by the three bars as indicated in the key. The error bars indicate 95% confidence intervals of the loads estimated by the bootstrap method. **(B)** Squared factor loadings (indicating the proportion to the total variance for the task accounted for by that component). Other conventions are the same as in **(A)**.

For all four lateralization tasks, the FL^2 values by PC1 were above 0.5. PC1 had positive loads on all the tasks (**Figure 5B**), implying that PC1 reflects the general ability of the listeners to conduct psychophysical tasks. Note, however, that the loads on the low- and high-frequency Time tasks were relatively small. Also, there were marked contributions of PC2 and PC3, depending on the task. For the low-frequency ITD task, PC2 could account for more than 30% of the variance. An examination of FLs revealed that PC2 was associated predominantly with the low-frequency Time task (**Figure 5B**), and the FLs on the low-frequency ITD and Time tasks had opposite signs (**Figure 5A**). This implies that PC2 reflects a factor that had opposing effects on the Pitch and ITD tasks at low frequency. PC3 had appreciable contributions to low-frequency ILD and high-frequency ITD tasks. PC3 was associated with the high-frequency Pitch task, which had the same sign as the FL on the high-frequency ITD task. To a lesser degree, PC3 also showed some association with the low-frequency Level task, which had the same sign as the FL on the low-frequency ILD task. Exclusion of listener 10 did not alter the general conclusions of the analysis.

DISCUSSION

The major findings of the present study were: positive correlations between the performance of pairs of lateralization tasks (i.e., ITD and ILD tasks) both within and across stimulus frequencies; a negative correlation for the low-frequency ITD and the Time tasks, revealed by the multiple-regression analysis; a positive correlation for the high-frequency ITD and the Time tasks; and a positive correlation for the low-frequency ILD and the Level tasks.

The mean thresholds obtained in the present study were generally at the same levels of those obtained by earlier comparative studies: ITD: Bernstein and Trahiotis (2002), Furukawa (2008); ILD: Grantham (1984), Furukawa (2008); Time: Plack and Carlyon (1995), Moore and Sek (2009); Level: Moore et al. (1997). Thresholds in the ITD task for the high frequency stimulus were greater than those for the low frequency stimulus by an order of magnitude. This quantitative difference is likely due to the difference in the tone and modulator frequencies and does not immediately indicate mechanistic difference between the frequencies: Typical threshold ITD for the 125-Hz tone, which is considered to be equivalent to the present transposed stimulus in terms of the peripheral phase locking, is comparable to the threshold for the transposed stimulus (see Bernstein and Trahiotis, 2002).

The significant positive correlations generally found between the performance of pairs of lateralization tasks indicate that some degree of inter-individual variation of performance could be accounted for by a common factor or mechanism that underlies lateralization based on both ITDs and ILDs over frequency regions. This notion is supported further by the fact that PC1 found in the PCA had large contributions to all the lateralization tasks. Furukawa (2008) found that the degree of ITD and ILD interaction is greater at high frequency than at low frequency, indicating that the dominance of a common mechanism depends on stimulus frequency or that different mechanisms for ITD and ILD processing are involved for low- and high-frequency stimulus. The present analyses regarding ITD-ILD relations, however, provided no indication of frequency-dependent processes for ITDs and ILDs: The correlation coefficients for the ITD and ILD pairs were not significantly different between low- and high-frequency stimuli ($p = 0.581$; t-test after the Fisher transformation of the correlation coefficients). One candidate for such a mechanism is a binaural mechanism that can process both ITDs and ILDs and can operate across frequency regions. Unfortunately, the present study cannot rule out another candidate, which is a non-sensory, higher-order factor related to the experimental procedure. It is possible that the inter-listener variability in the lateralization performance reflected predominantly the difference in procedure-specific skills. It was common across all the lateralization tasks that the listener had to identify the direction in which (toward left or right) intracranial images of two successive stimulus intervals changed. In the other tasks, on the other hand, the listener was asked to choose the interval that would contain changes in stimulus attributes.

The performance of the ITD task for the high frequency stimulus showed a significant positive correlation with that of the Time task. The following multiple-regression analyses also indicated a significant contribution of the high-frequency pitch task performance to account for the individual variability of the ITD performance. This tendency was captured in PC3 revealed by the PCA, suggesting that this positive correlation reflects a factor that is independent of another non-task-specific factor that determines the listener's overall psychophysical performance (expressed as PC1) or a factor that reflects the relationship of ITD and Time tasks (expressed as PC2; described later). This finding supports our initial hypothesis that the efficiency of neural phase locking to envelope of high frequency stimulus has a significant contribution to ITD-based lateralization performance.

For the low frequency stimulus, however, we failed to observe a positive correlation in the ITD and Time task pairs for the low frequency stimulus. This failure may be attributable to difference in the order of magnitude required for the two tasks: In the low-frequency Time task, a typical threshold of 10-Hz frequency shift of our SSMC stimulus is considered to correspond to difference in peak-to-peak time of TFS by about 100 μs (see Moore, 2012 pp. 220-223), which is an order of magnitude greater than a typical ITD threshold of 20 μs. For the high frequency, on the contrary, a typical threshold Δf_m of 4 Hz corresponds to change in the peak-to-peak interval of the modulation by about 250 μs, which falls in the range of ITD thresholds.

It is interesting that the across-frequency multiple-regression analysis with a variable selection procedure (**Table 2**) revealed that the low-frequency Time-task performance was a significant predictor of the low-frequency ITD-task performance, and it had a *negative* contribution. This negative relationship was observed also as the opposite signs of the FLs for the two tasks in PC2, an independent factor (**Figure 5**). This negative relationship not only was unexpected on the basis of our initial hypothesis but also appears to contradict to earlier reports on hearing-impaired or aged listeners (Strelcyk and Dau, 2009; Hopkins and Moore, 2011). This discrepancy among studies could be explained by postulating two factors that determine the listener's sensitivities to ITDs and the TFS: One factor, associated with the negative correlation, is dominant for normal-hearing listeners. As hearing impairment progresses, the other factor would dominate, resulting in a positive correlation in a population of normal- and hearing-impaired listeners.

One might be concerned about the listener's use of the excitation-pattern or spectral cue as a confounding factor for this negative relationship. Although the change in the excitation level for a typical threshold value (around $\Delta f/F_0 = 0.1$) was expected to be negligible (Moore and Sek, 2009), listeners who exhibited relatively high threshold might rely on the excitation pattern cue, which was usable for frequency shifts near their thresholds. Those listeners might be simply insensitive to the TFS information or might have adapted to placing more weights on the spectral cue than on the temporal cue in pitch judgments through their long-term experience (McLachlan et al., 2013). However, it is difficult to explain the negative correlation in terms of the use of the excitation-pattern cue: Listeners with general insensitivities to TFS would be expected to be insensitive to ITD also, leading to a positive correlation. We cannot think of obvious association between larger weighting on the place over the temporal cues and better (or poorer) performance in the ITD task.

One explanation for the puzzling negative correlation is that the listeners could use two types of ITD cues when conducting the ITD task, namely, envelope and TFS-based ITDs (since ITDs were imposed on both of those properties), and the performance depended on the relative weights placed on the two cues by individual listeners. It is possible that the envelope ITD of our stimulus was more reliably coded in the auditory system than the TFS-based ITD was. In the Time task, on the other hand, the TFS information could be the main cue for the judgments (although other types of information, such as distortion products by cochlear non-linearity and the excitation pattern, are also arguably potential cues, Oxenham et al., 2009; Micheyl et al., 2010), while the temporal envelope of the stimulus provided no useful cue, since it always had the same repetition rate (100 Hz). Therefore, a listener who places a greater weight on the envelope cue would tend to exhibit better and poor performance in the ITD and Pitch tasks, respectively. It should be noted that this explanation assumes that individual listeners applied more or less the same relative weights on the envelope and TFS invariantly in the Time and ITD tasks.

As for the relationship between the ILD and Level tasks, a significant positive correlation for the low-frequency stimulus supports our initial hypothesis that, at least for the low frequency stimulus, the inter-individual variability of ILD performance reflects the difference in the efficiency of intensity coding at a processing stage earlier than binaural interaction. One might be concerned that the listeners in the ILD task based their judgments primarily on the change of stimulus level within a single ear, and thus the ILD task measured essentially monaural sensitivity to level change. However, this is not likely, as supported by the suggestion of Bernstein (2004) that the listener's judgment is likely to be based on changes in the position of an intracranial image, not on the monaural cues.

AUTHOR CONTRIBUTIONS

Author Atsushi Ochi designed and conducted the experiments, analyzed the data, and prepared the manuscript. Tatsuya Yamasoba designed the experiments. Shigeto Furukawa conceived and designed the experiments, analyzed the data, and prepared the manuscript.

ACKNOWLEDGMENTS

This study was supported by internal research funding of NTT Corporation. Portions of the data were presented at the International Symposium on Hearing 2012 and have appeared in the conference book (Furukawa et al., 2013).

REFERENCES

Bernstein, L. R. (2001). Auditory processing of interaural timing information: new insights. *J. Neurosci. Res.* 66, 1035–1046. doi: 10.1002/jnr.10103

Bernstein, L. R. (2004). Sensitivity to interaural intensitive disparities: listeners' use of potential cues. *J. Acoust. Soc. Am.* 115, 3156–3160. doi: 10.1121/1.1719025

Bernstein, L. R., and Trahiotis, C. (2002). Enhancing sensitivity to interaural delays at high frequencies by using "transposed stimuli." *J. Acoust. Soc. Am.* 112, 1026–1036. doi: 10.1121/1.1497620

Burnham, K. P., and Anderson, D. R. (2002). *Model Selection and Multimodel Inference: A Practical Information-Theoretic Approach.* New York, NY: Springer-Verlag.

De Boer, E. (1956). Pitch of inharmonic signals. *Nature* 178, 535–536. doi: 10.1038/178535a0

Furukawa, S. (2008). Detection of combined changes in interaural time and intensity differences: segregated mechanisms in cue type and in operating frequency range? *J. Acoust. Soc. Am.* 123, 1602–1617. doi: 10.1121/1.2835226

Furukawa, S., Washizawa, S., Ochi, A., and Kashino, M. (2013). "How independent are the pitch and interaural-time-difference mechanisms that rely on temporal fine structure information?," in *Basic Aspects of Hearing*, eds B. C. J. Moore, R. D. Patterson, I. M. Winter, R. P. Carlyon, and H. E. Gockel (New York, NY: Springer), 91–99.

Grantham, D. W. (1984). Interaural intensity discrimination - insensitivity at 1000 Hz. *J. Acoust. Soc. Am.* 75, 1191–1194. doi: 10.1121/1.390769

Hacker, M. J., and Ratcliff, R. (1979). A revised table of *d'* for *M*-alternative forced choice. *Percept. Psychophys.* 26, 168–170. doi: 10.3758/BF03208311

Hopkins, K., and Moore, B. C. (2007). Moderate cochlear hearing loss leads to a reduced ability to use temporal fine structure information. *J. Acoust. Soc. Am.* 122, 1055–1068. doi: 10.1121/1.2749457

Hopkins, K., and Moore, B. C. (2011). The effects of age and cochlear hearing loss on temporal fine structure sensitivity, frequency selectivity, and speech reception in noise. *J. Acoust. Soc. Am.* 130, 334–349. doi: 10.1121/1.3585848

Levitt, H. (1970). Transformed up-down methods in psychoacoustics. *J. Acoust. Soc. Am.* 49, 467–477. doi: 10.1121/1.1912375

McLachlan, N. M., Marco, D. J., and Wilson, S. J. (2013). The musical environment and auditory plasticity: hearing the pitch of percussion. *Front. Psychol.* 4:768. doi: 10.3389/fpsyg.2013.00768

Micheyl, C., Dai, H., and Oxenham, A. J. (2010). On the possible influence of spectral- and temporal-envelope cues in tests of sensitivity to temporal fine structure. *J. Acoust. Soc. Am.* 127, 1809–1810. doi: 10.1121/1.3384106

Moore, B. C., Huss, M., Vickers, D. A., Glasberg, B. R., and Alcantara, J. I. (2000). A test for the diagnosis of dead regions in the cochlea. *Br. J. Audiol.* 34, 205–224. doi: 10.3109/03005364000000131

Moore, B. C. J. (2012). *An Introduction to the Psychology of Hearing.* Bingley: Emerald.

Moore, B. C., Peters, R. W., Kohlrausch, A., and Van De Par, S. (1997). Detection of increments and decrements in sinusoids as a function of frequency, increment, and decrement duration and pedestal duration. *J. Acoust. Soc. Am.* 102, 2954–2965. doi: 10.1121/1.420350

Moore, B. C., and Sek, A. (2009). Development of a fast method for determining sensitivity to temporal fine structure. *Int. J. Audiol.* 48, 161–171. doi: 10.1080/14992020802475235

Moore, G. A., and Moore, B. C. (2003). Perception of the low pitch of frequency-shifted complexes. *J. Acoust. Soc. Am.* 113, 977–985. doi: 10.1121/1.1536631

Oxenham, A. J., Bernstein, J. G., and Penagos, H. (2004). Correct tonotopic representation is necessary for complex pitch perception. *Proc. Natl. Acad. Sci. U.S.A.* 101, 1421–1425. doi: 10.1073/pnas.0306958101

Oxenham, A. J., Micheyl, C., and Keebler, M. V. (2009). Can temporal fine structure represent the fundamental frequency of unresolved harmonics? *J. Acoust. Soc. Am.* 125, 2189. doi: 10.1121/1.3089220

Plack, C. J., and Carlyon, R. P. (1995). Differences in frequency modulation detection and fundamental frequency discrimination between complex tones consisting of resolved and unresolved harmonics. *J. Acoust. Soc. Am.* 98, 1355–1364. doi: 10.1121/1.413471

Schouten, J., Ritsma, R. J., and Cardozo, B. (1962). Pitch of the Residue. *J. Acoust. Soc. Am.* 34, 1418–1424. doi: 10.1121/1.1918360

Strelcyk, O., and Dau, T. (2009). Relations between frequency selectivity, temporal fine-structure processing, and speech reception in impaired hearing. *J. Acoust. Soc. Am.* 125, 3328–3345. doi: 10.1121/1.3097469

Strouse, A., Ashmead, D. H., Ohde, R. N., and Grantham, D. W. (1998). Temporal processing in the aging auditory system. *J. Acoust. Soc. Am.* 104, 2385–2399. doi: 10.1121/1.423748

Van De Par, S., and Kohlrausch, A. (1997). A new approach to comparing binaural masking level differences at low and high frequencies. *J. Acoust. Soc. Am.* 101, 1671–1680. doi: 10.1121/1.418151

Zeng, F. G., Kong, Y. Y., Michalewski, H. J., and Starr, A. (2005). Perceptual consequences of disrupted auditory nerve activity. *J. Neurophysiol.* 93, 3050–3063. doi: 10.1152/jn.00985.2004

10

Sound localization with head movement: Implications for 3-d audio displays

Ken I. McAnally* and Russell L. Martin

Aerospace Division, Defence Science and Technology Organisation, Melbourne, VIC, Australia

Correspondence:
Ken I. McAnally, Aerospace Division, Defence Science and Technology Organisation, PO Box 4331, Melbourne, VIC 3001, Australia
e-mail: ken.mcanally@dsto.defence.gov.au

Previous studies have shown that the accuracy of sound localization is improved if listeners are allowed to move their heads during signal presentation. This study describes the function relating localization accuracy to the extent of head movement in azimuth. Sounds that are difficult to localize were presented in the free field from sources at a wide range of azimuths and elevations. Sounds remained active until the participants' heads had rotated through windows ranging in width of 2, 4, 8, 16, 32, or 64° of azimuth. Error in determining sound-source elevation and the rate of front/back confusion were found to decrease with increases in azimuth window width. Error in determining sound-source lateral angle was not found to vary with azimuth window width. *Implications for 3-d audio displays*: the utility of a 3-d audio display for imparting spatial information is likely to be improved if operators are able to move their heads during signal presentation. Head movement may compensate in part for a paucity of spectral cues to sound-source location resulting from limitations in either the audio signals presented or the directional filters (i.e., head-related transfer functions) used to generate a display. However, head movements of a moderate size (i.e., through around 32° of azimuth) may be required to ensure that spatial information is conveyed with high accuracy.

Keywords: audio displays, sound localization, auditory-vestibular integration

Three-dimensional (3-d) audio displays are designed to create an illusion of immersion in an acoustic environment by presenting via headphones the acoustic signals that would normally be present at a listener's ears (Wightman and Kistler, 1989). It has been proposed that such displays be included in a number of work environments, for example aviation (Begault, 1998), where spatial information could be imparted to operators by the direction of virtual acoustic sources. For virtual sound sources to appear stable in the world, the position and orientation of the listener's head must be tracked and head movement compensated for by updating the head-referenced, head-related transfer functions (HRTFs) that render virtual acoustic space.

There are at least three issues that may limit the utility of a 3-d audio display of directional information. The first is that listeners commonly mislocalize sounds to the incorrect front/back hemifield (Oldfield and Parker, 1984) and the rate of these errors is generally higher when listening to a 3-d audio display than when listening in the free field (e.g., Wightman and Kistler, 1989). The second is that spectral cues to source location (Shaw and Teranishi, 1968; Blauert, 1969/1970) are highly listener specific (Wenzel et al., 1993) and care must be taken to reproduce these cues accurately to ensure good localization performance. This may require the measurement of HRTFs for each individual listener. The third is that not all sounds can be well localized. For a sound to be well localized, it must have a broad bandwidth and a relatively flat spectrum that does not mask monaural spectral cues to location (King and Oldfield, 1997).

Cues to sound-source location also include interaural differences in the time of arrival (the interaural time difference, ITD) and level (the interaural level difference, ILD) of a sound. These cues are ambiguous and, to a first approximation, specify a cone-of-confusion centered on the interaural axis upon which a source lies (e.g., Mills, 1972). Monaural spectral cues resulting from the interaction of a sound wave with the external ear, head and torso can be used to specify the source elevation and front/back hemifield (see Carlile et al., 2005, for a review).

Wallach (1940) suggested that dynamic ITDs and ILDs associated with movement of the head should resolve confusion regarding the front/back hemifield of a sound source. Using speakers located in front of a listener, Wallach was able to simulate sources in the rear by manipulating the direction in which ITDs and ILDs changed as a listener's head rotated in azimuth. Macpherson (2013) has since shown that it is dynamic ITDs rather than ILDs that provide a strong cue to front/back hemifield. The role of head movement in resolving front/back confusion has also been confirmed by other studies in which the head was allowed to move during signal presentation (Thurlow et al., 1967; Perrett and Noble, 1997a; Wightman and Kistler, 1999; Iwaya et al., 2003). However, in many of these studies (Perrett and Noble, 1997a; Wightman and Kistler, 1999; Iwaya et al., 2003; Macpherson, 2013) confusions were not entirely eliminated by head movement.

Wallach (1940) also suggested that the rates of change of ITDs and ILDs with changes in head azimuth would provide a cue to sound-source elevation. ITDs and ILDs change most rapidly with changes in head azimuth when sources are on the horizon. For sources directly above or below a listener, they are unaffected by head azimuth. Wallach was able to simulate sound sources at different elevations by manipulating the rate at which the sound source was switched from one location on the horizon to another as the listener's head rotated in azimuth.

That head movement can improve localization in elevation has been confirmed by a number of subsequent studies (Thurlow and Runge, 1967; Perrett and Noble, 1997a,b; Kato et al., 2003). In one of those studies, Perrett and Noble (1997b) showed that dynamic ITD cues can compensate for the disruption of monaural spectral cues that results when tubes are inserted into the ear canals. Similarly, Kato et al. (2003) reported that head movement improves elevation localization when monaural spectral cues are disrupted by ear molds. These results suggest that dynamic interaural difference cues associated with head movement may compensate, at least in part, for the compromised spectral cues likely to be provided by 3-d audio displays generated using imperfect HRTFs.

Previous research, therefore, suggests that localization of sounds presented via 3-d audio displays may be improved by allowing listeners the opportunity to move their heads. While the previously described studies demonstrate that head movement can reduce the incidence of front/back confusion and the magnitude of elevation errors, the function relating sound localization accuracy to the extent of head movement has not been described. If large head movements are required to extract accurate directional information from a 3-d audio display, the display's utility would be limited in many situations, for example where operators are required to perform simultaneous visual tasks. The present study addresses this issue by examining the effect on localization accuracy of the availability of dynamic ITD and ILD cues associated with rotation of the head through windows ranging in width from 2 to 64° of azimuth. In order to simulate conditions where the HRTFs used to render a display are not of high fidelity and/or the sound to be localized has not been optimized for localization, monaural cues to sound-source elevation and front/back hemifield were reduced by randomizing the signal spectrum from trial to trial. The study was conducted in the free field, rather than a virtual acoustic environment, to ensure that the localization accuracy observed was not dependant on limitations in the fidelity of a particular 3-d audio display. In particular, it was desirable that the dynamic interaural difference cues made available by head movement were of high fidelity, and not limited by the quality of spatial interpolation between measured HRTFs.

METHODS

PARTICIPANTS

Eight volunteers (six men and two women) participated. Their average age was 34.5 years. All participants had normal hearing sensitivity (i.e., their absolute thresholds were no more than one standard deviation above age-relevant norms (Corso, 1963; Stelmachowicz et al., 1989) for seven pure tones ranging in frequency from 0.5 to 16 kHz). They also had substantial experience in localizing sound within the experimental setting. All participants gave informed consent.

DESIGN

Head movement was allowed in six conditions, in each of which the offset of the sound to be localized was triggered when the participant's head had rotated through a predefined window of azimuth. The width of this window was 2, 4, 8, 16, 32, or 64°, as measured using a head-worn magnetic-tracker receiver (Polhemus, 3Space Fastrak). The head tracker had an accuracy of 0.08 cm in translation and 0.15° in rotation. Each participant completed two sessions, each of 42 trials, for each of the six conditions. The order of conditions followed a randomized-blocks design.

STIMULUS GENERATION

The sound to be localized was broadband noise with a spectrum that varied randomly from trial to trial to reduce monaural spectral cues to source elevation and front/back hemifield. All stimuli were generated digitally at 50 kHz (Tucker-Davis Technologies system II). The spectrum of each random-spectrum noise comprised 42 bands centered on frequencies ranging from 0.013 to 19.7 kHz. The width of each band was one equivalent rectangular bandwidth (Glasberg and Moore, 1990). The level of each band was set to a random value within a 60-dB range. Rise and fall times were 40 ms. Stimuli were passed through a digital filter that compensated for variations in the response of the loudspeaker through which they were presented (Bose, FreeSpace tweeter) across the frequency range from 200 Hz to 20 kHz and were presented in the free field at about 65 dB SPL (A-weighted).

LOCALIZATION PROCEDURE

Participants sat on a swiveling chair in an anechoic chamber at the center of rotation of a motorized hoop on which the loudspeaker was mounted. The hoop allowed the loudspeaker to be placed at any azimuth and at any elevation between −50 and +80° with 0.1° accuracy. Their view of the loudspeaker was obscured by an acoustically transparent cloth sphere. Participants wore a headband upon which the magnetic-tracker receiver and a laser pointer were mounted. To begin each trial the participant placed his/her chin on a rest and oriented toward a light emitting diode at 0° of azimuth and elevation. When he/she pressed a hand-held button, the head's position and orientation were recorded. A stimulus was presented if the head was stationary and in the center of the hoop. Upon presentation of the stimulus, the participant was instructed to remove his/her chin from the rest and to turn his/her head and body in a direct manner in order to point the head-mounted laser pointer's beam at the location on the surface of the cloth sphere where he/she had perceived the sound source to be and then to press a hand-held button. Inspection of head motion trajectories confirmed that listeners complied with the instruction to orient directly to the perceived source. The azimuth and elevation of the location on the cloth sphere illuminated by the laser pointer, referenced to the center of the hoop, were calculated. The head's position and orientation were recorded at 25 Hz throughout each trial. No feedback was given with regard to localization performance.

Stimuli were presented from locations ranging from −180 to +180° of azimuth and from −50 to +80° of elevation. The location for any given trial was chosen pseudorandomly such that sound-source locations were distributed more-or-less evenly across the part-sphere in any given session. The loudspeaker was moved to a random location between successive trials so that the participant could not discern the sound-source location by listening to the motors controlling the hoop.

DATA ANALYSIS

Data analysis was restricted to trials in which the perceived azimuth was outside of the azimuth window. This was to ensure that the head had rotated through the desired range of azimuths and stimulus offset had been triggered. Analysis was also restricted to source locations with absolute azimuths greater than 64° in order to ensure that the distribution of sources was well matched across azimuth window conditions. These restrictions resulted in an average of 436 trials/condition (range from 432 to 440).

The proportion of trials in which a front/back confusion was made was calculated for each participant and condition. For a response to be considered a front/back confusion, the actual and perceived sound-source locations had to be in different front/back hemispheres and more than a criterion angle of azimuth (i.e., 7.5° divided by the cosine of the location's elevation to adjust for convergence of azimuth at the poles) from the plane separating the front and back hemispheres. Trials in which actual and/or perceived sound-source locations were close to that plane were excluded when calculating front/back confusion rate because it could not be concluded with confidence that a front/back confusion had occurred where this was the case. Localization errors comprising unsigned errors of lateral angle and elevation were calculated for all responses that were not classified as front/back confusions. Lateral angle is defined as the angle between a source and the median plane and indicates the cone of confusion upon which the source lies. Elevation is defined as the angle between a source and the interaural horizontal plane.

Results were analyzed using either one-way, repeated-measures analyses of variance (ANOVAs), incorporating Greenhouse–Geisser corrections for violations of the assumption of sphericity where appropriate (e.g., Keppel, 1991), or Friedman analyses of variance by ranks. Post-hoc comparisons were made using either paired-sample *t*-tests or Wilcoxon tests, correcting for the false discovery rate (Benjamini and Hochberg, 1995). Significant effects were further explored by regression analyses. An *a priori* alpha level of 0.05 was applied when interpreting all inferential statistics.

RESULTS

Mean lateral errors for individual participants, and averaged across participants, are shown in **Figure 1A**. A One-Way repeated-measures ANOVA revealed that the effect of azimuth window was not significant, $F_{(3.1,\ 21.9)} = 2.63$, $p = 0.07$, partial $\eta^2 = 0.27$.

Mean elevation errors for individual participants, and averaged across participants, are shown in **Figure 1B**. The overall mean elevation error was around 14 for the 2° azimuth window which confirms that spectral cues to elevation were reduced. [The mean elevation error is normally around 8° for a brief white noise stimulus (Martin et al., 2004)]. A One-Way repeated-measures ANOVA revealed a significant effect of azimuth window, $F_{(3.0,\ 21.1)} = 10.8$, $p < 0.001$, partial $\eta^2 = 0.61$. *Post-hoc* comparisons, controlling for the false discovery rate, revealed that mean elevation error for the 2° azimuth window was significantly larger than those for all windows greater than 8°, and that the mean elevation error for the 64° window was significantly

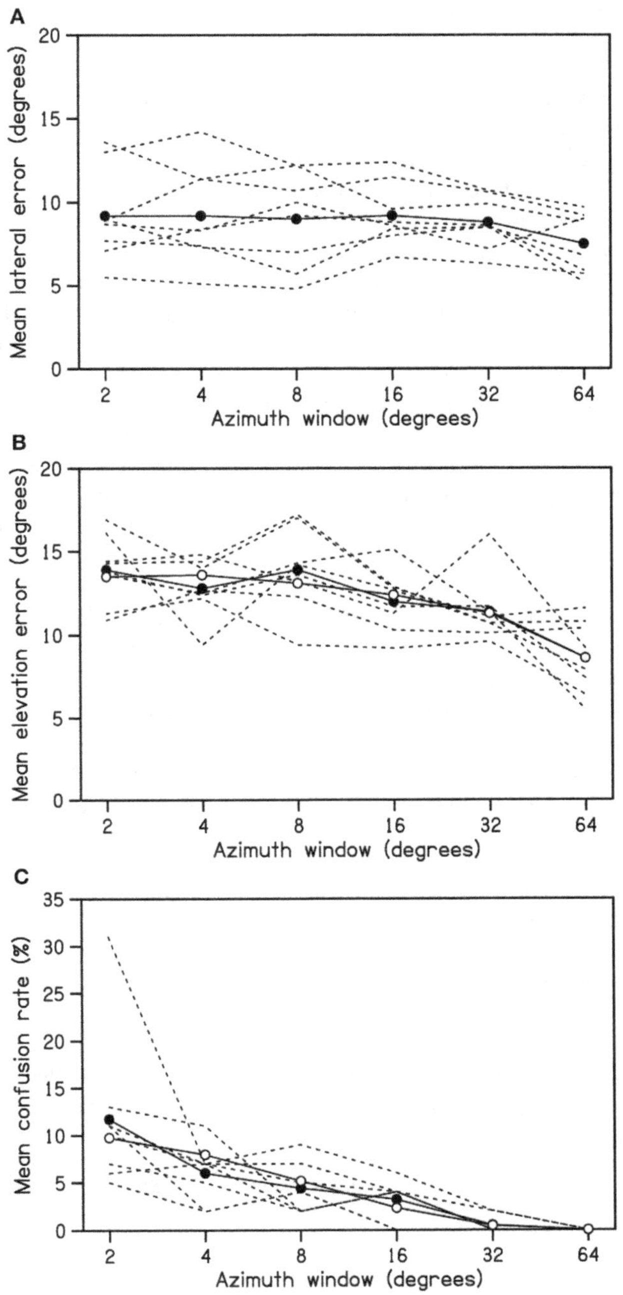

FIGURE 1 | Mean lateral error (A), elevation error (B), and front/back confusion rate (C) as functions of azimuth window width. Dashed lines represent means for individual participants. Solid symbols with solid lines represent means across participants. Open symbols with solid lines represent means predicted by the regression, partialling out the effects of duration and the extent of head rotation in elevation.

smaller than those for all windows less than 32°, $t_{(7)} \geq 2.92$, $p \leq 0.02$.

Mean rates of front/back confusion, shown in **Figure 1C**, decreased to zero with increasing azimuth window width. A Friedman analysis of variance by ranks revealed that the effect of azimuth window was significant, $\chi^2_{(5)} = 34.4, p < 0.001$. *Post-hoc* Wilcoxon tests, controlling for the false discovery rate, revealed that all comparisons were significant with the exception of 4 vs. 8°, 8 vs. 16°, and 32 vs. 64°, $Z \geq 2.33, p \leq 0.02$.

In addition to the extent of head rotation in azimuth during stimulus presentation, the width of the azimuth window could be expected to be correlated with both stimulus duration and the extent of head rotation in elevation[1]. That this was the case is confirmed by the data presented in **Table 1**, which show significant correlations between stimulus duration, the extent of head rotation in azimuth, and the extent of head rotation in elevation during signal presentation. It is therefore unclear which of these three variables was responsible for the above-described effects of azimuth window on elevation error and front/back confusion rate.

In order to determine which of these variables influenced elevation error, a multiple regression analysis was conducted. Stimulus duration, the extent of head rotation in azimuth, and the extent of head rotation in elevation were the predictor variables of interest. To facilitate the interpretation of relationships between elevation error and these variables, the absolute lateral angle and elevation of the sound source and the individual participant were added to the predictor variable list.

The complete regression model was found to explain 16.9% of the observed variance in elevation error. As shown in **Table 2**, all three predictors of interest explained a significant, unique component of this variance. Elevation error was found to decrease significantly with increasing head rotation in either azimuth or elevation. Of some surprise, elevation error was found to *increase* significantly with increasing stimulus duration. The mean elevation errors predicted by the regression, partialling out the effects of duration and the extent of head rotation in elevation, are plotted in **Figure 1B** (open symbols) and follow a similar form to the raw means.

A multiple logistic regression analysis predicting front/back confusion rate from the same list of variables was conducted to determine which of the three predictors of interest influenced this error measure. The complete logistic regression model was found to explain 26.3% of the observed variance in front/back confusion rate. As shown in **Table 3**, both stimulus duration and the extent of head rotation in azimuth explained a significant, unique component of this variance. Front/back confusion rate was found to increase significantly with increasing stimulus duration (odds ratio > 1) and decrease significantly with increasing head rotation in azimuth (odds ratio < 1). The extent of head rotation in elevation was found to have no significant unique influence on front/back confusion rate. The mean front/back confusion rates predicted by the regression, partialling out the effects of duration and the extent of head rotation in elevation, are plotted in

Table 1 | Pearson correlations between stimulus duration and the extents of head rotation in azimuth and elevation during stimulus presentation.

	Azimuth rotation	Elevation rotation
Duration	0.24	0.37
Azimuth rotation		0.57

Note: All p-values < 0.001.

Table 2 | Results of multiple regression predicting elevation errors for trials where a front/back confusion was not made.

Predictor	β	t	p
Participant 1	0.042	1.75	0.08
Participant 2	−0.001	−0.03	0.97
Participant 3	0.027	1.14	0.25
Participant 4	−0.031	−1.27	0.20
Participant 5	0.014	0.54	0.59
Participant 6	0.025	1.02	0.30
Participant 7	0.021	0.89	0.37
Source |lateral angle|	−0.127	−6.05	<0.001
Source |elevation|	0.298	13.89	<0.001
Duration	0.104	4.37	<0.001
Azimuth rotation	−0.111	−4.82	<0.001
Elevation rotation	−0.096	−3.86	<0.001

Table 3 | Results of multiple logistic regression predicting front/back confusion rates.

Predictor	Odds ratio	Wald	p
Participant 1	0.57	1.05	0.30
Participant 2	0.15	15.64	<0.001
Participant 3	0.59	0.92	0.34
Participant 4	0.58	1.01	0.31
Participant 5	0.23	8.35	0.004
Participant 6	0.29	6.02	0.014
Participant 7	0.39	3.35	0.07
Source |lateral angle|	1.02	7.66	0.006
Source |elevation|	1.05	50.01	<0.001
Duration	1.22	3.76	0.05
Azimuth rotation	0.89	38.34	<0.001
Elevation rotation	1.02	0.85	0.36

[1] It is important to note that the actual extent of head rotation in azimuth during stimulus presentation was not completely determined by the width of the azimuth window for two reasons. First, the azimuth windows were symmetric about the midline. Participants occasionally rotated their heads a little away from the source when exiting the chin rest. Second, stimulus offset was triggered when the head had rotated through the azimuth window but occurred with a slight delay because of the low sample rate of the head tracker. For these reasons, our regression analyses utilized the actual extent of head rotation in azimuth during signal presentation rather than azimuth window width. The extent of head rotation in azimuth was defined as the range of azimuth through which the head rotated during signal presentation. Similarly, the extent of head rotation in elevation was defined as the range of elevation through which the head rotated during signal presentation.

Figure 1C (open symbols) and follow a similar form to the raw means.

DISCUSSION

In many situations where a 3-d audio display could be applied it may not be possible or desirable for a listener to freely move his/her head in order to enhance sound localization. For example, the range of desirable head movements may be limited by concurrent visual tasks in the work environment. In order to predict the localization performance that can be expected in different situations, it is necessary to understand the manner in which the accuracy of sound localization varies as a function of the extent of head movement. The present study describes the function relating localization errors to the extent of head movement in greater detail than does any previous study. The extent of head movement was constrained by terminating the auditory stimulus when the participant's head had rotated through a predefined window of azimuth, and the nature of head movement was constrained by instructing the participant to orient directly toward the perceived location of the sound source. Head rotation through an azimuth window as narrow as 4° was found to significantly reduce the rate at which front/back confusions were made. In contrast, head rotation through an azimuth window of 16° was found to be required to significantly reduce elevation error. Head movement was not found to significantly affect lateral localization error.

Most previous studies of the effect of head movement on sound localization allowed free head movement, and controlled neither the range nor the manner of that movement (Thurlow and Runge, 1967; Perrett and Noble, 1997a; Wightman and Kistler, 1999; Iwaya et al., 2003; Kato et al., 2003). Although some previous studies included a condition in which the range of movement was constrained by verbal instruction, for example to between −30 and +30° of azimuth or to between two light emitting diodes (Perrett and Noble, 1997a,b), the small number of movement conditions in those studies does not allow a description of the function relating localization performance to the extent of head movement during stimulus presentation. In a recent study by Macpherson and Kerr (2008), sound onset and offset were gated with reference to head azimuth across a range of window widths. However, that study only examined localization in azimuth for sources on the horizon. The present study extended Macpherson and Kerr's study by examining localization in azimuth and elevation as well as front/back confusion for sources distributed across most of the sphere.

In this study, larger movements of the head were associated with longer stimulus durations. For example, the mean stimulus duration for the 2° azimuth window was 1.2 s, whereas that for the 64° azimuth window was 1.8 s. However, as we observed that stimulus duration was *positively* related to both elevation error magnitude and the rate of front/back confusion, it seems unlikely that the reductions in mean elevation error and front/back confusion rate that accompanied increases in azimuth window width were driven by the associated increases in stimulus duration. Rather, they appear to be attributable to the associated increases in the extents of head rotation during stimulus presentation. The fact that we found no evidence to indicate that localization accuracy improves as stimulus duration increases beyond a second or so is consistent with previous studies that have shown that functions relating localization or lateralization performance and stimulus duration are asymptotic at durations considerably less than one second (Tobias and Zerlin, 1957; Hofman and van Opstal, 1998). For example, Hofman and van Opstal inferred that the auditory localization system can form a stable estimate of sound-source azimuth and elevation on the basis of a sample of about 80 ms. The positive relationship we observed between stimulus duration and localization errors may be attributable to a tendency for participants to orient more slowly toward stimuli which were difficult to localize.

It has commonly been reported that although head movement reduces the incidence of front/back confusion, it does not necessarily eliminate such confusion (Perrett and Noble, 1997a; Wightman and Kistler, 1999; Iwaya et al., 2003; Macpherson and Kerr, 2008). For example, Macpherson and Kerr (2008) examined the effect of head rotation through 0, 2.6, 5, and 20° azimuth windows at a rate of 50°/s on localization in azimuth for sources of wide-band noise, low-frequency noise, and high-frequency noise. Low-frequency noise is the most comparable of their stimuli to the random-spectrum noise used in the present study because it would have provided robust interaural time difference (ITD) cues, including dynamic ITD cues, but poor monaural spectral cues to location. In the case of that stimulus, Macpherson and Kerr (2008) observed a marked reduction in the rate of front/back confusion for azimuth windows as narrow as 2.6°, but windows of around 20° were required to eliminate these confusions. In the present study, head movement through a 4° azimuth window significantly reduced the front/back confusion rate, but movement through a 32° azimuth window was required to almost eliminate these confusions.

Wallach (1940) showed that the rate of change of interaural difference cues with head rotation in azimuth provides a cue to (the absolute value of) a sound source's elevation. This is because the elevation of a source determines the rate at which its lateral angle changes as the head is rotated in azimuth. The negative relationship we observed between elevation error magnitude and the extent of head rotation in azimuth during stimulus presentation is thus consistent with Wallach's (1940) proposal that dynamic interaural difference cues are integrated with knowledge about head rotation in azimuth to help determine sound-source location. It can be seen from **Figure 1** that all listeners were similarly able to integrate vestibular and/or proprioceptive information about head rotation with dynamic auditory cues to improve sound localization.

The negative relationship we observed between elevation error magnitude and the extent of head rotation in elevation during stimulus presentation, in contrast, is suggestive of the presence of *dynamic spectral cues* to sound-source elevation. That is, it suggests that the way in which a sound's spectra at the ears changes as the head is rotated in elevation provides information concerning the elevation of its source. Because the source spectrum was constant within a trial, any such dynamic spectral cues would not be expected to be disrupted by the trial-to-trial spectral roving that was applied to the stimuli in order to reduce static spectral cues to source location.

In order to determine whether the information concerning head movement that participants integrate with dynamic interaural difference cues to refine localization judgements is derived from vestibular or proprioceptive sources, Kim et al. (2013) compared azimuthal sound localization under conditions of active head movement, passive head movement, and body movement with the head fixed. They concluded that vestibular information associated with head movement is both necessary and sufficient to improve sound localization. In contrast, they found that proprioceptive information does not improve localization.

We expect that the observed beneficial effects of head movement on sound localization will generalize to (i) other situations where audio signals (e.g., warnings) have spectra that are not optimal for localization and (ii) situations where a 3-d audio display is generated using imperfect HRTFs, such as those that have not been tailored for the particular listener. While small head movements were found to reduce the rate of front/back confusion, moderate movements (i.e., around 16–32°) were found to be required to significantly reduce elevation errors and to almost eliminate confusions. In situations where head movements of this magnitude are impractical, it will be necessary to optimize both the HRTFs used to generate a 3-d audio display and the signals presented through it in order to ensure that the display is of high spatial fidelity.

REFERENCES

Begault, D. R. (1998). Virtual acoustics, aeronautics, and communications. *J. Audio Eng. Soc.* 46, 520–530.

Benjamini, Y., and Hochberg, Y. (1995). Controlling the false discovery rate: a practical and powerful approach to multiple testing. *J. R. Stat. Soc.* 57, 289–300.

Blauert, J. (1969/1970). Sound localization in the median plane. *Acustica* 22, 205–213.

Carlile, S., Martin, R., and McAnally, K. (2005). Spectral information in sound localization. *Int. Rev. Neurobiol.* 70, 399–434. doi: 10.1016/S0074-7742(05)70012-X

Corso, J. F. (1963). Age and sex differences in pure-tone thresholds. *Arch. Otolaryngol.* 77, 385–405. doi: 10.1001/archotol.1963.00750010399008

Glasberg, B. R., and Moore, B. C. J. (1990). Derivation of auditory filter shapes from notched-noise data. *Hear. Res.* 47, 103–138. doi: 10.1016/0378-5955(90) 90170-T

Hofman, P. M., and van Opstal, A. J. (1998). Spectro-temporal factors in two-dimensional human sound localization. *J. Acoust. Soc. Am.* 103, 2634–2648. doi: 10.1121/1.422784

Iwaya, Y., Suzuki, Y., and Kimura, D. (2003). Effects of head movement on front-back error in sound localization. *Acoust. Sci. Technol.* 24, 322–324. doi: 10.1250/ast.24.322

Kato, M., Uematsu, H., Kashino, M., and Hirahara, T. (2003). The effect of head motion on the accuracy of sound localization. *Acoust. Sci. Technol.* 24, 315–317. doi: 10.1250/ast.24.315

Keppel, G. (1991). *Design and Analysis: a Researcher's Handbook.* Englewood Cliffs, NJ: Prentice Hall.

Kim, J., Barnett-Cowan, M., and Macpherson, E. A. (2013). "Integration of auditory input with vestibular and neck proprioceptive information in the interpretation of dynamic sound localization cues," in *Proceedings of Meetings on Acoustics,* Vol. 19 (Montreal, QC), 050142.

King, R. B., and Oldfield, S. R. (1997). The impact of signal bandwidth on auditory localization: implications for the design of three-dimensional audio displays. *Hum. Factors* 39, 287–295. doi: 10.1518/001872097778 543895

Macpherson, E. A. (2013). "Cue weighting and vestibular mediation of temporal dynamics in sound localization via head rotation," in *Proceedings of Meetings on Acoustics,* Vol. 19 (Montreal, QC), 050131.

Macpherson, E. A., and Kerr, D. M. (2008). "Minimum head movements required to localize narrowband sounds," in *American Audiology Society 2008 Annual Meeting* (Scottsdale, AZ).

Martin, R. L., Paterson, M., and McAnally, K. I. (2004). Utility of monaural spectral cues is enhanced in the presence of cues to sound-source lateral angle. *J. Assoc. Res. Otolaryngol.* 5, 80–89. doi: 10.1007/s10162-003-3003-8

Mills, A. W. (1972). "Auditory localization," in *Foundations of Modern Auditory Theory,* Vol. 2, ed J. V. Tobias (New York, NY: Academic Press), 303–348.

Oldfield, S. R., and Parker, S. P. A. (1984). Acuity of sound localization: a topography of auditory space. I. Normal hearing conditions. *Perception* 13, 581–600. doi: 10.1068/p130581

Perrett, S., and Noble, W. (1997a). The contribution of head motion cues to localization of low-pass noise. *Percept. Psychophys.* 59, 1018–1026. doi: 10.3758/BF03205517

Perrett, S., and Noble, W. (1997b). The effect of head rotations on vertical plane sound localization. *J. Acoust. Soc. Am.* 102, 2325–2332. doi: 10.1121/1.419642

Shaw, E. A. G., and Teranishi, R. (1968). Sound pressure generated in an external-ear replica and real human ears by a nearby point source. *J. Acoust. Soc. Am.* 44, 240–249. doi: 10.1121/1.1911059

Stelmachowicz, P. G., Beauchaine, K. A., Kalberer, A., and Jesteadt, W. (1989). Normative thresholds in the 8- to 20-kHz range as a function of age. *J. Acoust. Soc. Am.* 86, 1384–1391. doi: 10.1121/1.398698

Thurlow, W. R., Mangels, J. W., and Runge, P. S. (1967). Head movements during sound localization. *J. Acoust. Soc. Am.* 42, 489–493. doi: 10.1121/1.1910605

Thurlow, W. R., and Runge, P. S. (1967). Effect of induced head movements on localization of direction of sounds. *J. Acoust. Soc. Am.* 42, 480–488. doi: 10.1121/1.1910604

Tobias, J., and Zerlin, S. (1957). Effect of stimulus duration on lateralization threshold. *J. Acoust. Soc. Am.* 29, 774–775. doi: 10.1121/1.1918837

Wallach, H. (1940). The role of head movements and vestibular and visual cues in sound localization. *J. Exp. Psychol.* 27, 339–368. doi: 10.1037/h0054629

Wenzel, E. M., Arruda, M., Kistler, D. J., and Wightman, F. L. (1993). Localization using nonindividualized head-related transfer functions. *J. Acoust. Soc. Am.* 94, 111–123. doi: 10.1121/1.407089

Wightman, F. L., and Kistler, D. J. (1989). Headphone simulation of free-field listening. I. Stimulus synthesis. *J. Acoust. Soc. Am.* 85, 858–867. doi: 10.1121/1.397557

Wightman, F. L., and Kistler, D. J. (1999). Resolution of front-back ambiguity in spatial hearing by listener and source movement. *J. Acoust. Soc. Am.* 105, 2841–2853. doi: 10.1121/1.426899

11

Do you hear where I hear?: Isolating the individualized sound localization cues

Griffin D. Romigh * and Brian D. Simpson

Air Force Research Laboratory, Dayton, OH, USA

Correspondence:
Griffin D. Romigh, Air Force Research Laboratory, 2610 Seventh St., Wright-Patterson AFB, Dayton, OH 45433, USA
e-mail: griffin.romigh@us.af.mil

It is widely acknowledged that individualized head-related transfer function (HRTF) measurements are needed to adequately capture all of the 3D spatial hearing cues. However, many perceptual studies have shown that localization accuracy in the lateral dimension is only minimally decreased by the use of non-individualized head-related transfer functions. This evidence supports the idea that the individualized components of an HRTF could be isolated from those that are more general in nature. In the present study we decomposed the HRTF at each location into average, lateral and intraconic spectral components, along with an ITD in an effort to isolate the sound localization cues that are responsible for the inter-individual differences in localization performance. HRTFs for a given listener were then reconstructed systematically with components that were both individualized and non-individualized in nature, and the effect of each modification was analyzed via a virtual localization test where brief 250 ms noise bursts were rendered with the modified HRTFs. Results indicate that the cues important for individualization of HRTFs are contained almost exclusively in the intraconic portion of the HRTF spectra and localization is only minimally affected by introducing non-individualized cues into the other HRTF components. These results provide new insights into what specific inter-individual differences in head-related acoustical features are most relevant to sound localization, and provide a framework for how future human-machine interfaces might be more effectively generalized and/or individualized.

Keywords: head-related transfer function, spatial hearing, individual differences, auditory display

INTRODUCTION

It has long been the desire of auditory scientists to discover and map how specific physical features of the sound arriving at the two ears translate to distinct locations in perceptual space. While much progress has been made toward accomplishing this feat, the highly-individual nature of high-frequency spectral cues used for localization in the vertical and front-back dimensions has thwarted most efforts to create a universally accepted feature-based model for localization in these dimensions.

All of the physical cues available to a listener for making spatial judgments are captured in a listener's head-related transfer function, which describes the transformation a sound undergoes as it travels from a specific location in space, interacts with the listener's head, shoulders, and outer ears and arrives at a listener's eardrums (Mehrgardt and Mellert, 1977). These transfer functions can be calculated for a specific sound source direction by outfitting a listener with binaural microphones and recording the arrival of a known signal presented from the desired location (Mehrgardt and Mellert, 1977; Wightman and Kistler, 1989a). Once measured for an individual, this transfer function can be used to impart spatial information on an arbitrary single-channel sound to create the perceptual illusion that the sound originates from an actual position out in space when presented over headphones (Wightman and Kistler, 1989b; Bronkhorst, 1995; Brungart et al., 2009).

While virtual auditory displays (VADs) based on this technology have been employed in many applications including entertainment, gaming, virtual reality (Travis, 1996) and navigational aids for pilots (Simpson et al., 2007), high fidelity performance, or more specifically accurate localization in the vertical and front-back dimensions, requires that the HRTF be measured on the specific user utilizing the display, limiting their widespread implementation. Several authors have shown that when VADs use HRTFs measured on a different individual or acoustic mannequin, localization performance is severely degraded, resulting in especially poor elevation localization and frequent confusions about the front-back hemisphere of the target sound (Wenzel et al., 1993; Middlebrooks, 1999a; Brungart and Romigh, 2009).

The cues believed to be responsible for localization in these dimensions are found in the high-frequency (above 4 kHz) region of the right and left monaural HRTF magnitude spectra (Hebrank and Wright, 1974; Asano et al., 1990). This region of the HRTF is also impacted greatly by the effect of head shadow on the contralateral ear, a feature that leads to the interaural level cue used for lateral location judgments (Blauert, 1997). This means that the physical cues for both lateral localization judgments and vertical and front-back judgments are combined in the high-frequency HRTF spectrum. While much work has been done to better understand localization cues in the vertical and front-back dimensions (Blauert, 1969; Hebrank and Wright, 1974; Asano

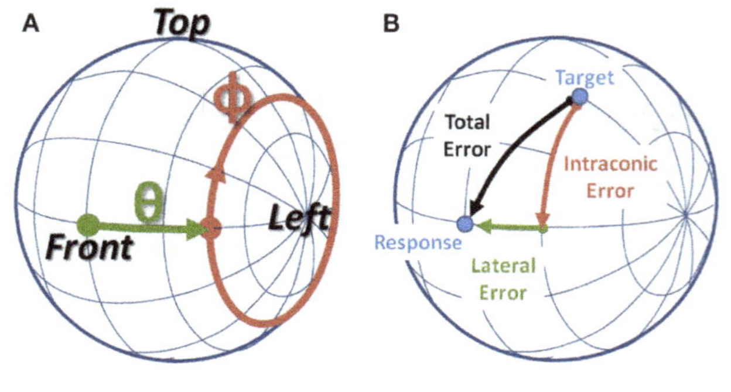

FIGURE 1 | (A) Interaural-Polar coordinate system. **(B)** Example of a localization error broken down into lateral and intraconic components.

et al., 1990; Langendijk and Bronkhorst, 2002), without a method to effectively isolate the influence of the two cues, it remains unclear what spectral features require individualization.

The current work presents a method for decomposing an HRTF into a series of components that are believed to be perceptually separable. With this decomposition, it is believed that the physical features governing localization in the vertical and front-back dimensions reside only in a subset of the resulting components. If such a subset exists, utilizing this decomposition technique should allow more focused efforts in future works designed to identify relevant spectral cues and model localization in these dimensions.

MATERIALS AND METHODS

SPECTRAL DECOMPOSITION

In order to separately address the cues believed to mediate sound localization, the interaural-polar coordinate system was adopted and employed for both the HRTF decomposition and for depicting the behavioral data. In the interaural polar coordinate system, depicted in **Figure 1A**, one can define a lateral angle ($-90^o \leq \theta \leq 90^o$) along the interaural axis, and the intraconic angle ($-180^o < \phi \leq 180^o$), where intraconic was chosen to highlight the fact that the parameter approximately describes the angular path along the cone-of-confusion for a given lateral angle. In addition, henceforth, the term "HRTF" will be used to refer to the entire set of spatial filters, while "sample HRTF" will be used to indicate a spatial filter corresponding to a single location.

The spectral decomposition technique requires that sample HRTFs be measured at (or interpolated to) a semi-regular spacing in the interaural-polar coordinate system. For simplicity, it will be assumed that the baseline HRTF was sampled every five degrees in both the lateral dimension, $\theta_s = \{-90, -85, \ldots, 0, \ldots, 85, 90\}$, and intraconic dimension, $\phi_s = \{-175, -170, \ldots, 0, \ldots, 175, 180\}$. First, the average HRTF spectrum across all locations is subtracted from each sample HRTF to create directional spectra. Then, for each lateral angle measured, a lateral spectrum is computed by finding the median spectrum of all the directional spectra measured at that lateral angle. Finally, intraconic spectra are computed by taking the difference between the directional spectrum at each location and the corresponding lateral spectrum.

Figure 2 provides a graphical example of the decomposition stages (rows) for locations along the intraconic dimension at three different lateral angles (columns). In each panel, heat maps are plotted that show the left-ear spectra for a single listener as a function of frequency (ordinate, kHz) and intraconic angle (abscissa, indicated positions are relative to listener). Color indicates the decibel level of each frequency-space bin and contour lines are drawn every 9 dB. This figure illustrates the fact that while the full spectra, the directional spectra, and the intraconic spectra are different for each location, the average spectra and the lateral spectra are constant across all locations and across all intraconic angles of a specific lateral angle, respectively.

The original spectrum at any sampled location can be reconstructed by adding together the average spectrum, the lateral spectrum corresponding to the lateral angle, and the intraconic spectrum from the sampled location. A spatial filter can then be reconstructed by converting the full spectra into the time domain using minimum phase assumptions, and delaying the resulting contralateral impulse response by the interaural time-difference (ITD) value. Alternatively, individual components from one HRTF can be swapped out for the components from a different HRTF measurement before reconstruction to create novel HRTFs constructed with components from two different measurements. In the current study, we examine the importance of having individualized HRTF measurements on a component-by-component basis by constructing HRTFs that have some individualized components and some components from an HRTF measured on a KEMAR acoustic mannequin.

EXPERIMENTAL METHODS

Subjects

Nine paid listeners (4 males, 5 females) with audiometric thresholds in the normal range (less than 20 dB HL from 150 to 8 kHz) participated in the study over the course of several weeks. All subjects had completed both free-field and virtual localization studies prior to the start of the experiment.

Facility

All of the behavioral research was conducted in the Auditory Localization Facility (ALF), located at the Air Force Research Laboratory, Wright Patterson AFB, OH (**Figure 3**). The ALF consists of a large anechoic chamber with 4-foot fiberglass wedges on all six surfaces and a suspended floor. Inside the chamber is a 7-foot-radius geodesic sphere with Bose loudspeakers positioned at each one of its 277 vertices. The sphere is also outfitted with a 6-DOF ultrasonic tracker (Intersense IS 900) and a cluster of 4 LEDs at the face of each loudspeaker. During measurement and testing, listeners stand on a small platform inside the sphere with their interaural axis aligned vertically with the center of the sphere.

HRTF Collection

For each individual listener and a KEMAR acoustic mannequin, an HRTF was measured at the beginning of the study according to the methods described in Brungart et al. (2009). In short, subjects were outfitted with binaural microphones that blocked off, and sat flush with, the entrance of the ear canal while broadband signals (periodic chirps) were presented from each ALF loudspeaker

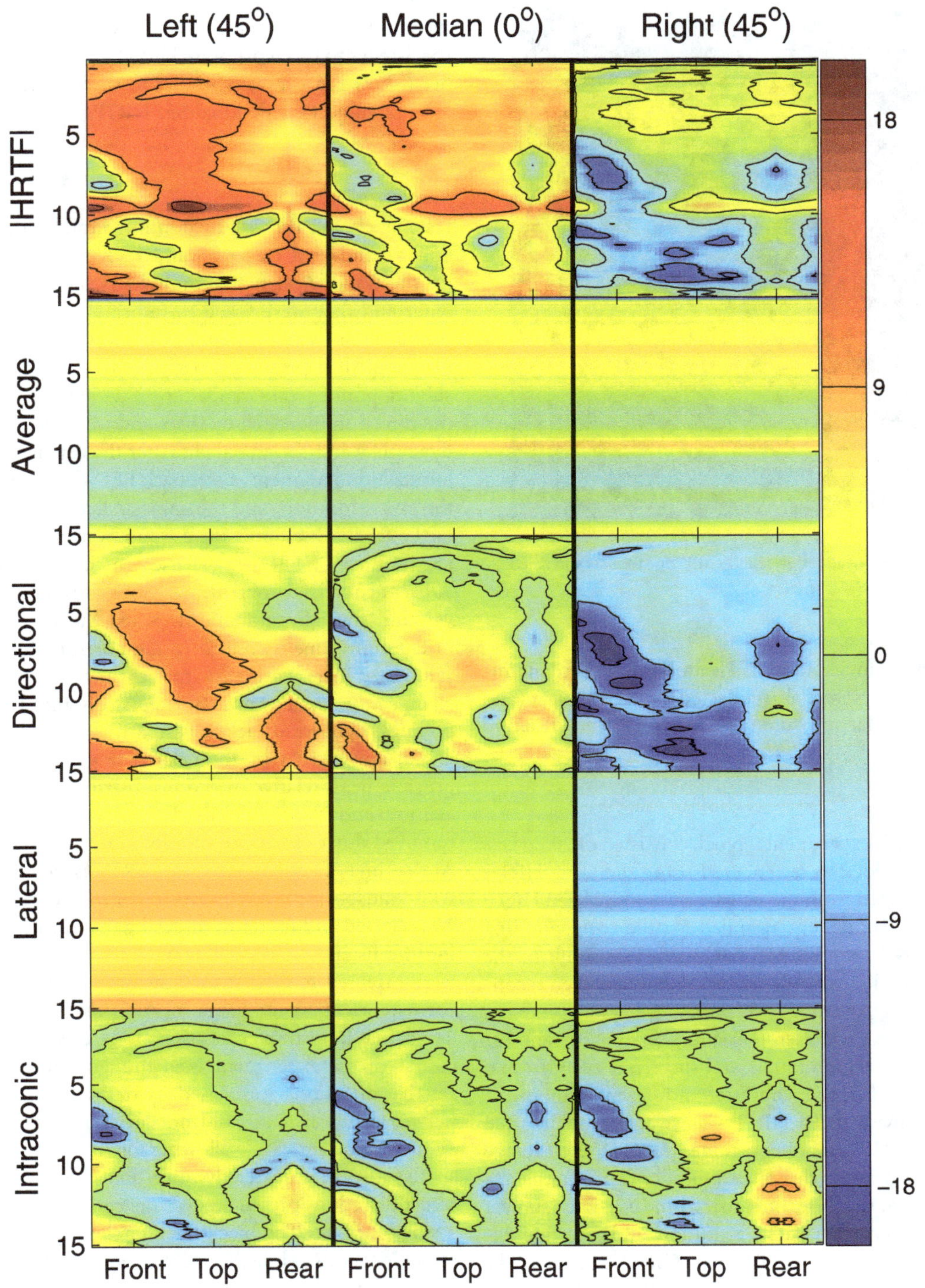

FIGURE 2 | Illustration of HRTF decomposition into individual components (rows) and three different lateral angles (columns). Each panel represents a spectral component around the correspondin cone of confusion as a function of frequency in kHz (ordinate) and intraconic angle (abscissa). Color represents absolute level in decibels.

location and recorded binaurally. A similar process was used for the KEMAR mannequin, but utilized the built-in ear-canal microphones (GRAS 46AO). The resulting recordings were subsequently used to calculate a sample HRTF for each location in the form of 256 Discrete Fourier Transform magnitude coefficients for each ear and a corresponding ITD. ITDs were found by taking the difference in slope of the best-fit lines to the unwrapped low-frequency (300–1500 Hz) phase response of each ear. Magnitude responses were then converted to the decibel scale and decomposed into average, lateral, and intraconic components using

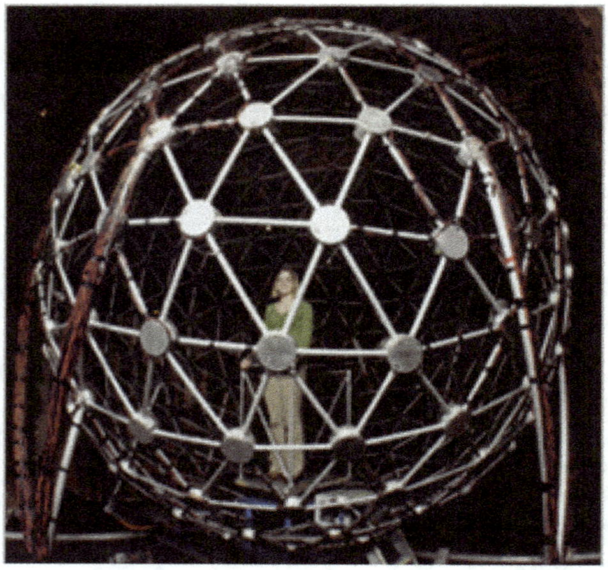

FIGURE 3 | The auditory localization facility at Wright-Patterson AFB, OH.

the method described in Section 2.1. Headphone (Beyerdynamic DT990) correction filters were also collected for each subject (and KEMAR) using a similar measurement technique (described in Brungart et al., 2009).

Stimuli

During the study, each experimental block consisted of 205 trials. All stimuli within a block were rendered using the same HRTF, which was reconstructed from the listener's individualized HRTF with up to a single component swapped for the corresponding component measured on KEMAR. For example, stimuli in the "Lat" condition were filtered with an HRTF that had been reconstructed with the ITD, average spectrum, intraconic spectrum, and headphone correction filter measured on the current listener, but with the corresponding lateral spectrum taken from a KEMAR HRTF. In each HRTF condition a different component of the listener's individualized HRTF was swapped out for the corresponding KEMAR component; none, the ITD, the average spectrum (Ave), the headphone correction filter (HpTF), the lateral spectrum (Lat), or the intraconic spectrum (IC). Each subject completed two blocks of each HRTF condition, and the presentation order was randomized across listeners. On 90% of the trials, the raw stimulus (i.e., before being filtered with an HRTF) consisted of a 250-ms noise burst, bandpass filtered between 200 and 15 kHz. On the remaining 10% of the trials the same stimulus was extended out to 10 s in duration to allow for exploratory head movements. The presentation order for the stimulus duration was randomized across trials. In a follow-up experiment listeners completed similar blocks with HRTFs constructed from a complete KEMAR HRTF, and a KEMAR HRTF where the IC spectrum was swapped to match the listener's measured IC spectrum.

For all conditions, the virtual stimuli were rendered in real-time using SLAB, a software based virtual acoustic environment rendering system (Miller and Wenzel, 2002). The current implementation of the software allows for real-time head movements of the listener to be incorporated into the virtual rendering, and has been shown in previous studies to support accurate localization when a subject's individualized HRTFs are employed (Brungart et al., 2009).

Procedure

Listeners began the task by donning headphones, a head-tracker and a hand-held tracked wand then pressing a trigger button on the wand. A virtual stimulus was then presented to the listener and they were asked to indicate the perceived location of the stimulus by pointing the wand at the perceived source location, and then pressing a response button on the wand. As the subject pointed the wand, the LEDs on the speaker closest to the direction indicated by the wand were illuminated, creating a dynamic wand-slaved cursor. After the listener responded with a localization judgment, a feedback LED cluster was illuminated at the target location, and the subjects had to acknowledge receipt of the feedback by pressing a wand button that corresponded to the number of LEDs (1–4) used in the feedback presentation. Subsequent trials progressed without a fixed inter-stimulus interval, and started automatically when the subject's head-tracked orientation came within 5° of the horizontal plane and became stationary. Here, stationary implies the head's orientation did not change more than 3° in total angular distance between successive pollings of the headtracker, 1 s apart.

On any given trial the desired target direction was 1 of 41 possible head-relative directions distributed throughout 360° in azimuth and from −45° to +90° in elevation. Low elevations were removed due to potential interference with the subject platform. At the time of presentation, the HRTF associated with the actual ALF loudspeaker location closest to the desired target direction was selected and used for rendering the virtual stimuli. By allowing the listeners freedom about what azimuthal direction they were oriented toward at the start of a trial, rather then having them reorient to the same location at the start of every trial, 245 actual loudspeaker locations were used as targets across the course of the experiment even though only 41 different head-relative directions were used as desired target locations. This helped ensure listeners did not learn a specific subset of loudspeaker locations, while allowing for repeated testing of the same small subset of head-relative directions. **Figure 4** shows the actual target directions presented over the course of the whole study for a single subject. The black filled circles represent the 41 desired target locations, while the green open circles represent tested target locations. Black rings show a 10° angular distance around each desired location to act as a distance reference under the stretching that occurs toward the poles when the spherical coordinates are plotted on a rectangular grid. As can be seen, the resulting tested target locations end-up tightly clustered and evenly distributed around the desired locations, and almost all tested locations fell within 10° of the desired location.

RESULTS

Figures 5, 6 show average angular errors computed over subject and target location. Localization errors are broken down in

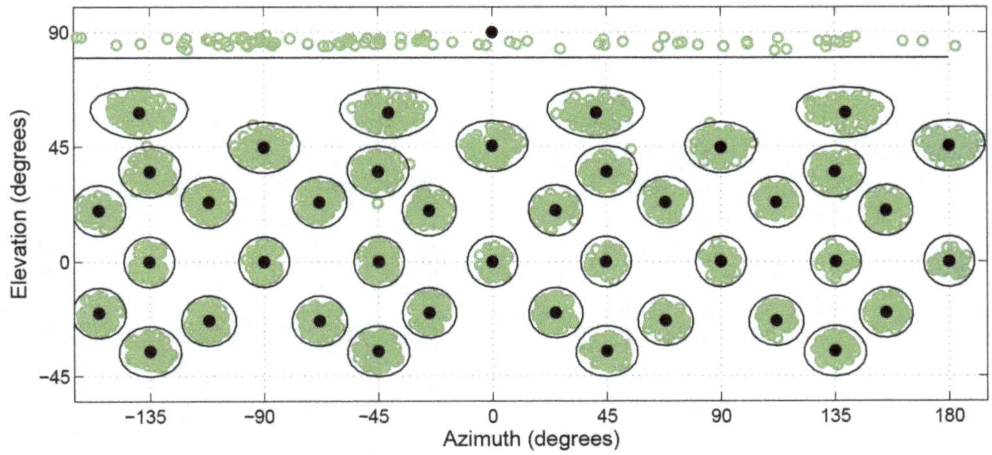

FIGURE 4 | Actual head-relative target directions (green circles) relative to desired target directions (black circles) for a single subject over the course of the entire study. Black lines enclose regions within 10° of desired target directions.

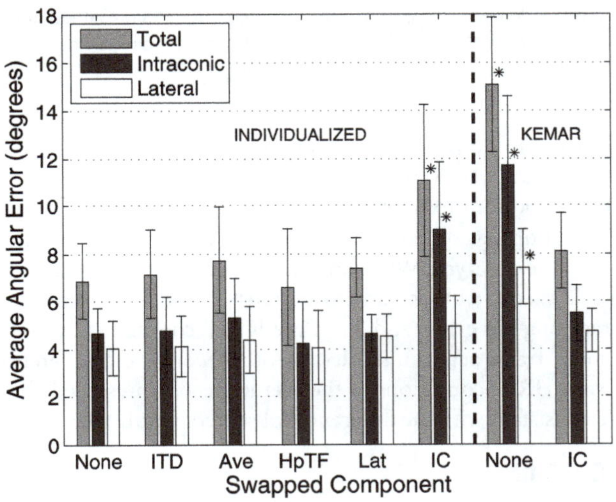

FIGURE 5 | Average localization errors with 10-s stimuli for each HRTF condition averaged over all subjects. Errors reported in terms of average total, lateral, and intraconic localization errors. Error bars represent 95% confidence intervals. *Result is statistically different from baseline (indicated in text) ($p < 0.005$, paired t-test).

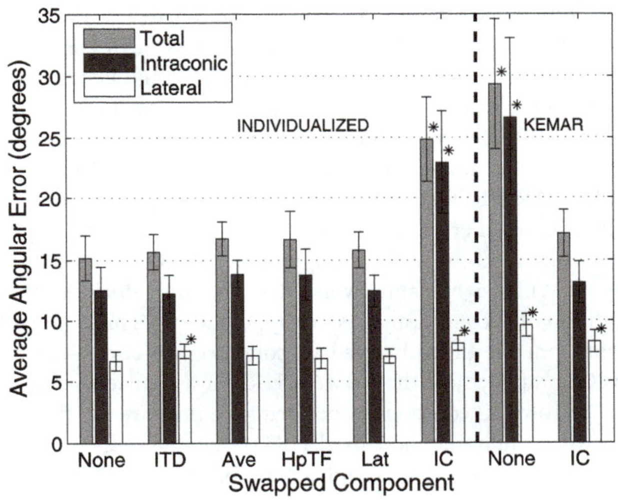

FIGURE 6 | Average localization errors with 250-ms stimuli for each HRTF condition averaged over all subjects. Errors reported in terms of average total, lateral, and intraconic localization errors. Error bars represent 95% confidence intervals. *Result is statistically different from baseline (indicated in text) ($p < 0.005$, paired t-test).

terms of the total angular, intraconic, and lateral components (depicted in **Figure 1B**), and plotted as separate color-coded bars. Each group of bars to the left of the line, labeled "Individualized" represent the first set of conditions in which isolated components (indicated on the abscissa) of the listener's individualized HRTF were swapped out for the corresponding KEMAR component. The two groups of bars to the right of the line, labeled "KEMAR," represent the two additional conditions in which a full KEMAR HRTF (None), or a KEMAR HRTF with the IC component for the listener's individualized IC component, were used. For example, INDIVIDUALIZED-None is a fully individualized HRTF and KEMAR-None is a full KEMAR HRTF. In all conditions, error bars represent 95% confidence intervals for the means, and asterisks indicate a statistically significant difference ($p < 0.05$) from the baseline condition (Individualized-None) in a paired t-test.

The left side of **Figure 5** shows the average localization results for the 10-s stimuli for the first experiment. In this condition the stimuli were long enough in duration to allow for exploratory head-motion which likely accounts for the fact that no difference in average angular error was seen when any of components of the HRTF, except the IC component, were swapped. The largest total angular error for any of the individualized HRTF conditions occurred when the IC component was swapped with KEMAR, and resulted in a significant difference in terms of total angular error. As expected most of this error was an increase in intraconic error relative to the none condition (black bars). In contrast, switching out other individualized components resulted in only negligible changes (within 1°) in lateral error.

The left side of **Figure 6** utilizes the same format for representing the average results for the 250 ms stimuli. Here, localization errors across all conditions are generally about twice as large as the corresponding conditions with 10-s stimuli (note the change in scale of the vertical axis). This is likely due to the fact that the 250-ms stimuli are too brief to allow listeners to utilize exploratory head movements. As seen in all HRTF conditions this also leads to a larger amount of the total error occurring in the intraconic dimension. Again, there was significant increase in the amount of total angular error when the IC component of the individualized HRTF was swapped out for the KEMAR IC component (25°) compared to the Individualized-None condition (15°), similar to the results with longer stimuli. The results also indicate a significant difference in the lateral error between the None and ITD conditions, as well as between the None and the IC condition, though the overall magnitude of the difference remains quite small (1°–2°).

Based on the results of the initial experimental conditions, two additional conditions were run to investigate how the earlier results compared to performance with a full KEMAR HRTF, and whether performance with a KEMAR HRTF could be improved significantly by swapping out only the IC component for the subject's own. Results from those two conditions are represented to the right of the dashed line in **Figures 5, 6.** Not surprisingly, the full KEMAR HRTF condition led to the worst performance for all three types of error with an average of about 15° total angular error with the 10-s stimuli, and approximately 28° for the 250-ms stimuli. While significantly worse than the Individualized-None condition, this condition does not appear to be significantly different from the Individualized-IC condition. In contrast, when the IC component of the KEMAR HRTF was replaced with the listener's own IC component, performance improved to the level seen with a fully-individualized HRTF (i.e., the individualized-none condition) for both stimulus durations and error types, with the exception of the lateral error with the 250-ms stimulus.

A common occurrence when using virtual audio with non-individualized HRTFs is a large increase in the rate of front-back reversals, trials in which virtual sound sources are perceived to be in the opposite front-back hemisphere to the target location. **Figure 7** shows the percentage of trials in which a front-back reversal occurred for the 250-ms stimuli, averaged over subjects. Here, all of the conditions in which there was an individualized IC component resulted in front-back reversals on about 10% of the trials, while the two conditions with a KEMAR IC spectral component resulted in front-back reversals on 20% of the trials.

Average localization results for the 250-ms stimuli for each subject from the first experiment are shown in **Figure 8.** Performance is seen to vary considerably between listeners and across the different HRTF conditions. In the baseline condition, in which no individualized components were swapped for KEMAR components (None), the best total angular error (11°) was achieved by listener 1436, while the worst performer (19°) was listener 1496. Consistent with the average results, all listeners had the worst performance in the IC condition where the listener's own intraconic spectra were replaced with those of KEMAR;

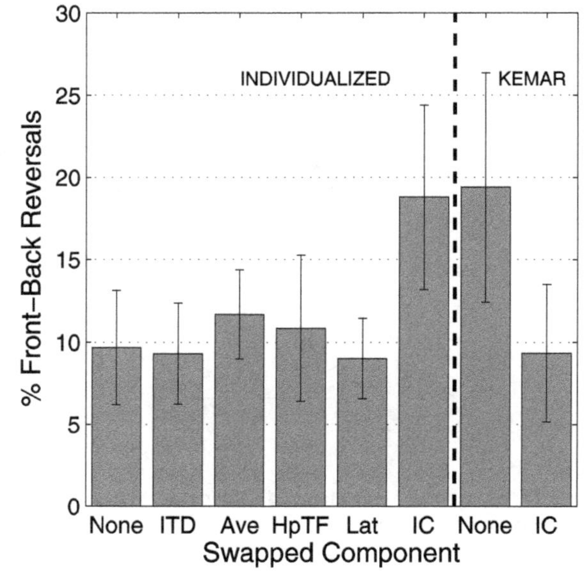

FIGURE 7 | Percentage of front-back reversals with 250-ms stimuli for each HRTF condition averaged over all subjects. Error bars represent 95% confidence intervals.

however, this modification seemed to hinder some listeners (e.g., 1581) more than others (e.g., 1564).

It is important to note, that although feedback about the target's location was provided on every trial, no significant learning effects were observed. When analyzed separately the first and fifth quintile in each block showed at most 4° of improvement in average angular error, and all of the HRTF conditions exhibited a similar trend across quintiles. In other words, the differences between HRTF conditions in the average results presented above were consistent with the differences observed in quintile averages.

DISCUSSION

Overall, the localization results agree well with published results for similar experiments using virtual stimuli both from our lab (Brungart and Romigh, 2009; Brungart et al., 2009; Romigh, 2012), and other laboratories (Wenzel et al., 1993; Bronkhorst, 1995; Middlebrooks, 1999b). In fact, in a recent meta-analysis of combined data from more than 82,000 trials collected across 161 listeners in five different laboratories, Best et al. (2011) showed a free-field localization performance of 15.6° total angular error for brief sounds, which corresponds well with the virtual performance seen in the current study with the fully individualized HRTFs. These results suggest that the baseline virtual representation was adequate to preserve all of the relevant localization cues.

Most interesting, the results indicate that the IC spectral component is the component of the HRTF that is most important to maintain virtual localization accuracy comparable to performance with fully individualized HRTFs (and potentially free-field sources). This conclusion comes from the results of both experiments which, taken together, showed that differences between performance with a fully individualized HRTF and a full KEMAR HRTF could be diminished by swapping only the IC component.

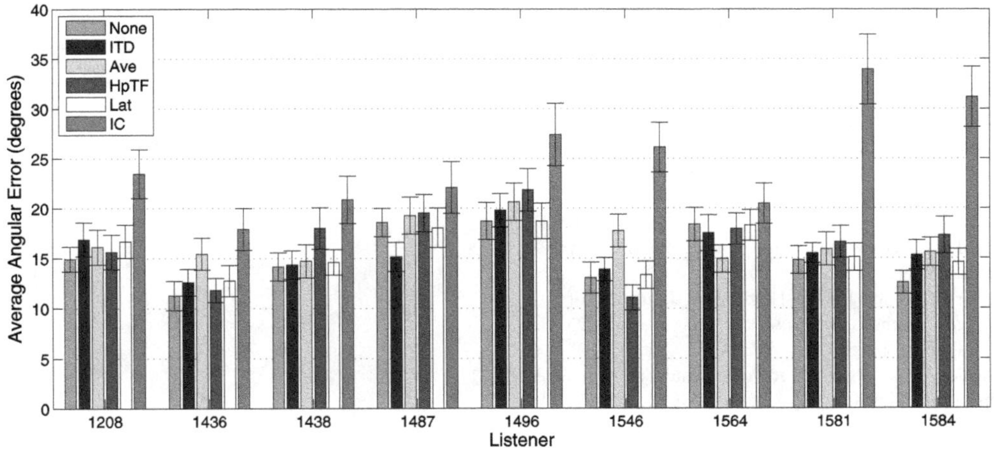

FIGURE 8 | Average total absolute localization error with 250-ms stimuli for each HRTF condition by subjects. Error bars represent 95% confidence intervals.

What this means for future work is that studies focusing on the differences between the HRTFs of individual subjects can be focused on a single component of the HRTF. Moreover, in combination with the previous discussion point, studies geared toward modeling localization in the intraconic dimension can focus their analysis toward only the physical cues contained in the IC component.

The negligible difference seen in localization performance when the other individualized components were replaced with KEMAR equivalents suggests that, for most subjects, generalized values for these components are sufficient for maintaining localization accuracy. Relating the behavioral results back to the anthropometric cause of these cues may suggest that, in terms of acoustical influence, anthropometric properties like head-size, which directly affects the ITD and lateral spectral component (Algazi et al., 2002), may be more consistent across subjects than the pinna shapes that are responsible for the contours of the IC spectral component (Algazi et al., 2001). Conversely, the differences may result from the non-linear nature of the mapping between spectral cues and intraconic location. In other words, a small change to the ITD or lateral spectrum will likely result in a perceptual image near the original, while it is much less predictable where a stimulus with a small spectral modification might be perceived spatially.

The lack of effect seen when swapping out the headphone correction (HpTF component) or the spectral average component suggests that these effects, which in some cases caused severe changes to the resulting HRTF spectrum, are ignored or compensated for when making a localization judgment. Since both of these components would have been consistent for every trial within each block, it is likely that their effects were incorporated into the listener's internal representation of the source spectrum, and therefore treated as directionally uninformative. It is important to note that despite their lack of effect on localization, initial testing by the authors confirmed that very noticeable timbrel differences were apparent when these components were exchanged, which may be of consequence for some types of auditory displays.

REFERENCES

Algazi, V. R., Duda, R. O., Duraiswami, R., Gumerov, N. A., and Tang, Z. (2002). Approximating the head-related transfer function using simple geometric models of the head and torso. *J. Acoust. Soc. Am.* 112, 2053–2064. doi: 10.1121/1.1508780

Algazi, V. R., Duda, R. O., Morrison, R. P., and Thompson, D. M. (2001). "Structural composition and decomposition of HRTFs," in *Proceedings of the IEEE Workshop the Applications of Signal Processing to Audio and Acoustics* (New Paltz, NY), 103–106.

Asano, F., Suzuki, Y., and Sone, T. (1990). Role of spectral cues in median plane localization. *J. Acoust. Soc. Am.* 88, 159–168. doi: 10.1121/1.399963

Best, V., Brungart, D., Carlile, S., Jin, C., Macpherson, E. A., Martin, R. L., et al. (2011). "A meta analysis of localization errors made in the Anechoic free-field," in *Principles and Applications of Spatial Hearing*, eds Y. Suzuki, D. Brungart, Y. Iwaya, K. Lida, D. Cabrera, and H. Kato (Hackensack, NJ: World Scientific Publishing Company), 14–23. doi: 10.1142/9789814299312-0002

Blauert, J. (1969). Sound localization in the median plane. *Acustica* 22, 205–213.

Blauert, J. (1997). *Spatial Hearing.* Cambridge, MA: The MIT Press.

Bronkhorst, A. W. (1995). Localization of real and virtual soubd sources. *J. Acoust. Soc. Am.* 98, 2542–2553. doi: 10.1121/1.413219

Brungart, D. S., and Romigh, G. D. (2009). "Spectral HRTF enhancement for improved vertical-polar auditory localization," in *IEEE Workshop on Applications of Signal Processing to Audio and Acoustics* (New Paltz, NY: IEEE WASPAA).

Brungart, D. S., Romigh, G. D., and Simpson, B. D. (2009). "Rapid collection of HRTFs and comparison to free-field listening," in *International Workshop on the Principles and Applications of Spatial Hearing* (New Paltz, NY).

Hebrank, J., and Wright, D. (1974). Spectral cues used in the localization of sound sources on the median plane. *J. Acoust. Soc. Am.* 56, 1829–1834. doi: 10.1121/1.1903520

Langendijk, E. H. A., and Bronkhorst, A. W. (2002). Contribution of spectral cues to human sound localization. *J. Acoust. Soc. Am.* 112, 1583–1596. doi: 10.1121/1.1501901

Mehrgardt, S., and Mellert, V. (1977). Transformation of the external human ear. *J. Acoust. Soc. Am.* 61, 1567–1576. doi: 10.1121/1.381470

Middlebrooks, J. C. (1999a). Individual differences in external-ear transfer functions reduced by scaling in frequency. *J. Acoust. Soc. Am.* 106, 1480–1491. doi: 10.1121/1.427176

Middlebrooks, J. C. (1999b). Virtual localization improved by scaling nonindividualized external-ear transfer functions in frequency. *J. Acoust. Soc. Am.* 106, 1493–1510. doi: 10.1121/1.427147

Miller, J. D., and Wenzel, E. M. (2002). "Recent developements in SLAB: a software-based system for interactive spatial sound synthesis," in *Proceedings of the 2002 International Conference on Auditory Display* (Kyoto).

Romigh, G. D. (2012). *Individualized Head-Related Transfer Functions: Efficient Modeling and Estimation from Small Sets of Spatial Samples.* PhD thesis, Carnegie Mellon University, Pittsburgh, PA.

Simpson, B. D., Brungart, D. S., Dallman, R. C., Yasky, R. J., Romigh, G. D., and Raquet, J. F. (2007). "In-flight navigation using head-coupled and aircraft-coupled spatial audio cues," in *Proceedings of the Human Factors and Ergonomics Society 51st Annual Meeting* (San Francisco, CA).

Travis, C. (1996). Virtual reality perspective on headphone audio. *J. Aud. Eng. Soc.* 4354, 1–13.

Wenzel, E. M., Arruda, M., Kistler, D. J., and Wightman, F. L. (1993). Localization using nonindividualized head-related transfer functions. *J. Acoust. Soc. Am.* 93, 111–123. doi: 10.1121/1.407089

Wightman, F. L., and Kistler, D. J. (1989a). Headphone simulation of free-field listening. I: stimulus synthesis. *J. Acoust. Soc. Am.* 85, 111–123. doi: 10.1121/1.397557

Wightman, F. L., and Kistler, D. J. (1989b). Headphone simulation of free-field listening. II: psychophysical validation. *J. Acoust. Soc. Am.* 85, 868–878. doi: 10.1121/1.397558

12

Acoustic and non-acoustic factors in modeling listener-specific performance of sagittal-plane sound localization

Piotr Majdak*, Robert Baumgartner and Bernhard Laback

Psychoacoustics and Experimental Audiology, Acoustics Research Institute, Austrian Academy of Sciences, Wien, Austria

Correspondence:
Piotr Majdak, Psychoacoustics and Experimental Audiology, Acoustics Research Institute, Austrian Academy of Sciences, Wohllebengasse 12-14, Wien 1040, Austria
e-mail: piotr@majdak.com

The ability of sound-source localization in sagittal planes (along the top-down and front-back dimension) varies considerably across listeners. The directional acoustic spectral features, described by head-related transfer functions (HRTFs), also vary considerably across listeners, a consequence of the listener-specific shape of the ears. It is not clear whether the differences in localization ability result from differences in the encoding of directional information provided by the HRTFs, i.e., an acoustic factor, or from differences in auditory processing of those cues (e.g., spectral-shape sensitivity), i.e., non-acoustic factors. We addressed this issue by analyzing the listener-specific localization ability in terms of localization performance. Directional responses to spatially distributed broadband stimuli from 18 listeners were used. A model of sagittal-plane localization was fit individually for each listener by considering the actual localization performance, the listener-specific HRTFs representing the acoustic factor, and an uncertainty parameter representing the non-acoustic factors. The model was configured to simulate the condition of complete calibration of the listener to the tested HRTFs. Listener-specifically calibrated model predictions yielded correlations of, on average, 0.93 with the actual localization performance. Then, the model parameters representing the acoustic and non-acoustic factors were systematically permuted across the listener group. While the permutation of HRTFs affected the localization performance, the permutation of listener-specific uncertainty had a substantially larger impact. Our findings suggest that across-listener variability in sagittal-plane localization ability is only marginally determined by the acoustic factor, i.e., the quality of directional cues found in typical human HRTFs. Rather, the non-acoustic factors, supposed to represent the listeners' efficiency in processing directional cues, appear to be important.

Keywords: sound localization, localization model, sagittal plane, listener-specific factors, head-related transfer functions

INTRODUCTION

Human listeners use monaural spectral cues to localize sound sources in sagittal planes (e.g., Wightman and Kistler, 1997; van Wanrooij and van Opstal, 2005). This includes the ability to assign the vertical position of the source (e.g., Vliegen and van Opstal, 2004) and to distinguish between front and back (e.g., Zhang and Hartmann, 2010). Spectral cues are caused by the acoustic filtering of the torso, head, and pinna, and can be described by means of head-related transfer functions (HRTFs; e.g., Møller et al., 1995). The direction-dependent components of the HRTFs are described by directional transfer functions (DTFs, Middlebrooks, 1999b).

The ability to localize sound sources in sagittal planes, usually tested in psychoacoustic experiments as localization performance, varies largely across listeners (Middlebrooks, 1999a; Rakerd et al., 1999; Zhang and Hartmann, 2010). A factor contributing to the variability across listeners might be the listeners' morphology. The ear shape varies across the human population (Algazi et al., 2001) and these differences cause the DTF features to vary across individuals (Wightman and Kistler, 1997). One might expect that different DTF sets provide different amounts of cues available for the localization of a sound. When listening with DTFs of other listeners, the performance might be different, an effect we refer to in this study as the *acoustic factor* in sound localization.

The strong effect of training on localization performance (Majdak et al., 2010, Figure 7) indicates that in addition to the acoustic factor, also other listener-specific factors are involved. For example, a link between the listener-specific sensitivity to the spectral envelope shape and the listener-specific localization performance has been recently shown (Andéol et al., 2013). However, other factors like the ability to perform the experimental task, the attention paid to the relevant cues, or the accuracy in responding might contribute as well. In the present study, we consolidate all those factors to a single factor which we refer to as the *non-acoustic factor*.

In this study, we are interested in the contribution of the acoustic and non-acoustic factors to sound localization performance. As for the acoustic factor, its effect on localization performance has already been investigated in many studies (e.g., Wightman and Kistler, 1997; Middlebrooks, 1999a; Langendijk and Bronkhorst, 2002). However, most of those studies investigated *ad-hoc* listening with modified DTFs without any re-calibration of the spectral-to-spatial mapping in the auditory system (Hofman et al., 1998). By testing the *ad-hoc* localization performance to modified DTFs, two factors were simultaneously varied: the directional cues in the incoming sound, and their mismatch to the familiarized (calibrated) mapping. The acoustic factor of interest in our study, however, considers changes in the DTFs of the *own* ears, i.e., changes of DTFs without any mismatch between the incoming sound and the calibrated mapping. A localization experiment testing such a condition would need to minimize the mismatch by achieving a re-calibration. Such a re-calibration is indeed achievable in an extensive training with modified DTFs, however, the experimental effort is rather demanding and requires weeks of exposure to the modified cues (Hofman and van Opstal, 1998; Majdak et al., 2013). Note that such a long-term re-calibration is usually attributed to perceptual adaptation, in contrast to the short-term learning found to take place within hours (Zahorik et al., 2006; Parseihian and Katz, 2012).

Using a model of the localization process, the condition of a complete re-calibration can be more easily achieved. Thus, our study is based on predictions from a model of sagittal-plane sound localization (Baumgartner et al., 2013). This model assumes that listeners create an internal template set of their specific DTFs as a result of a learning process (Hofman et al., 1998; van Wanrooij and van Opstal, 2005). The more similar the representation of the incoming sound compared to a template, the larger the assumed probability of responding at the polar angle corresponding to that template (Langendijk and Bronkhorst, 2002). The model from Baumgartner et al. (2013) uses a method to compute localization performance based on probabilistic predictions and considers both acoustic factors in terms of the listener-specific DTFs and non-acoustic factors in terms of an uncertainty parameter U. In Baumgartner et al. (2013), the model has been validated under various conditions for broadband stationary sounds. In that model, the role of the acoustic factor can be investigated by simultaneously modifying DTFs of both the incoming sound and the template sets. This configuration allows to predict sound localization performance when listening with others' ears following a complete re-calibration to the tested DTFs.

In the following, we briefly describe the model and revisit the listener-specific calibration of the model. Then, the effect of the uncertainty representing the non-acoustic factor, and the effect of the DTF set representing the acoustic factor, are investigated. Finally, the relative contributions of the two factors are compared.

MATERIALS AND METHODS

MODEL

In this study, we used the model proposed by Baumgartner et al. (2013). The model relies on a comparison between an internal representation of the incoming sound and an internal template set (Zakarauskas and Cynader, 1993; Hofman and van Opstal, 1998; Langendijk and Bronkhorst, 2002; Baumgartner et al., 2013). The internal template set is assumed to be created by means of learning the correspondence between the spectral features and the direction of an acoustic event based on feedback from other modalities (Hofman et al., 1998; van Wanrooij and van Opstal, 2005). The model is implemented in the Auditory Modeling Toolbox as `baumgartner2013` (Søndergaard and Majdak, 2013).

Figure 1 shows the basic structure of the model from Baumgartner et al. (2013). Each block represents a processing stage of the auditory system in a functional way. The target sound is processed in order to obtain an internal (neural) representation. This target representation is compared to an equivalently processed internal template set consisting of the DTF representations for the given sagittal plane. This comparison process is the basis of a spectral-to-spatial mapping, which yields the prediction probability for responding at a given polar angle.

In general, in this study, we used the model configured as suggested in Baumgartner et al. (2013). In the following, we summarize the model stages and their configuration, focusing on the acoustic and non-acoustic factors in the localization process.

Peripheral processing

In the model, the same peripheral processing is considered for the incoming sound and the template. The peripheral processing stage aims at modeling the effect of human physiology while focusing on directional cues. The effect of the torso, head and pinna are considered by filtering the incoming sound by a DTF.

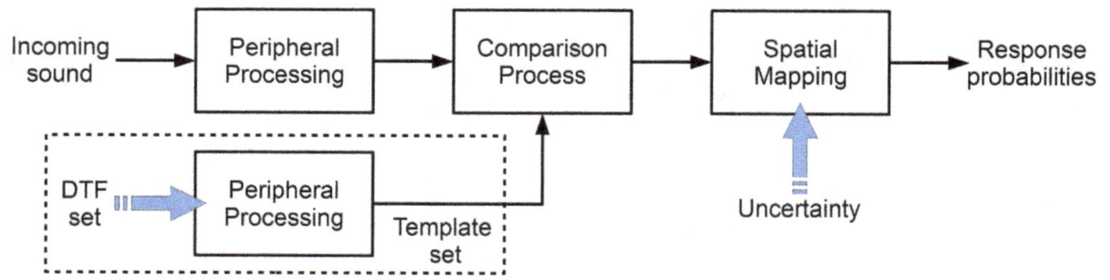

FIGURE 1 | Structure of the sound localization model from Baumgartner et al. (2013). The incoming target sound is peripherally processed and the result is compared to an internal template set. The comparison result is mapped yielding the probability for responding at a given polar angle. The blue arrows indicate the free parameters of the corresponding sections. In the model, the DTF set and the uncertainty represent the acoustic and non-acoustic factors, respectively.

The effect of the cochlear filtering was considered as linear Gammatone filter bank (Patterson et al., 1988). The filter bank produces a signal for each frequency band. 28 frequency bands were considered in the model, determined by the lowest frequency of 0.7 kHz, the highest frequency of 18 kHz, and the frequency spacing of the bands corresponding to one equivalent rectangular bandwidth (Glasberg and Moore, 1990). In the model, the output of each frequency band is half-wave rectified and low-pass filtered (2nd-order Butterworth filter, cut-off frequency of 1 kHz) in order to simulate the effect of the inner hair cells (Dau et al., 1996). The filtered outputs are then temporally averaged in terms of root-mean-square (RMS) amplitude, resulting in the internal representation of the sound.

Comparison stage

In the comparison stage, the internal representation of the incoming sound is compared with the internal template set. Each template is selected by a polar angle denoted as template angle. A distance metric is calculated as a function of the template angle and is interpreted as a descriptor contributing to the prediction of the listener's response.

In the model, the distance metric is represented by the standard deviation (SD) of the inter-spectral differences between the internal representation of the incoming sound and a template calculated across frequency bands. The SD of inter-spectral differences is robust against changes in overall level and has been shown to be superior to other metrics like the inter-spectral cross-correlation coefficient (Langendijk and Bronkhorst, 2002).

Spatial mapping

In the model, a probabilistic approach is used for the mapping of the distance metric to the predicted response probability. For a particular target angle, response angle, and ear, the distance metric is mapped by a Gaussian function to a similarity index (SI), interpreted as a measure reflecting the response probability for a response angle.

The mapping function actually reflects the *non-acoustic factor* of the localization process. In the model, the width of the Gaussian function was considered as a property of an individual listener. Baumgartner et al. (2013) assumed that a listener being more precise in the response to the same sound would need a more narrow mapping than a less precise listener. Thus, the width of the mapping function was interpreted as a listener-specific uncertainty, U. In the model, it accounted for listener-specific localization performance and was a free parameter in the calibration process. In Langendijk and Bronkhorst (2002), the uncertainty parameter has actually also been used (their S), however, it was considered to be constant for all listeners, thus representing a rather general property of the auditory system. The impact of the uncertainty U, representing the non-acoustic factor responsible for the listener variability on the predicted localization performance is described in the following sections.

In the model, the contribution of the two ears was considered by applying a binaural weighting function (Morimoto, 2001; Macpherson and Sabin, 2007), which reduces the contribution of the contralateral ear with increasing lateral angle of the target sound. The binaural weighting function is applied to each monaural SI, and the sum of the weighted monaural SIs yields the binaural SI.

In the model, for a given target angle, the binaural SIs are calculated as a function of the response angle, i.e., for all templates. The SI as a function of response angle is scaled to a sum of one in order to be interpreted as a probability mass vector (PMV), i.e., a discrete version of a probability density function. Such a PMV describes the listener's response probability as a function of the response angle for a given incoming sound.

EXPERIMENTAL CONDITIONS FOR CALIBRATION

In Baumgartner et al. (2013), the model was calibrated to the actual performance of a pool of listeners for the so-called baseline condition, for which actual data (DTFs and localization responses) were collected in two studies, namely in Goupell et al. (2010) and Majdak et al. (2013). In both studies, localization responses were collected using virtual stimuli presented via headphones. While localization performance seems to be better when using free-field stimuli presented via loudspeakers (Middlebrooks, 1999b), we used virtual stimuli in order to better control for cues like head movements, loudspeaker equalization, or room reflections. In this section, we summarize the methods used to obtain the baseline conditions in those two studies.

Subjects

In total, 18 listeners were considered for the calibration. Eight listeners were from Goupell et al. (2010) and 13 listeners were from Majdak et al. (2013), i.e., three listeners participated in both studies. None of them had indications of hearing disorders. All of them had thresholds of 20-dB hearing level or lower at frequencies from 0.125 to 12.5 kHz.

HRTFs and DTFs

In both Goupell et al. (2010) and Majdak et al. (2013), HRTFs were measured individually for each listener. The DTFs were then calculated from the HRTFs. Both HRTFs and DTFs are part of the ARI HRTF database (Majdak et al., 2010).

Twenty-two loudspeakers (custom-made boxes with VIFA 10 BGS as drivers) were mounted on a vertical circular arc at fixed elevations from −30° to 80°, with a 10° spacing between 70° and 80° and 5° spacing elsewhere. The listener was seated in the center point of the circular arc on a computer-controlled rotating chair. The distance between the center point and each speaker was 1.2 m. Microphones (Sennheiser KE-4-211-2) were inserted into the listener's ear canals and their output signals were directly recorded via amplifiers (FP-MP1, RDL) by the digital audio interface.

A 1729-ms exponential frequency sweep from 0.05 to 20 kHz was used to measure each HRTF. To speed up the measurement, for each azimuth, the multiple exponential sweep method was used (Majdak et al., 2007). At an elevation of 0°, the HRTFs were measured with a horizontal spacing of 2.5° within the range of ±45° and 5° otherwise. With this rule, the measurement positions for other elevations were distributed with a constant spatial angle, i.e., the horizontal angular spacing increased with the elevation. In total, HRTFs for 1550 positions within the full 360° horizontal span were measured for each listener. The measurement procedure lasted for approximately 20 min. The acoustic influence of the equipment was removed by equalizing the HRTFs with the transfer functions of the equipment. The equipment transfer functions were derived from reference measurements in which the microphones were placed at the center point of the circular arc and the measurements were performed for all loudspeakers.

The DTFs (Middlebrooks, 1999b) were calculated. The magnitude of the common transfer function (CTF) was calculated by averaging the log-amplitude spectra of all HRTFs for each individual listener and ear. The phase spectrum of the CTF was set to the minimum phase corresponding to the amplitude spectrum. The DTFs were the result of filtering HRTFs with the inverse complex CTF. Finally, the impulse responses of all DTFs were windowed with an asymmetric Tukey window (fade in of 0.5 ms and fade out of 1 ms) to a 5.33-ms duration.

Stimulus

In Majdak et al. (2013), the experiments were performed for targets in the lateral range of ±60°. In Goupell et al. (2010), the experiments were performed for targets in the lateral range of ±10°. The direction of a target is described by the polar angle ranging from −30° (front, below eye-level) to 210° (rear, below eye-level).

The audio stimuli were Gaussian white noise bursts with a duration of 500 ms, which were filtered with the listener-specific DTFs corresponding to the tested condition. The level of the stimuli was 50 dB above the individually measured absolute detection threshold for that stimulus, estimated in a manual up-down procedure for a frontal eye-leveled position. In the experiments, the stimulus level was randomly roved for each trial within the range of ±5 dB in order to reduce the possibility of using overall level cues for localization.

Apparatus

In both studies, Goupell et al. (2010) and Majdak et al. (2013), the virtual acoustic stimuli were presented via headphones (HD 580, Sennheiser) in a semi-anechoic room. Stimuli were generated using a computer and output via a digital audio interface (ADI-8, RME) with a 48-kHz sampling rate. A virtual visual environment was presented via a head-mounted display (3-Scope, Trivisio). It provided two screens with a field of view of 32° x 24° (horizontal x vertical dimension). The virtual visual environment was presented binocularly with the same picture for both eyes. A tracking sensor (Flock of Birds, Ascension), mounted on the top of the listener's head, captured the position and orientation of the head in real time. A second tracking sensor was mounted on a manual pointer. The tracking data were used for the 3-D graphic rendering and response acquisition. More details about the apparatus are provided in Majdak et al. (2010).

Procedure

For the calibration, the data were collected in two studies using the same procedure. In Goupell et al. (2010), the data were the last 300 trials collected within the acoustic training, see their Sec. II. D. In Majdak et al. (2013), the data were the 300 trials collected within the acoustic test performed at the beginning of the pre-training experiments, see their Sec. II. D. In the following, we summarize the procedure used in the two studies.

In both studies, the listeners were immersed in a spherical virtual visual environment (for more details see Majdak et al., 2010). They were standing on a platform and held a pointer in their right hand. The projection of the pointer direction on the sphere's surface, calculated based on the position and orientation of the tracker sensors, was visualized and recorded as the perceived target position. The pointer was visualized whenever it was in the listeners' field of view.

Prior to the acoustic tests, listeners participated in a visual training procedure with the goal to train them to point accurately to the target. The visual training was a simplified game in the first-person perspective in which listeners had to find a visual target, point at it, and click a button within a limited time period. This training was continued until 95% of the targets were found with an RMS angular error smaller than 2°. This performance was reached within a few hundred trials.

In the acoustic experiments, at the beginning of each trial, the listeners were asked to align themselves with the reference position, keep the head direction constant, and click a button. Then, the stimulus was presented. The listeners were asked to point to the perceived stimulus location and click the button again. Then, a visual target in the form of a red rotating cube was shown at the position of the acoustic target. In cases where the target was outside of the field of view, arrows pointed towards its position. The listeners were asked to find the target, point at it, and click the button. At this point in the procedure, the listeners had both heard the acoustic target and seen the visualization of its position. To stress the link between visual and acoustic location, the listeners were asked to return to the reference position and listen to the same acoustic target once more. The visual feedback was intended to trigger a procedural training in order to improve the localization performance within the first few hundred of trials (Majdak et al., 2010). During this second acoustic presentation, the visual target remained visualized in the visual environment. Then, while the target was still visualized, the listeners had to point at the target and click the button again. An experimental block consisted of 50 targets and lasted for approximately 15 min.

DATA ANALYSIS

In the psychoacoustic experiments, the errors were calculated by subtracting the target angles from the response angles. We separated our data analysis into confusions between the hemifields and the local performance within the correct hemifield. The rate of confusions was represented by the quadrant error (QE), which is the percentage of responses where the absolute polar error exceeded 90° (Middlebrooks, 1999b). In order to quantify the local performance in the polar dimension, the local polar RMS error (PE) was calculated, i.e., the RMS of the polar errors calculated for the data without QEs.

The listener-specific results from both Goupell et al. (2010) and Majdak et al. (2013) were pooled. Only responses within the lateral range of ±30° were considered because (1) most of the localization responses were given in that range, (2) Baumgartner et al. (2013) evaluated the model using only that range, and (3) recent evaluations indicate that predictions for that range seem to be slightly more accurate than those for more lateral ranges (Baumgartner et al., 2014). For the considered data, the average

QE was 9.3% ± 6.0% and the average PE was 34° ± 5°. This is similar to the results from Middlebrooks (1999b) who tested 14 listeners in virtual condition using DTFs. His average QE was 7.7% ± 8.0% and the average PE was 29° ± 5°.

In the model, targets in the lateral range of ±30° were considered in order to match the lateral range of the actual targets from the localization experiments. For each listener, PMVs were calculated for three lateral segments with a lateral width of 20° each, and these PMVs were evaluated corresponding to the actual lateral target angles. The QE was the sum of the corresponding PMV entries outside the local polar range for which the response-target distance exceeded 90°. The PE was the discrete expectancy value within the local polar range. Both errors were calculated as the arithmetic averages across all polar target angles considered.

RESULTS AND DISCUSSION

MODEL CALIBRATION

In Baumgartner et al. (2013), the model was calibrated individually for each listener by finding the uncertainty U providing the smallest residual in the predictions as compared to the actual performance obtained in the localization experiments.

In our study, this calibration process was revisited. For each listener and all target directions, PMVs were calculated for varying uncertainty U ranging from 0.1 to 4.0 in steps of 0.1. Listener-specific DTFs were used for both the template set and incoming sound. **Figure 2** shows PMVs and the actual localization responses for four exemplary listeners and exemplary uncertainties.

For each listener, the predicted PEs and QEs were calculated from the PMVs, and the actual PEs and QEs were calculated from the experimental results. **Figure 3** shows the predicted QEs and PEs as a function of the uncertainty for the four exemplary listeners. The symbols show the actual QEs and PEs.

In Baumgartner et al. (2013), the uncertainty yielding the smallest squared sum of residues between the actual and predicted performances (PE and QE) was considered as optimal. Using the same procedure, the optimal uncertainties U_k were calculated for each listener k and are shown in **Table 1**. For the

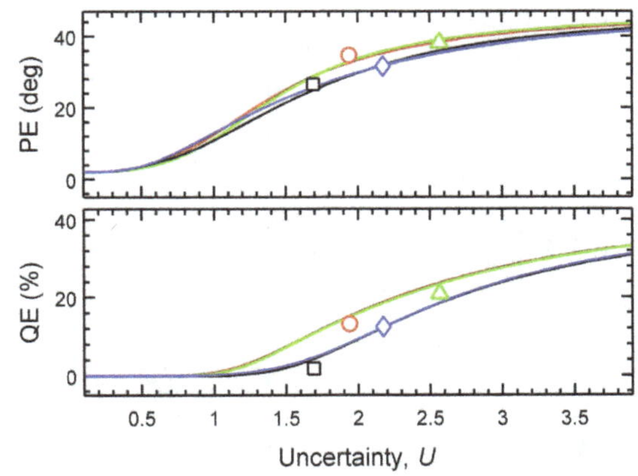

FIGURE 3 | Predicted localization performance depends on the uncertainty. PEs and QEs are shown as functions of U for four exemplary listeners ($k = 3$: blue squares, $k = 9$: red triangles, $k = 12$: green diamonds, $k = 15$: black circles). Lines show the model predictions. Symbols show the actual performance obtained in the localization experiment (placement on the abscissa corresponds to the optimal listener-specific uncertainty U_k).

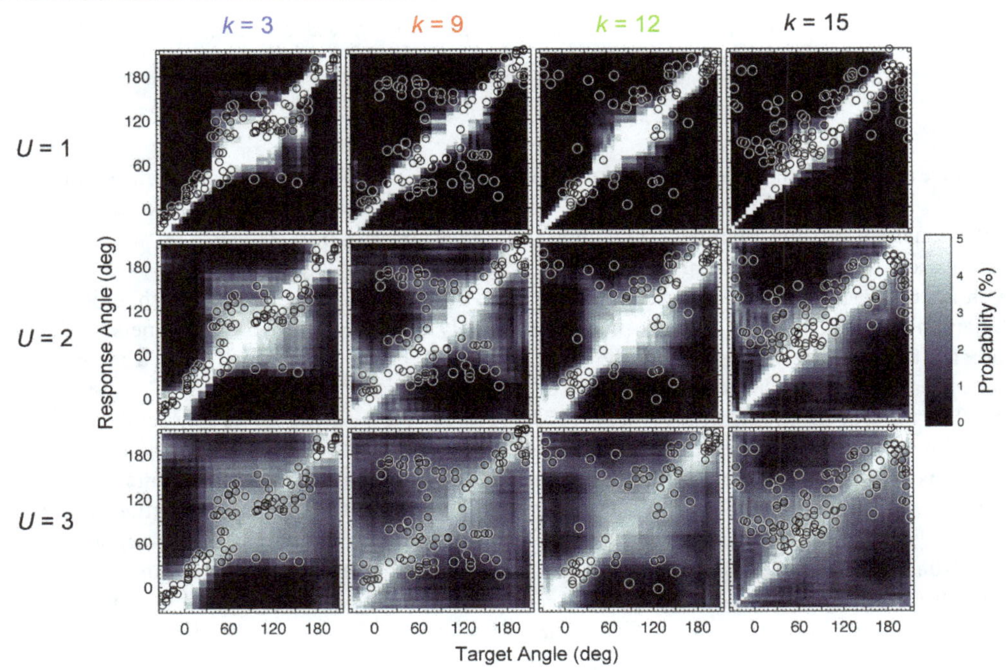

FIGURE 2 | Actual and modeled localization. Actual localization responses (circles) and modeled response probabilities (PMVs, brightness encoded) calculated for three uncertainties U and four exemplary listeners indexed by k.

Table 1 | Uncertainty U_k of individual listener with index k.

k	1	2	3	4	5	6	7	8	9	10	11	12	13	14	15	16	17	18
x	58	53	12	42	46	43	15	21	22	71	55	64	72	68	33	39	62	41
U	1.48	1.63	1.68	1.74	1.75	1.83	1.85	1.91	1.94	2.01	2.12	2.22	2.24	2.29	2.33	2.35	2.47	3.05

Listener indexed by k is identified in the ARI HRTF database by NHx_k. The listeners are sorted by k corresponding to ascending U_k.

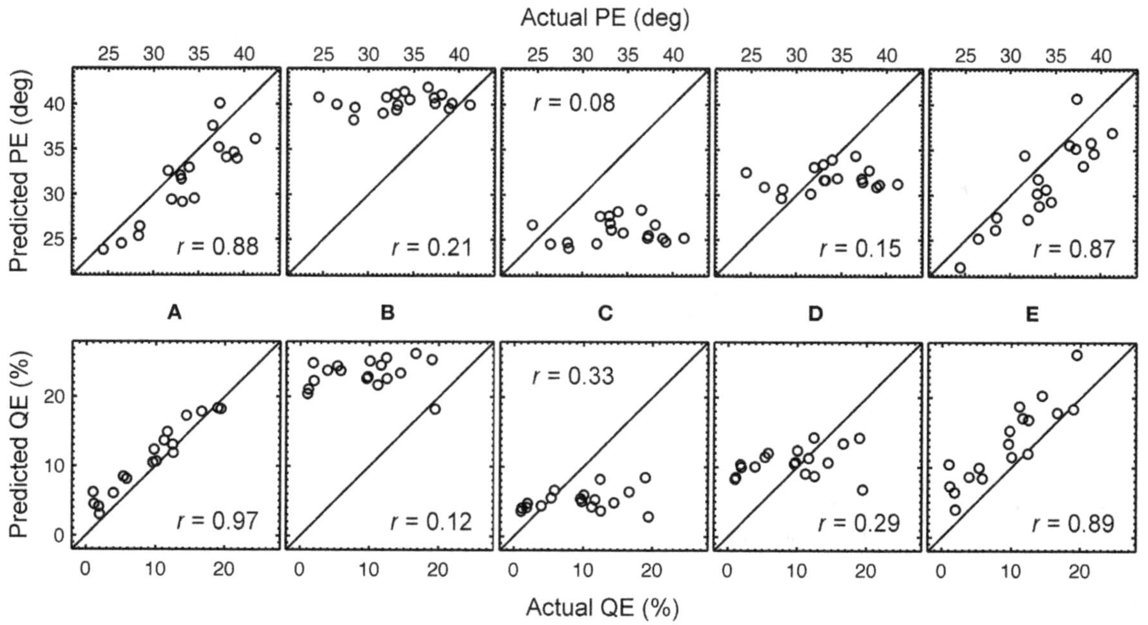

FIGURE 4 | Predicted versus actual localization performance. Predicted PEs and QEs are shown as functions of the actual PEs and QEs, respectively, for each listener. **(A)** Optimal listener-specific uncertainties U_k. **(B)** Listener-constant uncertainty yielding best correlation for PE, $U = 2.89$. **(C)** Listener-constant uncertainty yielding best correlation for QE, $U = 1.87$. **(D)** Listener-constant uncertainty from (Langendijk and Bronkhorst, 2002), $U = 2.0$. **(E)** Listener-specific uncertainties U_k and the same DTF set ($k = 14$) for all listeners (see Section 3.3 for more details). The correlation coefficient is denoted by r.

listener group, the average listener-specific uncertainty amounted to 2.05 ($SD = 0.37$).

With the optimal listener-specific uncertainties from **Table 1**, predictions were compared to the actual localization performances. **Figure 4A** shows the correspondence between the actual and predicted QEs and PEs of all listeners when using those listener-specific uncertainties. For the listener group, the correlation coefficient between actual and predicted localization errors was 0.88 for PE and 0.97 for QE. In Baumgartner et al. (2013), the model calibrated with those optimal uncertainties was evaluated in further conditions involving DTF modifications yielding correlation coefficients in the range of 0.75.

3.2. NON-ACOUSTIC FACTOR: LISTENER-SPECIFIC UNCERTAINTY

In Baumgartner et al. (2013), the optimal listener-specific uncertainties were assumed to yield most accurate performance predictions. In Langendijk and Bronkhorst (2002), the effect of spectral cues was modeled by using a parameter corresponding to our uncertainty. Interestingly, that parameter was constant for all listeners and the impact of this listener-specific uncertainty is not clarified yet. Thus, in this section, we investigate the effect of uncertainty being listener-specific as compared to uncertainty being constant for all listeners, when using the model from Baumgartner et al. (2013).

Predictions were calculated with a model calibrated to uncertainty being constant for all listeners. Three uncertainties were used: (1) $U = 2.89$, which yielded largest correlation with the actual PEs of the listeners, (2) $U = 1.87$, which yielded largest correlation with the actual QEs, and (3) $U = 2.0$, which corresponds to that used in Langendijk and Bronkhorst (2002). The DTFs used for the incoming sound and the template set were still listener-specific, representing the condition of listening with own ears. The predictions are shown in **Figures 4B–D**. The corresponding correlation coefficients are shown as insets in the corresponding panels. From this comparison and the comparison to that for listener-specific uncertainties (**Figure 4A**), it is evident that listener-specific calibration is required to account for the listener-specific actual performance.

Our findings are consistent with the results from Langendijk and Bronkhorst (2002) who used a constant calibration for all listeners. The focus of that study was to investigate the change in predictions caused by the variation of spectral cues. Thus, prediction changes for different conditions *within* an individual listener were important, which, in the light of the model from Baumgartner et al. (2013), correspond to the variation of the DTFs used for the incoming sound and not to the variation of the uncertainty. $U = 2.0$ seems to be indeed an adequate choice for predictions for an "average listener". This is supported by the similar average uncertainty of our listener group ($U = 2.05$). It is further supported by the performance predicted with $U = 2.0$, which was similar to the actual group performance. For acurate listener-specific predictions, however, listener-specific uncertainty is required.

The listener-constant uncertainty seems to have largely reduced the predicted performance variability in the listener group. In order to quantify this observation, the group SDs were calculated for predictions with listener-constant U from 1.1 to 2.9 in steps of 0.1 for each listener. For PE, the group SD was $0.96° \pm 0.32°$. For QE, the group SD was $1.34\% \pm 0.87\%$. For comparison, the group SD for predictions with listener-*specific* uncertainties was 4.58° and 5.07% for PE and QE, respectively, i.e., three times larger than those for predictions with the listener-constant uncertainties.

In summary, the listener-specific uncertainty seems to be vital to obtain accurate predictions of the listeners' actual performance. The listener-constant uncertainty drastically reduced the correlation between the predicted and actual performance. Further, the listener-constant uncertainty reduced the group variability in the predictions. Thus, as the only parameter varied in the model, the uncertainty seems to determine to a large degree the baseline performance predicted by the model. It can be interpreted as a parameter calibrating the model in order to represent a good or bad localizer; the smaller the uncertainty, the better the listeners' performance in a localization task. Notably, uncertainty is not associated with any acoustic information considered in the model, and thus, it represents the non-acoustic factor in modeling sound localization.

3.3. ACOUSTIC FACTOR: LISTENER-SPECIFIC DIRECTIONAL CUES

In the previous section, the model predictions were calculated for listeners' own DTFs in both the template set and the incoming sound; a condition corresponding to listening with own ears. With the DTFs of other listeners but own uncertainty, their performance might have been different.

For the investigation of that effect, one possibility would be to vary the quality of the DTF sets along a continuum simultaneously in both the incoming sound and the template set, and analyze the corresponding changes in the predictions. Such an investigation would be, in principle, similar to that from the previous section where the uncertainty was varied and the predicted performance was analyzed. While U represents a measure of the uncertainty, a similar metric would be required in order to quantify the quality differences between two DTF sets. Finding an appropriate metric is challenging. A potentially useful metric is the spectral SD of inter-spectral differences (Middlebrooks, 1999b; Langendijk and Bronkhorst, 2002) as used in the model from (Baumgartner et al., 2013) as the distance metric and thus as basis for the predictions. Being a part of the model, however, this metric is barred from being an independent factor in our investigation.

In order to analyze the DTF set variation as a parameter without any need for quantification of the variation, we systematically replaced the listeners' own DTFs by DTFs from other listeners from this study. The permutation of the DTF sets and uncertainties within the same listener group allowed us to estimate the effect of directional cues relative to the effect of uncertainty on the localization performance of our group.

For each listener, the model predictions were calculated using a combination of DTF sets and uncertainties of all listeners from the group. Indexing each listener by k, predicted PEs and QEs as functions of U_k and D_k were obtained, with U_k and D_k being the uncertainty and the DTF set, respectively, of the k-th listener. **Figure 5** shows the predicted PEs and QEs for all combinations of U_k and D_k. The listener group was sorted such that the uncertainty increases with increasing k and the same sorting order was used for D_k. This sorting order corresponds to that from **Table 1**.

The results reflect some of the effects described in the previous sections. The main diagonal represents the special case of identical k for D_k and U_k, corresponding to listener-specific performance, i.e., predictions for each listener's actual DTFs and optimal listener-specific uncertainty from the calibrated model described

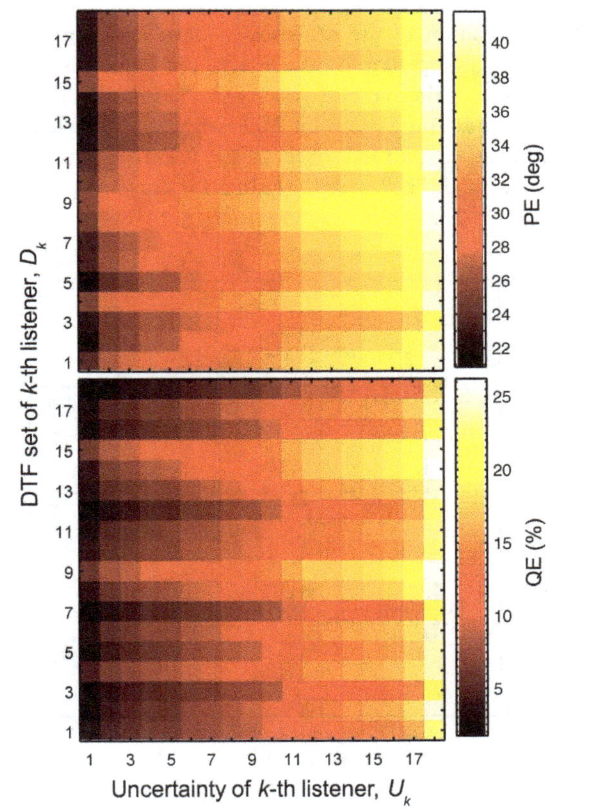

FIGURE 5 | Localization performance depends on the uncertainty and DTF set. Predicted PEs and QEs as functions of the uncertainty of k-th listener (U_k) and DTF set of k-th listener (D_k).

in Section 3.1. Each row, i.e., constant D_k but varying U_k, represents the listener-specific effect of the uncertainty described in Section 3.2, i.e., listening with own ears but having different uncertainties.

In this section, we focus on the results in the columns. Each column describes results for a constant U_k but varying D_k, representing the listener-specific effect of the DTF set. While the predictions show a variation across both columns and rows, i.e., substantial effects of both uncertainty and DTF set, some DTF sets show clear differences to others across all uncertainties. This analysis is, however, confounded by the different baseline performance of each listener and can be improved by considering the performance relative to the listener-specific performance. **Figure 6** shows ΔPEs and ΔQEs, i.e., PEs and QEs relative to the listener-specific PEs and QEs, respectively, averaged over all uncertainties for each DTF set D_k. Positive values represent the performance amount by which our listener group would deteriorate when listening with the DTF set of k-th listener (and being fully re-calibrated). For example, the DTF sets of listeners $k = 9$ and $k = 15$ show such deteriorations. Those DTF sets seem to have provided less accessible directional cues. Further, DTF sets improving the performance for the listeners can be identified, see for example, the DTF sets of listeners $k = 3$ and $k = 12$. These DTF sets seem to have provided more accessible directional cues. The effect of those four DTF sets can be also examined in **Figure 2** by comparing the predictions for constant uncertainties, i.e., across rows.

Thus, variation of the DTF sets had an effect on the predictions suggesting that it also affects the comparison of the predictions with the actual performance. This leads to the question to what extend a constant DTF set across all listeners can explain the actual performances? It might even be the case that listener-specific DTFs are not required for accurate predictions.

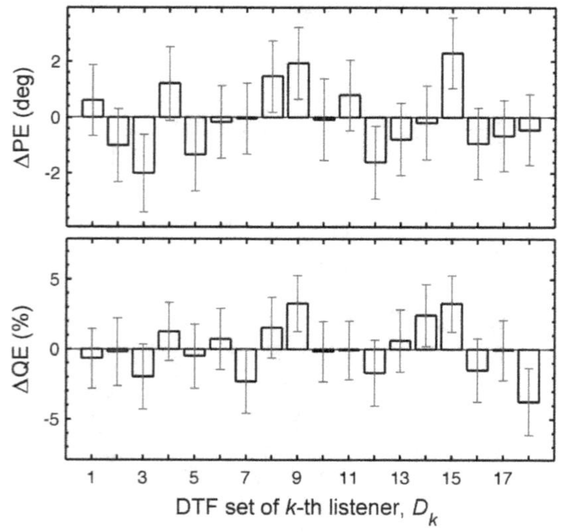

FIGURE 6 | Listener-specific performance depends on the DTF set used in the model. ΔPEs and ΔQEs averaged over all U_ks as a function of D_k. ΔPEs and ΔQEs are the PEs and QEs relative to the listener-specific PEs and QEs, respectively. The whiskers show ±1 SD.

Thus, similarly to the analysis from Section 3.2 where the impact of listener-specific uncertainty was related to that of a listener-constant uncertainty, here, we compare the impact of listener-specific DTF sets relative to that of a listener-constant DTF set. To this end, predictions were calculated with a model calibrated to the same DTF set for all listeners but with a listener-specific uncertainty. All DTF sets from the pool of available listeners were tested. For each of the DTF sets, correlation coefficients between the actual and predicted performances were calculated. The correlation coefficients averaged over all DTF sets were 0.86 ($SD = 0.007$) for PE and 0.89 ($SD = 0.006$) for QE. Note the extremely small variability across the different DTF sets, indicating only little impact of the DTF set on the predictions. The DTF set from listener $k = 14$ yielded the largest correlation coefficients, which were 0.87 for PE and 0.89 for QE. The corresponding predictions as functions of the actual performance are shown in **Figure 4E**. Note the similarity to the predictions for the listener-specific DTF sets (**Figure 4A**). These findings have a practical implication when modeling the baseline performance of sound localization: for an arbitrary listener, the DTFs of another arbitrary listener, e.g., NH68 ($k = 14$), might still yield listener-specific predictions.

Recall that in our investigation, both the incoming sound and the template set were filtered by the same DTF set, corresponding to a condition where the listener is completely re-calibrated to those DTFs. The highest correlation found for NH68's DTF set does not imply that this DTF set is optimal for *ad-hoc* listening.

In summary, the predicted localization performance varied by a small amount depending on the directional cues provided by the different DTF sets, even when the listener-specific uncertainty was considered. Note that full re-calibration was simulated. This finding indicates that some of the DTF sets provide better access to directional cues than others. Even though the acoustic factor might contribute to the variability in localization performance across listeners, the same DTF set of a single listener (here, NH68) for modeling performance of all listeners yielded still a good prediction accuracy.

RELATIVE CONTRIBUTIONS OF ACOUSTIC AND NON-ACOUSTIC FACTORS

Both the DTF set and the uncertainty had an effect on the predicted localization performance. However, a listener-constant DTF set provided still acceptable predictions, while a listener-constant uncertainty did not. In this section, we aim at directly comparing the relative contributions of the two factors to localization performance. To this end, we compare the SDs in the predictions as a function of each of the factors. The factor causing more variation in the predictions is assumed to have more impact on sound localization.

We used PEs and QEs predicted for all combinations of uncertainties and DTF sets, as shown in **Figure 5**. For each listener and each performance metric, two SDs were calculated: (1) as a function of the listener-specific DTF set D_k for all available uncertainties, i.e., calculating the SDs across a column separately for each row; and (2) as a function of the listener-specific uncertainty U_k for all available DTF sets, i.e. calculating the SD across

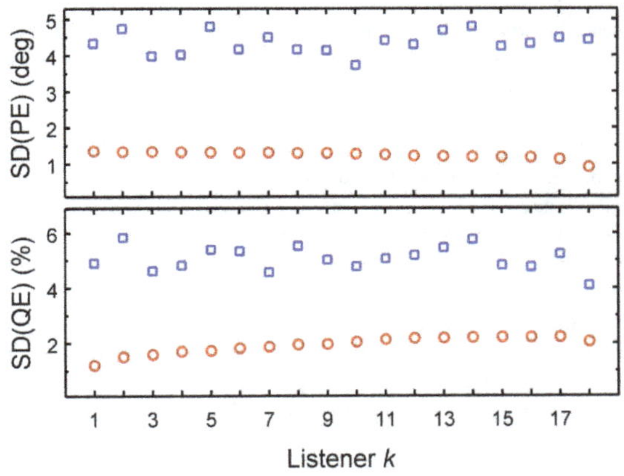

FIGURE 7 | DTF set contributes less than uncertainty to the performance variability of the group. PE SDs and QE SDs as functions of either listener-constant DTF set calculated for listener-specific uncertainties (U_k varied, blue squares) or the listener-constant uncertainty calculated for listener-specific DTF sets (DTF varied, red circles). The abscissa is sorted by the ascending listener-specific uncertainty U_k.

a row separately for each column. **Figure 7** shows these SDs as functions of the k-th listener, sorted by ascending listener-specific uncertainty. When U_k was varied, the average SD across listeners was 4.4° ± 0.3° and 5.1% ± 0.4% for PE and QE, respectively. When the DTF set was varied, the average SD was 1.2° ± 0.1° and 1.9% ± 0.3% for PE and QE, respectively. On average, the factor uncertainty caused more than twice as much variability as the factor DTF set.

This analysis shows that while both listener-specific uncertainty and listener-specific DTF set were important for the accuracy in predicted localization performance, the uncertainty affected the performance much more than the DTF set. This indicates that the non-acoustic factor, uncertainty, contributes more than the acoustic factor, DTF set, to the localization performance. This is consistent with the observations of Andéol et al. (2013), where localization performance correlated with the detection thresholds for spectral modulation, but did not correlate with the prominence of the HRTF's spectral shape. The directional information captured by the spectral shape prominence corresponds to the acoustic factor in our study. The sensitivity to the spectral modulations represents the non-acoustic factor in our study. Even though the acoustic factor (DTF set) contributed to the localization performance of an individual listener, the differences *between* the listeners seem to be more determined by a non-acoustic factor (uncertainty).

Note that the separation of the sound localization process into acoustic and non-acoustic factors in our model assumes a perfect calibration of a listener to a DTF set. It should be considered, though, that listeners might actually be calibrated at different levels to their own DTFs. In such a case, the potentially different levels of calibration would be implicitly considered in the model by different uncertainties, confounding the interpretation of the relative contribution of the acoustic and non-acoustic factors. While the general capability to *re*-calibrate to a new DTF set has been investigated quite well (Hofman and van Opstal, 1998; Majdak et al., 2013), the level of calibration to the own DTF set has not been clarified yet.

CONCLUSIONS

In this study, a sound localization model predicting the localization performance in sagittal planes (Baumgartner et al., 2013) was applied to investigate the relative contributions of acoustic and non-acoustic factors to localization performance in the lateral range of ±30°. The acoustic factor was represented by the directional cues provided by the DTF sets of individual listeners. The non-acoustic factor was represented by the listener-specific uncertainty considered to describe processes related to the efficiency of processing the spectral cues. Listener-specific uncertainties were estimated in order to calibrate the model to the actual performance when localizing broadband noises with own ears. Then, predictions were calculated for the permutation of DTF sets and uncertainties across the listener group. Identical DTF sets were used for the incoming sound and the template set, which allowed to simulate the listeners being completely re-calibrated to the tested DTF sets, a condition nearly unachievable in psychoacoustic localization experiments.

Our results show that both the acoustic and non-acoustic factors affected the modeled localization performance. The non-acoustic factor had a strong effect on the predictions, and accounted very well for the differences between the individual listeners. In comparison, the acoustic factor had much less effect on the predictions. In an extreme case of using the same DTF set for modeling performance for all listeners, an acceptable prediction accuracy was still obtained.

Note that our investigation considered only targets positioned in sagittal planes of ±30° around the median plane. Even though we do not have evidence for contradicting conclusions for more lateral sagittal planes, one should be careful when applying our conclusions to more lateral targets. Further, the model assumes direction-static and stationary stimuli presented in the free field. In realistic listening situations, listeners can move their head, the acoustic signals are temporally fluctuating, and reverberation interacts with the direct sound.

An unexpected conclusion from our study is that, globally, i.e., on average across all considered directions, all the tested DTF sets encoded the directional information similarly well. It seems like listener-specific DTFs are not necessarily required for predicting the global listener-specific localization ability in terms of distinguishing between bad and good localizers. What seems to be required, however, is an accurate estimate of the listener-specific uncertainty. One could speculate that, given a potential relation between the uncertainty and a measure of spectral-shape sensitivity, in the future, the global listener-specific localization ability might be predictable by obtaining a measure of the listener-specific uncertainty in a non-spatial experimental task without any requirement of listener-specific localization responses.

ACKNOWLEDGMENTS

We thank Christian Kasess for fruitful discussions on data analysis. This work was supported by the Austrian Science Fund (FWF, projects P 24124–N13 and M1230).

REFERENCES

Algazi, V. R., Avendano, C., and Duda, R. O. (2001). Elevation localization and head-related transfer function analysis at low frequencies. *J. Acoust. Soc. Am.* 109, 1110–1122. doi: 10.1121/1.1349185

Andéol, G., Macpherson, E. A., and Sabin, A. T. (2013). Sound localization in noise and sensitivity to spectral shape. *Hear. Res.* 304, 20–27. doi: 10.1016/j.heares.2013.06.001

Baumgartner, R., Majdak, P., and Laback, B. (2013). "Assessment of sagittal-plane sound localization performance in spatial-audio applications," in *The Technology of Binaural Listening, Modern Acoustics and Signal Processing*, ed J. Blauert (Berlin; Heidelberg: Springer), 93–119.

Baumgartner, R., Majdak, P., and Laback, B. (2014). *Modeling Sound-Source Localization in Sagittal Planes for Human Listeners.* Available online at: http://www.kfs.oeaw.ac.at/research/Baumgartner_et_al_2014.pdf. (Last modified April 10, 2014).

Dau, T., Püschel, D., and Kohlrausch, A. (1996). A quantitative model of the "effective" signal processing in the auditory system. I. Model structure. *J. Acoust. Soc. Am.* 99, 3615–3622. doi: 10.1121/1.414959

Glasberg, B. R., and Moore, B. C. J. (1990). Derivation of auditory filter shapes form notched-noise data. *Hear. Res.* 47, 103–138. doi: 10.1016/0378-5955(90)90170-T

Goupell, M. J., Majdak, P., and Laback, B. (2010). Median-plane sound localization as a function of the number of spectral channels using a channel vocoder. *J. Acoust. Soc. Am.* 127, 990–1001. doi: 10.1121/1.3283014

Hofman, P. M., and van Opstal, J. (1998). Spectro-temporal factors in two-dimensional human sound localization. *J. Acoust. Soc. Am.* 103, 2634–2648. doi: 10.1121/1.422784

Hofman, P. M., van Riswick, J. G. A., and van Opstal, J. (1998). Relearning sound localization with new ears. *Nat. Neurosci.* 1, 417–421. doi: 10.1038/1633

Langendijk, E. H. A., and Bronkhorst, A. W. (2002). Contribution of spectral cues to human sound localization. *J. Acoust. Soc. Am.* 112, 1583–1596. doi: 10.1121/1.1501901

Macpherson, E. A., and Sabin, A. T. (2007). Binaural weighting of monaural spectral cues for sound localization. *J. Acoust. Soc. Am.* 121, 3677–3688. doi: 10.1121/1.2722048

Majdak, P., Balazs, P., and Laback, B. (2007). Multiple exponential sweep method for fast measurement of head-related transfer functions. *J. Audio. Eng. Soc.* 55, 623–637.

Majdak, P., Goupell, M. J., and Laback, B. (2010). 3-D localization of virtual sound sources: effects of visual environment, pointing method, and training. *Atten. Percept. Psycho.* 72, 454–469. doi: 10.3758/APP.72.2.454

Majdak, P., Walder, T., and Laback, B. (2013). Effect of long-term training on sound localization performance with spectrally warped and band-limited head-related transfer functions. *J. Acoust. Soc. Am.* 134, 2148–2159. doi: 10.1121/1.4816543

Middlebrooks, J. C. (1999a). Individual differences in external-ear transfer functions reduced by scaling in frequency. *J. Acoust. Soc. Am.* 106, 1480–1492. doi: 10.1121/1.427176

Middlebrooks, J. C. (1999b). Virtual localization improved by scaling nonindividualized external-ear transfer functions in frequency. *J. Acoust. Soc. Am.* 106, 1493–1510. doi: 10.1121/1.427147

Møller, H., Sørensen, M. F., Hammershøi, D., and Jensen, C. B. (1995). Head-related transfer functions of human subjects. *J. Audio. Eng. Soc.* 43, 300–321.

Morimoto, M. (2001). The contribution of two ears to the perception of vertical angle in sagittal planes. *J. Acoust. Soc. Am.* 109, 1596–1603. doi: 10.1121/1.1352084

Parseihian, G., and Katz, B. F. G. (2012). Rapid head-related transfer function adaptation using a virtual auditory environment. *J. Acoust. Soc. Am.* 131, 2948–2957. doi: 10.1121/1.3687448

Patterson, R., Nimmo-Smith, I., Holdsworth, J., and Rice, P. (1988). *An Efficient Auditory Filterbank Based on the Gammatone Function.* Cambridge: APU

Rakerd, B., Hartmann, W. M., and McCaskey, T. L. (1999). Identification and localization of sound sources in the median sagittal plane. *J. Acoust. Soc. Am.* 106, 2812–2820. doi: 10.1121/1.428129

Søndergaard, P., and Majdak, P. (2013). "The auditory modeling toolbox," in *The Technology of Binaural Listening, Modern Acoustics and Signal Processing*, ed J. Blauert (Berlin; Heidelberg: Springer), 33–56.

van Wanrooij, M. M., and van Opstal, J. (2005). Relearning sound localization with a new ear. *J. Neurosci.* 25, 5413–5424. doi: 10.1523/JNEUROSCI.0850-05.2005

Vliegen, J., and van Opstal, J. (2004). The influence of duration and level on human sound localization. *J. Acoust. Soc. Am.* 115, 1705–1703. doi: 10.1121/1.1687423

Wightman, F. L., and Kistler, D. J. (1997). Monaural sound localization revisited. *J. Acoust. Soc. Am.* 101, 1050–1063. doi: 10.1121/1.418029

Zahorik, P., Bangayan, P., Sundareswaran, V., Wang, K., and Tam, C. (2006). Perceptual recalibration in human sound localization: learning to remediate front-back reversals. *J. Acoust. Soc. Am.* 120, 343–359. doi: 10.1121/1.2208429

Zakarauskas, P., and Cynader, M. S. (1993). A computational theory of spectral cue localization. *J. Acoust. Soc. Am.* 94, 1323–1331. doi: 10.1121/1.408160

Zhang, P. X., and Hartmann, W. M. (2010). On the ability of human listeners to distinguish between front and back. *Hear. Res.* 260, 30–46. doi: 10.1016/j.heares.2009.11.001

13

Brain dynamics that correlate with effects of learning on auditory distance perception

Matthew G. Wisniewski[1,2]*, Eduardo Mercado III[2], Barbara A. Church[2], Klaus Gramann[3] and Scott Makeig[4]

[1] 711th Human Performance Wing, U. S. Air Force Research Laboratory, Wright-Patterson Air Force Base, OH, USA
[2] Department of Psychology, University at Buffalo, The State University of New York, Buffalo, NY, USA
[3] Biological Psychology and Neuroergonomics, Berlin Institute of Technology, Berlin, Germany
[4] Swartz Center for Computational Neuroscience, Institute for Neural Computation, University of California, San Diego, San Diego, CA, USA

Correspondence:
Matthew G. Wisniewski, 711th Human Performance Wing, U.S. Air Force Research Laboratory, Building 441, Area B, Wright Patterson Air Force Base, OH 45433, USA
e-mail: matt.g.wisniewski@gmail.com

Accuracy in auditory distance perception can improve with practice and varies for sounds differing in familiarity. Here, listeners were trained to judge the distances of English, Bengali, and backwards speech sources pre-recorded at near (2-m) and far (30-m) distances. Listeners' accuracy was tested before and after training. Improvements from pre-test to post-test were greater for forward speech, demonstrating a learning advantage for forward speech sounds. Independent component (IC) processes identified in electroencephalographic (EEG) data collected during pre- and post-testing revealed three clusters of ICs across subjects with stimulus-locked spectral perturbations related to learning and accuracy. One cluster exhibited a transient stimulus-locked increase in 4–8 Hz power (theta event-related synchronization; ERS) that was smaller after training and largest for backwards speech. For a left temporal cluster, 8–12 Hz decreases in power (alpha event-related desynchronization; ERD) were greatest for English speech and less prominent after training. In contrast, a cluster of IC processes centered at or near anterior portions of the medial frontal cortex showed learning-related enhancement of sustained increases in 10–16 Hz power (upper-alpha/low-beta ERS). The degree of this enhancement was positively correlated with the degree of behavioral improvements. Results suggest that neural dynamics in non-auditory cortical areas support distance judgments. Further, frontal cortical networks associated with attentional and/or working memory processes appear to play a role in perceptual learning for source distance.

Keywords: electroencephalography (EEG), perceptual learning, familiarity, independent component analysis (ICA), ranging, event-related spectral perturbation (ERSP)

INTRODUCTION

Most of what is currently known about human auditory distance perception comes from research focused on variations in acoustic cues produced by propagation, and on how degrading or altering such cues affects distance judgments. This work has shown that listeners utilize intensity, spectral, binaural, and direct-to-reverberant energy features to judge distances and that judgments can be altered by interfering with feature perception (for review, see Zahorik et al., 2005; Fluitt et al., 2013). For example, changing the ambient properties of listening environments can make sources sound nearer or farther than they actually are (e.g., Mershon et al., 1989).

Interestingly, auditory distance perception also depends on experience, even between sounds with similar acoustic properties. Coleman (1962) had listeners judge distances of noise bursts and found that on the first experimental trial judgments were unreliable. In later trials accuracy improved, presumably as participants learned to gauge the intensities of the sound source via feedback (Coleman, 1962). Blind individuals discriminate auditory source distance better than normally sighted individuals (Voss et al., 2004; Kolarik et al., 2013), possibly reflecting learning-induced cortical plasticity in areas normally devoted to vision (e.g., Gougoux et al., 2004; Voss et al., 2011). Also, the source distance of speech played forward is more accurately judged than the same speech played backwards (McGregor et al., 1985; Brungart and Scott, 2001; Banks et al., 2007; Wisniewski et al., 2012). Because the known acoustic cues to distance are well matched between stimuli played forward and time-reversed (McGregor et al., 1985; Brungart and Scott, 2001), better performance for forward speech suggests that central cognitive processes play a significant role in distance perception. Important to note is that in all the above studies acoustic distance cues were identical or quite similar across conditions, demonstrating that auditory distance perception cannot be fully understood by focusing solely on the impact of cue alteration and degradation on distance judgments.

Cognitive neuroscience has advanced our understanding of the mechanisms involved in the azimuthal localization of sounds (e.g., Zatorre et al., 2002; Salminen et al., 2010) and may potentially be able to play a similar role in understanding the processes involved in auditory distance perception and effects of learning. However, research on the neural bases of distance perception has been limited. Some studies suggest a reliance on right lateralized auditory areas when intensity is a useful distance cue (Mathiak et al., 2003; Altmann et al., 2013). The left posterior superior temporal gyrus and planum temporale may be important for processing intensity independent cues, at least when sounds are presented on the right side of the inter-aural axis (Kopčo et al., 2012). There is also some evidence that judging distance of ecologically relevant sound sources involves cortical networks outside of traditional auditory areas. For instance, Seifritz et al. (2002) found that processing rising intensity (approaching or looming sources) compared to falling intensity sounds led to greater blood oxygen level-dependent (BOLD) signals in right parietal, motor, and premotor areas, in addition to left and right superior temporal sulci and middle temporal gyri.

We recently observed a distributed cortical network involved in auditory distance perception using electroencephalography (EEG). In that study, participants were tested on their ability to discriminate the distances of intensity normalized English and Bengali forwards and backwards speech prerecorded at near (2 m) and far (30 m) distances (Wisniewski et al., 2012). Replicating previous behavioral results, accuracy was higher for forward than backwards speech. Independent component analysis (ICA), a blind source separation method that finds spatially fixed and temporally independent component (IC) processes in multichannel EEG data, identified several cortical sources of EEG (cf. Makeig et al., 2004). Clusters of IC processes localized to a range of cortical areas including the medial frontal cortex, left and right superior temporal gyri, and parietal areas, showed significant event-related changes in oscillatory dynamics associated with making distance judgments.

There were also quantitative differences related to processing distance cues from different types of speech. For the left temporal IC process cluster, English speech trials showed the strongest event-related desynchronization (ERD) of the alpha rhythm (i.e., decreases in 8–12 Hz power). As alpha ERD can be considered to reflect a break from resting-state neural synchrony (for review see Pfurtscheller and Lopes da Silva, 1999) and/or a state of cortical excitation (Weisz et al., 2011), ERD in the left temporal cluster of ICs may have reflected the use of left-lateralized cortical speech areas for processing familiar speech (Boatman, 2004; Hickok and Poeppel, 2007) or enhanced processing of intensity independent distance cues (Kopčo et al., 2012). For IC processes localized at or near medial frontal cortex, event-related power increases (Event-related synchronization; ERS) in the high-alpha/low-beta range (10–16 Hz) were largest for accurately judged Bengali speech. In contrast, poorly perceived backwards speech samples induced relatively large transient ERS in the theta range (4–8 Hz) for a separate cluster of IC processes. ICs in this cluster showed scalp projections similar to scalp maps seen for late auditory-evoked potential (AEP) components (i.e., strong projection to central electrodes), suggesting that transient ERS was at least partially related to typically observed obligatory responses to auditory stimulation.

Medial frontal brain regions such as the anterior cingulate cortex have been implicated in sustained auditory attention (Paus et al., 1997; Zatorre et al., 1999; Benedict et al., 2002) and EEG work suggests that sources localized to nearby regions show sustained ERS that indexes cognitive demands placed on these frontal networks (Onton et al., 2005; Ahveninen et al., 2013). In contrast, transient ERS and concurrent ERP features have been linked to orienting (Barry et al., 2012), novelty processing (Debener et al., 2005), and auditory distraction (Schröger, 1996). That medial frontal source activities correlate with performance bolsters arguments that non-auditory brain regions have a significant role to play in auditory distance perception (Seifritz et al., 2002). Furthermore, the differences seen between speech categories in medial frontal, left temporal, and other possible AEP/ERP sources, suggest that analyses of larger scale brain dynamics are needed to understand the mechanisms driving learning-related effects. To date, little work has been done in this area. Learning-related effects have instead been attributed to "cognitive factors," often with no attempt to explore what those factors may be or how they relate to processing in cortical areas outside of the canonical auditory system (Zahorik et al., 2005).

The current work builds on our earlier study by examining how training impacts accuracy and cortical processing across speech categories. A pre-/post-test design was employed wherein participants were initially tested on their distance perception accuracy, subsequently trained on the task, and then tested again. English, Bengali, and backwards samples of English and Bengali speech were used as stimuli. We expected that training would improve the accuracy of distance perception across speech categories and that the degree of improvement would be related to speech familiarity. It was also expected that the comparison of pre- and post-test EEG would clarify how the cortical networks described above are involved in auditory distance perception (Seifritz et al., 2002; Wisniewski et al., 2012). Specifically, we hypothesized that EEG dynamics previously associated with successful task performance (e.g., upper-alpha/low-beta ERS and alpha ERD) would be more evident in post-test than pre-test EEG. EEG features associated with speech categories showing poor distance perception accuracy should be less evident (e.g., large transient theta ERS for backwards speech). Although the current study was designed to measure how within-experiment learning interacts with speech familiarity, we also expected that the findings of the previous study, which focused exclusively on familiarity effects, would be replicated here. Specifically, we predicted that the quantitative differences in ERS/ERD patterns that we previously observed would be evident in the post-test. Although our main interest was in processes related to auditory distance perception learning, the study was not meant to identify features in EEG that are specialized for distance perception. EEG correlates of performance and learning in distance perception tasks may very well correlate with behavior in other non-distance-related and non-spatial listening tasks. A secondary goal of the study was thus to identify features in EEG that could potentially be explored in other, non-spatial tasks involving auditory perceptual learning. Most past studies of human auditory perceptual learning have focused on transient EEG features associated with AEPs rather than the time-frequency features we explored here.

MATERIALS AND METHODS

ETHICS STATEMENT

The Human Research Protections Program of the University of California, San Diego approved the study. All participants signed an informed consent form before participating.

PARTICIPANTS

The same 17 participants from our original study (Wisniewski et al., 2012) were paid to participate in additional training and post-test phases. All phases were run in a single session. Participants were fluent speakers of English with no fluency in Bengali. Two participants' data were dropped from analyses due to errors that occurred in data collection.

STIMULI

One male speaker, fluent in English and Bengali, was recorded in the lab producing several English and Bengali phrases. Recordings were made on a Sony MD Walkman MZ-NH900 digital recorder (Sony Corporation of America, New York, NY) with an AKG D9000 microphone (frequency range: 20–20 kHz; AKG Acoustics, Austria). The microphone was placed ~15 cm from the speaker's mouth. Backwards speech tokens were created from a subset of English and Bengali phrases (italicized in **Table 1**) by reversing the speech waveforms. The selections of stimuli used for backwards speech tokens were based on previous behavioral work (McGregor et al., 1985; Brungart and Scott, 2001; Banks et al., 2007). English is the most familiar speech category as it is lexically and phonetically familiar to our sample of listeners. Bengali is less familiar than English due to no knowledge of word meaning, but is more familiar than backwards speech because of some phonetic content that overlaps with English (Barman, 2009).

All recordings were then broadcast from a SUNN speaker (Model 1201, Fender Musical Instruments Corporation, Scottsdale, AZ) in an open grass field at 2 m (near) or 30 m (far) away from the microphone using the same equipment as the original recordings. Recordings were made at night to minimize environmental noise. The mean amplitudes of recordings were normalized to ~ -10 dB FS. The final stimulus set contained 20 tokens in each of the three speech categories (10 near, 10 far), yielding a total of 60 stimuli[1].

Figure 1 shows mean spectra for each speech category and distance. Spectra were analyzed in 5 single-octave bands (100–200 Hz, 200–400 Hz 400–800 Hz, 800–1600 Hz, and 1600–3200 Hz) to test for possible differences in cues to distance across speech categories in the stimulus set. A mixed-model 2 (Distance) × 3 (Speech Category) × 5 (Octave) ANOVA, treating Speech Category as a between subjects factor, found significant main effects of Distance [$F_{(1,\ 27)} = 55.25, p < 0.001, \eta_p^2 = 0.67$], and Octave [$F_{(4,\ 108)} = 213.70, p < 0.001, \eta_p^2 = 0.88$]. The main effect of distance trended such that power was lower for far sounds (i.e., the dashed lines in **Figure 1** are on average lower than the solid lines). The main effect of octave relates to a drop in power with increasing frequency. There was also a significant Distance × Octave interaction [$F_{(4,\ 108)} = 97.21, p < 0.001, \eta_p^2 = 0.78$], possibly related, in part, to a greater rate of attenuation of higher frequencies with increasing distance (Zahorik et al., 2005). Another factor contributing to the interaction is differences in spectral peaks and notches. This difference between near and far distances may reflect decreased signal-to-noise ratio in recordings at far distances (cf. Zahorik et al., 2005). Because the amplitude normalization process increased the amplitude of far recordings, background noise was amplified along with speech signals, making it more evident in far recordings. The signal-to-noise ratio difference between near and far recordings, although amplified here, is an effective distance cue under more naturalistic conditions (Fluitt et al., 2013). No main effects or interactions with the Speech Category Factor were found ($p > 0.55$). The durations of stimuli (**Table 1**) are also similar across speech categories[2]. Overall, the stimulus set analysis shows that there are spectral cues to distance when overall amplitude cues are minimized, and that cue presence is comparable across speech categories. Although the current stimulus set does not contain all natural cues to distance perception (e.g., binaural cues), similar stimulus sets have proved informative for examining learning-related effects in distance perception (McGregor et al., 1985).

Table 1 | Phrases recorded by a speaker that were later recorded at distances of 2 m and 30 m.

Speech sequence	Duration (ms)
Don't ask me to carry an oily rag like that.	2544
How far away do you think I am?	1591
Threat.	277
Warning.	501
Emergency.	666
Look out.	500
Over here.	530
Caution.	561
Hello.	290
Goodbye.	520
Amaka ooghta tooltaa bolonah.	1734
Aa kha nae.	531
Aloo.	364
Kawla.	344
Choo noo dau.	632
Shaub dhan ah.	728
Aamee kau tou dor ah ache.	1589
Mo mosh Kar.	707
Hah.	408
Nah.	355

Backwards stimuli were made from italicized phrases.

APPARATUS

Experimental procedures were executed using the ERICA software platform (Delorme et al., 2011) running on Windows XP. Stimuli were presented over computer speakers in a closed room placed ~1 m in front of subjects at a level not exceeding 75 dB SPL. Speakers were used to avoid interference from head or earphones in the placement of electrodes and collection of data from our high-density electrode array. Room and speaker arrangements were identical for each participant and did not change throughout the experiment. Any effects seen in behavior or EEG

[1]A subset of environmental sounds were recorded and also tested, but data associated with these sounds are not discussed due to drastic acoustic differences between these environmental sounds and speech.

[2]A One-Way ANOVA on stimulus durations showed no significant effect of Speech Category ($p > 0.70$).

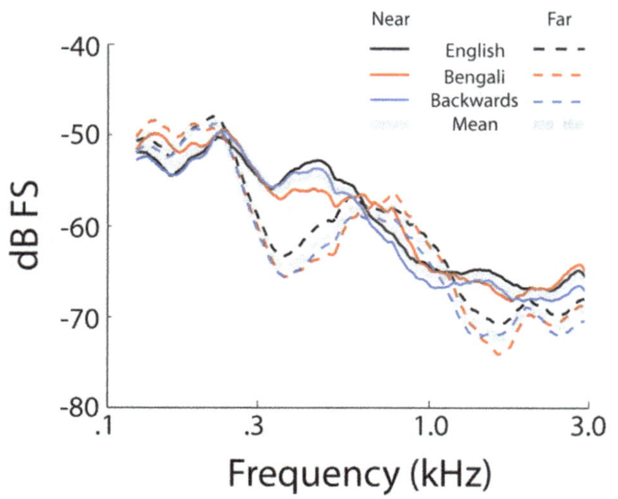

FIGURE 1 | Stimulus set spectra. Mean spectra for each speech category at each level of distance. Solid lines represent near recordings and dashed lines represent far.

between conditions can therefore not be explained by differences in room acoustics. Listeners responded via a computer keyboard. Feedback was presented on a computer screen.

BEHAVIORAL PROCEDURES

In a single-interval, two-alternative forced choice task (1i-2afc), participants were instructed to indicate whether a presented sound was near (2 m) or far (30 m) using only two fingers of their right hand, which were to remain on the keyboard near the "j" and "k" keys. Keys were labeled "N" (for near) and "F" (for far), respectively. Participants were made aware that the sounds were speech sounds recorded at different distances and then equalized in amplitude so that overall intensity was not a valid cue to distance.

There were three phases of the experiment: pre-test, training, and post-test. All phases employed the task described above and contained three blocks of 60 trials (one trial for each individual stimulus; see **Table 1**). The order of trials was randomized within a block. Feedback of correctness was presented during training. During the pre- and post-tests no feedback was provided.

EEG ACQUISITION AND ICA DECOMPOSITION

During the pre- and post-tests EEG was recorded from 248 channels at 24-bit A/D resolution, sampled at 512 Hz, and referenced to CMS-DRL of a Biosemi ActiveTwo system (Biosemi, Netherlands). A custom whole head electrode montage was used, the 3-D positions of which were recorded for each individual (Polhemus Inc, Colchester, VT). Water-based conductive gel was inserted into wells of the cap before placing electrodes in those wells. Voltage offsets for electrodes were brought within $\pm$ 20 μV, or were rejected from analysis when this criterion could not be met.

All offline analyses were conducted using the open source EEGLAB toolbox (Delorme and Makeig, 2004; http://sccn.ucsd.edu/eeglab) and custom scripts written in MATLAB (Mathworks, Natick, MA). Recorded EEG data was first re-sampled to 250 Hz, high-pass filtered (1 Hz), and then low-pass filtered (100 Hz). Channels containing excessive artifacts were rejected from analysis. Data segments containing high-amplitude, high-frequency muscle noise were rejected as well. Data was then re-referenced to the average voltage of the retained channels (134–224 channels per subject; $M = 186$, $SD = 32$).

EEG reflects a sum of brain and non-brain processes (e.g., muscle noise, eye movement artifact, line noise, etc.). To find maximally independent component processes in EEG, full-rank extended infomax ICA was applied to each individual's data using the *binica()* function in EEGLAB. Extended infomax ICA is a blind source separation algorithm that, under favorable circumstances, decomposes linearly mixed processes contributing to the EEG at scalp channels. An ICA decomposition of EEG data returns a spatially fixed and maximally temporally independent set of component processes without relying on *a priori* assumptions about the spatial distributions and temporal dynamics of those processes. The event-related dynamics of ICs can be analyzed with the same methods used to analyze event-related dynamics in channel data. For further information on the application of ICA in EEG research see Makeig et al. (1997, 2004).

ICs were fit with single equivalent current dipole models using each individual's recorded electrode locations fit to a template boundary element head model and then localized in the template brain using the *dipfit()* function in EEGLAB. ICs retained for later clustering (described below) were those for which the estimated equivalent current dipole was in the brain volume and for which the scalp projection of the equivalent dipole accounted for more than 85% of the variance in the IC scalp projection. An average of 19 ICs ($SD = 7$) were retained per participant. ICs identified as blinks, lateral eye-movements, or muscle-related artifacts were removed from channel data.

EVENT-RELATED SPECTRAL PERTURBATIONS (ERSPs)

Following ICA decomposition, 4-s epochs (from 1 s before to 3 s after stimulus onsets) were extracted from the continuous data. A time-frequency approach to analysis was taken by examining ERSPs (Makeig, 1993). The *newtimef()* function of the EEGLAB toolbox was used to compute each IC's event-related spectrum using Morlet wavelets in a frequency range between 2 and 20 Hz (2 cycles at the lowest frequency to 10 cycles at the highest). Following this computation single trials were linearly time-warped to produce equal numbers of data points between stimulus onset and key presses in each trial. The mean spectrum from the pre-stimulus period (calculated using all epochs) was used as a divisive baseline (Gain model; see Grandchamp and Delorme, 2011) to determine relative power. The same method was used to compute ERSPs for channel data.

Single-trial time-frequency decompositions were also computed. For each trial a one-dimensional vector of spectral power within a specified frequency window was extracted from ERSPs (exact frequency bands given below). Then, all trials (combined across within-cluster ICs) were sorted by stimulus offset or response time (RT), smoothed over trials, and plotted. Both the time-warped ERSPs and single-trial sorting served to determine whether relative power within a time-frequency region of interest was related more strongly to stimulus processing (aligned to stimulus onset) or to stimulus offsets and key presses. For further detail on time-frequency decompositions and sorting see Supplementary Materials.

AEPs

Although not critically related to our hypotheses, transient ERS is often associated with components of the AEP. Given that we expected to observe transient ERS, we computed AEP waveforms for Cz and its nearest neighboring 8 channels using data back-projected from: (1) all non-artifactual ICs and (2) the cluster of IC processes showing the clearest transient ERS. Channels surrounding Cz were selected on the basis of fronto-central scalp distributions for AEP components and the scalp projection of ICs within the cluster showing clear transient theta ERS at stimulus onset. Baseline correction used the 100 ms preceding the onset of stimuli. Waveform peaks were extracted by taking the maximal voltage deflections within the following time-windows: N1 (80–160 ms), P2 (160–260 ms).

CLUSTER SELECTION, STATISTICS, AND PLOTTING

An automated K-means procedure was used to identify ICs within and across participants having similar scalp map topographies, equivalent current dipole locations, ERSPs, and mean log power spectra. A detailed description of clustering procedures is given in Supplementary Material.

Each IC's mean time-warped ERSP image was masked to reflect only significant perturbations from baseline (bootstrap resampling, $p < 0.01$). Displayed time-warped ERSPs represent an average of the masked individual ICs within an IC process cluster, masked further using a binomial test at each time-frequency point ($p < 0.01$; see Onton et al., 2005). To limit Type I error, we formally analyzed only IC clusters previously shown to be of interest and in time-frequency windows close to those in which we previously found differences between speech categories (Wisniewski et al., 2012). Analyses thus focused on a Central Midline cluster showing transient theta ERS (0.15–0.6 s; 4–8 Hz), a Frontal Midline cluster showing sustained upper-alpha/low-beta ERS (0.4–1.7 s; 10–16 Hz), and a Left Temporal cluster showing alpha ERD (0.5–2.45 s; 8–12 Hz). No attempt was made to optimize time-frequency windows. Pending determination of stimulus-related responses in time-warped and smoothed single-trial ERSPs, mean relative power measures within these windows were entered into 3 (Speech Category: English, Bengali, Backwards) × 2 (Test: Pre-test, Post-test) repeated measures ANOVAs.

To further characterize how changes in ERSPs from pre- to post-test related to perceptual learning for distance, Pearson correlations were calculated between behavioral improvement scores for each speech category and associated relative power changes. Both behavioral and EEG change measures were computed by subtracting pre-test from post-test measures. Some participants contributed more ICs per IC process cluster. When this was the case, the mean relative power change across an individual's ICs was entered into correlations.

We did not expect to see differences between near and far trials in ERSPs. Most studies reporting differences in electro/magnetic responses to acoustically similar stimuli employ oddball paradigms to get responses to some oddball stimulus that differ from a frequently presented one (for a distance-related study of this type, see Mathiak et al., 2003). We did not use such a task here because our goal was to characterize brain dynamics associated with processes of making distance judgments rather than to track responses related to representational differences along the dimension of distance (cf. Altmann et al., 2013; Kopčo et al., 2012; Mathiak et al., 2003). Nevertheless, we examined potential differences between near and far trials using 2 (Test: Pre-test, Post-test) × 2 (Distance: Near, Far) repeated measures ANOVAs. The factor of Distance was analyzed separately from Speech Category, because breaking up the analysis into all factors left a limited number of trials per condition.

When necessary for interpreting main effects or interactions, *post-hoc* paired-sample *t*-tests were conducted and interpreted with a false discovery rate (FDR) procedure ($\alpha = 0.05$)[3]. Corrected *p*-values are reported. The same FDR procedure was used for interpreting correlations.

RESULTS

BEHAVIOR

Behavior was analyzed using a signal detection measure for sensitivity according to the formula: $d' = z(H) - z(F)$. Correct responses to near stimuli were counted as "Hits" (H) and incorrect responses to far stimuli as false alarms (F) (see Macmillan and Creelman, 1991). **Figure 2** shows d' for each speech category at pre- (white bars) and post-test (gray bars). A 3 (Speech Category) × 2 (Test) ANOVA revealed a main effect of Speech Category [$F_{(2,28)} = 31.23$, $p < 0.001$, $\eta_p^2 = 0.69$] stemming from differences in perceptual sensitivity. *Post-hoc* paired comparisons revealed that both English [$t_{(14)} = 6.95$, $p < 0.001$, $r^2 = 0.79$] and Bengali [$t_{(14)} = 6.38$, $p < 0.001$, $r^2 = 0.76$] were judged more accurately than backwards speech. Mean accuracies for English and Bengali speech were not significantly different ($p > 0.47$).

The main effect of Test [$F_{(1,14)} = 11.60$, $p = 0.004$, $\eta_p^2 = 0.45$] and the Speech Category × Test interaction were also significant [$F_{(2,28)} = 5.10$, $p = 0.013$, $\eta_p^2 = 0.27$]. Accuracy was greater in the post- than the pre-test for English [$t_{(14)} = 3.06$, $p = 0.018$, $r^2 = 0.40$], Bengali [$t_{(14)} = 3.20$, $p = 0.02$, $r^2 = 0.42$], and Backwards speech [$t_{(14)} = 2.74$, $p = 0.028$, $r^2 = 0.35$]. Although learning related to perceptual sensitivity occurred for each speech category, the interaction suggests differential learning across speech categories. To further examine this, improvement scores were analyzed

[3]An FDR procedure introduced by Benjamini and Hochberg (1995) was used wherein the false discovery rate for hypothesis k is bounded by $\frac{np(k)}{k} \leq 0.05$. Here, n is the number of tests, k denotes the rank of the p value being corrected (from small to large), and $p(k)$ is the k-th smallest of the p values. In the results, p values are reported as corrected by the left side of the equation. FDR was applied separately for each family of post-hoc comparisons. For example, paired comparisons on data from one cluster of ICs were treated as a family separate from other clusters.

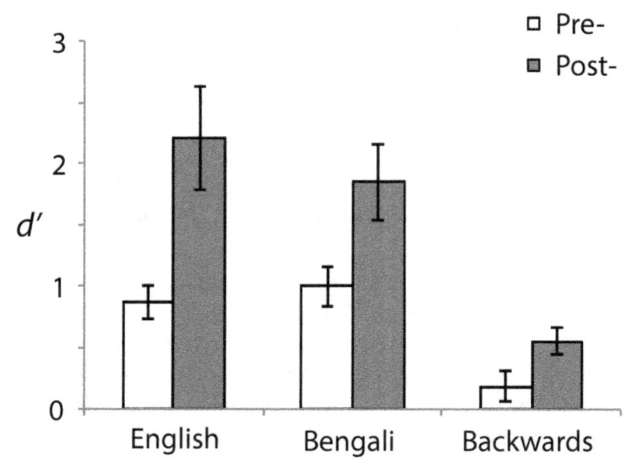

FIGURE 2 | Perceptual sensitivity (*d*′). Sensitivities to distance differences are shown for each speech category and test. Error bars show standard errors of means.

(Post-test minus Pre-test sensitivity). Mean improvements in d' were as follows: English = 1.34 (SE = 44), Bengali = 0.85 ($SE = 0.27$), and backwards = 0.37 ($SE = 0.13$). Improvements were significantly greater for English [$t_{(14)} = 2.47$, $p = 0.041$, $r^2 = 0.30$], and Bengali [$t_{(14)} = 2.29$, $p = 0.049$, $r^2 = 0.27$], relative to backwards speech. The difference in learning between English and Bengali speech was not significant ($p > 0.11$).

In regards to distance judgment accuracy, behavioral data shows that: (1) sensitivity to differences in distance improved from pre- to post-test across speech categories; (2) English and Bengali speech were perceived more accurately than backwards speech; and (3) there was a learning advantage for English and Bengali over backwards speech[4].

ELECTROPHYSIOLOGY - CHANNEL DATA

We first describe qualitatively the ERSPs at channels Fz, Cz, and Pz before presenting detailed analyses of IC process clusters derived from ICA decomposition of channel data. **Figure 3** shows mean ERSPs (averaged across participants) at each of these channels for the pre- and post-test. For clarity, ERSPs represent data averaged across speech categories (English, Bengali, and backwards), and distance (near and far). Differences across these factors were either not apparent, or appear as quantitative differences in similar ERS/ERD patterns discussed below. In these images, red indicates an increase in power relative to baseline (ERS), green indicates no change, and blue indicates a decrease in power (ERD). Because images reflect time-warped ERSPs, the relative power before mean RT (vertical pink lines) indicates activity occurring prior to key presses.

[4]The c signal detection parameter was calculated using Hit and False Alarm rates across all trials to determine if there was a bias to respond near or far. There existed a slight bias to respond "Near" ($M = -0.20$, $SE = 0.06$) that was significant [$t(14) = 3.50, p = 0.004, r^2 = 0.47$]. Bias did not change from pre- to post-test, $t < 1$.

Note that the event-related dynamics of frequency bands vary across channels. For instance, the transient theta ERS (~4–8 Hz) observed during pre-test recordings, possibly in part related to components of the AEP, is strongest at Cz. Similarly, there appears to be a band of low-beta (~13–16 Hz) ERS that is present at Fz, but absent in the more posterior channels. Alpha ERD (blue portion of ERSPs near 10 Hz) is clearly present at Fz, Cz, and Pz.

In regards to possible correlates of learning, channel data provide some evidence in support of our initial hypotheses and some evidence to the contrary. Based on the original study in which accurately judged Bengali speech showed the greatest upper-alpha/low-beta ERS (Wisniewski et al., 2012), we hypothesized that this feature would increase as a result of learning. Visual comparison of low-beta ERS at Fz between pre- and post-tests seems to suggest that this was the case. We hypothesized that alpha ERD would be enhanced after learning since accurately judged English speech previously showed the greatest alpha ERD in a left temporal IC process cluster (Wisniewski et al., 2012). Channel data actually suggest the opposite. It also looks as though transient theta ERS fades from pre- to post-test, consistent with our hypothesis that this response should decrease with learning.

ERSPs derived from channel data should be interpreted with caution. One alternative explanation of increased low-beta power is that brain sources contributing to alpha ERD, possibly more so in the pre-test, are masking ERS in the low-beta band. In this case, masking release resulting from reduced alpha ERD might appear as increases in low-beta power, even if low-beta power remains stable. Additionally, several cortical sources generate theta, alpha, and beta rhythms (for review, see Buzsáki, 2006), making it difficult to relate channel data to the cortical networks generating these rhythms, some of which were specific to our hypotheses. We therefore focused primarily on analyses of ERSPs derived from IC processes.

ELECTROPHYSIOLOGY - IC PROCESS CLUSTERS

Figure 4A shows scalp maps of IC process clusters of interest. Central midline, Frontal Midline, and Left Temporal clusters of IC processes were identified. Scalp projections of these clusters were similar to those previously observed (Wisniewski et al., 2012). Cluster centroids (large spheres) and best-fit equivalent current dipoles for each IC (small spheres) are shown in **Figure 4B**. Centroids were located near posterior portions of the medial frontal gyrus (Central Midline cluster; blue sphere), the left anterior cingulate cortex (Frontal Midline cluster; green sphere), and left superior temporal gyrus (Left Temporal cluster; red sphere)[5] . The absence of an individualized head model, varying numbers of electrodes between participants, and differences in the co-registration of electrode locations can greatly increase estimation error in dipole locations (Akalin Acar and Makeig, 2013). Additionally, the Central Midline cluster shows a scalp map similar to late components of AEPs, which are partly generated by sources in the temporal lobes (e.g., Debener et al., 2008). To avoid undue specification of anatomical regions,

[5]Locations listed in the text refer to the gray matter nearest to cluster centroids.

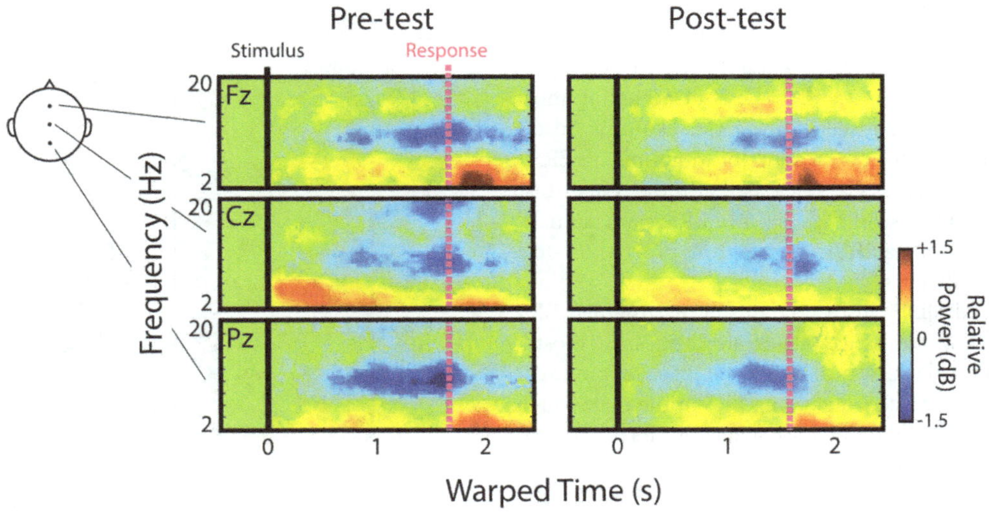

FIGURE 3 | Channel ERSPs. ERSPs at channels Fz, Cz, and Pz at pre- and post-test.

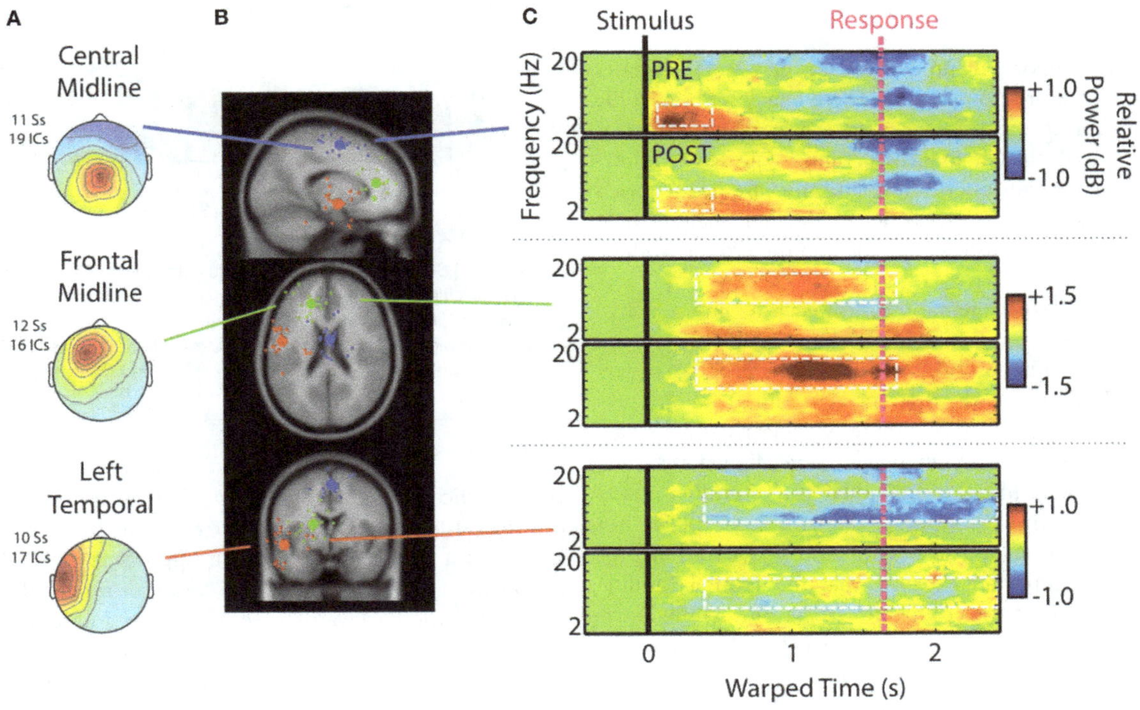

FIGURE 4 | Cluster characteristics. (A) Scalp maps, **(B)** centroids of IC process clusters, and **(C)** time-warped ERSPs averaged across speech categories and participants. In **(B)**, the blue, green, and red spheres represent Central Midline, Anterior Midline, and Left Temporal clusters respectively. Rows of **(C)** show ERSPs for these different clusters. In **(C)**, the top panels show ERSPs for the pre-test and the bottom panels show ERSPs for the post-test. The white boxes indicate time-frequency windows drawn from our previous study (Wisniewski et al., 2012) and designated as regions of interest in the current analysis. These windows are: Central Midline cluster (0.15–0.6 s; 4–8 Hz), Frontal Midline cluster (0.4–1.7 s; 10–16 Hz), and Left Temporal cluster (0.5–2.45 s; 8–12 Hz).

we refer to these clusters by their scalp distribution. Also, source estimates within medial cortical areas may be more susceptible to errors in lateralization due to their proximity to the boundary between hemispheres. Thus, we refrained from making any claims regarding lateralization in midline clusters.

Figure 4C shows time-warped ERSPs averaged across speech categories for the pre- (top) and post-tests (bottom) for each IC process cluster[6]. Dashed white boxes outline time-frequency windows designated for analysis (see Materials and Methods). The Central Midline cluster shows transient ERS occurring shortly after stimulus onsets between 2 and 10 Hz, but occurring most strongly in the theta range between 4 and 8 Hz. That this cluster shows a strong projection to central scalp locations and an ERSP feature similar to that seen at Cz, suggests that these ICs at least partially contribute to transient theta seen in ERSPs at channels. Note also that transient theta ERS decreases from pre- to post-test as it does in channel data.

For the Frontal Midline cluster, there is clear sustained ERS in the upper-alpha/low-beta range (10–16 Hz), appearing mostly between the stimulus (black vertical line) and response (pink vertical line). There is also an accompanying ERS in the theta range (cf., Onton et al., 2005). High-alpha/low-beta appears to increase from pre- to post-test as seen in ERSPs at Fz. Cluster ERSPs suggest that there was some masking of sustained ERS in channel data by alpha ERD. That is, sustained ERS in the cluster ERSPs appears within a wider frequency range that extends into alpha (10–16 Hz). However, the low-beta power increase from pre- to post-test seen in channels is not merely a cause of decreased alpha-masking, as it appears in the cluster ERSPs with little or no alpha ERD.

For the Left Temporal IC process cluster there were decreases in alpha ERD from pre- to post-test. There may have been some changes from pre- to post-test in theta and low-beta bands for the Left Temporal cluster, but these time-frequency windows did not satisfy our analysis criterion, and thus are not reported on. For the same reason we also do not further analyze some ERSP features of other clusters (e.g., theta in the Frontal Midline cluster).

Single trials (all experimental trials for each IC, in each cluster, and smoothed over trials) sorted by stimulus offset and RT are shown in **Figure 5**. The two midline IC process clusters showed that ERS in the theta (Central Midline) and upper-alpha/low-beta ranges (Frontal Midline) was clearly time-locked to stimulus onsets. Increases in power were aligned vertically instead of diagonally like the individual trial stimulus offsets and RTs (pink lines). This suggests that observed ERS is not related to sound offset or response planning/preparation processes. It is also important to note that the Frontal Midline cluster shows sustained upper-alpha/low-beta ERS in single trials and that this ERS sustains longer in trials with longer RTs. That is, longer RT trials show ERS up to ~1.8 s in the RT sorted plot, whereas short RTs generally show little ERS past ~1 s. Single-trial sorted alpha power for the Left Temporal cluster is less clearly aligned to stimulus onsets. However, there does appear to be some evidence of vertical alignment of alpha ERD around 0.4–1 s.

Figure 6 shows mean relative power for each speech category within the time-frequency windows of interest. For the Central Midline cluster there was a main effect of Test [$F_{(1,\ 18)} = 6.23$, $p = 0.022$, $\eta_p^2 = 0.26$], demonstrating a decrease in theta ERS from pre- to post-test. The main effect of Speech Category was also significant [$F_{(2,\ 36)} = 3.73$, $p = 0.034$, $\eta_p^2 = 0.17$]. In our previous study we observed larger transient ERS for backwards speech in a similar cluster, which appears to be replicated in the post-test here. *Post-hoc* paired comparisons (FDR corrected) found that the backwards speech category induced marginally significant greater theta ERS than English [$t_{(18)} = 2.21$, $p = 0.060$, $r^2 = 0.21$] and Bengali speech [$t_{(18)} = 2.60$, $p = 0.054$, $r^2 = 0.27$]. The difference between English and Bengali speech was not significant ($p > 0.65$). The Speech Category x Test interaction was not significant ($p > 0.45$).

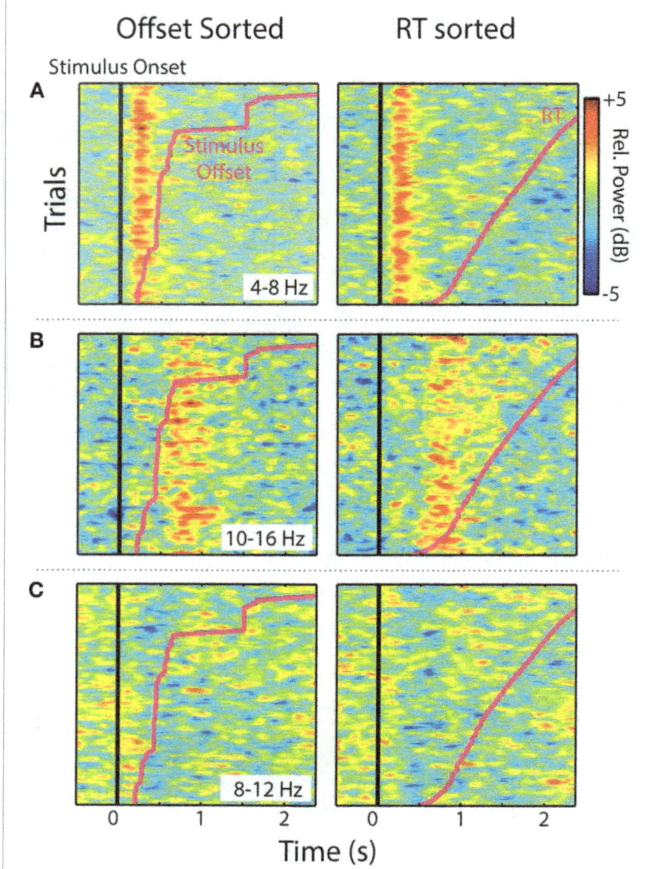

FIGURE 5 | Sorted single-trials. Stimulus offset and RT-sorted power within specified frequency ranges for IC process clusters (all trials for all participants). Images show relative power smoothed across a moving-average 80-trial window for **(A)** Central Midline theta (4–8 Hz), **(B)** Frontal Midline upper-alpha/low-beta (10–16 Hz), and **(C)** Left Temporal alpha (8–12 Hz).

For the Frontal Midline cluster's upper-alpha/low-beta, there was a significant main effect of Test [$F_{(1,\ 15)} = 6.97$, $p = 0.019$, $\eta_p^2 = 0.032$], showing that ERS in the upper-alpha/low-beta range increased from pre- to post-test. The main effect of Speech Category and Speech Category × Test interaction were not significant ($p > 0.40$).

For the Left Temporal cluster there was a main effect of Test [$F_{(1,\ 16)} = 12.75$, $p = 0.003$, $\eta_p^2 = 0.44$], indicating that alpha ERD decreased from pre- to post-test. There was also a significant effect of Speech Category [$F_{(2,\ 32)} = 8.66$, $p = 0.001$, $\eta_p^2 = 0.35$],

[6]Unmasked and non-time-warped ERSPs are shown in Supplementary Material.

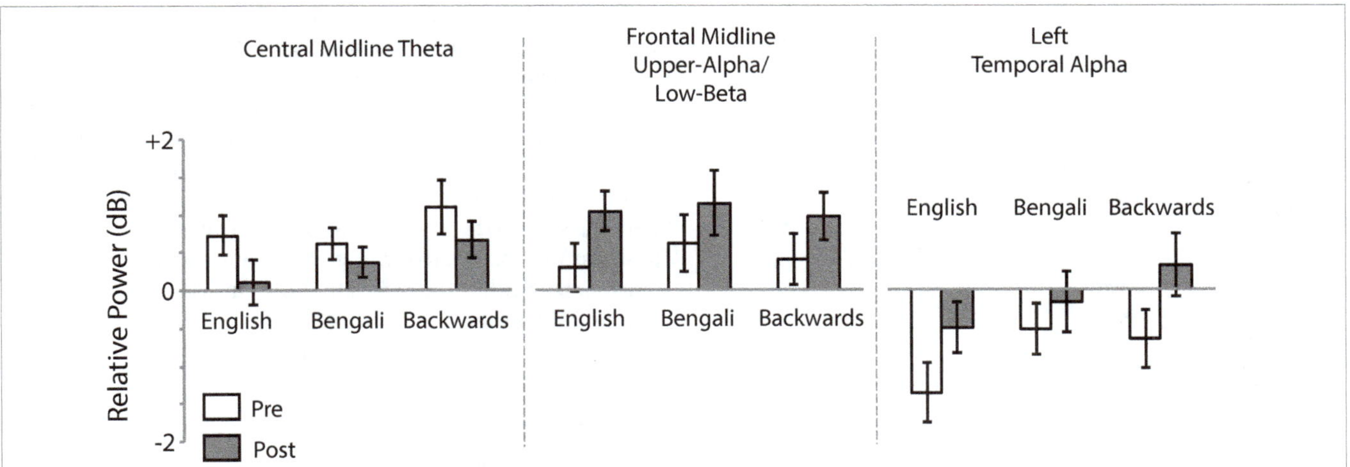

FIGURE 6 | Mean relative power. Relative power within time-frequency windows of interest for the Central Midline, Frontal Midline, and Left Temporal IC process clusters. Error bars show standard errors of means.

relating to our previous report of the largest ERD having been for English speech. Indeed, *post-hoc* paired *t*-tests revealed that English speech induced greater alpha ERD than Bengali [$t_{(16)} = 3.48$, $p = 0.009$, $r^2 = 0.43$] and backwards speech [$t_{(16)} = 3.03$, $p = 0.012$, $r^2 = 0.36$]. The Speech Category x Test interaction was only marginally significant [$F_{(2, 32)} = 3.11$, $p = 0.058$, $\eta_p^2 = 0.16$].

Analysis of Near vs. Far stimuli revealed only main effects of Test for each 2 (Test) × 2 (Distance) ANOVA, replicating those above ($p < 0.05$). No significant main effects of Distance or Distance × Test interactions were found for any IC process cluster ($p > 0.15$).

ELECTROPHYSIOLOGY - AEPs

As noted above, the Central Midline cluster shows a scalp map very similar to that of AEP components N1 and P2. Using ICA to decompose high-density EEG recordings from an auditory oddball task, Debener et al. (2005) observed a similar central midline cluster of IC processes that showed N1, P2, and an additional P3 component. The transient theta ERS observed here could be related to any one or all of these features.

Figure 7 shows the ERP at channels surrounding Cz, combining all non-artifactual sources in backprojection (**Figure 7A**). These AEPs represent typical waveforms after removing eye- and movement-related artifacts form the data. ERPs produced after backprojecting only ICs in the Central Midline cluster are also shown (**Figure 7B**). Waveforms show N1 and P2 peaks for both backprojections. P1 appears in the data after backprojecting all non-artifactual sources, but is less apparent in the data backprojecting only ICs within the Central Medial cluster.

As with transient theta ERS, it appears as though N1 and P2 decrease from pre- to post-test, with the largest amplitudes for backwards speech. That is, the solid lines show larger peaks than the dashed lines, and the blue lines (backwards speech) generally show greater amplitudes than the red (Bengali) and black (English) lines. This is evident in both backprojections. However, no significant effects were found in 3 (Speech Category) × 2 (Test) ANOVAs for N1 or P2 components for waveforms obtained using Central Midline cluster ICs ($p > 0.10$). Also, note that these time-domain features do not extend into the full range of ERS seen in ERSPs (up to ~600 ms) and likely do not fully account for ERS seen in the Central Midline cluster (Makeig et al., 2004).

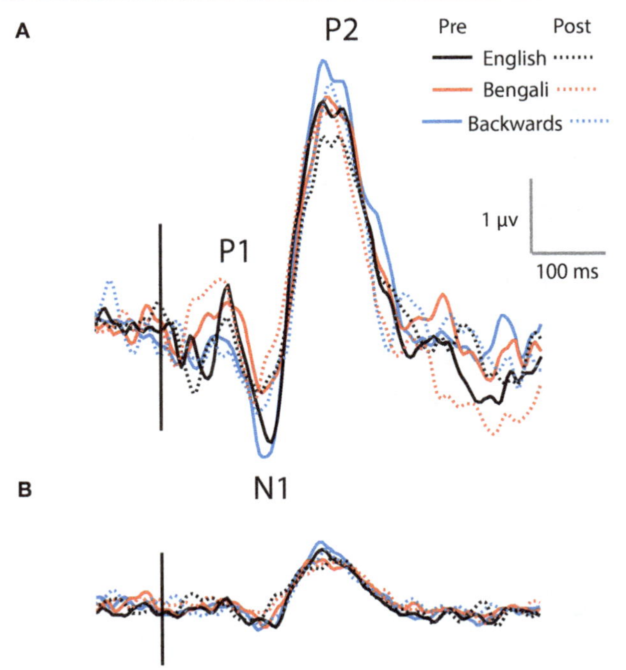

FIGURE 7 | AEPs. AEPs for data backprojected to channels surrounding Cz from all non-artifactual ICs **(A)** and ICs within the Central Midline IC process cluster **(B)**.

RELATIONSHIP OF EEG TO BEHAVIOR

Figure 8 shows changes in Central Midline theta, Anterior Midline high-alpha/low-beta, and Left Temporal alpha plotted as a function of d' improvement scores (Post-Pre-test d').

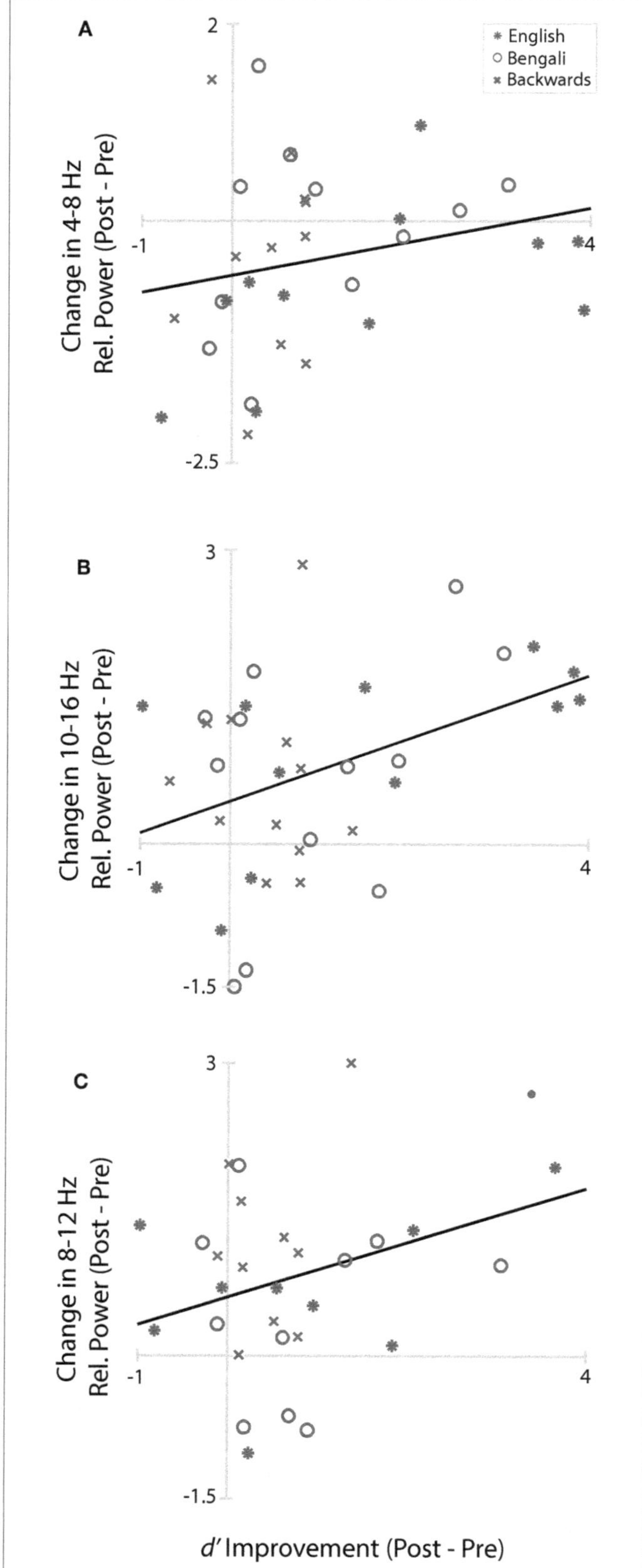

FIGURE 8 | Learning/EEG correlations. Scatterplots of improvement scores and changes in relative power from pre- to post-test in each cluster and time-frequency window. Asterisks mark English, circles mark Bengali, and Xs mark backwards speech.

Solid black lines in the figure depict linear fits. Positive values on the y-axis indicate greater power within the designated time-frequency window in the post-test. Positive values on the x-axis depict improvements in perceptual sensitivity to distance. The only significant relationship was between changes in Frontal Midline cluster high-alpha/low-beta and improvement scores, $r_{(34)} = 0.42$, $p = 0.033$. The relationship was positive, trending such that greater increases in relative power from pre- to post-test were associated with greater improvements in distance judgments. Neither the correlation of improvement scores with Central Midline theta, $r_{(31)} = 0.22$, $p = 0.221$, nor Left Temporal alpha, $r_{(28)} = 0.34$, $p = 0.104$, reached significance.

DISCUSSION

In the current study, we examined how perceptual training with speech sounds differing in familiarity altered distance perception accuracy and event-related spectral dynamics of EEG. An ICA approach to EEG analysis was used to characterize how independent and distributed brain processes relate to variations in distance perception accuracy. In part, the study served to determine whether or not EEG features shown to correlate with speech familiarity effects (Wisniewski et al., 2012) relate to within-experiment learning effects on distance perception. It was also intended to extend neuroimaging studies of human auditory distance perception beyond investigations of representational differences for near and far sounds in canonical auditory processing regions of cortex (cf., Mathiak et al., 2003; Kopčo et al., 2012; Altmann et al., 2013). We hoped to characterize how the cortical dynamics involved in active listening for distance cues changed with training.

Training led to more accurate distance perception across English, Bengali, and backwards speech categories, with greater improvement for familiar speech sounds (i.e., forwards speech). Replicating previous EEG work (Wisniewski et al., 2012), speech familiarity was related to differences in spectral perturbation patterns in Central Midline and Left Temporal clusters of IC processes. In the Central Midline cluster, backwards speech appeared to lead to the greatest transient theta ERS. English led to the greatest alpha ERD in a Left Temporal cluster. Perceptual learning in all speech categories was associated with a reduction in both of these cortical responses. In contrast, sustained upper-alpha/low-beta ERS localized at or near anterior regions of the medial frontal cortex was amplified after training. Furthermore, increases in this sustained ERS were positively correlated with learning.

The advantage of forward over backwards speech in terms of auditory distance perception has been previously reported (McGregor et al., 1985; Brungart and Scott, 2001; Wisniewski et al., 2012), but the present data seems to be the first evidence for a learning advantage. This advantage cannot be explained based on general auditory processing enhancements (e.g., Voss et al., 2004; Kolarik et al., 2013), because the different speech categories contained comparable known acoustic cues to distance. Furthermore, if performance differences were driven by global increases in auditory sensitivity, the dynamics of the left temporal IC cluster should have been most clearly related to changes in performance given its nearness to traditional auditory processing regions (Recanzone et al., 1993; Weinberger,

2007). Left temporal alpha ERD actually decreased from pre- to post-test, suggesting decreased involvement of this region after training. A similar trend was qualitatively observable in AEPs, which decreased in amplitude rather than increased as is typically associated with auditory perceptual learning (e.g., Orduña et al., 2012).

The advantage of learning associated with forward speech might actually reflect a disadvantage for learning backwards speech. For instance, listeners' initial difficulty judging differences between near and far backwards speech might have interfered in some way with their ability to benefit from training. Learning does tend to be limited for stimulus contrasts that are difficult to discriminate before training in comparison to contrasts that are easier (e.g., Lawrence, 1952; Orduña et al., 2012; Church et al., 2013). However, in past studies difficulty has typically been manipulated by modifying physical stimulus differences. Although acoustic features within speech sounds were not identical across speech categories, available cues to distance were highly similar (see **Figure 1**). Differences in learning, even if related to pre-training difficulty, thus are more likely to reflect differences in processing inherent to judging forward vs. backwards speech sounds[7].

Why is it then that listeners were better able to learn to distinguish the distances of sound sources producing forward speech? EEG data provide some clues. First, greater transient theta ERS was predictive of poor auditory distance perception performance in both the current and previous study. Specifically, relatively large transient ERS was associated with less accurate perception of backwards speech sounds, and decreases in this transient response accompanied increases in performance from pre- to post-test. One possibility is that transient ERS may be a sign of processing that is irrelevant or counterproductive for performing the auditory distance judgment task. Several ERP studies of auditory distraction have shown that novelty and orienting responses, such as MMN (e.g., Schröger, 1996) and P3 (e.g., Berti, 2013) components, are associated with decreases in performance on some primary perceptual task. For instance, even though participants may be instructed to ignore a task-irrelevant auditory stream, oddball sounds within that stream lead to both an increase in RT for a primary visual task, and a larger amplitude P3 in the ERP time-locked to auditory events (Berti, 2013). Other work analyzing time-frequency features of EEG have associated transient theta ERS to novelty/orienting responses in similar oddball paradigms, and have suggested that such responses reflect obligatory "attention switching" caused by obtrusive sensory events (Dietl et al., 1999; Barry et al., 2012). The transient ERS seen here may be related to these types of obligatory processes, especially for unfamiliar and unnatural sounding backwards speech, making it harder for listeners to execute the primary task of determining distance from relevant acoustic cues. A decrease in such novelty-driven interference occurring after multiple stimulus presentations (i.e., habituation; Friedman et al., 2001) may make it easier for participants to devote resources to the task at hand (Schröger, 1996; Berti, 2013). This interpretation makes the yet to be tested prediction that individuals with extensive experience localizing backward speech should perform as well at localizing backwards speech as forward speech, and should show comparable cortical activation patterns for either stimulus type.

While transient theta ERS decreased after training, sustained upper-alpha/low-beta ERS attributed to the medial frontal cortex increased. In one study analyzing the spectral dynamics of a similar frontal midline cluster of IC processes, both sustained theta and low-beta power increased as more items were held in working memory (Onton et al., 2005). There are also several fMRI and PET studies of auditory attention that show greater activation in prefrontal and anterior cingulate areas in tasks requiring increased attentional (Zatorre et al., 1999; Benedict et al., 2002; Janata et al., 2002; Mulet et al., 2007; Ahveninen et al., 2013; Uhlig et al., 2013) or memory resources (Zatorre et al., 1994). Others have reported increased activation in similar regions when specific acoustic features need to be tracked over time (Janata et al., 2002; Uhlig et al., 2013). Sustained upper-alpha/low-beta ERS may similarly relate to higher-level processing important for either sustained attention-related effects on auditory perception or working-memory related processes important for the integration, extraction, and/or retention of multiple acoustic cues to distance. Learning may involve increased engagement of these networks during listening.

We cannot provide a clear answer as to why sustained ERS features increase in parallel to decreases in transient ERS. Although a reduction in orienting/novelty processing might make it easier to sustain task-related processing in other regions, it is also possible that the relationship is reversed. For instance, some data suggests that increasing working memory demands can decrease ERP signatures of involuntary orienting to distracting sounds (Lv et al., 2010). In this vein, EEG signatures of orienting may be reduced because listeners are engaging more in sustained processing. Another possibility is that it takes training over several trials for listeners to reliably use appropriate listening strategies and that there is no causal relationship between the observed transient and sustained responses. Rather, there is only a transition in processing because listeners discovered that a sustained attentional or memory related strategy was effective. Regardless, in this study activity in frontal cortical networks seem to be more closely related to performance and learning than cortical networks ostensibly viewed as "auditory processing" regions.

[7] An alternative hypothesis is that audiospatial learning for speech and non-speech stimuli involve different mechanisms (Loebach and Pisoni, 2008), but the current data provide no support for this possibility. Rather, differences in EEG between speech categories appear to reflect quantitative differences in cortical activity. Another possibility is that backwards speech is processed differently because of its more graded onsets (He, 2001). However, distance cues within the speech sounds, such as SNR-related differences between near and far stimuli, were present throughout the duration of each stimulus. Furthermore, explicit training produces comparable perceptual learning curves for features occurring at sound onsets and offsets (Mossbridge et al., 2006, 2008), suggesting that the presence or absence of particular time domain features within speech sounds is unlikely to strongly constrain an individual's ability to learn to differentiate auditory distance cues. Although there are acoustic differences between forward and backwards speech, all known acoustic distance cues are comparable between these two categories. If other acoustic features that differ between forward and backwards speech are useful for distance perception, they have yet to be tested experimentally. However, if they exist, they could in principle affect the ease with which one can learn.

PSYCHOPHYSIOLOGICAL INVESTIGATIONS INTO AUDITORY LEARNING

By far, most psychophysiological studies of human auditory learning have employed evoked-potential methods. For instance, there exist several studies reporting that N1, P2, and MMN components of the AEP are plastic, showing changes in amplitude and latency with learning (e.g., Tremblay et al., 2001; Atienza et al., 2002; Gottselig et al., 2004; Boaz et al., 2010; Orduña et al., 2012). Learning-related modifications to these evoked responses are generally observed less than 500 ms post-stimulus onset. In contrast, we found that the strongest correlate of learning was induced ERS in an upper-alpha/low-beta frequency band. The presence of this ERS sustained well past typical evoked-potential latencies (~1700 ms post-stimulus onset). Familiarity with English speech was also associated with a sustained EEG feature. Namely, greater alpha ERD at time points exceeding 500 ms. These features would go undetected in a typical ERP study of auditory learning.

It is common to observe sustained ERS and ERD features during listening. Pesonen et al. (2006) asked listeners to indicate whether or not a spoken probe word was presented in a previous set of spoken words. Not only did the probe induce alpha ERD from 400 to ~1000 ms after probe onset, but theta and low-beta ERS was present up to ~1400 ms. Furthermore, words in the memory set did not induce low-beta ERS, suggesting that this feature was related to auditory recognition rather than encoding. In one recent study, the degree of alpha ERD corresponded with perception of a tone as high or low, even when the physical stimuli accompanying these perceptions were identical (Hartmann et al., 2012). Others have found that alpha ERD precedes the presentation of informative auditory stimuli, suggesting a relationship between oscillatory activity and anticipatory attention (e.g., Bastiaansen and Brunia, 2001). These studies are only a sample of demonstrated long-duration event-related modulations of the EEG spectrum during listening tasks (for review, see Krause, 2006; Weisz et al., 2011).

The evoked-potential approach to studying auditory learning assumes that non-phase locked spectral perturbations in EEG are noise, and that learning is mostly related to changes in evoked activity that occur close in time to stimulus onset. Although evoked–potential changes likely play an important role in auditory learning, these measures may fail to capture many learning processes. Because oscillatory dynamics of EEG seem to be related to auditory memory (Pesonen et al., 2006), subjective impressions of physically identical sounds (Hartmann et al., 2012), and active listening (Bastiaansen and Brunia, 2001), it seems likely that their examination could be informative in understanding how training leads to changes in perceptual acuity. The data reported here show that sustained phase-independent EEG features do change with learning. Future auditory learning studies may benefit from consideration of how both evoked-potential and oscillatory dynamics of EEG relate to learning-induced cortical plasticity.

FURTHER CONSIDERATIONS AND CAVEATS

Both the current and our earlier study represent initial attempts to characterize neural correlates of auditory distance perception in the oscillatory dynamics of EEG attributed to a distributed network of brain regions. Previous neuroimaging research has focused mainly on responses attributed to temporal brain regions (Mathiak et al., 2003; Kopčo et al., 2012; Altmann et al., 2013). Given the absence of data to support strong hypotheses regarding the activity of other cortical circuits that might contribute to auditory distance perception, a data-driven analysis approach was taken. We first identified clusters of IC processes that were related to performance and that showed clear event-related spectral dynamics (Wisniewski et al., 2012). Expanding on that original work, oscillatory dynamics of those processes were examined before and after training. Although portions of the data are consistent with prior work (i.e., temporal clusters of ICs show task-related dynamics; Mathiak et al., 2003; Kopčo et al., 2012; Altmann et al., 2013), previously ignored non-auditory cortical networks were found to relate most clearly to learning-related improvements in distance perception. Future hypothesis-driven studies are needed to validate the effects and interpretations presented here. Our identification of a distributed cortical network involved in auditory distance perception and learning should facilitate the development of such experiments.

Our work does not directly support several previous proposals regarding how learning impacts distance perception, but these proposals should not be dismissed. It remains possible that more subtle modifications to perceptual processing (e.g., Voss et al., 2004; Kolarik et al., 2013) indexed by higher-frequency spectral dynamics (Ahveninen et al., 2013), phase-locked responses (Orduña et al., 2012), or receptive fields of single neurons (Weinberger, 2007), contribute to performance improvements. Similarly, speech vs. non-speech representational differences in the brain may be related to performance, and detectable with other neuroimaging methodologies that are better suited for exploring neural processing with finer spatial resolution.

We collected no data verifying that listeners perceived stimuli as differing along a spatial dimension. That is, even though listeners discriminated far from near sounds, they may have perceived them as varying along some other dimension (e.g., background noisiness or timbre). Our intensity-normalized sounds also differ from most natural situations in which intensity differences are highly salient indicators of source distance (Coleman, 1963). This likely reduced the degree to which our stimulus set sounded natural. However, given that sounds contained viable cues to distance and that participants picked up on these cues (i.e., they performed at above chance levels), it seems likely that the sounds were perceived as varying in distance. Furthermore, the data show that listeners utilized distance cues, and learned about them, regardless of whether or not they truly perceived sounds as coming from sources at near or far locations.

As a final caveat, we have not compared processing during performance of the auditory distance perception task to processing during other auditory discrimination or spatial judgment tasks. The findings reported here may not be specific to distance perception. In fact, evidence that the strongest EEG correlates of performance are in non-auditory regions with spectral dynamics similar to those observed by others in non-auditory tasks would suggest that they are not. We do not see this as a weakness of the study, but rather a departure from previous approaches that serves to more fully characterize human brain dynamics during listening and distance judgment. One might also be concerned by the lack of clear differences in cortical activity induced by the processing of near and far sounds, given several studies suggesting that near and far distances are represented differently in the brain (e.g., Mathiak et al., 2003; Kopčo et al., 2012; Altmann et al., 2013). The EEG dynamics reported here are correlated with accuracy in distance perception even though they are not correlated with the dimension of distance. Our particular methodology may have either been insensitive to the detection of differences between near and far, or there exist large differences between individuals in regards to how they deal with this level of detail, making it difficult to detect differences in averaged data (cf. Wisniewski et al., 2014).

CONCLUSIONS

In two studies we have found task-related EEG oscillatory dynamics attributed to sources at or near both auditory and non-auditory brain regions. The earliest published neuroimaging work on human auditory distance perception suggested involvement of a distributed network of brain processes (Seifritz et al., 2002). However, most of the following work did not analyze activity in non-auditory brain regions (Mathiak et al., 2003; Kopčo et al., 2012; Altmann et al., 2013), instead restricting analyses to regions of interest in temporal cortex. The clearest conclusion that comes out of our studies is that activity in non-auditory cortical networks is associated with, and likely contributes to, auditory distance perception accuracy. These networks may be particularly important when effects on perception cannot be accounted for by the presence, absence, or manipulation of acoustic cues to distance. Given that we observed learning-related modifications to sustained ERS/ERD features, auditory perceptual learning research may benefit from explorations into how these non-phase dependent EEG dynamics relate to learning. Future work in both auditory distance perception and learning may find it useful to look beyond AEPs, which capture only a portion of the event-related processes observable in EEG (Makeig et al., 2004).

AUTHOR CONTRIBUTIONS

Conceived and designed the experiment: Eduardo Mercado III, Barbara A. Church, Matthew G. Wisniewski. Performed the experiment: Matthew G. Wisniewski, Klaus Gramann. Analyzed the data: Matthew G. Wisniewski. Contributed reagents/materials/analysis tools: Scott Makeig, Klaus Gramann. Wrote the paper: Matthew G. Wisniewski.

ACKNOWLEDGMENTS

This work was supported by NSF Grant No. SBE 0542013 to the Temporal Dynamics of Learning Center, SBE 0835976 to CELEST, a BRC grant from the Office of Naval Research and by a gift from The Swartz Foundation (Old Field, NY). Part of this research was performed while Matthew G. Wisniewski held a National Research Council Research Associateship Award at the Air Force Research Laboratory. The funders had no role in study design, data collection and analysis, decision to publish, or preparation of the manuscript. We thank Patchouly Banks for recording of stimuli and Arnaud Delorme for advice on EEG analysis. We also thank Max Goder-Reiser, Alexandria Zakrzewski, Ben Sawyer, and Itzel Orduña for comments on earlier versions of this manuscript.

REFERENCES

Ahveninen, J., Huang, S., Belliveau, J. W., Chang, W.-T., and Hämäläinen, M. (2013). Dynamic oscillatory processes governing cued orienting and allocation of auditory attention. *J. Cogn. Neurosci.* 25, 1926–1943. doi: 10.1162/jocn_a_00452

Akalin Acar, Z., and Makeig, S. (2013). Effects of forward model errors on EEG source localization. *Brain Topogr.* 26, 378–396. doi: 10.1007/s10548-012-0274-6

Altmann, C. F., Ono, K., Callan, A., Matsuhashi, M., Mima, T., and Fukuyama, H. (2013). Environmental reverberation affects processing of sound intensity in right temporal cortex. *Eur. J. Neurosci.* 38, 3210–3220. doi: 10.1111/ejn.12318

Atienza, M., Cantero, J. L., and Dominguez-Marin, E. (2002). The time course of neural changes underlying auditory perceptual learning. *Learn. Mem.* 9, 138–150. doi: 10.1101/lm.46502

Banks, P. N., Church, B. A., and Mercado, E. III. (2007). "The role of familiarity and reproducibility in auditory distance perception," in *Paper Presented at the 48th Annual Meeting of the Psychonomic Society* (Long Beach, CA).

Barman, B. (2009). A contrastive analysis of English and Bengla phonemics. *Dhaka Univ. J. Linguist.* 2, 19–42.

Barry, R. J., Steiner, G. Z., and De Blasio, F. M. (2012). Event-related EEG time-frequency analysis and the orienting reflex to auditory stimuli. *Psychophysiology* 49, 744–755. doi: 10.1111/j.1469-8986.2012.01367.x

Bastiaansen, M. C. M., and Brunia, C. H. M. (2001). Anticipatory attention: an event-related desynchronization approach. *Int. J. Psychophysiol.* 43, 91–107. doi: 10.1016/S0167-8760(01)00181-7

Benedict, R. H., Shucard, D. W., Santa Maria, M. P., Shucard, J. L., Abara, J. P., Coad, M. L., et al. (2002). Covert auditory attention generates activation in the rostral/dorsal anterior cingulate cortex. *J. Cogn. Neurosci.* 14, 637–645. doi: 10.1162/08989290260045765

Benjamini, Y., and Hochberg, Y. (1995). Controlling the false discovery rate: a practical and powerful approach to multiple testing. *J. R. Stat. Soc. Ser. B* 57, 289–300.

Berti, S. (2013). The role of auditory transient and deviance processing in distraction of task performance: a combined behavioral and event-related brain potential study. *Front. Hum. Neurosci.* 7:352. doi: 10.3389/fnhum.2013.00352

Boatman, D. (2004). Cortical bases of speech perception: evidence from functional lesion studies. *Cognition* 92, 47–65. doi: 10.1016/j.cognition.2003.09.010

Boaz, M. B. D., Campeanu, S., Tremblay, K. L., and Alain, C. (2010). Auditory evoked potentials dissociate rapid perceptual learning from task repetition without learning. *Psychophysiology* 48, 797–807.

Brungart, D. S., and Scott, K. R. (2001). The effects of production and presentation level on the auditory distance perception of speech. *J. Acoust. Soc. Am.* 110, 425–440. doi: 10.1121/1.1379730

Buzsáki, G. (2006). *Rhythms of the Brain.* New York, NY: Oxford University Press. doi: 10.1093/acprof:oso/9780195301069.001.0001

Church, B. A., Mercado, E. III., Wisniewski, M. G., and Liu, E. H. (2013). Temporal dynamics in auditory perceptual learning: impacts of sequencing and incidental learning. *J. Exp. Psychol.* 39, 270–276. doi: 10.1037/a0028647

Coleman, P. D. (1962). Failure to localize the source distance of an unfamiliar sound. *J. Acoust. Soc. Am.* 34, 345–346. doi: 10.1121/1.1928121

Coleman, P. D. (1963). An analysis of cues to auditory depth perception in free space. *Psychol. Bull.* 60, 302–315. doi: 10.1037/h0045716

Debener, S., Hine, J., Bleeck, S., and Eyles, J. (2008). Source localization of auditory evoked potentials after cochlear implantation. *Psychophysiology* 45, 20–24. doi: 10.1111/j.1469-8986.2007.00610.x

Debener, S., Makeig, S., Delorme, A., and Engel, A. K. (2005). What is novel in the novelty oddball paradigm? Functional significance of the novelty P3 event-related potential as revealed by independent component analysis. *Cogn. Brain Res.* 22, 309–321. doi: 10.1016/j.cogbrainres.2004.09.006

Delorme, A., and Makeig, S. (2004). EEGLAB: an open source toolbox for analysis of single-trial EEG dynamics including independent components analysis. *J. Neurosci. Methods* 134, 9–21. doi: 10.1016/j.jneumeth.2003.10.009

Delorme, A., Mullen, T., Kothe, C., Akalin Acar, Z., Bigdely-Shamlo, N., Vankov, A., et al. (2011). EEGLAB, SIFT, NFT, BCILAB, and ERICA: new tools for advanced EEG processing. *Comput. Intell. Neurosci.* 2011:130714. doi: 10.1155/2011/130714

Delorme, A., Westerfield, M., and Makeig, S. (2007). Medial prefrontal theta bursts precede rapid motor responses during visual selective attention. *J. Neurosci.* 27, 11949–11959. doi: 10.1523/JNEUROSCI.3477-07.2007

Dietl, T., Dirlich, G., Vogl, L., Lechner, C., and Strian, F. (1999). Orienting response and frontal midline theta activity: a somatosensory spectral perturbation study. *Clin. Neurophysiol.* 110, 1204–1209. doi: 10.1016/S1388-2457(99)00057-7

Fluitt, K. F., Mermagen, T., and Letowski, T. (2013). *Auditory Perception in Open Field: Distance Estimation (ARL-TR-6520).* Aberdeen Proving Ground, MD: Army Research Laboratory.

Friedman, D., Cycowicz, Y. M., and Gaeta, H. (2001). The novelty P3: an event-related brain potential (ERP) sign of the brain's evaluation of novelty. *Neurosci. Biobehav. Rev.* 25, 355–373. doi: 10.1016/S0149-7634(01)00019-7

Gottselig, J. M., Brandeis, D., Hofer-Tinguely, G., Borbély, A. A., and Achermann, P. (2004). Human central auditory plasticity associated with tone sequence learning. *Learn. Mem.* 11, 162–171. doi: 10.1101/lm.63304

Gougoux, F., Lepore, F., Lassonde, M., Voss, P., Zatorre, R. J., and Belin, P. (2004). Pitch discrimination in the early blind. *Nature* 430:309. doi: 10.1038/430309a

Grandchamp, R., and Delorme, A. (2011). Single-trial normalization for event-related spectral decomposition reduces sensitivity to noisy trials. *Front. Psychol.* 2:236. doi: 10.3389/fpsyg.2011.00236

Hartmann, T., Schlee, W., and Weisz, N. (2012). It's only in your head: expectancy of aversive auditory stimulation modulates stimulus-induced auditory cortical alpha desynchronization. *Neuroimage* 60, 170–178. doi: 10.1016/j.neuroimage.2011.12.034

He, J. (2001). ON and OFF Pathways segregated at the auditory thalamus of the guinea pig. *J. Neurosci.* 21, 8672–8679.

Hickok, G., and Poeppel, D. (2007). The cortical organization of speech processing. *Nat. Rev. Neurosci.* 8, 393–402. doi: 10.1038/nrn2113

Janata, P., Tillmann, B., and Bharucha, J. J. (2002). Listening to polyphonic music recruits domain-general attention and working memory circuits. *Cogn. Affect. Behav. Neurosci.* 2, 121–140. doi: 10.3758/CABN.2.2.121

Kolarik, A. J., Cirstea, S., and Pardhan, S. (2013). Evidence for enhanced discrimination of virtual auditory distance among blind listeners using level and direct-to-reverberant cues. *Exp. Brain Res.* 224, 623–633. doi: 10.1007/s00221-012-3340-0

Kopčo, N., Huang, S., Belliveau, J. W., Raij, T., Tengshe, C., and Ahveninen, J. (2012). Neuronal representations of distance in human auditory cortex. *Proc. Natl. Acad. Sci. U.S.A.* 109, 11019–11024. doi: 10.1073/pnas.1119496109

Krause, C. M. (2006). "Cognition- and memory-related ERD/ERS responses in the auditory stimulus modality," in *Event-Related Dynamics of Brain Oscillations. Progress in Brain Research,* eds C. Neuper and W. Klimesch (London: Elsevier), 197–207.

Lawrence, D. H. (1952). The transfer of a discrimination along a continuum. *J. Comp. Physiol. Psychol.* 45, 511–516. doi: 10.1037/h0057135

Loebach, J. L., and Pisoni, D. B. (2008). Perceptual learning of spectrally degraded speech and environmental sounds. *J. Acoust. Soc. Am.* 123, 1126–1139. doi: 10.1121/1.2823453

Lv, J.-Y., Wang, T., Qiu, J., Feng, S.-H., Tu, S., and Wei, D.-T. (2010). The electrophysiological effect of working memory load on involuntary attention in an auditory-visual distraction paradigm: an ERP study. *Exp. Brain Res.* 205, 81–86. doi: 10.1007/s00221-010-2360-x

Macmillan, N. A., and Creelman, C. D. (1991). *Detection Theory: a User's Guide.* New York, NY: Cambridge University Press.

Makeig, S. (1993). Auditory event-related dynamics of the EEG spectrum and effects of exposure to tones. *Electroencephalogr. Clin. Neurophysiol.* 86, 283–293. doi: 10.1016/0013-4694(93)90110-H

Makeig, S., Debener, S., Onton, J., and Delorme, A. (2004). Mining event-related brain dynamics. *Trends Cogn. Sci.* 8, 204–210. doi: 10.1016/j.tics.2004.03.008

Makeig, S., Jung, T.-P., Bell, A. J., Ghahremani, D., and Sejnowski, T.J. (1997). Blind separation of auditory event-related brain responses into independent components. *Proc. Natl. Acad. Sci.* 94, 10979–10984. doi: 10.1073/pnas.94.20.10979

Mathiak, K., Hertrich, I., Kincses, W. E., Riecker, A., Lutzenberger, W., Ackermann, H., et al. (2003). The right supratemporal plane hears the distance of objects: neuromagnetic correlates of virtual reality. *Neuroreport* 14, 307–311. doi: 10.1097/00001756-200303030-00002

McGregor, P., Horn, A. G., and Todd, M. A. (1985). Are familiar sounds ranged more accurately? *Percept. Mot. Skills* 61, 1082. doi: 10.2466/pms.1985.61.3f.1082

Mershon, D. H., Ballenger, W. L., Little, A. D., McMurtry, P. L., and Buchanan, J. L. (1989). Effects of room reflectance and background noise on perceived auditory distance. *Perception* 18, 403–416. doi: 10.1068/p180403

Mossbridge, J. A., Fitzgerald, M. B., O'Connor, E. S., and Wright, B. A. (2006). Perceptual learning evidence for separate processing of asynchrony and order tasks. *J. Neurosci.* 26, 12708–12716. doi: 10.1523/JNEUROSCI.2254-06.2006

Mossbridge, J. A., Scissors, B. N., and Wright, B. A. (2008). Learning and generalization on asynchrony and order tasks at sound offset: implications for underlying neural circuitry. *Learn. Mem.* 15, 13–20. doi: 10.1101/lm.573608

Mulet, B., Valero, J., Gutiérrez-Zotes, A., Montserrat, C., Cortés, M. J., Jariod, M., et al. (2007). Sustained and selective attention deficits as vulnerability markers to psychosis. *Eur. Psychiatry* 22, 171–176. doi: 10.1016/j.eurpsy.2006.07.005

Onton, J., Delorme, A., and Makeig, S. (2005). Frontal midline EEG dynamics during working memory. *Neuroimage* 27, 341–356. doi: 10.1016/j.neuroimage.2005.04.014

Orduña, I., Liu, E. H., Church, B. A., Eddins, A. C., and Mercado, E. III. (2012). Evoked-potential changes following discrimination learning involving complex sounds. *Clin. Neurophysiol.* 123, 711–719. doi: 10.1016/j.clinph.2011.08.019

Paus, T., Zatorre, R. J., Hofle, N., Caramanos, Z., Gotman, J., Petrides, M., et al. (1997). Time-related changes in neural systems underlying attention and arousal during the performance of an auditory vigilance task. *J. Cogn. Neurosci.* 9, 392–408. doi: 10.1162/jocn.1997.9.3.392

Pesonen, M., Björnberg, C. H., Hämäläinen, H., and Krause, C. M. (2006). Brain oscillatory 1-30 Hz EEG ERD/ERS responses during the different stages of an auditory memory search task. *Neurosci. Lett.* 399, 45–50. doi: 10.1016/j.neulet.2006.01.053

Pfurtscheller, G., and Lopes da Silva, F. H. (1999). Event-related EEG/MEG synchronization and desychronization: basic principles. *Clin. Neurophysiol.* 110, 1842–1857. doi: 10.1016/S1388-2457(99)00141-8

Recanzone, G. H., Schreiner, C. E., and Merzenich, M. M. (1993). Plasticity in the frequency representation of primary auditory cortex following discrimination training in adult owl monkeys. *J. Neurosci.* 13, 87–103.

Salminen, N. H., Tiitinen, H., Miettinen, I., Alku, P., and May, P. J. C. (2010). Asymmetrical representation of auditory space in human cortex. *Brain Res.* 1306, 93–99. doi: 10.1016/j.brainres.2009.09.095

Schröger, E. (1996). A neural mechanism for involuntary attention shifts to changes in auditory stimulation. *J. Cogn. Neurosci.* 8, 527–539. doi: 10.1162/jocn.1996.8.6.527

Seifritz, E., Neuhoff, J. G., Bilecen, D., Scheffler, K., Mustovic, H., Schächinger, H. ä., et al. (2002). Neural processing of auditory looming in the human brain. *Curr. Biol.* 12, 2147–2151. doi: 10.1016/S0960-9822(02)01356-8

Tremblay, K., Kraus, N., McGee, T., Ponton, C., and Otis, B. (2001). Central auditory plasticity: changes in the N1-P2 complex following speech-sound training. *Ear Hear.* 22, 79–90. doi: 10.1097/00003446-200104000-00001

Uhlig, M., Fairhurst, M. T., and Keller, P. E. (2013). The importance of integration and top-down salience when listening to complex multi-part musical stimuli. *Neuroimage* 77, 52–61. doi: 10.1016/j.neuroimage.2013.03.051

Voss, P., Lassonde, M., Gougoux, F., Fortin, M., Guillemot, J. P., Lepore, F., et al. (2004). Early- and late-onset blind individuals show supra-normal auditory abilities in far-space. *Curr. Biol.* 14, 1734–1738. doi: 10.1016/j.cub.2004.09.051

Voss, P., Lepore, F., Gougoux, F., and Zatorre, R. J. (2011). Relevance of spectral cues for auditory spatial processing in the occipital cortex of the blind. *Front. Psychol.* 2:48. doi: 10.3389/fpsyg.2011.00048

Weinberger, N. M. (2007). Auditory associative memory and representational plasticity in the primary auditory cortex. *Hear. Res.* 229, 54–68. doi: 10.1016/j.heares.2007.01.004

Weisz, N., Hartmann, T., Müller, N., and Obleser, J. (2011). Alpha rhythms in audition: cognitive and clinical perspectives. *Front. Psychol.* 2:73. doi: 10.3389/fpsyg.2011.00073

Wisniewski, M. G., Church, B. A., and Mercado, E. III. (2014). Individual differences during acquisition predict shifts in generalization. *Behav. Processes* 104, 26–34. doi: 10.1016/j.beproc.2014.01.007

Wisniewski, M. G., Mercado, E. III., Gramann, K., and Makeig, S. (2012). Familiarity with speech affects cortical processing of auditory distance cues and increases acuity. *PLoS ONE* 7:e41025. doi: 10.1371/journal.pone.0041025

Zahorik, P., Brungart, D. S., and Bronkhorst, A. W. (2005). Auditory distance perception in humans: a summary of past and present research. *Acta Acustica United Acoust.* 91, 409–420.

Zatorre, R. J., Bouffard, M., Ahad, P., and Belin, P. (2002). Where is "where" in the human auditory cortex? *Nat. Neurosci.* 5, 905–909. doi: 10.1038/nn904

Zatorre, R. J., Evans, A. C., and Myer, E. (1994). Neural mechanisms underlying melodic perception and memory for pitch. *J. Neurosci.* 14, 1908–1919.

Zatorre, R. J., Mondor, T. A., and Evans, A. C. (1999). Auditory attention to space and frequency activates similar cerebral systems. *Neuroimage* 10, 544–554. doi: 10.1006/nimg.1999.0491

14

Single-sided deafness and directional hearing: Contribution of spectral cues and high-frequency hearing loss in the hearing ear

Martijn J. H. Agterberg[1,2], Myrthe K. S. Hol[2], Marc M. Van Wanrooij[1,2], A. John Van Opstal[1] and Ad F. M. Snik[1,2]*

[1] Department of Biophysics, Donders Institute for Brain, Cognition and Behaviour, Radboud University Nijmegen, Nijmegen, Netherlands
[2] Department of Otorhinolaryngology, Donders Institute for Brain, Cognition and Behaviour, Radboud University Medical Center, Nijmegen, Netherlands

Correspondence:
Martijn J. H. Agterberg, Department of Biophysics, Donders Institute for Brain, Cognition and Behaviour, Radboud University Nijmegen, Heyendaalseweg 135, 6525 AJ Nijmegen, Netherlands
e-mail: m.agterberg@donders.ru.nl

Direction-specific interactions of sound waves with the head, torso, and pinna provide unique spectral-shape cues that are used for the localization of sounds in the vertical plane, whereas horizontal sound localization is based primarily on the processing of binaural acoustic differences in arrival time (interaural time differences, or ITDs) and sound level (interaural level differences, or ILDs). Because the binaural sound-localization cues are absent in listeners with total single-sided deafness (SSD), their ability to localize sound is heavily impaired. However, some studies have reported that SSD listeners are able, to some extent, to localize sound sources in azimuth, although the underlying mechanisms used for localization are unclear. To investigate whether SSD listeners rely on monaural pinna-induced spectral-shape cues of their hearing ear for directional hearing, we investigated localization performance for low-pass filtered (LP, <1.5 kHz), high-pass filtered (HP, >3kHz), and broadband (BB, 0.5–20 kHz) noises in the two-dimensional frontal hemifield. We tested whether localization performance of SSD listeners further deteriorated when the pinna cavities of their hearing ear were filled with a mold that disrupted their spectral-shape cues. To remove the potential use of perceived sound level as an invalid azimuth cue, we randomly varied stimulus presentation levels over a broad range (45–65 dB SPL). Several listeners with SSD could localize HP and BB sound sources in the horizontal plane, but inter-subject variability was considerable. Localization performance of these listeners strongly reduced after diminishing of their spectral pinna-cues. We further show that inter-subject variability of SSD can be explained to a large extent by the severity of high-frequency hearing loss in their hearing ear.

Keywords: azimuth, head-shadow effect, mold, single-sided deaf(ness), spectral pinna-cues

INTRODUCTION

Listeners with total single-sided deafness (SSD) lack the ability to localize sounds on the basis of interaural differences in time (ITD) and sound level (ILD). As a result, SSD listeners encounter significant problems with the processing of auditory information in daily life (Van Wieringen et al., 2011; Lieu, 2013), and demonstrate impaired sound-localization abilities (Humes et al., 1980; Colburn, 1982; Slattery and Middlebrooks, 1994; Bosman et al., 2003; Van Wanrooij and Van Opstal, 2004; Wazen et al., 2005). Similar effects have been reported for unilateral plugged control listeners (McPartland et al., 1997; Van Wanrooij and Van Opstal, 2007; Kumpik et al., 2010; Irving and Moore, 2011; Agterberg et al., 2012), and unilateral plugged experimental animals (Keating et al., 2013; Kral et al., 2013). Several studies, in which sound levels were fixed or varied over a small range, have demonstrated sound-localization abilities of SSD listeners (Batteau, 1967; Colburn, 1982; Häusler et al., 1983; Slattery and Middlebrooks, 1994; Wightman and Kistler, 1997). When stimuli are presented at a single sound level, SSD listeners could rely on the perceived sound level at the hearing ear because of the azimuth-dependent attenuation produced by the head-shadow effect (HSE). Van Wanrooij and Van Opstal (2004) demonstrated that the HSE indeed contributes to sound localization abilities of SSD listeners. Furthermore, the possibility that these listeners have learned to use monaural pinna-induced spectral-shape cues of their hearing ear for localization in azimuth, has been postulated (Batteau, 1967; Colburn, 1982; Häusler et al., 1983; Slattery and Middlebrooks, 1994; Wightman and Kistler, 1997; Van Wanrooij and Van Opstal, 2004; Shub et al., 2008; Kumpik et al., 2010; Rothpletz et al., 2012). The studies mentioned above did not take into account the hearing loss of the better ear, and included only subjects with a normal hearing ear (i.e., hearing thresholds ≤25 dB HL at frequencies between 0.25 and 8 kHz). Especially when stimuli contain high-frequencies information,

Abbreviations: BB, broadband; HP, high-pass; HRTFs, head-related transfer functions; HSE, head-shadow effect; ILDs, interaural level differences; ITDs, interaural time differences; LP, low-pass; MAE, mean absolute error; SSD, single-sided deaf(ness).

monaural pinna-induced spectral-shape cues can be beneficial for localization (Best et al., 2005). Recently it has been reported that older listeners (63–80 years) with hearing loss above 5 kHz demonstrated deteriorated sound localization in elevation as compared to normal hearing listeners (Otte et al., 2013). High-frequency hearing loss did not affect sound localization abilities in azimuth. These results show that with advancing age and subsequent increasing high-frequency hearing loss, listeners lose the access to spectral-shape information for the localization of broadband (BB) stimuli in elevation. The loss of this ability might be of importance for listeners with SSD.

Animal studies have indicated that early onset of unilateral deafness results in a unilateral aural preference, reflected by local field potentials recorded from the cortical surface (Kral et al., 2013). Others, demonstrated that the ability to use spectral localization cues diminished as soon as normal hearing was experienced (Keating et al., 2013). As it is unclear whether a critical period for this auditory plasticity might also be present in humans, and it is postulated that the etiology of subjects with SSD may be unrelated to their localization abilities (Colburn, 1982), we investigated whether the onset of unilateral deafness (congenital vs. acquired) affects sound-localization performance in azimuth and elevation when tested at a later age.

Listeners with SSD demonstrate a large variability in their localization performance and it is not clear whether this variation is related to hearing loss, pinna-induced spectral shape cues, or to the onset of unilateral deafness. In the present study we investigated to what extent high-frequency hearing loss in the hearing ear of SSD listeners affects their use of spectral-shape cues to localize sounds in azimuth. Furthermore, for SSD patients who are seeking hearing revalidation an improved number of treatment options have become available. It is important to identify the factors affecting sound localization abilities of SSD listeners. This information is helpful for clinicians in the search for the best possible treatment for listeners with monaural hearing.

METHODS

LISTENERS WITH SSD AND CONTROL LISTENERS

Nineteen listeners with complete SSD (16–67 years; mean $\pm$ *SD* : 40.7 $\pm$ 16.7 years) and 15 control listeners (22–61 years; mean $\pm$ *SD* : 30.9 $\pm$ 12.4 years) participated in the present study. **Table 1** lists the characteristics of listeners with SSD and indicates which listeners experienced listening with a bone-conduction device. To assess hearing loss in the better ear, we performed pure-tone audiometry at 0.125, 0.25, 0.5, 1, 2, 4, and 8 kHz. Hearing thresholds were thus obtained using standard procedures and standard equipment (Interacoustics AC 40 clinical audiometer, Interacoustics A/S, Assens, Denmark).

MOLD IN THE BETTER EAR

The SSD listeners were tested in two hearing conditions that were presented in randomized order: (i) monaural hearing; (ii) monaural hearing with a custom-made mold, fabricated from rubber casting material (Otoform Otoplastik—K/c; Dreve, Unna, Germany), inserted in the pinna of the better-hearing ear without obstructing the ear canal.

All control listeners were tested under normal hearing conditions, and after altering their pinna-cues with custom-made molds in both pinna.

STIMULI

Listeners were asked to localize (i) low-pass (LP; 0.5–1.5 kHz); (ii) high-pass (HP; 3–20 kHz), and (iii) broadband (BB; 0.5–20 kHz) filtered Gaussian white noises. Spectral cues are minimal for LP noises (Middlebrooks and Green, 1991; Middlebrooks, 1992; Frens and Van Opstal, 1995; Blauert, 1997; Van Wanrooij and Van Opstal, 2004, 2007), and we therefore hypothesized that LP noises could not be localized in azimuth at all by SSD listeners.

BB and HP stimuli were chosen to maximize the use of potential spectral-shape cues provided by the pinna of the better-hearing ear. BB and HP stimuli had randomly-selected sound levels in the range 45–65 dB SPL. LP noises were interleaved with the BB and HP stimuli, and only presented at a level of 55 dB SPL. To minimize measurement time and because the attenuation of sound level by the head is not very effective for LP noises, we decided not to rove the levels of the LP stimuli.

All stimuli had 150-ms duration, 5-ms sine- and cosine-squared on- and offset ramps and a flat spectrum level within their pass bands. Sounds were digitally generated in Matlab (The MathWorks) at a sampling rate of 50 kHz, and were delivered through a BB loudspeaker, moved by a computer-controlled motorized system at a distance of 1.15 m from the listener's head. Stimulus coordinates for BB and HP stimuli ranged from −85° to +85° in azimuth and from −30° to +30° in elevation. LP stimuli were presented at 0° in elevation.

Table 1 | Audiometric characteristics of the listeners with SSD.

SSD patients	Age (y)	Side HL	Congenital acquired	Gender	Threshold dB HL 8 kHz
P1	32	L	Congenital	M	0
P2	22	L	Congenital	M	10
P3	22	L	Congenital	M	5
P4	24	R	Congenital	V	10
P5	51	L	Congenital	M	65
P6*	46	L	Congenital	V	10
P7*	27	R	Congenital	M	5
P8	46	L	Congenital	V	5
P9*	16	L	Congenital	M	0
P10*	34	L	Congenital	M	35
P11	20	L	Congenital	V	0
P12	67	L	Acquired	M	70
P13	38	R	Acquired	V	20
P14*	53	R	Acquired	V	40
P15*	63	L	Acquired	V	5
P16	34	L	Acquired	M	30
P17	51	L	Acquired	M	40
P18	67	R	Acquired	M	55
P19	60	L	Acquired	M	60

**Indicates listeners who experienced listening with a bone-conduction device.*

SETUP

For a detailed description of the setup see Bremen et al. (2010). Briefly, we ensured that listeners could only use acoustic information to localize sounds by testing directional hearing in a completely dark, sound-attenuated room. Horizontal and vertical head-movement components were recorded with the magnetic search-coil induction technique (Robinson, 1963; Hofman and Van Opstal, 1998). Listeners pointed with a head-fixed laser pointer, which projected onto a small (1 cm^2) black plastic plate positioned in front (40 cm) of the listener's eyes. Listeners were asked to point the laser dot as fast and as accurately as possible in the perceived sound direction after stimulus exposure. Listeners were observed continuously by the experimenter with an infrared camera, but did not receive any feedback about their performance during the experiments.

PARADIGM

The experimental session started with a brief visual calibration experiment to establish the off-line mapping of the coil signals onto known target locations. After this, listeners performed a brief practice session containing 10 trials to become familiar with the head-movement response procedure.

During the sound-localization experiments the listener first fixated on an LED that was located at 0° azimuth and 0° elevation and then triggered the start of the trial by pressing a button. Between 150 and 300 ms the LED disappeared, and 200 ms later the sound stimulus was presented. After stimulus exposure the listener had to direct the head-fixed laser pointer as fast and accurately as possible, by making a rapid head movement toward the apparent sound direction.

DATA ANALYSIS

We analyzed the azimuth (α) responses separately for each stimulus condition (LP, HP, and BB noises) and for each listener. We determined the best linear fit (based on the mean-squared error criterion) of the stimulus-response relationship (pooled across presentation levels and elevation angles for HP and BB noises):

$$\alpha_{RESP} = b + g \cdot \alpha_{STIM} \quad (1)$$

where α_{RESP} is the response azimuth (in degrees), α_{STIM} is the stimulus azimuth (in degrees), b is the response bias (in degrees), and g the response gain (dimensionless). We also computed Pearson's correlation coefficient between fit and data, as well as the coefficient of determination (r^2). To dissociate the potential contribution of the proximal sound level, L, from that of the actual stimulus location, we performed a partial correlation analysis:

$$\widehat{\alpha}_{RESP} = p \cdot \widehat{\alpha}_{STIM} + q \cdot \hat{L} \quad (2)$$

with p as the dimensionless azimuth coefficient and q as the dimensionless proximal sound-level coefficient; each determines to what extent sound-source azimuth or proximal sound level explains the observed responses. Variables α_{RESP}, α_{STIM} and L were transformed into their (dimensionless) z-scores $\hat{x}$:

$$\hat{x} \equiv \frac{x - \mu_x}{\sigma_x} \quad (3)$$

with x the variable to be z-transformed, μ_x its mean, and σ_x its standard deviation (resulting in $\widehat{\alpha}_{RESP}$, $\widehat{\alpha}_{STIM}$, and $\hat{L}$). We determined proximal sound level L by correcting the free-field presentation levels of the stimuli with the frequency- and azimuth-dependent attenuation produced by the HSE.

The HSE was derived for BB noises from the best fit of free-field HSE measurements of four listeners (Van Wanrooij and Van Opstal, 2004). For HP and BB noises the HSE can vary between −15 and +15 dB over the entire azimuth range, for LP noises the HSE is less pronounced.

For the elevation (ε) responses to BB and HP noises the best linear fits of the stimulus-response relationships were also determined.

$$\varepsilon_{RESP} = b + g \cdot \varepsilon_{STIM} \quad (4)$$

ε_{RESP} and ε_{STIM} are the response elevation and stimulus elevation in degrees, b is the response bias (in degrees) and g the response gain (dimensionless).

RESULTS

HIGH-FREQUENCY HEARING LOSS

Normal hearing thresholds (defined as 20 dB HL or better) in the functioning ear were confirmed in all listeners with SSD ($n = 19$) for frequencies up to 4 kHz. At 8 kHz 11 SSD listeners demonstrated normal hearing. The other SSD listeners demonstrated thresholds ≥20 dB HL, with six listeners demonstrating thresholds ≥40 dB HL (see **Table 1**).

In the group of control listeners ($n = 15$), two older listeners (age 56 and 61 years) suffered from a symmetric hearing loss at 8 kHz (thresholds ≥ 40 dB HL). All other control listeners demonstrated normal hearing thresholds between 500 Hz and 4 kHz, and thresholds of 40 dB HL, or better, for 8 kHz.

EFFECT OF STIMULUS BANDWIDTH

Figure 1A shows the stimulus-response relations in azimuth for a control listener (C1), and two listeners with SSD at their left side (P3 and P12), for BB, LP, and HP stimuli. For the BB and HP stimuli responses for the presentation levels (45, 55, and 65 dB SPL) were pooled. The dashed lines represent the best-fit linear regression lines (Equation 1) on the azimuth response components. The control listener (right-hand column) could accurately localize stimuli for all conditions as is indicated by r^2 values and gains close to 1. Note that perfect localization would mean that all individual responses would exactly be on the diagonal with slope +1.0 (with parameters: $r^2 = 1, g = 1, b = 0$). Listener P3 with SSD demonstrated good localization performance for BB and HP stimuli ($r^2 > 0.79$; $g > 0.72$; b between 0° and 4°). In contrast, listener P12 with SSD demonstrated poor sound-localization abilities. This listener perceived the stimuli mainly at the hearing side, which resulted in a considerable leftward bias ($b = 80°$ for BB stimuli), and small coefficients of determination ($r^2 < 0.10$) for all stimuli and conditions. The hearing thresholds

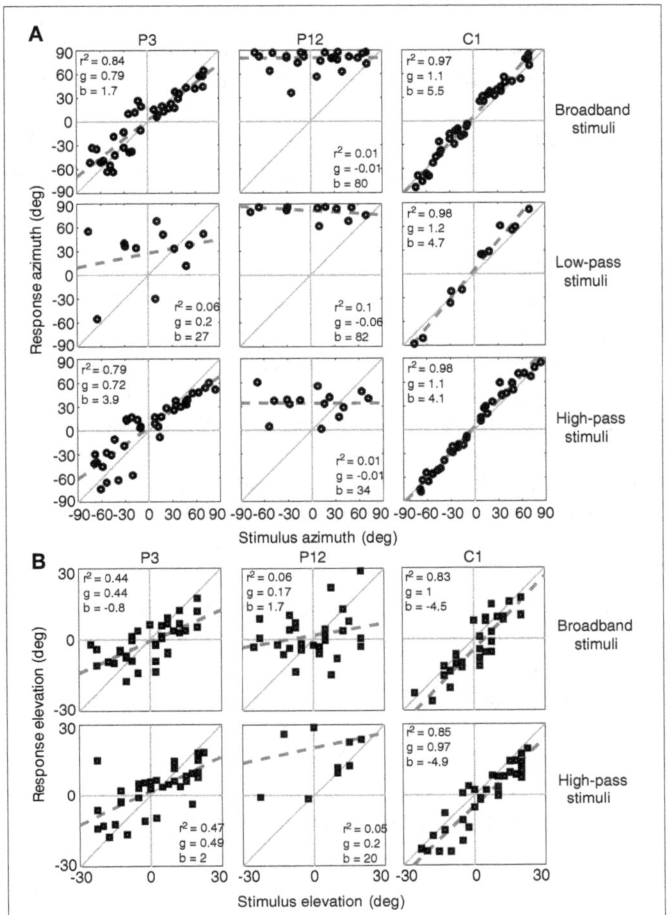

FIGURE 1 | Sound-localization responses for SSD listener with a thresholds at 8 kHz < 40 dB HL (P3), a SSD listener with a thresholds at 8 kHz ≥ 40 dB HL (P12) and a control listener (C1). Responses are plotted for the BB, HP, and LP stimuli in azimuth **(A)** and elevation **(B)**. The dashed gray line denotes the linear regression fit. Note the high degree of variation in monaural localization abilities of the listeners with SSD. Listener P3 had fairly good localization of BB and HP stimuli. r^2, coefficient of determination, *g*, response gain, *b*, bias.

at 8 kHz in the better ear are listed in **Table 1**. Listener P3 demonstrated a 8 kHz hearing threshold of 5 dB HL, P12 demonstrated a 8 kHz threshold of 70 dB HL. Because of the high-frequency hearing loss listener P12 did not detect all stimuli.

Figure 1B shows the stimulus-response relations in elevation (Equation 4) for the same listeners. Listener P3, with better horizontal sound localization abilities than listener P12, demonstrated also better elevation performance ($g > 0.44$ vs. $g < 0.2$).

Figure 2 shows the pooled azimuth stimulus-response relations of all control listeners ($n = 15$), all SSD listeners with 8 kHz thresholds below 40 dB HL ($n = 13$), and SSD listeners with 8 kHz thresholds higher than 40 dB HL ($n = 6$), for BB, LP and HP stimuli. If the right ear was the deaf ear, data are presented without modification. If the left ear was the deaf ear, data of left and right ears were swapped before pooling the data. The figure demonstrates that listeners without high-frequency hearing loss outperformed listeners with 8 kHz thresholds higher than 40 dB HL, for BB and HP sounds. The figure hints at the possibility

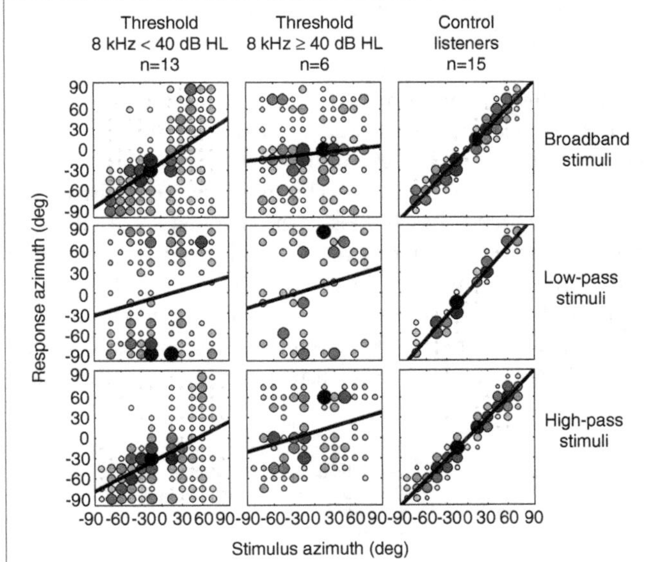

FIGURE 2 | Azimuth stimulus-response relationships for BB, LP, and HP noise burst pooled for SSD listeners with 8 kHz thresholds below 40 dB HL (left hand column), SSD listeners with 8 kHz thresholds higher than 40 dB HL (middle column), and control listeners (right hand column). Black bold lines denote best-fit regression lines over the pooled data. Grayscale and size of the data points indicates the number of responses on that location. Black indicates a larger number of responses than white.

that SSD listeners with 8 kHz thresholds below 40 dB HL were able to use spectral pinna-cues, as they could localize the BB and HP stimuli in azimuth, but were not able to localize the LP sounds. Listeners with 8 kHz thresholds higher than 40 dB HL were equally poor in localization of BB, LP, and HP stimuli.

Figure 3 shows the pooled stimulus-response relations in elevation. Listeners with 8 kHz thresholds below 40 dB HL outperformed listeners with 8 kHz thresholds higher than 40 dB HL. The figure shows that SSD listeners with 8 kHz thresholds below 40 dB HL were able to use spectral pinna-cues for the localization of BB and HP stimuli in elevation. Listeners with 8 kHz thresholds higher than 40 dB HL were equally poor in localization of BB and HP stimuli. Two control listeners with high-frequency hearing loss (threshold 8 kHz > 40 dB HL) were not included in the pooled elevation stimulus-response relations (right hand column).

CONTRIBUTION OF SPECTRAL CUES

Figure 4 plots response azimuth localization gains for BB stimuli against response elevation gains for 13 SSD listeners with 8 kHz thresholds in the hearing ear below 40 dB HL (filled symbols), six SSD listeners with 8 kHz thresholds above 40 dB HL (open circles), and the 15 control listeners (crosses).

Figure 4A shows the gains for the listeners with SSD in the monaural condition, and for the normal hearing control listeners (spectral-shape cues are available). Listeners with SSD demonstrated considerable variability in performance, and there was a clear correlation between azimuth gains and elevation gains ($r = 0.83$, $p < 0.01$). The SSD listeners with 8 kHz thresholds below

40 dB HL demonstrated higher azimuth and elevation gains than the SSD listeners with thresholds above 40 dB HL. The latter group of listeners had both gains close to zero, indicating poor directional hearing performance in both azimuth and elevation. The r^2 were also small (<0.4, data not shown). The far majority of control listeners had azimuth and elevation gains that were close to the ideal value of one. The two older control listeners with high-frequency hearing loss demonstrated small elevation gains, confirming earlier reports of deteriorated vertical sound localization performance in the elderly (Otte et al., 2013).

Figure 4B shows the resulting azimuth and elevation gains when the molds reduced the spectral-shape cues ($r = 0.2$, $p = 0.87$). Note that the SSD listeners with a relatively low high-frequency hearing loss demonstrated a clear deterioration in their sound localization performance in both directions. Molds in the pinnae of control listeners only affected their elevation performance. This deterioration of sound localization abilities in elevation, after altering the pinna-cues with custom-made molds in both pinna, has been reported previously (Oldfield and Parker, 1984).

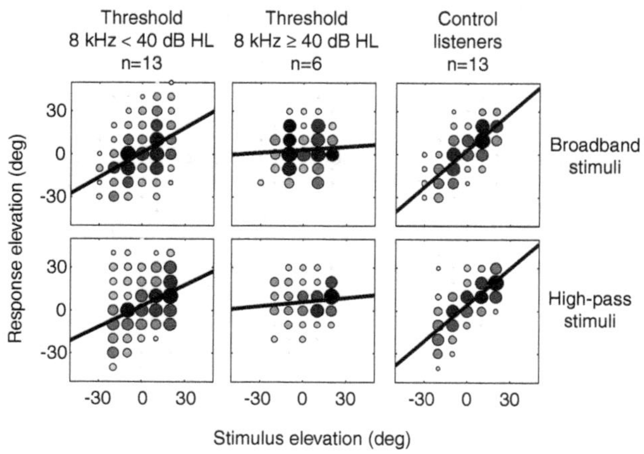

FIGURE 3 | Elevation stimulus-response relationships for BB and HP noise burst pooled for SSD listeners with 8 kHz thresholds below 40 dB HL (left hand column), SSD listeners with 8 kHz thresholds higher than 40 dB HL (middle column) and control listeners ($n = 13$, right hand column). Black bold lines denote best-fit regression lines over the pooled data. Grayscale and size of the data points indicates the number of responses on that location. Black indicates a larger number of responses than white.

CONTRIBUTION OF HIGH-FREQUENCY HEARING LOSS

Figure 5 illustrates the effect of high-frequency (8 kHz) hearing loss on the localization performance, of BB noises, of SSD listeners in the horizontal plane. When the hearing loss at 8 kHz exceeds about 30 dB HL the azimuth gains are always small ($g < 0.4$). Good high-frequency hearing in the only hearing ear appears to be an important requirement for adequate sound localization performance. The variation in localization performance is not explained by the onset of unilateral deafness (congenital vs. acquired). In addition we also included the data of 9 listeners with SSD from the study of Van Wanrooij and Van Opstal (2004; squares). This figure clearly shows that almost half of the subjects with 8 kHz thresholds below 40 dB HL demonstrate poor sound localization abilities.

Elevation gains also clearly deteriorate with increasing high-frequency hearing loss. For all subjects with 8 kHz thresholds above 40 dB HL elevation gains were small.

EFFECT OF SOUND LEVEL ON LOCALIZATION PERFORMANCE

Figure 6 shows the partial correlation coefficients for azimuth (p in Equation 2) and for the proximal sound level (q in Equation 2) for the BB stimuli, for SSD listeners (circles) and control listeners (crosses). These partial correlation coefficients reveal the relative contributions of the actual target azimuth and the perceived sound level at the hearing ear to their azimuth localization responses. For SSD listeners with an 8 kHz threshold below 40 dB, the contribution of proximal sound level varied systematically with the azimuth coefficient. Responses were more influenced by sound level when the (spectrally derived) estimate of azimuth

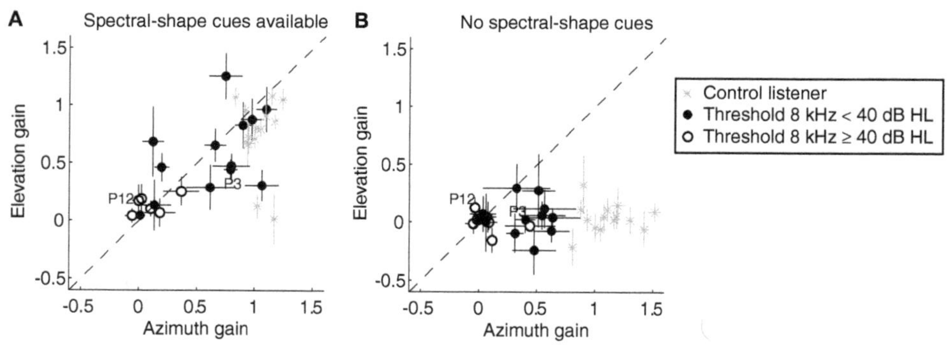

FIGURE 4 | Response elevation gain for BB stimuli plotted against the azimuth gain. Data from all control listeners (gray crosses), listeners with SSD with 8 kHz thresholds below 40 dB HL (filled circles) and SSD listeners with 8 kHz thresholds higher than 40 dB HL (open circles) are presented when spectral-shape cues were available **(A)**, and when spectral-shape cues were reduced by molds **(B)**. Error bars denote ± 1 SE of the azimuth and elevation regression coefficients. Data points from the two SSD listeners depicted in **Figure 1** (P3 and P12), are indicated in the figure. Data are pooled across presentation levels. Note the two clear outliers in the control group. These two listeners demonstrated bilateral high-frequency hearing loss (8 kHz thresholds higher than 40 dB HL).

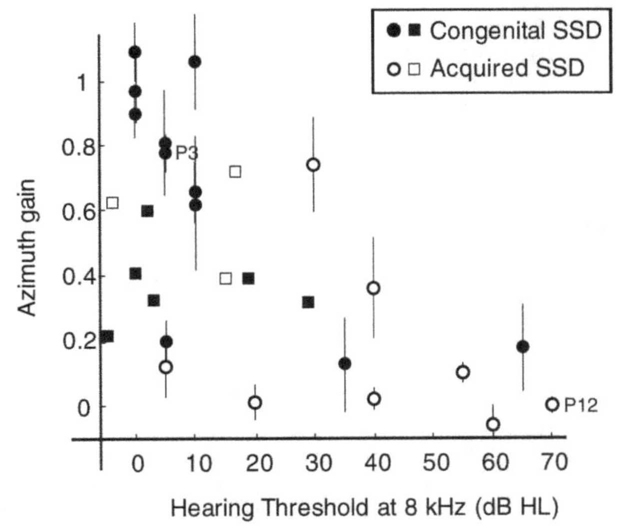

FIGURE 5 | Response azimuth gain for BB stimuli plotted against the hearing threshold at 8 kHz for listeners with congenital SSD (filled circles) and listeners with acquired SSD (open circles). Error bars denote ± 1 SE of the azimuth regression coefficient. Data points from SSD listeners P3 and P12 are emphasized in the figure. For comparison data (squares) of nine listeners with SSD from a study performed by Van Wanrooij and Van Opstal (2004) are plotted in the figure.

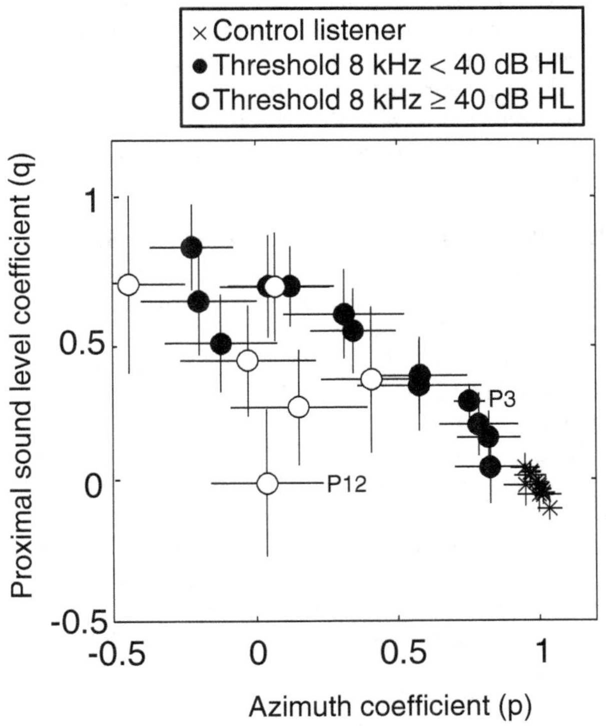

FIGURE 6 | Multiple linear regression analysis of azimuth localization performance for BB stimuli of SSD listeners with 8 kHz thresholds below 40 dB HL (filled circles), SSD listeners with 8 kHz thresholds higher than 40 dB HL (open circles) and control listeners (crosses). The coefficients for proximal sound level (q in Equation 2) and azimuth (p in Equation 2) are plotted against one another for each listener. Error bars denote ± 1 *SD* of the azimuth and intensity regression coefficients, respectively. Data points from SSD listeners P3 and P12 are emphasized in the figure. For clarity, some data points are slightly shifted.

was poor. Indeed, those SSD listeners typically perceived louder sounds on their hearing side. A similar effect of sound level on localization performance in cochlear-implant listeners has been reported by Majdak et al. (2011).

Listener P12 is the listener with the most severe high-frequency hearing loss (see **Table 1**). This listener did not detect all BB stimuli and therefore proximal sound level did not contribute to the localization performance.

Control listeners had their azimuth coefficients close to the ideal value of one, and the proximal sound level coefficient close to zero. When listeners can localize sounds on the basis of binaural difference cues they rely less on the HSE cue.

DISCUSSION

INDIVIDUAL DIFFERENCES IN SOUND LOCALIZATION PERFORMANCE

The present study demonstrates that SSD listeners without severe high-frequency hearing loss in their hearing ear can localize BB noises in the horizontal plane. Our data indicate that the amount of high-frequency hearing loss greatly influences the directional hearing abilities of SSD listeners (**Figure 5**). Colburn (1982) postulated that the etiology of subjects with unilateral total deafness (e.g., congenital vs. acquired), may be irrelevant for their localization abilities. In support of this idea, our data indicate that the variability in localization performance of SSD listeners can to a large extent be attributed to high-frequency hearing loss, and not to the onset of unilateral deafness (congenital vs. acquired). However, good high-frequency hearing (8 kHz thresholds <40 dB HL) does not always ensure good sound localization abilities. Even in the group of SSD listeners with 8 kHz thresholds below 40 dB HL almost half of the subjects demonstrate poor sound localization. This variation in sound localization performance can be related to several factors. Recently, Andéol et al. (2013) and Majdak et al. (2014) demonstrated that in listeners with normal hearing, non-acoustic factors like the perceptual ability to discriminate spectral shapes had a larger impact on the sound localization performance in elevation than cues provided by the listener-specific pinna-induced spectral-shape cues. These non-acoustic factors might also play a role in the azimuthal localization abilities of SSD listeners.

PINNA-INDUCED SPECTRAL-SHAPE CUES

Some listeners with SSD were able to use the spectral-pinna cues of their hearing ear for localization in azimuth. When the possibility to use spectral cues was disrupted by filling the pinna of their hearing ear with a mold, azimuthal localization deteriorated (**Figure 4B**). The spectral cues are specific for an individual listener and appear above about 4 kHz (Batteau, 1967; Middlebrooks and Green, 1991). BB noises can be localized in the vertical plane, because the brain can dissociate the elevation dependent pinna-induced spectral shape cues. Apparently, azimuth dependent changes in the spectral cues are used when the auditory system is deprived from binaural cues. Recently Otte et al. (2013) demonstrated that the pinna-induced spectral shape cues are changing during life because the ears keep growing, and that listeners adapt to this changing cues. A limitation of the present study is that we did not measure the spectral cues in terms of head-related transfer functions (HRTFs) or non-acoustic factors like the perceptual ability to discriminate spectral shapes (Andéol et al., 2013; Majdak et al., 2014) of the SSD listeners.

INCREASING NUMBER OF TREATMENT OPTIONS FOR SSD

Studies have shown that children with SSD demonstrate worse language scores compared to their normal-hearing peers, and that they are at risk for learning problems in school (Lieu, 2013). There is increasing evidence that adults with SSD experience problems in social settings because of their disability in binaural processing (Wie et al., 2010).

The criteria for treatment of SSD are expanding, and more treatment options become available. One treatment option is to provide a contralateral routing of sound (CROS) device. These devices transmit sounds presented at the deaf side to the hearing ear. Currently, the two most commonly applied CROS interventions are the wireless conventional CROS hearing aid, and the percutaneous bone-conduction hearing device (Bosman et al., 2003). Although listeners with SSD have only a single functioning cochlea, and therefore bone-conduction would not restore binaural hearing, the bone-conduction device is offered more often as an option for rehabilitation (Spitzer et al., 2002; Hol et al., 2004; Newman et al., 2008; Grantham et al., 2012; Nicolas et al., 2012; Battista et al., 2013).

In several countries cochlear implantation has become a treatment option (Arndt et al., 2011; Kamal et al., 2012; Arnoldner and Lin, 2013), and it is even proposed to implant children with congenital SSD already at a young age (Tzifa and Hanvey, 2013). Potentially, this option can lead to binaural hearing.

CONCLUSION

The present study emphasizes the importance of a precise evaluation of the monaural hearing abilities of listeners with SSD, especially at the higher frequencies for which the spectral-shape cues become unambiguous for sound localization. Some SSD listeners were using monaural pinna-induced spectral-shape cues of their hearing ear, for localization of BB noises in both azimuth and elevation. Because spectral cues are minimal for LP noises (Middlebrooks, 1992; Blauert, 1997) these stimuli could not be localized by SSD listeners. For clinicians it might be important to understand the factors affecting the localization performance of SSD listeners in order to give the hearing impaired the best advice in case of desired treatment.

ACKNOWLEDGMENTS

This research was funded by the William Demants og Hustru Ida Emilies Fond (Martijn J. H. Agterberg), the Radboud University Nijmegen (A. John Van Opstal), the Donders Institute for Brain, Cognition and Behaviour (Martijn J. H. Agterberg, Marc M. Van Wanrooij), and the Department of Otorhinolaryngology at the Radboud University Medical Centre Nijmegen (Ad F. M. Snik, Myrthe K. S. Hol). We thank Chris-Jan Beerendonk and Gunter Windau for their technical support.

REFERENCES

Agterberg, M. J., Snik, A. F., Hol, M. K., Van Wanrooij, M. M., and Van Opstal, A. J. (2012). Contribution of monaural and binaural cues to sound localization in patients with unilateral conductive hearing loss; improved directional hearing with a bone-conduction device. *Hear. Res.* 286, 9–18. doi: 10.1016/j.heares.2012.02.012

Andéol, G., Macpherson, E. A., and Sabin, A. T. (2013). Sound localization in noise and sensitivity to spectral shape. *Hear. Res.* 304, 20–27. doi: 10.1016/j.heares.2013.06.001

Arndt, S., Aschendorff, A., Laszig, R., Beck, R., Schild, C., Kroeger, S., et al. (2011). Comparison of pseudobinaural hearing to real binaural hearing rehabilitation after cochlear implantation in patients with unilateral deafness and tinnitus. *Otol. Neurotol.* 32, 39–47. doi: 10.1097/MAO.0b013e3181fcf271

Arnoldner, C., and Lin, V. Y. (2013). Expanded selection criteria in adult cochlear implantation. *Cochlear Implants Int.* 14(Suppl. 4), 10–13. doi: 10.1179/1467010013Z.000000000123

Batteau, D. W. (1967). The role of the pinna in human localization. *Proc. R. Soc. Lond. B Biol. Sci.* 168, 158–180. doi: 10.1098/rspb.1967.0058

Battista, R. A., Mullins, K., Wiet, R. M., Sabin, A., Kim, J., and Rauch, V. (2013). Sound localization in unilateral deafness with the Baha or TransEar device. *JAMA Otolaryngol. Head Neck Surg.* 139, 64–70. doi: 10.1001/jamaoto.2013.1101

Best, V., Carlile, S., Jin, C., and van Schaik, A. (2005). The role of high frequencies in speech localization. *J. Acoust. Soc. Am.* 118, 353–363. doi: 10.1121/1.1926107

Blauert, J. (1997). *Spatial Hearing. The Psychophysics of Human Sound Localization.* Cambridge, MA: MIT.

Bosman, A. J., Hol, M. K., Snik, A. F., Mylanus, E. A., and Cremers, C. W. (2003). Bone-anchored hearing aids in unilateral inner ear deafness. *Acta Otolaryngol.* 123, 258–260. doi: 10.1080/00016580310001105

Bremen, P., Van Wanrooij, M. M., and Van Opstal A. J. (2010). Pinna cues determine orienting response modes to synchronous sounds in elevation. *J. Neurosci.* 30, 194–204. doi: 10.1523/JNEUROSCI.2982-09.2010

Colburn, H. S. (1982). Binaural interaction and localization with various hearing impairments. *Scand. Audiol. Suppl.* 15, 27–45.

Frens, M. A., and Van Opstal, A. J. (1995). A quantitative study of auditory-evoked saccadic eye movements in two dimensions. *Exp. Brain Res.* 107, 103–117. doi: 10.1007/BF00228022

Grantham, D. W., Ashmead, D. H., Haynes, D. S., Hornsby, B. W., Labadie, R. F., and Ricketts, T. A. (2012). Horizontal plane localization in single-sided deaf adults fitted with a bone-anchored hearing aid (Baha). *Ear Hear.* 33, 595–603. doi: 10.1097/AUD.0b013e3182503e5e

Häusler, R., Colburn, S., and Marr, E. (1983). Sound localization in subjects with impaired hearing. Spatial-discrimination and interaural-discrimination tests. *Acta Otolaryngol. Suppl.* 400, 1–62. doi: 10.3109/00016488309105590

Hofman, P. M., and Van Opstal, A. J. (1998). Spectro-temporal factors in two-dimensional human sound localization. *J. Acoust. Soc. Am.* 103, 2634–2648. doi: 10.1121/1.422784

Hol, M. K., Bosman, A. J., Snik, A. F., Mylanus, E. A., and Cremers, C. W. (2004). Bone-anchored hearing aid in unilateral inner ear deafness: a study of 20 patients. *Audiol. Neurootol.* 9, 274–281. doi: 10.1159/000080227

Humes, L. E., Allen, S. K., and Bess, F. H. (1980). Horizontal sound localization skills of unilaterally hearing-impaired children. *Audiology* 19, 508–518. doi: 10.3109/00206098009070082

Irving, S., and Moore, D. R. (2011). Training sound localization in normal hearing listeners with and without a unilateral ear plug. *Hear. Res.* 280, 100–108. doi: 10.1016/j.heares.2011.04.020

Kamal, S. M., Robinson, A. D., and Diaz, R. C. (2012). Cochlear implantation in single-sided deafness for enhancement of sound localization and speech perception. *Curr. Opin. Otolaryngol. Head Neck Surg.* 20, 393–397. doi: 10.1097/MOO.0b013e328357a613

Keating, P., Dahmen, J. C., and King, A. J. (2013). Context-specific reweighting of auditory spatial cues following altered experience during development. *Curr. Biol.* 23, 1291–1299. doi: 10.1016/j.cub.2013.05.045

Kral, A., Hubka, P., Heid, S., and Tillein, J. (2013). Single-sided deafness leads to unilateral aural preference within an early sensitive period. *Brain* 136, 180–193. doi: 10.1093/brain/aws305

Kumpik, D. P., Kacelnik, O., and King, A. J. (2010). Adaptive reweighting of auditory localization cues in response to chronic unilateral earplugging in humans. *J. Neurosci.* 30, 4883–4894. doi: 10.1523/JNEUROSCI.5488-09.2010

Lieu, J. E. (2013). Unilateral hearing loss in children: speech-language and school performance. *B-ENT* 21, 107–115.

Majdak, P., Baumgartner, R., and Laback, B. (2014). Acoustic and non-acoustic factors in modeling listener-specific performance of sagittal-plane sound localization. *Front. Psychol.* 5:319. doi: 10.3389/fpsyg.2014.00319

Majdak, P., Goupell, M. J., and Laback, B. (2011). Two-dimensional localization of virtual sound sources in cochlear-implant listeners. *Ear Hear.* 32, 198–208. doi: 10.1097/AUD.0b013e3181f4dfe9

McPartland, J. L., Culling, J. F., and Moore, D. R. (1997). Changes in lateralization and loudness judgements during one week of unilateral ear plugging. *Hear. Res.* 113, 165–172. doi: 10.1016/S0378-5955(97)00142-1

Middlebrooks, J. C. (1992). Narrow-band sound localization related to external ear acoustics. *J. Acoust. Soc. Am.* 92, 2607–2624. doi: 10.1121/1.404400

Middlebrooks, J. C., and Green, D. M. (1991). Sound localization by human listeners. *Annu. Rev. Psychol.* 42, 135–159. doi: 10.1146/annurev.ps.42.020191.001031

Newman, C. W., Sandridge, S. A., and Wodzisz, L. M. (2008). Longitudinal benefit from and satisfaction with the Baha system for patients with acquired unilateral sensorineural hearing loss. *Otol. Neurotol.* 29, 1123–1131. doi: 10.1097/MAO.0b013e31817dad20

Nicolas, S., Mohamed, A., Yoann, P., Laurent, G., and Thierry, M. (2012). Long-term benefit and sound localization in patients with single-sided deafness rehabilitated with an osseointegrated bone-conduction device. *Otol. Neurotol.* 34, 111–114. doi: 10.1097/MAO.0b013e31827a2020

Oldfield, S. R., and Parker, S. P. (1984). Acuity of sound localisation: a topography of auditory space. II. Pinna cues absent. *Perception* 13, 601–617. doi: 10.1068/p130601

Otte, R. J., Agterberg, M. J., Van Wanrooij, M. M., Snik, A. F., and Van Opstal, A.J. (2013). Age-related hearing loss and ear morphology affect vertical but not horizontal sound-localization performance. *J. Assoc. Res. Otolaryngol.* 14, 261–273. doi: 10.1007/s10162-012-0367-7

Robinson, D. A. (1963). A method of measuring eye movements using a sclera search coil in a magnetic field. *IEEE Trans. Biomed. Eng.* 10, 137–145.

Rothpletz, A. M., Wightman, F. L., and Kistler, D. J. (2012). Informational masking and spatial hearing in listeners with and without unilateral hearing loss. *J. Speech Lang. Hear. Res.* 55, 511–531. doi: 10.1044/1092-4388(2011/10-0205)

Shub, D. E., Carr, S. P., Kong, Y., and Colburn, H. S. (2008). Discrimination and identification of azimuth using spectral shape. *J. Acoust. Soc. Am.* 124, 3132–3141. doi: 10.1121/1.2981634

Slattery, W. H. III., and Middlebrooks, J. C. (1994). Monaural sound localization: acute versus chronic unilateral impairment. *Hear. Res.* 75, 38–46. doi: 10.1016/0378-5955(94)90053-1

Spitzer, J. B., Ghossaini, S. N., and Wazen, J. J. (2002). Evolving applications in the use of bone-anchored hearing aids. *Am. J. Audiol.* 11, 96–103. doi: 10.1044/1059-0889(2002/011)

Tzifa, K., and Hanvey, K. (2013). Cochlear implantation in asymmetrical hearing loss for children: our experience. *Cochlear Implants Int.* 14(Suppl. 4), 56–61. doi: 10.1179/1467010013Z.000000000137

Van Wanrooij, M. M., and Van Opstal, A. J. (2004). Contribution of head shadow and pinna cues to chronic monaural sound localization. *J. Neurosci.* 24, 4163–4171. doi: 10.1523/JNEUROSCI.0048-04.2004

Van Wanrooij, M. M., and Van Opstal, A. J. (2007). Sound localization under perturbed binaural hearing. *J. Neurophys.* 97, 715–726. doi: 10.1152/jn.00260.2006

Van Wieringen, A., De Voecht, K., Bosman, A. J., and Wouters, J. (2011). Functional benefit of the bone-anchored hearing aid with different auditory profiles: objective and subjective measures. *Clin. Otolaryngol.* 36, 114–120. doi: 10.1111/j.1749-4486.2011.02302.x

Wazen, J. J., Ghossaini, S. N., Spitzer, J. B., and Kuller, M. (2005). Localization by unilateral BAHA users. *Otolaryngol. Head Neck Surg.* 132, 928–932. doi: 10.1016/j.otohns.2005.03.014

Wie, O. B., Pripp, A. H., and Tvete, O. (2010). Unilateral deafness in adults: effects on communication and social interaction. *Ann. Otol. Rhinol. Laryngol.* 119, 772–781.

Wightman, F. L., and Kistler, D. J. (1997). Monaural sound localization revisited. *J. Acoust. Soc. Am.* 101, 1050–1063. doi: 10.1121/1.418029

15

Cognitive processing load during listening is reduced more by decreasing voice similarity than by increasing spatial separation between target and masker speech

Adriana A. Zekveld[1,2,3], Mary Rudner[1,2], Sophia E. Kramer[3], Johannes Lyzenga[3] and Jerker Rönnberg[1,2]*

[1] Department of Behavioural Sciences and Learning, Linköping University, Linköping, Sweden
[2] Linnaeus Centre for Hearing and Deafness Research, The Swedish Institute for Disability Research, Linköping and Örebro Universities, Linköping, Sweden
[3] Section Audiology, Department of Otolaryngology-Head and Neck Surgery and EMGO Institute for Health and Care Research, VU University Medical Center, Amsterdam, Netherlands

***Correspondence:**
Adriana A. Zekveld, Section Audiology, Department of Otolaryngology-Head and Neck Surgery and EMGO Institute, VU University Medical Center, De Boelelaan 1118, PO Box 7057, 1081 HZ Amsterdam, Netherlands
e-mail: aa.zekveld@vumc.nl

We investigated changes in speech recognition and cognitive processing load due to the masking release attributable to decreasing similarity between target and masker speech. This was achieved by using masker voices with either the same (female) gender as the target speech or different gender (male) and/or by spatially separating the target and masker speech using HRTFs. We assessed the relation between the signal-to-noise ratio required for 50% sentence intelligibility, the pupil response and cognitive abilities. We hypothesized that the pupil response, a measure of cognitive processing load, would be larger for co-located maskers and for same-gender compared to different-gender maskers. We further expected that better cognitive abilities would be associated with better speech perception and larger pupil responses as the allocation of larger capacity may result in more intense mental processing. In line with previous studies, the performance benefit from different-gender compared to same-gender maskers was larger for co-located masker signals. The performance benefit of spatially-separated maskers was larger for same-gender maskers. The pupil response was larger for same-gender than for different-gender maskers, but was not reduced by spatial separation. We observed associations between better perception performance and better working memory, better information updating, and better executive abilities when applying no corrections for multiple comparisons. The pupil response was not associated with cognitive abilities. Thus, although both gender and location differences between target and masker facilitate speech perception, only gender differences lower cognitive processing load. Presenting a more dissimilar masker may facilitate target-masker separation at a later (cognitive) processing stage than increasing the spatial separation between the target and masker. The pupil response provides information about speech perception that complements intelligibility data.

Keywords: speech perception, pupil response, spatial cues, voice cues, interfering speech, cognitive abilities

INTRODUCTION

When speech perception is challenged by interfering speech signals, listening depends on both auditory factors and cognitive abilities like working memory capacity (Rönnberg, 2003; Rönnberg et al., 2013). The accumulating evidence for the role of cognitive abilities in speech perception (for reviews, see Akeroyd, 2008 and Besser et al., 2013 and see also Rönnberg, 2003; Kramer et al., 2009; Rönnberg et al., 2013) has resulted in an increase in research focused on the measurement of cognitive processing load during listening (Rabbitt, 1968; Rakerd et al., 1996; Gosselin and Gagné, 2011; Mackersie and Cones, 2011; Picou et al., 2011; Wild et al., 2012; Mishra et al., 2013a). In the present study, we applied pupillometry to assess cognitive processing load. The pupil size increases with increasing cognitive processing load induced by increasing task demands (e.g., Beatty, 1982; Engelhardt et al., 2010), including intelligibility level (Zekveld et al., 2010), sentence complexity (Piquado et al., 2010), visual context (Engelhardt et al., 2010), lexical competition (Kuchinsky et al., 2013) and masker type (Koelewijn et al., 2012a). Larger working memory capacity and better linguistic closure ability are associated with larger pupil dilation amplitude and a longer peak latency of the pupil response (Zekveld et al., 2011; Koelewijn et al., 2012b; Zekveld and Kramer, 2014), indicating that the allocation of larger amounts of cognitive capacity may come with more intensive mental processing in more difficult listening conditions (Ahern and Beatty, 1979; Van der Meer et al., 2010; Grady, 2012; Koelewijn et al., 2012b; Ng et al., 2013). Importantly, the cognitive processing load evoked by speech perception can be dissociated from the actual speech perception performance, as cognitive processing load can vary in conditions in which speech perception performance is similar (Mackersie and Cones, 2011; Koelewijn et al., 2012a).

The perception of speech in interfering sounds can be aided by different types of acoustic cues. For example, when female speech maskers are used for female target speech, talker-specific voice cues (e.g., voice-related pitch cues) distinguishing target and masker are less salient than when male speech maskers are used for female target speech. Less salient speech segregation cues generally result in reduced ability to perceive the target speech (Brungart et al., 2001). Additionally, if the target speech and interfering sounds come from different spatial locations, the speech reception thresholds (SRTs; the signal-to-noise ratio [SNR] required for a certain level of speech perception performance) of listeners with normal hearing can improve by as much as 18 dB SNR, depending on the amount of spatial separation between the sounds (Arbogast et al., 2002, 2005; Cameron et al., 2011). This benefit is referred to as spatial release from masking. The spatial release from masking is larger when the acoustic characteristics of the masker are more similar to those of the target speech (Arbogast et al., 2005; Best et al., 2012). The aim of the present study was to investigate the influence of target-masker similarity (i.e., differences in gender and spatial origin between the target and masker voices, and the interaction between these signal characteristics) on cognitive processing load indexed by the pupil response. We also studied the relation between individual differences in cognitive abilities, speech perception performance and the pupil response in different conditions.

Despite the fact that the relevance of cognitive abilities in speech perception has increasingly been acknowledged in the past decades (for a review, see Arlinger et al., 2009), only a few studies have assessed the role of cognitive abilities in spatially complex listening conditions. These studies (e.g., Neher et al., 2009, 2012; Glyde et al., 2013) suggest that better cognitive abilities are associated with better speech perception performances. The relation tended to be stronger when verbal measures of working memory are applied as compared to a more general cognitive screening instrument (Cognistat; Mueller et al., 2001) that measured eight cognitive functions (including attention, memory and language) with the aim of identifying cognitive deficits (Neher et al., 2009, 2012; Glyde et al., 2013). Also, the association was stronger when the origin of the maskers differed from that of the target speech as compared to co-located speech and maskers (Neher et al., 2009). Neher et al. (2009) argued that for the co-located target and masker condition presented in their study, listeners could basically only rely on level cues to segregate target and maskers. Consequently, performance was limited by the accessibility of auditory cues rather than top-down abilities. They also suggested that the relatively large amount of "*mental effort*" required to parse the target speech at the negative SNRs applied in the conditions with spatially separated target and masker speech could have driven the cognitive involvement in that condition. Similarly, Best et al. (2012) suggested that cognitive abilities play a larger role in speech perception when SNRs are negative. Gatehouse et al. (2003) also argued that it is important to take into account possible interactions between signal characteristics and cognitive abilities. These previous studies indicate that individual differences in cognitive abilities interact with the characteristics of the target and masker. It would be interesting to examine whether objective measures of *cognitive processing load* also reflect variations in target-masker similarity. For example, if spatial separation between the target and masker signals reduced cognitive processing load even when intelligibility levels were equalized, this would demonstrate an additional benefit of spatial cues that is not reflected by intelligibility data.

To our knowledge, no previous study has investigated the effect of voice characteristics and location differences between target and masker speech on the pupil response during listening. In the present study, we measured the pupil dilation response to listening to female speech masked by speech from either female or male speakers. Listeners rely on any differences in the characteristics of the voices (e.g., voice saliency or distinctiveness) to distinguish the target and masker voices, including level differences and a priori knowledge of the target voice characteristics (Brungart, 2001; Brungart et al., 2001). The method applied in the present study is similar to that of the LISN-S test (Cameron and Dillon, 2007). LISN-S measures the benefits due to voice and spatial cues, separately and combined. In the present study, we aimed to assess the influence of voice cues (female vs. male maskers) and spatial cues on speech perception performance and the pupil response. In a two- by two design giving four conditions, the similarity of the target voice and interfering speech maskers was varied, as well as the spatial separation between the masker and the target speech. We used HRTFs to manipulate the virtual spatial location of two streams of masker speech: these were perceived either from the same location as the target speech (0° azimuth) or from + and −90° (±90: one stream from the left of the listeners, and one from the right).

Furthermore, we assessed a range of cognitive functions known to be associated with speech perception performance when the listening takes place under adverse conditions (Kramer et al., 2009; Koelewijn et al., 2012a; Besser et al., 2013; Ellis and Munro, 2013) and the pupil response during listening to speech in background maskers (see Koelewijn et al., 2012b; Zekveld and Kramer, 2014). These were: working memory capacity (the reading span test [RSpan, Daneman and Carpenter, 1980; Rönnberg et al., 1989, 2013]) and the size comparison test [SicSpan, Sörqvist et al., 2010], information updating (the letter memory test; Morris and Jones, 1990), the ability to perceive degraded linguistic information [text reception threshold test (TRT, Zekveld et al., 2007)] and executive control abilities [the trail making test (Reitan, 1958)].

We expected, in line with the results of Neher et al. (2009) and Glyde et al. (2013), that better cognitive abilities would be associated with better speech perception. Also consistent with their findings, we expected this association to be strongest when cues distinguishing target from masker were maximized, that is when different-gender masker voices originated from a location different from that of the target. In these conditions, cognitive abilities can be used to benefit from the available cues. We expected that the pupil response would be larger with fewer voice and spatial cues available, as in these conditions, it is harder to segregate target speech from noise.

GENERAL METHODS

The test session started with pure-tone audiometry and near vision screening. Then, the reading span test (verbal working memory capacity) was presented. Participants performed a practice speech perception test, followed by the first speech perception block. In the speech perception tests, we employed a two-factor within-subjects factorial design, crossing two masker voices (male or female) with two spatial configurations (masker speech from 0° or ±90°). Then, participants performed the SicSpan test (verbal working memory capacity and inhibition), followed by a break, a second practice test and the second speech perception block. Subsequently, participants performed a practice TRT test and three additional TRT tests (linguistic closure). The test session was finished after performing the letter memory (information updating) and trail making (executive control ability) tests. The duration of the test session was 1.5 h with a 5-min-break halfway through the test session. The rationale for presenting two different tests of verbal working memory was that previous studies have shown that each of those tests can be differentially associated with speech perception performance and/or the pupil response evoked by different conditions (Koelewijn et al., 2012b; Sörqvist and Rönnberg, 2012; Besser et al., 2013).

PARTICIPANTS

Twenty-four young adults [20 women, 4 men; mean age 22 yrs, standard deviation (SD) = 2.8 yrs] with normal hearing thresholds participated. Flyers and advertisements were used to recruit students and employees of VU University and VU University Medical Centre. All participants were native Dutch speakers and had normal or corrected-to-normal vision as screened with a near vision test (Bailey and Lovie, 1980). Pure-tone hearing thresholds of the participants were measured to ensure that the thresholds of both ears were ≤20 dB HL at the octave frequencies between 125 and 8000 Hz. All participants had normal hearing thresholds; the mean pure-tone hearing thresholds were on average 7.2 dB HL (SD = 7.4 dB). The exclusion criteria were the following: dyslexia or other reading problems, or a history of a neurological or psychiatric disease. The project was approved by the Ethics Committee of the VU University Medical Center. All participants provided written informed consent.

STIMULI

The target and masker stimuli were selected from the meaningful, semantically neutral sentence material developed by Versfeld et al. (2000) and recorded with a sampling rate of 44100 Hz and a bit depth of 16 bits. Each sentence contained eight to nine syllables and no word contained more than three syllables. The individual words in the sentences were articulated at an average rate of 3.4 words per second across all sentences. An example sentence (translated into English) is: "the shop is within walking distance" (Versfeld et al., 2000). The target sentences were pronounced by a female speaker, and were always perceived from the front (0° azimuth) of the listener. The masker consisted of two independent streams of concatenated sentences that were played continuously, back-to-back, without silent gaps between the sentences. The onsets of target and masker sentences were not coordinated in time; the masker speech streams could start in the middle of a sentence. The two streams of masker speech were always from the same talker who was either male or female. The mean and range of the duration of the target sentences did not differ from that of the female and male masker sentences. On average, the mean sentence duration was 1.9 s, ranging from 1.3 to 3.0 s. The onset of the target sentence occurred 3000 ms after masker onset and target sentence offset was 4000 ms before masker offset. This allowed the measurement of the pupil response to masked speech while preventing the onset and offset of the masker stimulus from influencing the pupil dilation response between target-speech onset and the response of the listeners.The overall intensity of the target-masker mixture was fixed at 70 dB SPL; the SNR was varied by adapting both the level of the target speech and the level of the maskers.

Virtual target/masker separation (+90 and −90° azimuth; one stream from the left and the other from the right) and co-location (0° azimuth) were achieved using HRTFs that were developed using the KEMAR mannequin with the large pinnae (Algazi et al., 2001). We used the left-ear HRTFs in our tests, and used the mirror image of the left ear HRTFs for the right ear. Using HRTFs to manipulate the perceived location of sounds alters their frequency spectrum, therefore the spectrum of the masker speech will differ for presentation from 0 and ±90° azimuth. Such spectral differences may affect speech reception scores as indicated by the Speech-Intelligibility Index SII (ANSI, 1997). To prevent this, the long-term average frequency spectrums of the male and female masker speech in the 0-degree configuration were shaped using finite impulse response filtering to match those of the corresponding, combined, maskers from the +90 and −90° directions, in order to prevent any spectral differences between the masking stimuli from confounding the effects of spatial configuration on speech reception scores and pupil responses. The novel signals had a slightly different timbre and were evaluated by listening to them; no artifacts or changes in perceived location were observed. Prior to data collection, a pilot test was performed in which we asked five subjects to indicate the direction of the sound sources and evaluate the quality of the signals. The results indicated that the manipulation served its purposes and no further changes were required.

SET-UP

Test administration took place in a sound-attenuated room. The audiogram was made using an audiometer (Decos Systems B.V., software version 2010.2.6) connected to TDH 39 headphones. Auditory stimuli in the experimental tests were presented by an external soundcard (Creative Sound Blaster Audigy) through Sony MDR V900 headphones (Sony Corporation). Subjects were seated behind a SMI iView X RED remote eye-tracking system with spatial resolution of 0.03° and sampling frequency of 60 Hz. A PC screen was positioned on top of the pupillometric system, about 45 cm away from the subject's head. Subjects focused on a fixation dot presented in the middle of the screen.

PROCEDURE

In four conditions (2 masker voices × 2 spatial configurations), the SNR required for 50% correct sentence perception was estimated using an adaptive procedure. This entailed changing the

SNR for each sentence, based on the response to the previous sentence. The SNR of a sentence dropped by −2 dB following a single correct response, and increased by 2 dB following a single incorrect response. The SNR of the first sentence was −4 dB for the 0 degree condition and −10 dB for the ±90° condition. Subjects were asked to repeat the sentences aloud. They were instructed to wait until after masker offset (4 s after target speech offset) to make their response. The experimenter scored their answers. A sentence was scored correct if all words of the sentence were repeated in the correct order. In each condition, a list of 25 sentences was presented, as this allows a reliable estimation of the pupil response. The 25 sentences were randomly selected from 2 phonemically-balanced lists of 13 sentences created by Versfeld et al. (2000). The adaptive procedure resulted in a sentence intelligibility level of approximately 50% correct in each of the conditions. However, the SRTs (i.e., the average SNR of sentences 5–25) differed between the conditions. The rationale for this approach was that intelligibility differences have a large effect on the pupil response (Zekveld et al., 2010). Therefore, intelligibility should be controlled for when assessing the influence of other factors, such as masker characteristics. SNR differences itself are unlikely to have a major influence on the pupil response. For example, Koelewijn et al. (2012a) showed that stationary and fluctuating noise maskers evoked similar pupil dilation responses despite relatively large differences in SRT when sentence intelligibility was the same for the two maskers.

SRT testing was blocked by masker voice. Within blocks, the order of sentences from each of the two conditions (two spatial configurations) was pseudo-randomized with the restrictions that no more than two sentences from the same condition should be presented sequentially and that the difference in the cumulative number of sentences per condition should not exceed two at any point in the test block. This ensured that the procedures ran approximately in parallel, preventing any confounding order effects on performance or the pupil response. The order of masker voice blocks was counterbalanced across participants. The allocation of sentence lists to conditions was also counterbalanced across participants.

PUPILLOMETRY

The location and size of the pupil of the left eye were measured during each target-masker presentation (trial). Before the experiment started, the pupil size was measured in maximum illumination (100 lx) and in complete darkness. The room illumination was adapted individually such that the pupil size was around the middle of its dynamic range at the start of the experiment. This prevents ceiling and floor effects in the pupil response and makes the response independent of the baseline pupil size (Beatty and Lucero-Wagoner, 2000). The mean room illumination after individual adjustments across participants was 51 lux ($SD = 24$ lux).

The baseline pupil size in each trial was defined as the average pupil size during the first 1.0 s of the presentation of the masker, (between 3 s and 2 s prior to target-speech onset). The mean pupil diameter in each trial was calculated by averaging the pupil size between target speech onset and masker offset for the shortest sentence in the set (i.e., 5.3 s after target speech onset). Pupil diameters below 3 standard deviations of the mean diameter of each trial were coded as a blink. If the data contained more than 15% blinks between the start of the baseline and masker offset, the trial was excluded from data analysis. The pupil data were furthermore visually inspected for artifacts due to eye-movements. The pupil data for the first trial in each block were omitted from the analysis, as the adaptive SRT procedure commenced during this sentence. On average, the pupil data of 21 trials were included in each condition. Eye-blinks were replaced by linear interpolation starting 4 samples before and ending 8 samples after a blink. A 5-point moving average smoothing filter was passed over the selected and deblinked pupil data. Per trial, we determined the *peak pupil dilation* (peak dilation amplitude in mm) relative to the baseline pupil size in the same trial. Finally, the peak pupil dilation was averaged over trials, separately for each participant and condition.

TESTS ASSESSING COGNITIVE ABILITIES

Text reception threshold test

The TRT test measures the ability to perceive masked linguistic (text) information, also called "linguistic closure" ability (Besser et al., 2013). A total of 13 printed sentences (Versfeld et al., 2000) masked by a bar pattern were presented on a PC screen (see Zekveld et al., 2007). The sentences were different from those presented in SRT tests. The field background color was white, text color was red, and the color of the mask was black. At the start of each trial, the masker appeared with the text "behind" it in a word-by-word fashion. Display-onset of each word in the sentence was equal to the timing of the start of the utterance of each word in the corresponding audio file (Versfeld et al., 2000). The average duration of the audio utterance of the words was 281 ms, ranging from 44 to 854 ms. All words remained on the screen for 3500 ms after completion of the sentence. Participants were asked to read the sentences out loud. The experimenter scored whether the sentences were read entirely correctly. The masking percentage of the first sentence was 58% unmasked text. A 1-up-1-down adaptive procedure with a step-size of 6% was applied, targeting the percentage of unmasked text required to read 50% of the sentences correctly. The TRT was the average proportion of unmasked text for sentences 5–14; lower TRTs indicate better performance. The fourteenth sentence was not actually presented. However, the percentage of unmasked text for this sentence followed directly from the response to the previous sentence. We included this value in the calculation of the TRT to obtain a better estimate of the threshold (Plomp and Mimpen, 1979). Participants performed one practice and three regular TRT tests, and we used the TRT averaged over the three tests in the analysis.

Reading span test

The RSpan test (Daneman and Carpenter, 1980) measures verbal working memory capacity. In this test, 5-word Dutch sentences were presented visually. The materials were developed (Besser et al., 2013) to be equivalent to the Swedish version described by Rönnberg et al. (1989) and Andersson et al. (2001), in turn based on an English version (Baddeley et al., 1985). Half of the sentences are semantically incoherent (e.g., "The table sings a song.") and half are coherent (e.g., "The friend told a story"). First, three sets of three sentences were presented, followed by three sets of four sentences, three sets of five sentences, and three sets of six sentences. After each sentence, participants verbally indicated whether the sentence made sense or not. After each set of sentences, participants were asked to orally recall all first or all last nouns of the sentences in the set in serial order. The experimenter recorded the total number of words correctly recalled regardless of order. The maximum total score is 54.

Size comparison span

The size-comparison span (SicSpan) task (Sörqvist et al., 2010) measures verbal working memory capacity and also examines the ability to suppress irrelevant information. Sets of size-comparison questions like "is a BUSH larger than a TREE?" were presented on a PC screen. Then, a semantically related and to-be-remembered word like FLOWER was presented. Ten sets were presented in total; the set sizes ranged from 2 to 6 with each set size being presented twice. Within sets, nouns used in the questions and those to be remembered were from the same semantic category, but between sets these categories differed. Immediately after each question, participants responded to the question by pressing one of two buttons corresponding to "yes" or "no." After each set participants were asked to orally recall the to-be-remembered items. The SicSpan score was the total number of correctly recalled items regardless of order (maximum of 40), with higher scores reflecting better performance.

Letter memory test

To assess information updating, the visual letter memory task (Morris and Jones, 1990) was applied. A series of 5, 7, 9, or11 letters (consonants) was presented visually at the center of the screen for 2 s each using a DMDX platform (Forster and Forster, 2003). Each sequence length was presented three times, and the order of the sequence lengths presented was randomized. Two lists consisting of 7 and 9 letters each were presented as practice tests. Twelve lists were used in total. The participants were told that the presentation would end unexpectedly. They were asked to recall, in any order, the last four items presented. The total number of correctly recalled letters was scored (maximum score = 48).

Trail making

The trail making test (Reitan, 1958) consists of two parts. Part A is sensitive to visuo-perceptual abilities, and part B reflects working memory and task-switching ability. The difference in reaction times between the two parts (B–A) represents executive control abilities (Sánchez-Cubillo et al., 2009). In part A, a sheet of paper with 25 encircled numbers (1–25) was presented to the participant. In part B, a sheet of paper with 12 numbers (1–12) and 12 letters (A–L) was presented. For part A, participants had to draw lines sequentially connecting the numbers and for part B, they had to draw lines alternating between numbers and letters (e.g., 1, A, 2, B, 3, C, etc.). The amount of time required to complete each part was measured. We assume that control abilities are relevant for speech perception in the current study, because listeners need to focus on and follow the target speech while ignoring speech from two masker voices. Therefore, we used the B-A difference measure in the correlation analysis. This measure will be referred to as Trail-dif.

STATISTICAL ANALYSES

We assessed the influence of masker voice (male, female) and spatial configuration (0°, ±90°) on the SRTs in the adaptive conditions using repeated-measures analyses of variance (ANOVA). Repeated measures ANOVA with the same factors was also performed on the peak pupil dilation. Finally, we performed a correlation analysis to assess the strength of the associations between the TRT, RSpan, SicSpan, letter memory and Trail-dif performances on the one hand and the SRTs and peak pupil dilation amplitudes during the SRT tests on the other hand. We did not make adjustments for multiple comparisons in this correlation analysis.

RESULTS

DESCRIPTIVE STATISTICS: COGNITIVE TESTS

The descriptive statistics of the performances on the cognitive tests are presented in **Table 1**. The range in scores on the cognitive tests was comparable to that observed in other studies with similar subject groups (e.g., Zekveld et al., 2007; Besser et al., 2012, 2013; Mishra et al., 2013b; Zekveld and Kramer, 2014).

SPEECH PERCEPTION TEST RESULTS

The behavioral speech perception performance data are shown in **Figure 1**. The Figure shows that the estimated SNR required for 50% sentence perception thresholds is higher (worse) for the co-located (0 degree) as compared to the spatially separated (±90°) conditions. It also shows that the threshold is higher for the same-gender (female) as compared to the different-gender (male) masker in the 0° conditions, but that the threshold is higher for the different-gender as compared to the same-gender masker in the ±90° condition.

The repeated-measures ANOVA on the SRTs with independent variables masker voice (male, female), and spatial configuration (0°, ±90°) revealed a main effect of masker voice, such that estimated thresholds were lower (better) for the different-gender compared to the same-gender masker [$F_{(1, 23)} = 23.7$, $p < 0.001$]. The ANOVA also showed a main effect of spatial configuration, with lower thresholds in the spatially separated than in the co-located conditions [$F_{(1, 23)} = 573.0$, $p < 0.001$]. An interaction effect between masker voice and perceived spatial location was observed as well [$F_{(1, 23)} = 194.2$, $p < 0.001$]. *Post-hoc* paired *t*-tests indicated that for both the male and the female

Table 1 | Mean, standard deviation, and range of the performances on the cognitive tests.

	Mean	*SD*	Range (maximum score)
Reading span	21.7	5.4	12–34 (54)
Size comparison span	29.8	6.7	13–38 (40)
Text reception threshold	53.6%	2.9%	47.8–59.8%
Letter memory	41.6	3.8	35–47 (48)
Trail A	18.1 s	5.3 s	11.5–30.8 s
Trail B	37.3 s	16.9 s	20.3–83.9 s
Trail-dif	19.2 s	14.7 s	5.3–57.7 s

The maximum score on each test is indicated between parentheses.

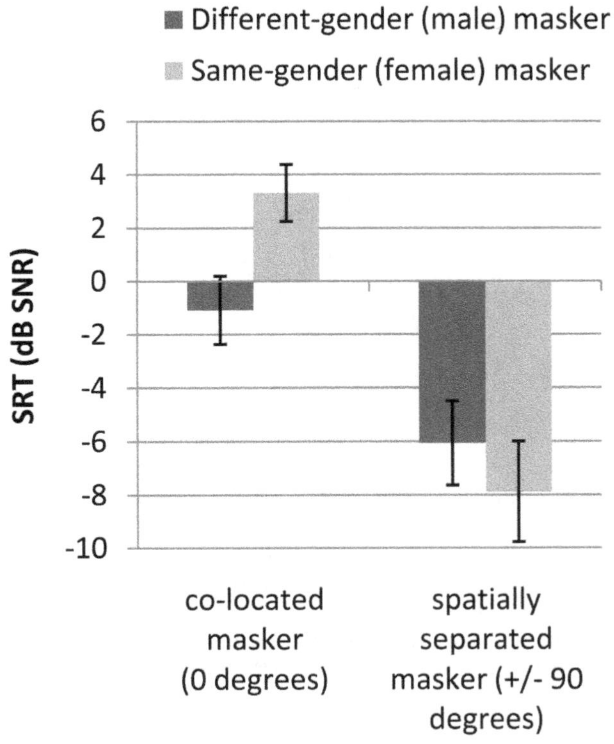

FIGURE 1 | Average speech reception thresholds (SRT) in dB signal-to-noise ratio (SNR). Error bars reflect standard deviations. Twenty-four participants were tested.

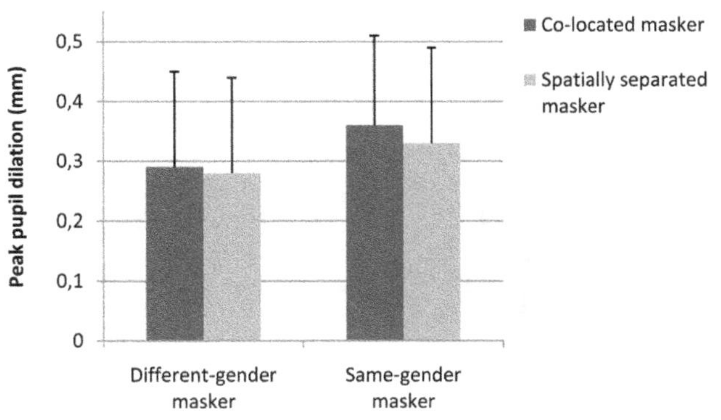

FIGURE 2 | Peak dilation amplitude of the pupil response during speech perception. Error bars reflect standard deviations. The pupil dilation is calculated relative to the baseline pupil size in the interval between 3 s and 2 s prior to the onset of the target speech. The peak dilation amplitude was the maximum pupil size in the nterval between target speech onset and masker offset for the shortest sentence in the set (i.e., 5.3 s after target speech onset). Twenty-four part cipants were tested.

maskers, the differences in SRTs between the 0 and ±90° configuration were statistically significant [$t_{(23)} = 13.9$, Bonferroni corrected $p < 0.00001$ and $t_{(23)} = 25.0$, Bonferroni corrected $p < 0.00001$, respectively]. For both the 0° and ±90° conditions, the difference in SRTs between the male and female maskers was statistically significant [$t_{(23)} = 14.9$, Bonferroni corrected $p < 0.00001$ and $t_{(23)} = 4.7$, Bonferroni corrected $p = 0.0004$, respectively]. The interaction effect indicates that the effect of different-gender maskers, as compared to same-gender maskers, is larger for co-located target speech and maskers and that the effect of spatial separation is larger for same-gender maskers.

RESULTS PUPILLOMETRY

Figures 2, 3 show the pupil response, in average peak amplitude and the time course of it, respectively. **Table 2** shows the baseline pupil size and peak pupil dilation in each of the four conditions. As shown in **Figures 2, 3**, the pupil dilation response was largest for the condition with same-gender masker and no spatial separation, followed by the condition with same-gender masker and spatial separation, and we observed smaller pupil responses for the conditions with different-gender maskers.

An ANOVA on the peak dilation amplitude (**Figures 2, 3**, **Table 2**) with independent variables masker voice and spatial configuration showed a main effect of masker voice [$F_{(1,\,23)} = 5.40$, $p = 0.029$], with larger pupil responses for the same-gender (female) masker than for the different-gender (male) masker. The effect of spatial configuration and the interaction effect between spatial configuration and masker voice were not statistically significant.

CORRELATION ANALYSIS

Table 3 shows the results of the Spearman correlation analysis between RSpan, SicSpan, letter memory, TRT, and Trail-diff performances on the one hand, and the SRTs and pupil responses on the other hand.

Higher SicSpan performance was associated with better (lower) SRTs in the condition with different-gender maskers and spatial separation. Better information updating ability (letter memory) was associated with lower (better) SRTs in the condition with same-gender maskers and no spatial separation. Finally, a larger Trail-dif score indicating poorer inhibition was associated with a higher (worse) SRT when different-gender maskers were presented with spatial separation. Note that none of the correlation coefficients are statistically significant when controlling for multiple comparisons (Bonferroni correction). Therefore, these correlation coefficients should be interpreted with caution. There were no statistically significant correlations between pupil response and cognitive variables.

The correlation analyses tentatively suggest that larger working memory capacity (SicSpan) and better control abilities (Trail-dif) are related to better speech perception when the masker voice is relatively dissimilar to the target voice (gender difference) and when spatial cues are available. In contrast, better information updating ability (letter memory) is associated with better speech perception when the masker voice is more similar to the target voice (same gender) and in the absence of spatial cues. Note that the results of the correlation analyses should be interpreted with caution due to the relatively small sample size.

DISCUSSION

In line with previous research (e.g., Brungart, 2001; Brungart et al., 2001; Neher et al., 2009, 2012), the current study showed that both spatial and voice cues help listeners to segregate target

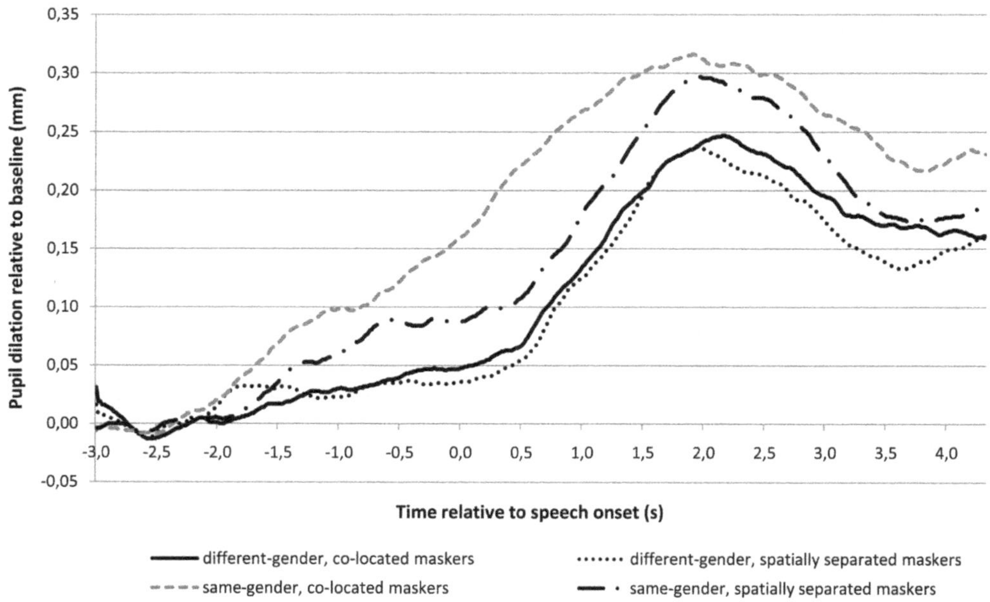

FIGURE 3 | Pupil response in the four speech reception threshold conditions as function of time relative to the onset of the target speech (time 0 s). The pupil dilation is calculated relative to the baseline pupil size in the interval between 3 s and 2 s prior to the onset of the target speech. Twenty-four participants were tested.

Table 2 | Mean peak dilation amplitude (mm) and baseline pupil size (mm) in each of the 4 conditions.

Procedure	Different-gender (male) masker		Same-gender (female) masker	
	Co-located masker	Spatially separated masker	Co-located masker	Spatially separated masker
Baseline (mm)	6.15 (0.65)	6.17 (0.63)	6.21 (0.68)	6.16 (0.70)
Peak dilation (mm)	0.29 (0.16)	0.28 (0.16)	0.36 (0.15)	0.33 (0.16)

Standard deviations are presented between parentheses.

Table 3 | Spearman correlation coefficients between text reception threshold (TRT), reading span, size comparison span (SicSpan), letter memory, trail making difference (Trail-diff), speech reception thresholds (SRTs), and the peak pupil dilation amplitude.

	SRTs				Peak dilation amplitude			
	M_0	M_{90}	F_0	F_{90}	M_0	M_{90}	F_0	F_{90}
TRT	0.10	0.34	0.38	−0.05	−0.21	−0.03	0.06	0.19
Reading span	−0.34	0.06	0.03	−0.25	0.16	0.23	0.32	0.21
SicSpan	−0.07	$r = -0.47$ $p = 0.021$	−0.21	−0.28	0.37	0.16	−0.18	0.13
Letter memory	−0.04	−0.25	$r = -0.53$ $p = 0.010$	−0.15	0.25	0.29	−0.10	−0.04
Trail−diff	0.07	$r = 0.64$ $p = 0.001$	0.31	0.22	−0.27	−0.10	−0.08	−0.08

Exact p-values are only provided for statistically significant ($p < 0.05$) correlation coefficients. Note that none of the correlation coefficients are statistically significant when controlling for multiple comparisons. M, male (different-gender) maskers; F, female (same-gender) maskers; 0, co-located maskers at 0°; 90, spatially separated maskers at ±90°.

speech from distracter speech. The effect of spatial configuration was larger when target speech was masked with same-gender as compared to different-gender speech. Also, the effect of masker voice (same-gender vs. different-gender) was larger for co-located target and masker speech than for spatially separated target and masker speech. This pattern of results is in line with those observed for the LISN-S test (Cameron et al., 2011). Surprisingly, speech recognition performance was better for the same-gender as compared to the different-gender masker when masker speech was spatially separated. However, pupil responses were larger, indicating greater cognitive load for the same-gender as compared to the different gender maskers. This finding of better performance accompanied by greater cognitive load may be explained by the stronger temporal fluctuations of the female masker speech as compared to the male masker speech [1]. These stronger fluctuations allow more listening into the masker dips which may improve SRTs. These temporal fluctuations come into play when target and masker are spatially separated but are smeared out for the 0° condition where the two masking voice streams are co-located.

The pupil response data were only partly in line with the behavioral data. The peak pupil amplitude was larger when the masker and target voices were more similar (same-gender as compared to different-gender voices). No effect of spatial configuration on the pupil response was observed, indicating that although the availability of the spatial cues enhanced performance (i.e., lowered the SRTs), this benefit did not affect cognitive processing load during listening. A masker voice less similar to the target voice improved the SRTs and reduced the cognitive processing load as reflected by the pupil response, whereas adding spatial separation between the target and masker only resulted in an improvement in SRTs. The present data are in line with the results of Koelewijn et al. (2012a). In that study, target speech masked by interfering speech resulted in larger pupil responses than target speech masked by fluctuating noise. The average peak dilation amplitude observed in that study for female speech masked with a single male speech stream (0.32 mm for young listeners with normal hearing) was similar to that observed in the current study for the female 2-talker speech masker. In general, this suggests that the pupil response is larger when the masker characteristics are more similar to the characteristics of the target speech, whereas the physical spatial characteristics of the target and masker do not influence the pupil response. Although speech perception can be improved either by decreasing the target-masker similarity or by increasing the spatial separation of the target and masker, the concomitant cognitive load is reduced more by the reduction of target-masker similarity. One possible interpretation is that spatial separation eases speech understanding at a more peripheral level of processing, perhaps subcortical, whereas voice cues have to be dealt with at the cortical level by using top-down processing.

The current results are in line with previous data showing that factors that do have a large effect on the SRT (e.g., presenting stationary vs. fluctuating noise maskers) do not necessarily influence the pupil response during listening. In general, this study shows that the measurement of the pupil response adds information about the effects of masker characteristics on the speech recognition process that is not evident from inspection of the behavioral results alone. The results are relevant for future studies focusing on the influence of talker and masker location on speech perception performance and cognitive processing load in clinical populations (e.g., listeners with hearing impairment) and studies using other measures of cognitive processing load (e.g., see Gosselin and Gagné, 2011; Mackersie and Cones, 2011; Picou et al., 2011; Mishra et al., 2013a).

The SRT procedure converged on an SNR that corresponded to 50% sentence intelligibility; SNRs differed between the conditions. SNR differences are not likely to explain the condition effects on the pupil response as the SNR was highest in the condition with the largest pupil response. In listeners with normal hearing, higher SNRs result in smaller pupil responses if intelligibility is not controlled for (Zekveld et al., 2010). Together with the present data, previous pupillometric studies suggest that other stimulus characteristics, such as the similarity between masker and target stimulus, have a larger effect on the pupil dilation response than SNR has when intelligibility is kept constant (e.g., Koelewijn et al., 2012a).

It is important to note that the current results only included a very limited selection of conditions in terms of points on the psychometric function (around 50% intelligibility) and characteristics of the maskers and spatial configuration. The results may differ when other conditions (e.g., other spatial configurations, other and/or a different number of masker voices) are applied. However, the current results provide an example of how measures of cognitive processing load can complement behavioral measures in speech perception research.

Importantly, the differences in pupil response between conditions may have been attenuated by our selection of the baseline interval. The presentation of the masker 3 s prior to target speech onset revealed the difficulty level of the upcoming trial, as it indicated both the identity and the spatial origin of the masker speech. We applied a baseline correction on the pupil dilation response based on the average pupil size between 3 and 2 s prior to target speech onset (i.e., the first second of the presentation of the masker signal). In speech perception research, the baseline pupil size is usually determined in the 1 s prior to target speech onset (Zekveld et al., 2010; Kuchinsky et al., 2013). We used the pupil size in the first second of the masking stimulus instead as any influence of the knowledge of the masker type likely increased during the progression of interval with masker speech only. Listeners may anticipate the difficulty level of the upcoming sentence which is revealed by the identity and location of the masker. However, the information regarding the identity and spatial location of the masker was apparent right from the onset of the masker so this knowledge may still have affected the baseline pupil size, and hence the baseline-corrected peak pupil dilation amplitude. This is suggested by the higher baseline pupil size in the condition with same-gender maskers from the front as compared to the baseline pupil size in any of the other conditions (see **Table 2**).

Individual cognitive abilities were related to speech perception performance (SRTs) when no corrections for multiple comparisons were applied. Better SicSpan performance and better trail-making ability were associated with relatively low SRTs in the condition with different-gender maskers that were spatially separated from the target speech. In line with our hypotheses and Neher et al. (2009) and Glyde et al. (2013), this tentatively indicates that when it is relatively easy to distinguish the masker and target speech signals, larger working memory performance and better executive control were associated with better speech

[1] To obtain an impression of the speech modulation strengths, we analyzed 10 concatenated sentences of equal RMS for both the male and the female speaker by calculating the, 30-Hz low-pass filtered, Hilbert transforms of both signals. Next, we estimated spectral levels for the modulations of both speakers by calculating the average spectrum of the low-pass filtered Hilbert transforms. We found that the average spectrum of the female modulations was parallel to and 1.3 dB higher than that of the male speaker.

perception performance. In these conditions, individual differences in working memory capacity and executive function may come into play.

Better letter memory performance (information updating ability) was related to better SRTs in the condition with same-gender maskers with no spatial separation. We suggest that the cognitive load revealed by the pupil response may be related to demands on the ability to keep working memory updated with relevant information when few voice cues are available to segregate target speech from masker. As stated in the Results section, the results of the present correlation analysis should be interpreted with caution and require follow-up confirmatory research.

We have previously shown that better TRTs and SicSpan performances tend to be associated with larger pupil responses in the SRT test (Zekveld et al., 2011; Koelewijn et al., 2012b). In contrast, in the present study, none of the cognitive tests was related to the peak dilation amplitude of the pupil response. This difference between the current and past studies may be related to the characteristics of the participants. In Zekveld et al. (2011) and Koelewijn et al. (2012b), some of the participants were middle-aged. In other recent studies in which only young normal hearing listeners were included, the relation between cognitive abilities and the pupil response was only present when speech perception performance was very low (Zekveld and Kramer, 2014). Interestingly, in the present study, the pupil response was not related to cognitive abilities even in the conditions in which the performance (SRT) was related to one of the cognitive tests. This may suggest that even when good cognitive abilities improve speech recognition performance, they do not reduce the pupil response (cognitive processing load). This in turn may suggest that applying cognitive abilities to speech processing to achieve good speech recognition is no less effortful than achieving mediocre speech recognition without the assistance of good cognitive capacity. In general, the influence of inter-individual differences may affect the relation between task characteristics and the pupil response. Future studies should pull apart external and internal factors influencing the pupil response, for example by introducing individual differences as between-groups manipulation. It would also be interesting to apply other measures that may be related to cognitive processing load in such future studies. For example, Picou et al. (2011) showed an association between better performances on a complex working memory test and larger benefit from the availability of visual information (a recording of the face of the speaker) in word recognition (paired associates recall task) in noise. The authors interpret these data as reflecting that larger cognitive resource capacity allows listeners to use visual information for reducing cognitive processing load (cf. Mishra et al., 2013b).

In conclusion, differences between target and masker speech in terms of voice characteristics and spatial origin substantially enhance speech perception when speech is masked by interfering 2-talker babble. However, the same is not true of the pupil response. Performance is better and the pupil response is smaller when target and masker voices are of different gender than when they are of the same gender. On the other hand, although performance is better when target and masker are spatially separated, there is no significant difference in pupil response. This indicates that even when performance is improved by spatial separation cognitive processing load is not reduced. This demonstrates that measures reflecting cognitive processing load can add information about the speech perception process not provided by speech perception performance measures. This has implications for the design of future studies focusing on cognitive processing load during listening. The current findings indicate that the mechanisms that allow listeners to use voice characteristics and spatial information to segregate speech and masking speech are complex and affect the cognitive processing load required during listening.

ACKNOWLEDGMENTS

We thank Hans van Beek for his assistance in the development of the test and analysis software. Thanks to Harleen van Rai for her assistance in the data collection. This work was financed from a grant of the Swedish Research Council.

REFERENCES

Ahern, S., and Beatty, J. (1979). Pupillary responses during information processing vary with scholastic aptitude test scores. *Science* 205, 1289–1292. doi: 10.1126/science.472746

Akeroyd, M. A. (2008). Are individual differences in speech reception threshold related to individual differences in cognitive ability? a survey of twenty experimental studies with normal and hearing-impaired adults. *Int. J. Audiol.* 47(Suppl. 2), S53–S71. doi: 10.1080/14992020802301142

Algazi, V. R., Duda, R. O., Thompson, D. M., and Avendano, C. (2001). "*The CIPIC HRTF Database*," in *Proceedings 2001 IEEE Workshop on Applications of Signal Processing to Audio and Electroacoustics* (New Paltz, NY: Mohonk Mountain House), 99–102.

Andersson, U., Lyxell, B., Rönnberg, J., and Spens, K.-E. (2001). Cognitive correlates of visual speech understanding in hearing-impaired individuals. *J. Deaf Stud. Deaf Educ.* 6, 103–116. doi: 10.1093/deafed/6.2.103

ANSI (1997). *ANSI S3.5-1997 American national standard methods for calculation of the speech intelligibility index.* New York, NY: American National Standards Institute.

Arbogast, T. L., Mason, C. R., and Kidd, G. Jr. (2002). The effect of spatial separation on informational and energetic masking of speech. *J. Acoust. Soc. Am.* 112, 2086–2098. doi: 10.1121/1.1510141

Arbogast, T. L., Mason, C. R., and Kidd, G. Jr. (2005). The effect of spatial separation on informational masking of speech in normal-hearing and hearing-impaired listeners. *J. Acoust.Soc. Am.* 117, 2169–2180. doi: 10.1121/1.1861598

Arlinger, S., Lunner, T., Lyxell, B., and Pichora-Fuller, M. K. (2009). The emergence of cognitive hearing science. *Scan. J. Psychol.* 50, 371–384. doi: 10.1111/j.1467-9450.2009.00753.x

Baddeley, A., Logie, R., Nimmo-Smith, I., and Brereton, N. (1985). Components of fluent reading. *J. Mem. Lang.* 24, 119–131. doi: 10.1016/0749-596X(85)90019-1

Bailey, I. L., and Lovie, J. E. (1980). The design and use of a near-vision chart. *Am. J. Optom. Physiol. Opt.* 57, 378–387. doi: 10.1097/00006324-198006000-00011

Beatty, J. (1982). Task-evoked pupillary responses, processing load, and the structure of processing resources. *Psychol. Bull.* 91, 276–292. doi: 10.1037/0033-2909.91.2.276

Beatty, J., and Lucero-Wagoner, B. (2000). "The pupillary system," in *Handbook of Psychophysiology, 2nd Edn.*, eds J. T. Cacioppo, L. G. Tassinary, and G. G. Berntson (New York, NY: Cambridge University Press), 142–162.

Besser, J., Koelewijn, T., Zekveld, A. A., Kramer, S. E., and Festen, J. M. (2013). How linguistic closure and verbal working memory relate to speech recognition in noise – a review. *Trends Amplif.* 17, 75–93. doi: 10.1177/1084713813495459

Besser, J., Zekveld, A. A., Kramer, S. E., Rönnberg, J., and Festen, J. M. (2012). New measures of masked text recognition in relation to speech-in-noise perception and their associations with age and cognitive abilities. *J. Speech Lang. Hear. Res.* 55, 194–209. doi: 10.1044/1092-4388(2011/11-0008)

Best, V., Marrone, N., Mason, C. R., and Kidd, G. Jr. (2012). The influence of non-spatial factors on measures of spatial release from masking. *J. Acoust. Soc. Am.* 131, 3103–3110. doi: 10.1121/1.3693656

Brungart, D. S. (2001). Informational and energetic masking effects in the perception of two simultaneous talkers. *J. Acoust. Soc. Am.* 109, 1101–1109. doi: 10.1121/1.1345696

Brungart, D. S., Simpson, B. D., Ericson, M. A., and Scott, K. T. (2001). Informational and energetic masking effects in the perception of multiple simultaneous talkers. *J. Acoust. Soc. Am.* 110, 2527–2538. doi: 10.1121/1.1408946

Cameron, S., and Dillon, H. (2007). Development of the listening in spatialized noise-sentences test (LISN-S). *Ear Hear.* 28, 196–211. doi: 10.1097/AUD.0b013e318031267f

Cameron, S., Glyde, H., and Dillon, H. (2011). Listening in spatialized noise – sentences test (LiSN-S): Normative and retest reliability data for adolescents and adults up to 60 years of age. *J. Am. Acad. Audiol.* 22, 697–709. doi: 10.3766/jaaa.22.10.7

Daneman, M., and Carpenter, P. A. (1980). Individual-differences in working memory and reading. *J. Verb.Learn. Verb Behav.* 19, 450–466. doi: 10.1016/S0022-5371(80)90312-6

Ellis, R. J. and Munro, K. J. (2013). Does cognitive function predict frequency compressed speech recognition in listeners with normal hearing and cognition? *Int. J. Audiol.* 52, 14–22. doi: 10.3109/14992027.2012.721013

Engelhardt, P. E., Ferreira, F., and Patsenko, E. G. (2010). Pupillometry reveals processing load during spoken language comprehension. *Q. J. Exp. Psychol.* 63, 639–645. doi: 10.1080/17470210903469864

Forster, K. I. and Forster, J. C. (2003). DMDX: a windows display program with millisecond accuracy. *Behav. Res. Methods Instrum. Comput.* 35, 116–124. doi: 10.3758/BF03195503

Gatehouse, S., Naylor, G., and Elberling, C. (2003). Benefits from hearing aids in relation to the interaction between the user and the environment. *Int. J. Audiol.* 42, S77–S85. doi: 10.3109/14992020309074627

Glyde, H., Cameron, S., Dillon, H., Hickson, L., and Seeto, M. (2013). The effects of hearing impairment and aging on spatial processing. *Ear Hear.* 34, 15–28. doi: 10.1097/AUD.0b013e3182617f94

Gosselin, P. A. and Gagné, J.-P. (2011). Older adults expend more effort than young adults recognizing speech in noise. *J. Speech Lang. Hear. Res.* 54, 944–958 doi: 10.1044/1092-4388(2010/10-0069)

Grady, C. (2012). The cognitive neuroscience of ageing. *Nat. Rev. Neurosci.*13, 491–505. doi: 10.1038/nrn3256

Koelewijn, T., Zekveld, A. A., Festen, J. M., and Kramer, S. E. (2012a). Pupil dilation uncovers extra listening effort in the presence of a single-talker masker. *Ear Hear.* 33, 291–300. doi: 10.1097/AUD.0b013e3182310019

Koelewijn, T., Zekveld, A. A., Festen, J. M., Rönnberg, J., and Kramer, S. E. (2012b). Processing load induced by informational masking is related to linguistic abilities. *Int. J. Otolaryngol.* 2012:865731. doi: 10.1155/2012/865731

Kramer, S. E., Zekveld, A. A., and Houtgast, T. (2009). Measuring cognitive factors in speech comprehension: the value of using the text reception threshold test as a visual equivalent of the SRT test. *Scand. J. Psychol.*50, 507–515. doi: 10.1111/j.1467-9450.2009.00747.x

Kuchinsky, S. E., Ahlstrom, J. B., Vaden, K. I. Jr., Cutre, S. L., Humes, L. E., Dubno, J. R., et al. (2013). Pupil size varies with word listening and response selection difficulty in older adults with hearing loss. *Psychophysiology* 50, 23–34. doi: 10.1111/j.1469-8986.2012.01477.x

Mackersie, C. L. and Cones, H. (2011). Subjective and psychophysiological indices of listening effort in a competing-talker task. *J. Am. Acad. Audiol.* 22, 113–122. doi: 10.3766/jaaa.22.2.6

Mishra, S., Lunner, T., Stenfelt, S., Rönnberg, J. and Rudner, M. (2013a). Seeing the talker's face supports executive processing of speech in steady state noise. *Front. Syst. Neurosci.* 7:96. doi: 10.3389/fnsys.2013.00096

Mishra, S., Lunner, T., Stenfelt, S., Rönnberg, J., and Rudner, M. (2013b). Visual information can hinder working memory processing of speech. *J. Speech Lang. Hear. Res.* 56, 1120–1132. doi: 10.1044/1092-4388(2012/12-0033)

Morris, N., and Jones, D. M. (1990). Memory updating in working memory: the role of the central executive. *Brit. J. Psychol.* 81, 111–121. doi: 10.1111/j.2044-8295.1990.tb02349.x

Mueller, J., Kiernan, R., and Langston, J. W. (2001). *Cognistat: The Neurobehavioral Cognitive Status Examination.* Fairfax, VA: The Northern Californian Neurobehavioral Group.

Neher, T., Behrens, T., Carlile, S., Jin, C., Kragelund, L., Specht Petersen, A., et al. (2009). Benefit from spatial separation of multiple talkers in bilateral hearing-aid users: Effects of hearing loss, age, and cognition. *Int. J. Audiol.* 48, 758–774. doi: 10.3109/14992020903079332

Neher, T., Lunner, T., Hopkins, K., and Moore, B. C. J. (2012). Binaural temporal fine structure sensitivity, cognitive function, and spatial recognition of hearing-impaired listeners (L). *J. Acoust. Soc. Am.* 131, 2561–2564. doi: 10.1121/1.3689850

Ng, E. H. N., Rudner, M., Lunner, T., and Rönnberg, J. (2013). Relationships between self-report and cognitive measures of hearing aid outcome. *Speech Lang. Hear.* 16, 197–207. doi: 10.1179/205057113X13782848890774

Picou, E., Ricketts, T. A., and Hornsby, B. W. Y. (2011). Visual cues and listening effort: individual variability. *J. Speech Lang. Hear. Res.* 54, 1416–1430. doi: 10.1044/1092-4388(2011/10-0154)

Piquado, T., Isaacowitz, D., and Wingfield, A. (2010). Pupillometry as a measure of cognitive effort in younger and older adults. *Psychophysiology* 47, 560–569. doi: 10.1111/j.1469-8986.2009.00947.x

Plomp, R., and Mimpen, A. M. (1979). Improving the reliability of testing the speech reception threshold for sentences. *Audiology* 18, 43–52. doi: 10.3109/00206097909072618

Rabbitt, P. M. A. (1968). Channel capacity, intelligibility and immediate memory. *Q. J. Exp. Psychol.* 20, 241–248. doi: 10.1080/14640746808400158

Rakerd, B., Seitz, P., and Whearty, M. (1996). Assessing the cognitive demands of speech listening for people with hearing loss. *Ear Hear.* 17, 97–106. doi: 10.1097/00003446-199604000-00002

Reitan, R. M. (1958). Validity of the trail making test as an indicator of organic brain damage. *Percept. Mot. Skills* 8, 271–276. doi: 10.2466/pms.1958.8.3.271

Rönnberg, J. (2003). Cognition in the hearing impaired and deaf as a bridge between signal and dialogue: a framework and a model. *Int. J. Audiol.* 42, S68–S76. doi: 10.3109/14992020309074626

Rönnberg, J., Arlinger, S., Lyxell, B., and Kinnefors, C. (1989). Visual evoked potentials: relation to adult speechreading and cognitive function. *J. Speech Hear. Res.* 32, 725–735.

Rönnberg, J., Lunner, T., Zekveld, A. A., Sörqvist, P., Danielsson, H., Lyxell, B., et al. (2013). The Ease of Language Understanding (ELU) model: theoretical, empirical, and clinical advances. *Front. Syst. Neurosci.*7:31. doi: 10.3389/fnsys.2013.00031

Sáñchez-Cubillo, I., Periáñez, J. A., Androver-Roig, D., Rodríguez-Sánchez, J. M., Ríos-Lago, M., Tirapu, J., et al. (2009). Construct validity of the trail making test: role of task-switching, working memory, inhibition/interference control, and visuomotor abilities. *J. Int. Neurospych. Soc.* 15, 438–450. doi: 10.1017/S1355617709090626

Sörqvist, P., Ljungberg, J. K., and Ljung, R. (2010). A sub-process view of working memory capacity: evidence from effects of speech on prose memory. *Memory* 18, 310–326. doi: 10.1080/09658211003601530

Sörqvist, P., and Rönnberg, J. (2012). Episodic long-term memory of spoken discourse masked by speech: What is the role for working memory capacity? *J. Speech Lang. Hear. Res.* 55, 210–218. doi: 10.1044/1092-4388(2011/10-0353)

Van der Meer, E., Beyer, R., Horn, J., Foth, M., Bornemann, B., ries, J., et al. (2010). Resource allocation and fluid intelligence: Insights from pupillometry. *Psychophysiology* 47, 158–169. doi: 10.1111/j.1469-8986.2009.00884.x

Versfeld, N. J., Daalder, L., Festen, J. M., and Houtgast, T. (2000). Method for the selection of sentence materials for efficient measurement of the speech reception threshold. *J. Acoust. Soc. Am.* 107, 1671–1684. doi: 10.1121/1.428451

Wild, C. J., Yusuf, A., Wilson, D. E., Peelle, J. E., Davis, M. H., and Johnsrude, I. S. (2012). Effortful listening: The processing of degraded speech depends critically on attention. *J. Neurosci.* 32, 14010–14021. doi: 10.1523/JNEUROSCI.1528-12.2012

Zekveld, A. A., George, E. L. J., Kramer, S. E., Goverts, S. T., and Houtgast, T. (2007). The development of the text reception threshold test: a visual analogue of the speech reception threshold test. *J. Speech Lang. Hear. Res.* 50, 576–584. doi: 10.1044/1092-4388(2007/040)

Zekveld, A. A. and Kramer, S. E. (2014). Cognitive processing load across a wide range of listening conditions: Insights from pupillometry. *Psychophysiology* 51, 277–284. doi: 10.1111/psyp.12151

Zekveld, A. A., Kramer, S. E., and Festen, J. M. (2010). Pupil response as an indication of effortful listening: The influence of sentence intelligibility. *Ear Hear.* 31, 480–490. doi: 10.1097/AUD.0b013e3181d4f251

Zekveld, A. A., Kramer, S. E., and Festen, J. M. (2011). Cognitive load during speech perception in noise: The influence of age, hearing loss, and cognition on the pupil response. *Ear Hear.* 32, 498–510. doi: 10.1097/AUD.0b013e31820512bb

16

The plastic ear and perceptual relearning in auditory spatial perception

Simon Carlile *

School of Medical Sciences and Bosch Institute, University of Sydney, Sydney, NSW, Australia

Correspondence:
Simon Carlile, School of Medical Sciences and Bosch Institute, University of Sydney, F13, Anderson Stuart Building, Sydney, NSW 2006, Australia
e-mail: simonc@physiol.usyd.edu.au

The auditory system of adult listeners has been shown to accommodate to altered spectral cues to sound location which presumably provides the basis for recalibration to changes in the shape of the ear over a life time. Here we review the role of auditory and non-auditory inputs to the perception of sound location and consider a range of recent experiments looking at the role of non-auditory inputs in the process of accommodation to these altered spectral cues. A number of studies have used small ear molds to modify the spectral cues that result in significant degradation in localization performance. Following chronic exposure (10–60 days) performance recovers to some extent and recent work has demonstrated that this occurs for both audio-visual and audio-only regions of space. This begs the questions as to the teacher signal for this remarkable functional plasticity in the adult nervous system. Following a brief review of influence of the motor state in auditory localization, we consider the potential role of auditory-motor learning in the perceptual recalibration of the spectral cues. Several recent studies have considered how multi-modal and sensory-motor feedback might influence accommodation to altered spectral cues produced by ear molds or through virtual auditory space stimulation using non-individualized spectral cues. The work with ear molds demonstrates that a relatively short period of training involving audio-motor feedback (5–10 days) significantly improved both the rate and extent of accommodation to altered spectral cues. This has significant implications not only for the mechanisms by which this complex sensory information is encoded to provide spatial cues but also for adaptive training to altered auditory inputs. The review concludes by considering the implications for rehabilitative training with hearing aids and cochlear prosthesis.

Keywords: auditory spatial perception, spectral cues, auditory accommodation, auditory-motor integration, adult functional plasticity

INTRODUCTION

The developing central nervous system, at first exuberant in its connectivity, is tamed and shaped by the experiences of youth to produce the fully formed and functional mature brain. This functionally plastic period of development allows the incredibly detailed connectivity of the brain to respond to the environment in which it finds itself rather than be bound and restricted by the limits of a single genetic program.

There was a time when it was believed that once organized, this developmental fluidity in the central nervous system, or "critical period," was shut down and the mature brain was to some extent fixed in form and function. The textbook studies included those looking at the development of the visual system and the impact of optical anomalies on the subsequent development of visual cortex. To avoid the negative impact of astigmatism on subsequent visual acuity, major visual screening programs in early school age children were instituted across the Western World resulting in many small children in the school playgrounds sporting thick framed glasses.

Over the last few decades much evidence has accumulated that demonstrates that the central nervous system is far more plastic in the mature state than previously believed. Of course this makes a lot of sense when considering the environments in which mature animals live. While the body never has to again go through the explosive changes associated with its initial development, there are many changes associated with maturity and aging that still need to be accounted for to maintain a veridical perception of the environment. Moreover, some activities can have a significant impact on the structure and function of the nervous system—for instance, there is a growing body of evidence on the effects of a lifelong practice of music on some pretty basic auditory perceptual processes (for review see Strait and Kraus, 2014). Rehabilitative medicine is, to a great extent, also predicated on the functional plasticity of the mature brain.

In the context of this short review we will look at a much smaller question: how the auditory system adapts to the changes in the shape of the outer ear that occurs over a lifetime. While a small example of plasticity in the mature auditory system, one hope in pursuing this line of research is that a deeper understanding of these model systems can uncover principles that can be applied more generally. This review will conclude with some discussion of the implications of this process for training and rehabilitation, particularly in the context of hearing impairment.

SPECTRAL CUES OF THE OUTER EAR

The shapes of the outer ear vary from person to person and it has long been argued that the precise morphology is sufficiently individualized to provide a strong form of biometric identification (see Mamta and Hanmandlu, 2013). The complexly convoluted shape of the outer ear results in a complex pattern of sound resonances and diffractions that filter the sound. Relatively small variations in the morphological characteristics of the outer ear can lead to perceptually significant differences in the spectrum of the pressure entering the ear canal (see **Figure 1**). So it's not just the shape of the ears that are individualized but also the spectral filtering of the sound provided to the brain. Another important acoustical property of the outer ear is that coupling of the various acoustic mechanisms with the sound field is dependent on the angle of incidence of the wave front (review Shaw, 1974). Of course this also means that the spectral filtering not only changes as a function of the relative location of the sound source but also in a manner that uniquely reflects the individual geometry of the ear.

The head-related transfer functions (HRTFs) shown in **Figure 1** have been band passed from 500 Hz to 16 kHz and represent the output of the microphones placed at the opening of the ear canal for sound sources located directly in front of the listener (mid sagittal plane or midline). The precise frequencies of the sharp dips or notches reflects the complex interactions of different acoustic modes at wavelengths that are of similar size or smaller than the different morphological features of the outer ear itself. It is the differences in the distribution and interaction of these modes produced by subtle differences in the dimensions of the cavities and folds that results in the inter-individual differences of the transfer functions (see for instance Shaw and Teranishi, 1968). These subtleties are encoded in the auditory nerve despite the filtering by the cochlea (Carlile and Pralong, 1994) and are perceptually significant: For instance, it has been known for some time that listening through other peoples ears (i.e., using non-individualized spectral cues) often results in a significant degradation in sound localization performance (Wenzel et al., 1993).

In addition to the spectral cues to sound location, the auditory system utilizes the information from both ears—the binaural cues to location (see Carlile, 1996 for a review). The separation of the ears by the head means that, for sound locations off the midline, there is a difference in the time of arrival of the sound to each ear—the interaural time difference (ITD) cue to azimuth or horizontal location. Likewise, the reflection and refraction of the sound by the head gives rise to an interaural level difference (ILD), also dependent on the horizontal location of the source. The head acts as a particularly effective obstacle for sound waves when the wavelengths are smaller than the head, so ILD cues are generally thought to operate at the middle to high frequencies of human hearing. Conversely, the auditory system is most sensitive to the phase of low frequency sounds and ITD cues are particularly important for low frequencies. This observation was

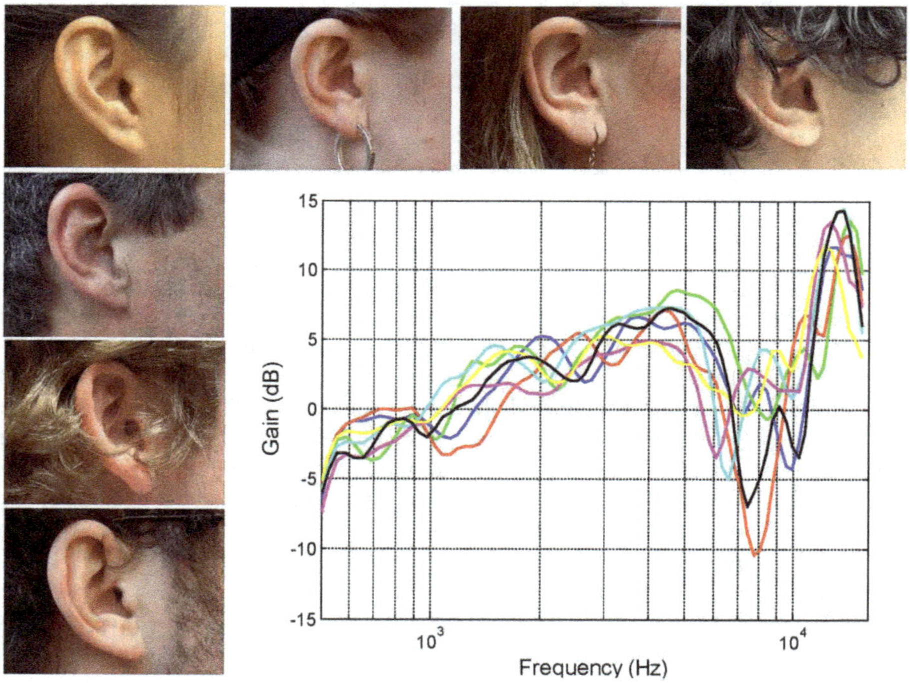

FIGURE 1 | The right ears of seven subjects together with their associated head-related transfer functions (HRTFs) recorded using a small microphone placed at the opening of the auditory canal (see Pralong and Carlile, 1994; Hammershoi and Moller, 2002). Note that the variations between the transfer functions remain small (<2 dB) up to around 5 kHz however, at higher frequencies, the frequencies of the prominent spectral notches and peaks results in a substantial inter-individual differences.

first made by Rayleigh (1907) and has come to be known as the duplex theory (see also Mills, 1958, 1972). These binaural cues to location, however, are ambiguous because of the symmetry of the placement of the ears on the head and can only be used to specify the sagittal plane containing the source. It is the location-dependent changes in the monaural filter functions that provide the cue to the location of the source on this so-called "cone of confusion" (Carlile et al., 2005; but see also Shinn-Cunningham et al., 2000).

The pattern of changes in the spectral cues around a single cone of confusion is illustrated in **Figure 2**. Plotted as a contour plot, several salient features (peaks and notches) can be seen in the HRTF for any one location but, more importantly, as the location of the source is varied from the front to the back of the listener, the frequency of these features change systematically over a range of an octave or more. For instance, when a sound source is located at the front there is a broad peak at around 4 kHz followed by a sharp notch at 8 kHz and a sharp peak at 12 kHz. When the source is located on the audio-visual (A-V) horizon but in the back, the peak is around 8 kHz and flanked by notches at 6 and 12 kHz.

While there is plenty of anecdotal evidence that the shape of the ears generally changes with age (just look at the collection of ears next time you are on public transport), the differences between ages have recently been quantified (Otte et al., 2013). Two morphological measures (ear size and conchal height) were found to be significantly different across three age cohorts: 6–11, 20–35, and >63 years. Importantly, this study also recorded the HRTFs from ears in each of the age groups. These HRTFs had substantial differences which were far larger than those seen in an age matched cohort such as those shown in **Figure 1**.

Some studies have look directly at the consequences of aging on sound localization performance. Reduced audibility resulting from age-related hearing loss can clearly produce a significant deterioration in performance (e.g., Noble et al., 1997). When audibility is controlled for, modest declines in performance for horizontal plane localization have been reported (e.g., Abel et al., 2000; Babkoff et al., 2002; Savel, 2009) evident principally in the front-back confusion rates (10–15%; Abel et al., 2000). In two recent studies (Dobreva et al., 2011, 2012), age-related decreases in precision (increased variance of the responses) are reported for both horizontal and vertical dimensions in the frontal hemisphere. Accounting for potential hearing loss and using different band-pass stimuli, the general consensus is that these declines represented changes in central processing of ITD and spectral cues. This is consistent with an age-related decrease in ITD sensitivity using click trains presented over headphones (Babkoff et al., 2002). Not all studies, however, have found age-related effects for horizontal localization in the frontal hemisphere (Savel, 2009; Otte et al., 2013).

In the context of the present review, while these studies generally suggest modest changes to localization performance with age, these are much less than might be expected based on the extent of the age-related change in the spectral cues produced by the changing shape of the ears (Otte et al., 2013). This suggests that the auditory system is capable of recalibrating to the progressive changes in spectral cues that occur over one's lifetime that would otherwise degrade localization performance.

ADAPTIVE CHANGE IN THE ADULT AUDITORY SYSTEM

Developmental plasticity is a fundamental feature of the brain. Precise neuronal interconnections and patterns of activity are sculpted by early experience to produce an incredibly complex computational system, which is tuned to its specific environment. Of interest here, though, is the level and range of plasticity in the adult auditory system.

There has been a significant amount of work looking at the plasticity of frequency tuning in the adult. Here, we are more focussed on adaptation to changing spatial cues but several general and very useful observations should be made (for an excellent and detailed review of overall auditory plasticity see Keuroghlian and Knudsen, 2007). First, the extent of plasticity seen in the adult state is not as large as that seen in the developing animal during the so-called "critical period" of development. Second, to effectively drive long-term plastic change, the stimulus generally has to have behavioral relevance such as being paired with positive or negative reinforcement or with some form of deep

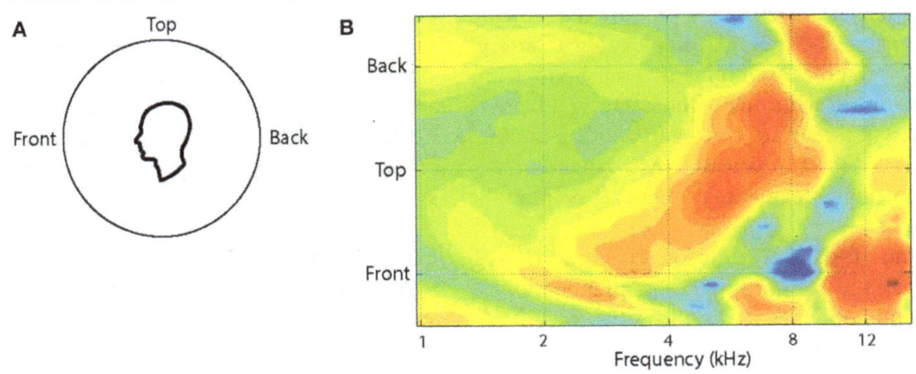

FIGURE 2 | The variation in the HRTF is shown as a function of location along a cone of confusion on the midline for the left ear of one subject (A). The HRTFs have been recorded at roughly 10° intervals and interpolated to provide the surface plot **(B)**. Recordings were not done for locations greater than 45° below the audio-visual horizon. The colors of the contours indicate the amplitude of the function at each frequency, location conjunction and extend from 12 dB (dark red) to −15 dB (dark blue).

brain micro-stimulation (presumably triggering such reinforcement mechanisms). Third, most of these studies have focussed on auditory cortex and generally found that cortical tuning can be adjusted independently for a range of parameters including frequency, level, and temporal selectivity. Fourth, previous training induced changes can be preferentially selected depending on the behavioral context of the task at hand (see also in particular Fritz et al., 2003, 2005; Keating et al., 2013).

Relatively fewer, but no less important studies, have examined the plasticity induced by changes to the auditory spatial localization cues (review Wright and Zhang, 2006). The simplest method of varying the binaural cues has been to insert an ear plug in one ear (Bauer et al., 1966; Florentine, 1976; Musicant and Butler, 1980; Butler, 1987; Slattery and Middlebrooks, 1994; McPartland et al., 1997; Kumpik et al., 2010). This approach produces relatively straight-forward changes in the sound level in the plugged ear although the effects on ITD are more complex and dependent on the conditions of the plugging (e.g., Hartley and Moore, 2003; Lupo et al., 2011).

Before proceeding with a more detailed discussion of these results, an important methodological issue needs to be considered. When studying the binaural cues to sound location, the stimulus of choice is often restricted in frequency range—low frequencies for ITD studies and middle to high frequencies for ILD studies. This reflects the different frequency ranges that these cues are thought to operate over (the so called duplex theory of localization processing discussed above). On the other hand, the greater bulk of the research examining auditory localization has used broadband noise as the stimulus. This is motivated principally by the fact that such stimuli contain the full range of acoustic localization cues and in particular, the spectral cues are necessarily dependent on a broad frequency range. An important distinction therefore is that stimuli with a relatively restricted frequency range are designed to probe the contributions of a single cue while a broad spectrum stimulus will provide the full range of acoustic cues to a sounds location.

Returning to the ear plugging experiments, when sound localization performance was measured immediately after inserting the ear plug, performance was significantly reduced and then recovered to a certain extent over a period of days [Bauer et al., 1966 (2–3 days); Kumpik et al., 2010 (~7 days)]. No recovery was found for shorter 24-h periods of plugging (Slattery and Middlebrooks, 1994). Studies examining ILD sensitivity with one ear plug are more mixed with one demonstrating adaptive change in ILD sensitivity (Florentine, 1976) and another finding only modest changes in a subset of listeners (McPartland et al., 1997) and another reporting no evidence of binaural adaptation (Kumpik et al., 2010).

Other studies have modified the binaural ITD cue using a hearing aid in one ear (Javer and Schwarz, 1995), a "pseudophone" (an arrangement of 2 microphones feeding into two ear pieces that could be manipulated independently of the head orientation: Held, 1955) or headphones presenting stimuli in virtual auditory space (sounds filtered with HRTFs but with changes in the normal ITDs: Shinn-Cunningham et al., 1998). Using localization performance as the metric these studies all report initial biases in localization consistent with the binaural change and subsequent reduction in bias following several (3–5) days (Javer and Schwarz, 1995), several (~7) hours of exposure (Held, 1955) or even repeated, relatively short (2 h) training sessions repeated over 2–6 weeks (Shinn-Cunningham et al., 1998), although adaptation was never complete.

Importantly, the work of Kumpik et al. (2010) mentioned above was one of the few studies that demonstrated adaptive change in auditory localization following ear plugging but intriguingly, found no changes in binaural sensitivity in parallel with those changes. Rather, these authors attribute the adaptive change to a relative reweighting of the binaural and monaural spectral cues to location (see also Kacelnik et al., 2006; Van Wanrooij and Van Opstal, 2007). The range of difference in the results of the previous studies could then be explained by reweighting of the different cues available in each study or other practice effects (Musicant and Butler, 1980; Butler, 1987).

This turns our focus to the monaural cues, which in ecological terms, are the more likely cues to be modified by the progressive changes in pinna shape over a lifetime. Around the turn of the twentieth century, Hofman et al. (1998) demonstrated that the adult auditory system was able to accommodate to substantial changes in the filter functions of the outer ears. Elevation localization was significantly disrupted when the HRTFs of human listeners were modified by inserting small molds in the concha (**Figure 3**). For the four listeners who wore the molds continuously, elevation localization improved significantly over periods ranging from 19 to 39 days. Furthermore, once the molds were removed, localization performance was the same as their performance before wearing the molds. This indicated that accommodation to the "new" cues did not interfere with representation of the "old" cues. The changes in spectral cues induced by the molds were both substantial and abrupt and unlike the slow, progressive changes that would occur through life. Nonetheless, this was a critical study that demonstrated the adaptive capability of the adult auditory system to changes in the shape of the outer ear.

Although there were only four subjects in that study, two other interesting observations can be made. First, there were significant individual differences in the rate of accommodation—the shortest being 19 days and the longest twice as long at 39 days. Second, the localization performance of three subjects approached that of pre-mold baseline, while the fourth subject fell somewhat short. One inter-subject variable may have been different environmental opportunities to relearn their new filter functions over the accommodation period. In ferrets (Kacelnik et al., 2006) and humans (Kumpik et al., 2010), King and colleagues demonstrated that unilateral ear plugs disrupted the azimuthal sound localization as discussed above but that, over a period of seven or more days, performance improved with training. Although an ear plug principally disrupts the binaural cues it will also produce distortions to the spectral cues in one ear, however, the principal point of interest here is the effect of experience on the accommodation. The amount of training *per se* did not appear to be a principal driver as performance improvements were only evident when the training was spread over the 7 days rather than simply delivered as a single large block of training.

A second inter-subject variable in the Hofman et al., study could have been the magnitude of the changes to HRTFs

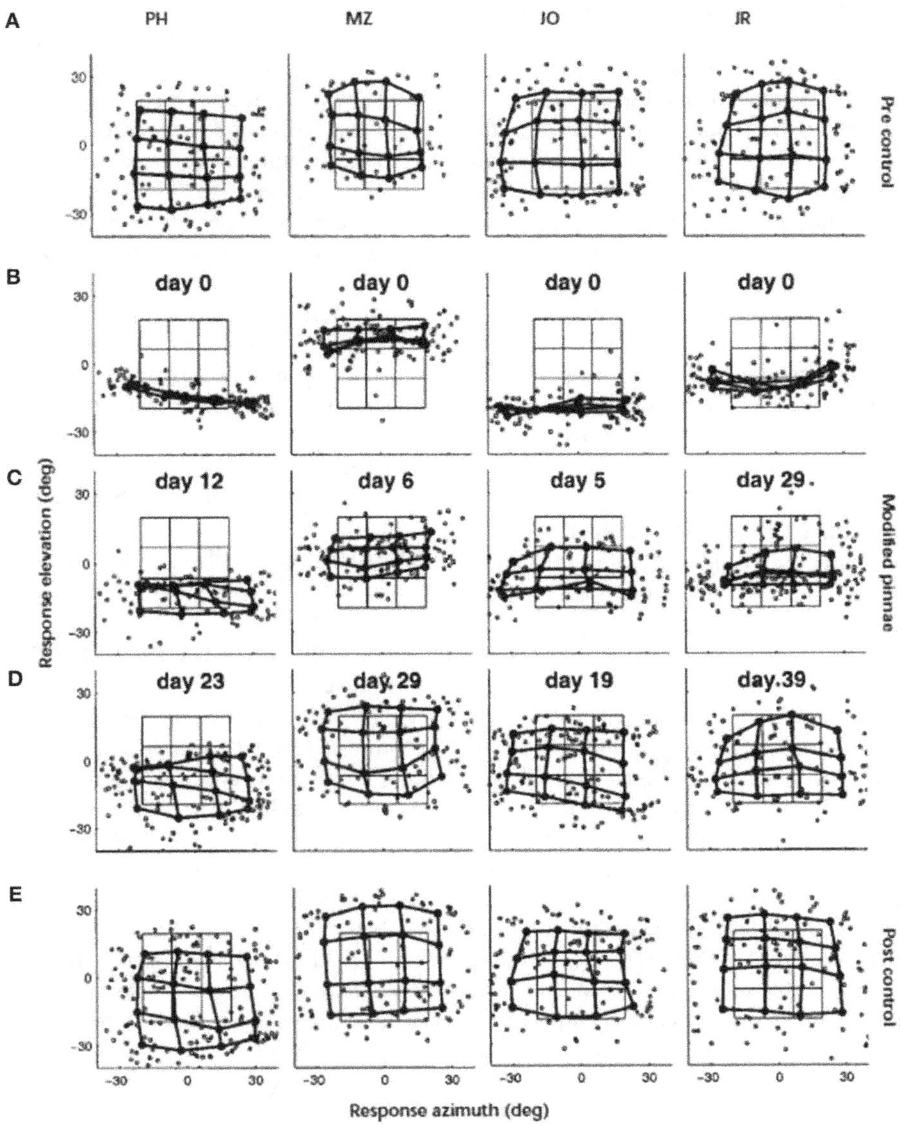

FIGURE 3 | Adaptation to altered spectral cues. Localization behavior of four subjects (from left to right) before, during, and immediately after the adaptation period. Day 0 marks the start of the adaptation experiment. The panels show, for each subject, the individual saccade vector endpoints in the azimuth–elevation plane (symbol °). In addition, the saccade vectors were also averaged for targets belonging to similar directions by dividing the target space into 16 half-overlapping sectors. Averaged data points (solid circle) from neighboring stimulus sectors are connected by thick lines. In this way, a regular response matrix indicates that the subject's saccade endpoints capture the actual spatial distribution of the applied target positions. The target matrix, computed in the same way as the saccade matrix, has been included for comparison (thin lines). **(A)** Results of the preadaptation control experiment on day 0, immediately preceding the application of the molds. **(B)** Localization responses immediately after inserting the molds (day 0). Note the dramatic deficit in elevation responses for all subjects. **(C)** Results during the adaptation period after 12 (PH), six (MZ), five (JO), and 29 (JR) days of continuously wearing the ear molds. **(D)** Results near the end of the adaptation period. Stable and reasonably accurate localization behavior has been established in all subjects. **(E)** Results of the control condition, immediately after removal of the molds. All subjects localized sounds with their original ears equally well as before the start of the experiment several weeks earlier. Figure 2 from Hofman et al. (1998).

produced by the molds. Consistent with this was the later finding that accommodation to monaural ear molds was dependent on the magnitude of the difference in the spectral cues between the bare ear and the mold ear (Van Wanrooij and Van Opstal, 2005). An overall similarity index (SI) was calculated from the standard deviations of the correlations between the HRTFs recorded from the anterior midline, with and without the molds. For 8 of 13 subjects, low similarity appeared to induce accommodation whereas the remaining five subjects, with only moderate differences between the mold and bare ear HRTFs, demonstrated oscillatory patterns in performance over the accommodation period rather than any progressive improvement.

In summary, modifying the binaural inputs by plugging one ear produces an acute decrease in auditory localization performance that recovers to some extent over a small number of days. This recovery does not seem to be accompanied by an adaptive variation in sensitivity to the binaural cues to location. Relatively subtle modifications to the monaural spectral cues also produce an initial reduction in localization performance in the elevation domain (on the cone of confusion) that also generally recovers to some extent over a period of 2–4 weeks. In the case of the ear plug, it is likely that the monaural cues provided by the plugged ear are also disrupted and the relatively rapid performance recovery has been attributed to a reweighting of the location cues to initially prioritize the veridical monaural cue provided by the unplugged ear. The differences in the accommodation times for the unilateral plugging compared to the bilateral molds is consistent with the idea that different processes might underlie the localization performance improvements in each case.

EFFECTS OF VISION ON AUDITORY SPATIAL TUNING

The role of visual input in guiding the development of the auditory spatial representation in the mammalian midbrain nucleus, the superior colliculus (SC) and its homolog the optic tectum of the barn owl, is well-documented. This is a particularly convenient nucleus to examine these interactions because of the topographic representation of auditory space and its spatial correspondence with the retinotopic visual representation. In an early developmental study using neonatal ferrets, a strabismus was induced in the one eye by cutting an extra-ocular muscle. The resultant shift in the visual representation in the SC induced a compensatory shift in the developing auditory representation, which maintained alignment of the two modalities (King et al., 1988). Similarly, shifting the visual field of the developing barn owl using optical prisms fixed in front of the eyes produced a similar shift in the auditory map in the optic tectum (Knudsen and Brainard, 1991). A range of other experimental manipulations have further underscored this developmental interaction (recent review: King, 2009).

However, vision is not necessary for the development of auditory spatial perception. Congenitally blind individuals are able to localize the source of a single sound with equal or even superior levels of performance compared to sighted individuals (e.g., Roder et al., 1999). There is, however, some evidence that congenitally blind localizers may be impaired perceiving more complex spatial relations between multiple sound sources (Gori et al., 2014).

There are also many examples of real-time audio-visual interaction in sound localization: Accuracy can be improved if the target is also visible (Shelton and Searle, 1980); Spatial disparities in synchronous audio-visual stimuli can result in the auditory location perceived as closer to the visual location (visual capture or the ventriloquist effect: e.g., Bertelson and Radeau, 1981); The ventriloquist after-effect can persist for minutes (e.g., Radeau and Bertelson, 1974; Woods and Recanzone, 2004).

Over a slightly longer time frame, conditioning the adult visual systems using distorting lenses for 3 days can lead to some compensatory distortion of auditory space (Zwiers et al., 2003). In a series of experiments using adult barn owls, Knudsen and colleagues examined the impact of shifting the visual field on the ITD tuning of neurons in the optic tectum. Prism lenses of increasing strength were used to incrementally shift the visual field. A progressive and corresponding shift in ITD tuning maintained the audio-visual coincidence in the neural representation (Linkenhoker and Knudsen, 2002). This incremental approach to retuning produced a five-fold greater change in neural tuning compared to a single large displacement of the visual field. Interestingly, owls that had accommodated progressively were able to later rapidly accommodate to a single large shift. In another experiment where owls were fitted with displacing prisms, hunting for live prey produced five-fold greater adaptive shift in ITD tuning in the optic tectum compared to owls that, under the same conditions, were fed dead mice. On the one hand this highlights the importance of bimodal stimulation in this accommodation (live mice are coincident auditory and visual targets) and a role for attention, arousal and behavioral relevance (reward). On the other hand, the audio-motor interactions involved in capturing live prey are far more complex than that for dead prey—this is a theme to which we will return in more detail.

VISUAL INPUT AND ACCOMMODATION TO PERTURBED SPECTRAL CUES

The first demonstration of adult auditory plasticity to perturbations in the spectral localization cues, discussed above (Hofman et al., 1998), used eye pointing to indicate the perceived location of a sound source. As a consequence, the possible range of locations was limited to ±30° from directly ahead. In a later study, the same group looked at the effects of monaural molds using eye pointing and this time the range of possible locations was ±70° (Van Wanrooij and Van Opstal, 2005). For locations within the visual field, any mismatch between the perceived auditory and visual locations of a sounding object could be used as a teacher signal as the auditory system recalibrates to the new spectral cues. This poses the interesting question as to whether the auditory system is even capable of retuning the spectral cues to locations outside the visual field in the absence of simultaneous visual input. Concurrent audio-visual inputs are not available for locations outside the visual field so, if the auditory system is able to accommodate to cues pointing to these locations, we might expect a different mechanism to be operating.

In a recent study in our laboratory we looked at the extent and rate of accommodation to new spectral cues for locations inside and outside the visual field (Carlile and Blackman, 2013). As in previous studies we used small bilateral ear molds to distort the spectral cues provided by the outer ear. The acoustic impact of the molds are shown for the left ear of one subject (**Figure 4**) and crucially, the molds can be seen to have modified the spectral cues for the posterior as well as the anterior hemispheres [see in particular panels (**F,I**)].

In contrast to previous studies we examined localization performance for 76 sound locations equally spaced around the listener. Insertion of the molds produced, on average, a seven fold increase in the number of front-back hemispheric confusions and a doubling of the polar angle (elevation) error (**Figures 5B,C**, 1st cf. 2nd columns). Subjects wore the molds continuously for 32 or more days (average 40.5 days) and showed an

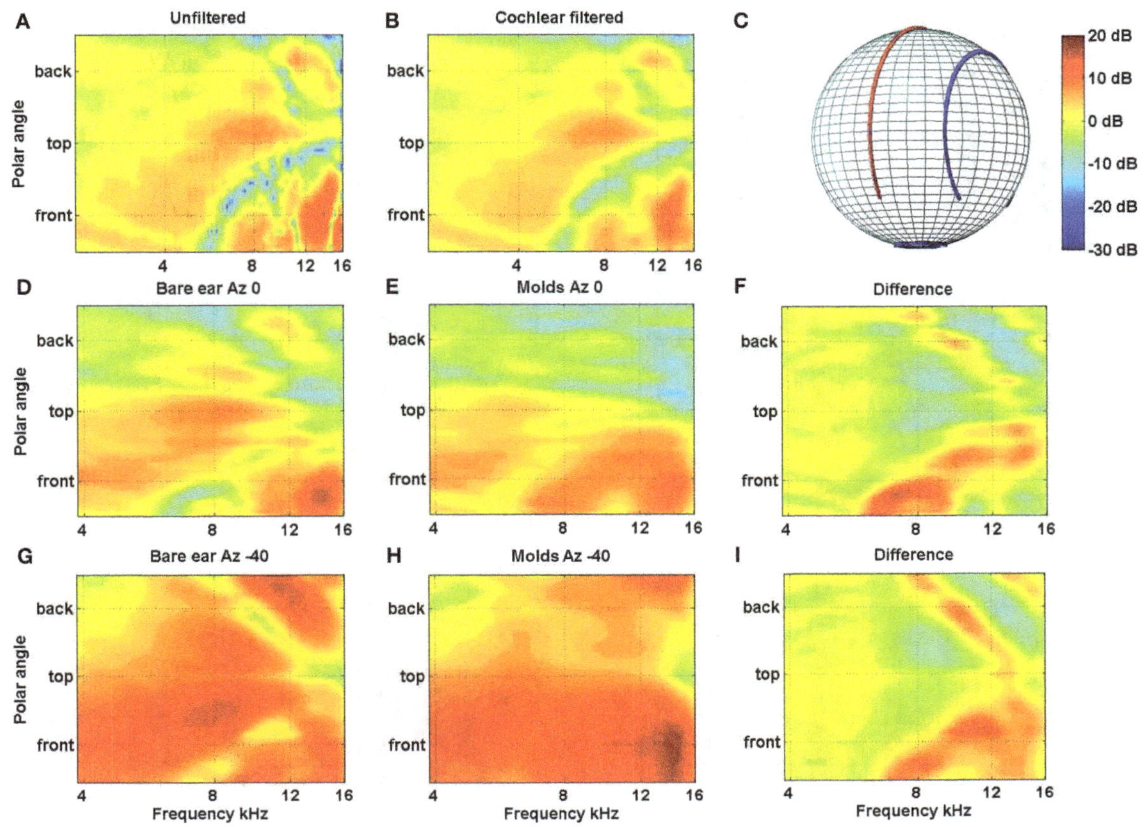

FIGURE 4 | (A) Filter functions of the left ear of one subject are plotted for the midline cone of confusion before and **(B)** after passing through a cochlear filter model. The features in **(B)** indicate that, despite the frequency filtering and spectral smoothing produced by the cochlear, substantial spectral features are preserved within the auditory nervous system. Filter functions for the left ear of a different subject are plotted for the midline [**D–F**: Azimuth 0°, cf. red line in **(C)**] and 40° off the midline [**G–I**: Azimuth −40°; cf. blue line in **(C)**] are plotted without molds **(D,G)** and with molds **(E,H)**. The data have been smoothed, as above, using the cochlear filter model. The differences between the bare ear and mold conditions for both lateral angles are plotted in **(F,I)** (Data from Carlile and Blackman, 2013).

improvement in performance toward pre-mold (control) values (**Figures 5B,C**, An cf. C). Critically, post accommodation (An) none of the performance parameters demonstrated a difference between locations within the audio-visual field [defined in this study as ±70° about the point directly ahead (gray bars)] and the audio only region [the rest of the sphere surrounding the listener (open bars)].

This indicates that (i) the system was able to accommodate to, or remap, new spectral cues in the absence of concurrent visual information and (ii) that the extent of accommodation was identical for both regions of space. That study also went on to examine the time course of accommodation and also found no differences in the rate of accommodation for the audio-visual compared to the audio-only regions of space. These latter findings are consistent with the idea of a single underlying process for both regions rather than one process that relies on vision and another that doesn't.

Removing the molds at the completion of the accommodation period resulted in an immediate return to control levels of performance (**Figure 5**, C cf. Post). This confirms the previous observation in a smaller group of subjects (Hofman et al., 1998) and indicates that despite more than a month of exposure and accommodation to the "new" spectral cues, the brain's representation of the "old" spectral cues was intact. Subjects also returned a week or more after the accommodation period, over which time they had not been wearing their molds. At this time, localization performance was tested with the molds reinserted and was not different from their accommodated performance (**Figure 5**, An cf. Ext). This suggests that following acquisition of the "new" cues, the auditory system was able to retain this mapping despite being chronically exposed once again to the "old" cues.

NON-AUDITORY INPUTS IN SOUND LOCALIZATION

A primary survival advantage provided by the auditory system is the detection and accurate localization of sources outside the listener's visual field. It therefore makes sense that the auditory system is able to effectively accommodate to changes in auditory cues that point to locations both inside and outside the visual field. At a minimum, maintaining the accurate calibration of the spectral cues resolving front from back on the cone-of-confusion would be essential to manage appropriate responses for example the approach of a predator. These data, together with the fact that congenitally blind individuals can localize sounds, raise the obvious question "if not vision, then what?"

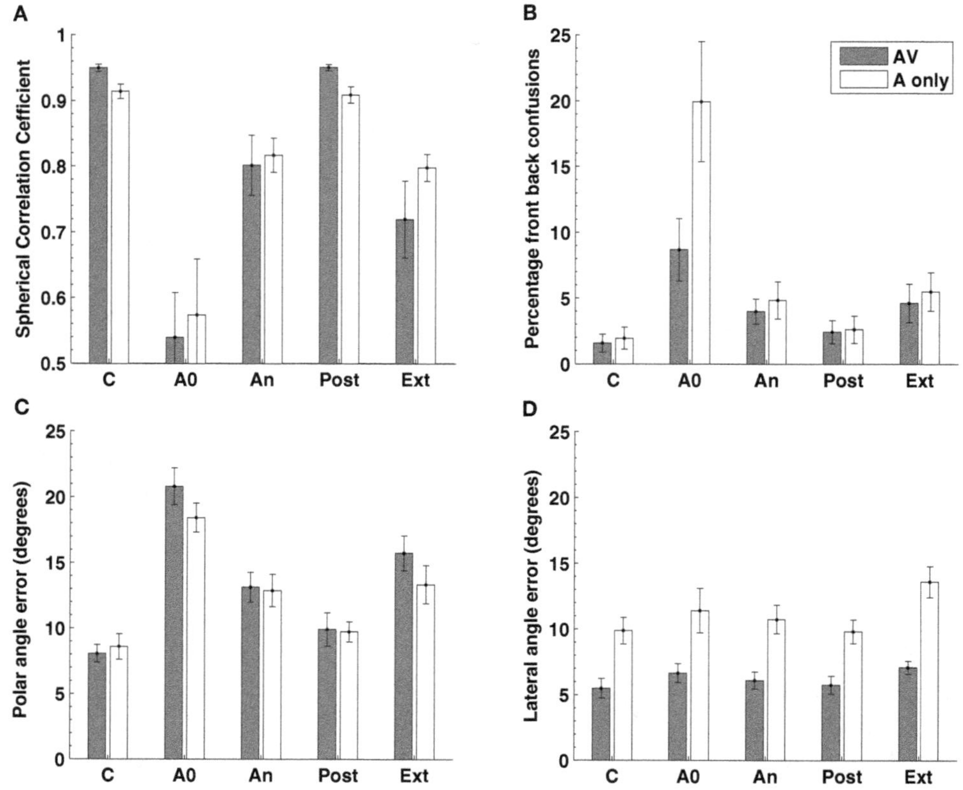

FIGURE 5 | Localization performance before, during, and after an accommodation period where spectrally distorting pinna molds were worn. Localization performance was measured using the **(A)** spherical correlation coefficient, **(B)** the percentage of front-back confusions, **(C)** the polar angle error (elevation error on the cone of confusion) and the **(D)** lateral angle (azimuth) error. The experimental manipulation is shown on the X-axis: C, control or baseline performance without the mold; A0 effect of acute placement of the mold; An, performance at the end of the accommodation period (mean 40.5 days); Post, performance immediately after removing the molds at the end of accommodation; Ext, performance on reinsertion of the molds more than a week after the end of accommodation. The gray bars represent data obtained from the audio-visual region of space (±70° from the midline) while the open bars represent data from the audio-only region outside these limits. Figure 2 from Carlile and Blackman (2013).

In answering that question we need to spend a little time looking at how we got here. Much of the work on auditory localization over the last century or so has followed in the excellent footsteps of Rayleigh (1907) and examined in some detail the relative contributions of the different acoustic cues to localization processing (reviews Middlebrooks and Green, 1991; Carlile, 1996; Carlile et al., 2005; Letowski and Letowski, 2012). On the one hand, these efforts have given us a good understanding of how we derive spatial information from the acoustics at each ear. On the other hand, the focus has primarily been on a single static sound source and speaks little to the manner in which this information is integrated with other non-auditory information to drive or guide action. The focus has largely been on pure tone or broadband noise stimuli presented under anechoic conditions and in silence and only recently have more real world stimuli such as speech (e.g., Best et al., 2005) been used in combination (Kopco et al., 2010) and in reverberant settings (Shinn-Cunningham et al., 2005; but see also Hartmann, 1983).

One important and related question is the spatial coordinates used in auditory localization processing. The ears of humans are relatively immobile and symmetrically placed on the head so that the coordinates of the acoustic cues to location are head-centered. In order to perceive and interact with the spatial location of sound sources, the location of the head with respect to the body needs to be taken into account. These sorts of questions have uncovered a wide range of important non-auditory influences on auditory localization performance.

In one study, using a sequence of an auditory then a visual stimulus, subjects first had to orientate to the (later) visual target and then to the (earlier) auditory stimulus. Although shifting the head to the later visual stimulus would change the head-centered coordinates of the auditory stimulus, subsequent orientation to the earlier auditory stimulus was still highly accurate (Goossens and Van Opstal, 1999). This suggests that the earlier auditory target was encoded in a body centered, rather than a head-centered, frame of reference. This study also suggested that head orientation had some influence on the localization of auditory target under static conditions. Another study using an ILD adjustment task, reported that shifts in the perceived midline of static stimuli were influenced by the right-left orientation of either the head or the eyes with the head fixed (Lewald and Ehrenstein, 1998). As the influence of both eye position and head position were about the same, they canceled out when the eyes were fixated on the auditory target, regardless of the head position. Similar results were obtained for both horizontal and vertical dimension using a laser pointing task to actual sound sources (Lewald and Getzmann, 2006). More recent detailed work has demonstrated that the spatial shift induced by eye position occurs in the absence of a visual target and also induces a shift in the perceived midline (Razavi et al., 2007; Cui et al., 2010). Vestibular stimulation has also been shown to influence the auditory spatial perception in the absence of change in the relative posture of the head (Lewald and Karnath, 2000; Dizio et al., 2001). This is far from an exhaustive review of this literature but the emerging picture suggests that a range of non-auditory inputs relating to the relative location of the head and eyes are also integrated with the acoustic cues to encode spatial location in body centered coordinates.

There are a range of sources of information about motor state including motor efference copy, proprioception and vestibular and visual information, all of which provide a dynamic, real time stream of data. If the head-eye position effects on auditory localization share the same mechanisms underlying similar effects in visual localization (see Hallet and Lightstone, 1976) then efference copy information regarding head position may be playing the driving role (see Guthrie et al., 1983). In a recent study in our laboratory, we have been looking at the ability to track a moving auditory stimulus using nose pointing (Leung et al., 2012). Listeners with schizophrenia, where motor efference copy mechanisms are thought to be severely disrupted (Ford et al., 2008), show significant deficits in this audio-motor tracking task (Burgess et al., 2014). In contrast, these patients did not show any deficits in the perception of the velocity of a moving auditory target *per se*, perceptual judgments that did not involve head movement. A role for motor efference in auditory spatial perception is also consistent with the distortions of auditory space that occur with rapid head saccades (Leung et al., 2008).

Whatever the mechanism, these experiments demonstrate that information about the motor state strongly influence the analysis of the acoustic information underlying the perception of space. From this perspective, sound localization is transformed from being a problem of the computational integration of the binaural and monaural acoustic cues to the static location of a sound source (a remarkable enough feat in itself) to a highly dynamic process involving a number of coordinate transformations and the disambiguation of source and self-motion. Consistent with this idea, it has been known for some time that, when a sound stimulus is of a duration that permits small head movements, multiple sampling of the sound field increases the localization performance, particularly in the context of resolving front-back confusions (Wightman and Kistler, 1999; see also Brimijoin and Akeroyd, 2012). More recently, the integration of self-motion information has also been shown to play an important role in the perception of an externalized sound source (Brimijoin et al., 2013).

At a theoretical level, it has recently been demonstrated that an auditory spatial representation can be established purely on the basis of audio-motor information. In a very important modeling study Aytekin et al. (2008) described a machine learning system that was able to construct a veridical representation of directional auditory space based on knowledge about (i) its own orientation movements and (ii) the auditory consequences of that movement. Put simply, their system made an "orientation movement" relative to some internal coordinate system and was then provided with two HRTFs that corresponded to that orientation. Over many pairs of movements and samples, the system built up an ordered list of the HRTF pairs that corresponded to the many different possible orientations from which the HRTFs were originally recorded. Their model was equally successful using human HRFTs taken from the CIPIC data base (Algazi et al., 2001) and on a collection of bat HRTFs. Other sensory-motor models of auditory localization have been subsequently developed (e.g., Bernard et al., 2012). Such models may provide a basis for understanding how auditory localization develops in the congenitally blind or how the mature auditory system is able to retune to spectral localization cues in the absence of visual input.

THE EFFECTS OF SENSORY-MOTOR FEEDBACK ON AUDITORY ACCOMMODATION

In the previous work showing accommodation to ear molds, we and others have found that there is a significant range of individual differences in both the extent and range of accommodation. Some subjects appear to asymptote in performance after a couple of weeks of wearing the molds, while others continue to improve over 4 or 5 weeks. Similarly, while most subjects show performance changes that approach their pre-mold, control levels, others improve far less (Hofman et al., 1998; Van Wanrooij and Van Opstal, 2005; Carlile and Blackman, 2013). Such difference could reflect individual differences in the capacity of the auditory system to adapt, although, given the relative homogeneity of the subject pool we feel this is unlikely. It is more likely, the inter-subject variance in accommodation could be caused by (i) different experiences and learning opportunities during the accommodation period and/or (ii) by differences in the acoustic distortion provided by the subjects' molds.

Taking the latter case first, acoustically related accommodation changes could result from differences in the extent of the distortion of the spectral cues produced by each mold. While the molds all looked fairly similar in size and shape, this is consistent with the large acoustic impact of relatively small differences in the sizes and shapes of normal outer ears (**Figure 1**; e.g., Shaw, 1974; Carlile and Pralong, 1994; Carlile, 1996). This could influence the size of the step change from the "old" to "new" spectral cues which may play a role in triggering and/or sustaining accommodation (Van Wanrooij and Van Opstal, 2005). In addition, the extent of performance improvements due to accommodation is also likely to be dependent on the spatial quality of the residual cues. For instance, near complete abolition of directionally dependent cues will provide very little acoustic spatial information for the auditory system to accommodate to.

We have recently completed an accommodation study where we first attempted to control for variations in the extent of spectral disruption produced by the mold and second, then focussed on the accommodation effects of training using sensory-motor feedback to source location. We found that a mold that filled the ear 40% by volume produced significant changes in localization performance when first inserted but retained elevation dependent acoustical changes in the frequencies of prominent spectral peaks and notches of the order an octave. We fitted these "standardized" molds to four groups of subjects and measured localization performance in response to different training regimes (Carlile et al., 2014).

The focus of the training regimes was to provide different levels of sensory and motor feedback each day of accommodation in addition to the subject's normal daily experiences. Given the theoretical modeling of the role of audio-motor feedback discussed above (Aytekin et al., 2008), we wanted to ensure a strong audio-motor component in the training regime. As before, localization testing and training was done in a darkened anechoic chamber. The first group received no performance feedback (Control) and just did three blocks of localization testing each day of accommodation; the second group received only visual feedback using a LED illuminated on the stimulus loudspeaker following each localization trial (Visual); the third group received visual and audio feedback where following each localization trial, the target loudspeaker pulsed at a rate inversely proportional to the nose-pointing error [Audio Visual Sensory Motor group (AVSM)]. In an attempt to maximize the audio-motor feedback, subjects were encouraged to explore the space around the target by moving their heads and to minimize the pointing error using this audio feedback before registering their corrected response; the fourth group used the AVSM paradigm with the room lights turned on during training. This provided subjects with an additional allocentric frame of reference over and above the body centered frame of reference provided by the endogenous audio-motor information [AVSM-Frame of Reference (AVSM-FOR)].

In contrast to previous studies, when compared to baseline, the acute effects of the molds were very similar for each group (**Figure 6**, Base cf. A0), confirming that the standardization of the spectral perturbation had to a large extent been successful. The difference in the feedback regimes can be seen most clearly in the front-back confusion rates by the tenth day of accommodation (**Figure 6**, top panel A10). While there was some improvement in the Control and Visual groups the most significant changes were for the groups receiving AVSM feedback. Similar improvement can also be seen with the elevation errors (PAE) although visual feedback alone was not significantly different to the AVSM feedback. The allocentric frame of reference (AVSM cf. AVSM-FOR) did not seem to confer further advantage, consistent with the idea that spatial location is coded in body-centered coordinates that does not require an external reference frame (Goossens and Van Opstal, 1999). Looking across the 10 days of accommodation it also appeared that AVSM feedback regimes produced a much quicker asymptote in performance at around 5–6 days (data not shown).

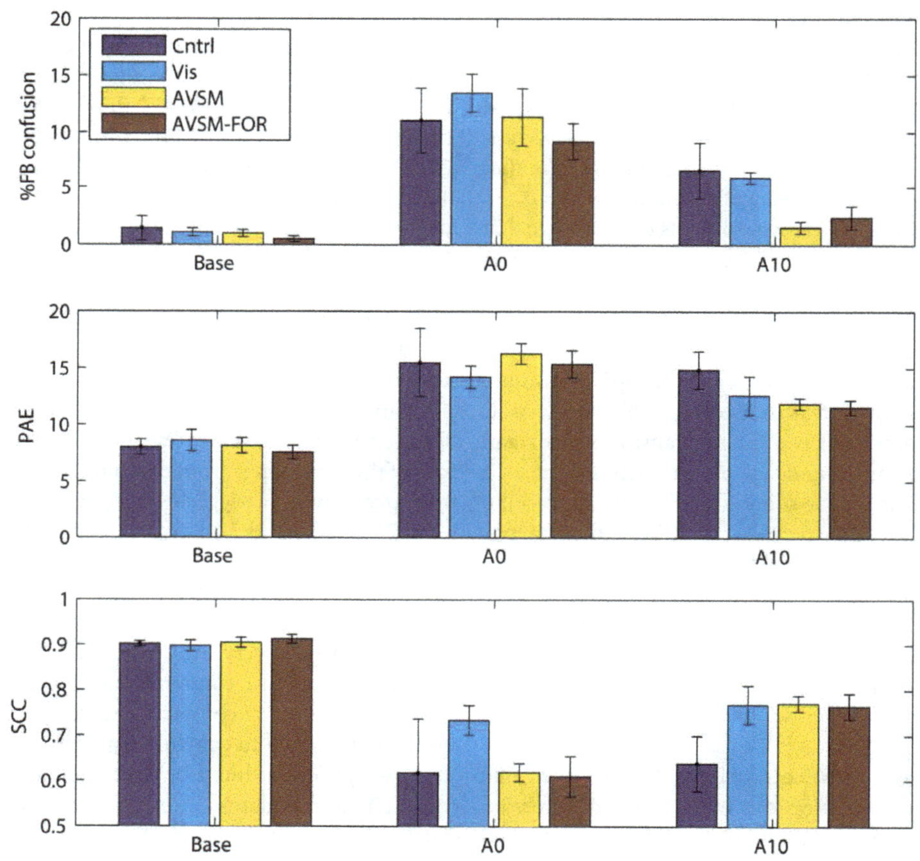

FIGURE 6 | The effects of training on accommodation to ear mold. Base: performance before accommodation with bare ears; A0: Performance on acute exposure to the mold; Acm10: performance following 10 days testing with feedback. PAE, Polar angle error; SCC, Spherical correlation coefficient. Data from Carlile et al. (2014).

Undoubtedly accommodation was occurring in the absence of any feedback-based training regime, presumably on the basis of the daily experience of the subject outside the laboratory, just as in the previous studies using ear molds. By contrast, however, AVSM feedback, in particular, resulted in an increased rate of and greater extent of accommodation. Three other studies have employed similar forms of sensory-motor feedback in assisting listeners to accommodate to non-individualized HRTFs used in virtual auditory displays (Zahorik et al., 2006; Parseihian and Katz, 2012; Majdak et al., 2013). Interaction with the sound objects in the display was a key part of each study and some improvements in front-back confusion rates were generally found after relatively short periods of training (Zahorik et al., 2006; Parseihian and Katz, 2012) however front-back confusion rates were still significantly higher than performance seen for subjects localizing in the free field with their own ears. With a longer period of training (21 days of 2 h sessions) improvements in both front-back confusion rates and elevation errors were reported (Majdak et al., 2013). A very interesting outcome of these studies, when compared to those employing molds, is that the auditory system appears to be able to accommodate to a different set of cues even though it does not experience a consistent exposure to the new cues over the full period of accommodation. In the case of the virtual display studies, as soon as the training session is complete the listeners are then listening through their own ears. By contrast, the molds listeners are encouraged to keep them in their ears during all waking hours (except when swimming or bathing).

CONCLUSIONS AND IMPLICATIONS

Investigations of auditory adaptation to changes in the spectral inputs have highlighted a number of interesting and important aspects of auditory localization processing. It seems likely that localizing sounds in the real world involves a range of non-auditory inputs, which may also be co-opted in the process of accommodating to changes in the auditory cues. Firstly, despite the early focus on the visual system's involvement in the development of auditory representation, it appears that visual input is not necessary for auditory accommodation to cue changes in the mature animal. There is a growing body of evidence that the motor state has an impact on the perception of auditory location. Again, the ecological problem of sound localization of even a single source is best characterized as a dynamic process involving the (i) transformation of the head-centered, acoustic cue coordinates to body-centered spatial coordinates and (ii) the disambiguation of source and self-motion. On-line information regarding motor state is critical to such processing—whether this represents motor efference copy information (as is the case for the visual system) or proprioceptive feedback or a combination of the two is very much an open question. Regardless of the mechanism, motor state information has also been shown to be, theoretically, sufficient to establish a veridical representation of auditory spatial information.

In this light, the demonstrated capacity to recalibrate to acoustic cues that point outside the immediate visual field and the impact of audio-motor training regimes on accommodation should not be that surprising. The range of individual differences seen in previous spectral accommodation studies using ear molds could also reflect the audio-motor training opportunities available to the individual. This of course raises the question of the capacity of such training regimes to promote, accelerate or complete accommodation to other forms spectral input changes including the application of hearing aids, changes to a hearing aid's processing or to the enhancement of the acoustic cues to location by the hearing aids. The role of attention and motivation in the perceptual learning of the altered spectral cues is likely to be a critical element in the success of any training regime (see Amitay et al., 2006; McGraw et al., 2009; Molloy et al., 2012). Although we have not been able to examine this literature in the course of this review there has also been much work in perceptual learning in the visual system (e.g., see Shams and Seitz, 2008; Deveau et al., 2014) that can also inform the development of effective auditory spatial training paradigms.

A recent study of the HRTFs obtained through different hearing aid styles (e.g., Completely in Canal vs. Behind the Ear) demonstrated substantial spectral cue differences associated with different form factors (Durin et al., in press). Moving from one hearing aid style to another would be expected to be the equivalent at least of fitting ear molds as described above. Real time signal processing also provides the potential for enhancement of spectral or other cues to spatial location which could aid in localization (Majdak et al., 2013) and/or the intelligibility of speech in noise (Jin et al., 2006). Clearly these kinds of enhancements would require the auditory system to accommodate to substantial changes in the localization cues and efficient means of driving such accommodation would aid substantially in their utility. Of course, the most substantial accommodation required of the auditory system follows the fitting of a cochlear prosthesis, which requires many months or years of training. The challenge here is to broaden research and discover whether the audio-motor interactions underlying the accommodation to spatial cues can also be applied more broadly to spectrally-temporally complex signals such as speech.

ACKNOWLEDGMENTS

Some of the work reported in this review was supported by the Australian Research Council Discovery Project grant (DP110104579). The author would like to acknowledge Martin Burgess for comments and discussion on a previous version of the manuscript.

REFERENCES

Abel, S. M., Giguere, C., Consoli, A., and Papsin, B. C. (2000). The effect of aging on horizontal plane sound localization. *J. Acoust. Soc. Am.* 108, 743–752. doi: 10.1121/1.429607

Algazi, V. R., Duda, R., Thompson, D. M., and Avendano, C. (2001). "The CIPIC HRTF database," in *IEEE Workshop on Applications of Signal Processing to Audio and Electroacoustics* (New Paltz, NY), 99–102.

Amitay, S., Irwin, A., and Moore, D. R. (2006). Discrimination learning induced by training with identical stimuli. *Nat. Neurosci.* 9, 1446–1448. doi: 10.1038/nn1787

Aytekin, M., Moss, C. F., and Simon, J. Z. (2008). A sensorimotor approach to sound localization. *Neural Comput.* 20, 603–635. doi: 10.1162/neco.2007.12-05-094

Babkoff, H., Muchnik, C., Ben-David, N., Furst, M., Even-Zohar, S., and Hildesheimer, M. (2002). Mapping lateralization of click trains in younger and older populations. *Hear. Res.* 165, 117–127. doi: 10.1016/S0378-5955(02)00292-7

Bauer, R. W., Matuzsa, J. L., Blackmer, R. F., and Glucksberg, S. (1966). Noise localization after unilateral attenuation. *J. Acoust. Soc. Am.* 40, 441–444. doi: 10.1121/1.1910093

Bernard, M., Pirim, P., De Cheveigne, A., and Gas, B. (2012). "Sensorimotor learning of sound localization from an auditory evoked behavior," in *2012 IEEE International Conference on Robotics and Automation* (St. Paul, MN), 91–96.

Bertelson, P., and Radeau, M. (1981). Cross-modal bias and perceptual fusion with auditory-visual spatial discordance. *Percept. Psychophys.* 29, 578–584. doi: 10.3758/bf03207374

Best, V., Carlile, S., Jin, C., and Van Schaik, A. (2005). The role of high frequencies in speech localization. *J. Acoust. Soc. Am.* 118, 353–363. doi: 10.1121/1.1926107

Brimijoin, W. O., and Akeroyd, M. A. (2012). The role of head movements and signal spectrum in an auditory front/back illusion. *Iperception* 3, 179–182. doi: 10.1068/i7173sas

Brimijoin, W. O., Boyd, A. W., and Akeroyd, M. A. (2013). The contribution of head movement to the externalsiaon and internalisation of sounds. *PLoS ONE* 8:e83068. doi: 10.1371/journal.pone.0083068

Burgess, M., Leung, J., and Carlile, S. (2014). "Auditory motion perception and tracking in Schizonphrenia," in *37th Midwinter Meeting of the Association for Research in Otolaryngology* (San Diego, CA), 250.

Butler, R. A. (1987). An analysis of the monaural displacement of sound in space. *Percept. Psychophys.* 41, 1–7.

Carlile, S. (ed.). (1996). "The physical and psychophysical basis of sound localization," in *Virtual Auditory Space: Generation and Applications*, Chapter 2 (Austin, TX: Landes), 27–77.

Carlile, S., Balachandar, K., and Kelly, H. (2014). Accommodating to new ears: the effects of sensory and sensory-motor feedback. *J. Acoust. Soc. Am.* 135, 2002–2011. doi: 10.1121/1.4868369

Carlile, S., and Blackman, T. (2013). Relearning auditory spectral cues for locations inside and outside the visual field. *J. Assoc. Res. Otolaryngol.* 15, 249–263. doi: 10.1007/s10162-013-0429-5

Carlile, S., Martin, R., and McAnnaly, K. (2005). "Spectral information in sound localisation," in *Auditory Spectral Processing*, eds D. R. F. Irvine and M. Malmierrca (San Diego, CA: Elsevier), 399–434.

Carlile, S., and Pralong, D. (1994). The location-dependent nature of perceptually salient features of the human head-related transfer function. *J. Acoust. Soc. Am.* 95, 3445–3459. doi: 10.1121/1.409965

Cui, Q. N., Razavi, B., Neill, W. E., and Paige, G. D. (2010). Perception of auditory, visual, and egocentric spatial alignment adapts differently to changes in eye position. *J. Neurophysiol.* 103, 1020–1035. doi: 10.1152/jn.00500.2009

Deveau, J., Ozer, D. J., and Seitz, A. R. (2014). Improved vision and on-field performance in baseball through perceptual learning. *Curr. Biol.* 24, R146–R147. doi: 10.1016/j.cub.2014.01.004

Dizio, P., Held, R., Lackner, J. R., Shinn-Cunningham, B., and Durlach, N. (2001). Gravitoinertial force magnitude and direction influence head-centric auditory localization. *J. Neurophysiol.* 85, 2455–2460.

Dobreva, M., O'Neill, W., and Paige, G. (2012). Influence of age, spatial memory, and ocular fixation on localization of auditory, visual, and bimodal targets by human subjects. *Exp. Brain Res.* 223, 441–455. doi: 10.1007/s00221-012-3270-x

Dobreva, M. S., O'Neill, W. E., and Paige, G. D. (2011). Influence of aging on human sound localization. *J. Neurophysiol.* 105, 2471–2486. doi: 10.1152/jn.00951.2010

Durin, V., Carlile, S., Guillon, P., Best, V., and Kalluri, S. (in press). Acoustic analysis of the monaural localization cues captured by five different hearing aid styles. *J. Acoust. Soc. Am.*

Florentine, M. (1976). Relation between lateralization and loudness in asymmetrical hearing losses. *J. Am. Audiol. Soc.* 1, 243–251.

Ford, J. M., Roach, B. J., Faustman, W. O., and Mathalon, D. H. (2008). Out-of-synch and out-of-sorts: dysfunction of motor-sensory communication in schizophrenia. *Biol. Psychiatry* 63, 736–743. doi: 10.1016/j.biopsych.2007.09.013

Fritz, J., Shamma, S., Elhilali, M., and Klein, D. (2003). Rapid task-related plasticity of spectrotemporal receptive fields in primary auditory cortex. *Nat. Neurosci.* 6, 1216–1223. doi: 10.1038/nn1141

Fritz, J. B., Elhilali, M., and Shamma, S. A. (2005). Differential dynamic plasticity of A1 receptive fields during multiple spectral tasks. *J. Neurosci.* 25, 7623–7635. doi: 10.1523/JNEUROSCI.1318-05.2005

Goossens, H. H., and Van Opstal, A. J. (1999). Influence of head position on the spatial representation of acoustic targets. *J. Neurophysiol.* 81, 2720–2736.

Gori, M., Sandini, G., Martinoli, C., and Burr, D. C. (2014). Impairment of auditory spatial localization in congenitally blind human subjects. *Brain* 137, 288–293. doi: 10.1093/brain/awt311

Guthrie, B. L., Porter, J. D., and Sparks, D. L. (1983). Corollary discharge provides accurate eye position information to the oculomotor system. *Science* 221, 1193–1195. doi: 10.1126/science.6612334

Hallet, P. E., and Lightstone, A. D. (1976). Saccadic eye movements towards stimuli triggered by prior saccades. *Vision Res.* 16, 99–106. doi: 10.1016/0042-6989(76)90083-3

Hammershoi, D., and Moller, H. (2002). Methods for binaural recording and reproduction. *Acta Acustica United with Acustica* 88, 303–311.

Hartley, D. E. H., and Moore, D. R. (2003). Effects of conductive hearing loss on temporal aspects of sound transmission through the ear. *Hear. Res.* 177, 53–60. doi: 10.1016/S0378-5955(02)00797-9

Hartmann, W. M. (1983). Localization of sound in rooms. *J. Acoust. Soc. Am.* 74, 1380–1391. doi: 10.1121/1.390163

Held, R. (1955). Shifts in binaural localization after prolonged exposures to atypical combinations of stimuli. *Am. J. Psychol.* 68, 526–548. doi: 10.2307/1418782

Hofman, P. M., Van Riswick, J. G., and Van Opstal, A. J. (1998). Relearning sound localization with new ears. *Nat. Neurosci.* 1, 417–421. doi: 10.1038/1633

Javer, A. R., and Schwarz, D. W. F. (1995). Plasticity in human directional hearing. *J. Otolaryngol.* 24, 111–117.

Jin, C., Van Schaik, A., Carlile, S., and Dillon, H. (2006). "Transposition of high frequency spectral information helps resolve the cocktail party problem in the mild to moderately hearing impaired listener," in *Proceedings of the Australian Neuroscience Society* (Sydney, NSW), 132.

Kacelnik, O., Nodal, F. R., Parsons, C. H., and King, A. J. (2006). Training-induced plasticity of auditory localization in adult mammals. *PLoS Biol.* 4:e71. doi: 10.1371/journal.pbio.0040071

Keating, P., Dahmen, J. C., and King, A. J. (2013). Context-specific reweighting of auditory spatial cues following altered experience during development. *Curr. Biol.* 23, 1291–1299. doi: 10.1016/j.cub.2013.05.045

Keuroghlian, A. S., and Knudsen, E. I. (2007). Adaptive auditory plasticity in developing and adult animals. *Prog. Neurobiol.* 82, 109–121. doi: 10.1016/j.pneurobio.2007.03.005

King, A. J. (2009). Visual influences on auditory spatial learning. *Philos. Trans. R. Soc. Lond. B Biol. Sci.* 364, 331–339. doi: 10.1098/rstb.2008.0230

King, A. J., Hutchings, M. E., Moore, D. R., and Blakemore, C. (1988). Developmental plasticity in the visual and auditory representations in the mammalian superior colliculus. *Nature* 332, 73–76. doi: 10.1038/332073a0

Knudsen, E. I., and Brainard, M. S. (1991). Visual instruction of the neural map of auditory space in the developing optic tectum. *Science* 253, 85–87. doi: 10.1126/science.2063209

Kopco, N., Best, V., and Carlile, S. (2010). Speech localisation in a multitalker mixture. *J. Acoust. Soc. Am.* 127, 1450–1457. doi: 10.1121/1.3290996

Kumpik, D. P., Kacelnik, O., and King, A. J. (2010). Adaptive reweighting of auditory localization cues in response to chronic unilateral earplugging in humans. *J. Neurosci.* 30, 4883–4894. doi: 10.1523/jneurosci.5488-09.2010

Letowski, T. R., and Letowski, S. T. (2012). *Auditory Spatial Perception: Auditory Localization.* Army Research Lab, Aberdeen Proving Ground, MD, DTIC Document.

Leung, J., Alais, D., and Carlile, S. (2008). Compression of auditory space during rapid head turns. *Proc. Natl. Acad. Sci. U.S.A.* 107, 6492–6497. doi: 10.1073/pnas.0710837105

Leung, J., Wei, V., and Carlile, S. (2012). "Dynamic of multisensory tracking," *in 35th Annual MidWinter Meeting of the Association for Research in Otolaryngology* (San Diego, CA).

Lewald, J., and Ehrenstein, W. H. (1998). Influence of head-to-trunk position on sound lateralization. *Exp. Brain Res.* 121, 230–238. doi: 10.1007/s00221 0050456

Lewald, J., and Getzmann, S. (2006). Horizontal and vertical effects of eye-position on sound localization. *Hear. Res.* 213, 99–106. doi: 10.1016/j.heares.2006.01.001

Lewald, J., and Karnath, H. O. (2000). Vestibular influence on human auditory space perception. *J. Neurophysiol.* 84, 1107–1111.

Linkenhoker, B. A., and Knudsen, E. I. (2002). Incremental training increases the plasticity of the auditory space map in adult barn owls. *Nature* 419, 293–296. doi: 10.1038/nature01002

Lupo, J. E., Koka, K., Thornton, J. L., and Tollin, D. J. (2011). The effects of experimentally induced conductive hearing loss on spectral and temporal aspects of sound transmission through the ear. *Hear. Res.* 272, 30–41. doi: 10.1016/j.heares.2010.11.003

Majdak, P., Walder, T., and Laback, B. (2013). Effect of long-term training on sound localization performance with spectrally warped and band-limited head related transfer functions. *J. Acoust. Soc. Am.* 134, 21482159. doi: 10.1121/1.4816543

Mamta, and Hanmandlu, M. (2013). Robust ear based authentication using Local Principal Independent Components. *Expert Syst. Appl.* 40, 6478–6490. doi: 10.1016/j.eswa.2013.05.020

McGraw, P. V., Webb, B. S., and Moore, D. R. (2009). Sensory learning: from neural mechanisms to rehabilitation. *Philos. Trans. R. Soc. Lond. B Biol. Sci.* 364, 279–283. doi: 10.1098/rstb.2008.0274

McPartland, J. L., Culling, J. F., and Moore, D. R. (1997). Changes in lateralization and loudness judgements during one week of unilateral ear plugging. *Hear. Res.* 113, 165–172. doi: 10.1016/S0378-5955(97)00142-1

Middlebrooks, J. C., and Green, D. M. (1991). Sound localization by human listeners. *Annu. Rev. Psychol.* 42, 135–159. doi: 10.1146/annurev.ps.42.020191.001031

Mills, A. W. (1958). On the minimum audible angle. *J. Acoust. Soc. Am.* 30, 237–246. doi: 10.1121/1.1909553

Mills, A. W. (ed.). (1972). *Foundations of Modern Auditory Theory*. New York, NY: Academic Press.

Molloy, K., Moore, D. R., Sohoglu, E., and Amitay, S. (2012). Less is more: latent learning is maximized by shorter training sessions in auditory perceptual learning. *PLoS ONE* 7:e36929. doi: 10.1371/journal.pone.0036929

Musicant, A. D., and Butler, R. A. (1980). Monaural localization: an analysis of practice effects. *Percept. Psychophys.* 28, 236–240. doi: 10.3758/BF03204379

Noble, W., Byrne, D., and Ter-Horst, K. (1997). Auditory localization, detection of spatial separateness, and speech hearing in noise by hearing impared listeners. *J. Acoust. Soc. Am.* 102, 2343–2352.

Otte, R. J., Agterberg, M. J. H., Van Wanrooij, M. M., Snik, A. F. M., and Van Opstal, A. J. (2013). Age-related hearing loss and ear morphology affect vertical but not horizontal sound-localization performance. *J. Assoc. Res. Otolaryngol.* 14, 261–273. doi: 10.1007/s10162-012-0367-7

Parseihian, G., and Katz, B. F. G. (2012). Rapid head-related transfer function adaptation using a virtual auditory environment. *J. Acoust. Soc. Am.* 131, 2948–2957. doi: 10.1121/1.3687448

Pralong, D., and Carlile, S. (1994). Measuring the human head-related transfer functions: a novel method for the construction and calibration of a miniature "in-ear" recording system. *J. Acoust. Soc. Am.* 95, 3435–3444.

Radeau, M., and Bertelson, P. (1974). The after-effects of ventriloquism. *Q. J. Exp. Psychol.* 26, 63–71. doi: 10.1080/14640747408400388

Rayleigh, L. (1907). On our perception of sound direction. *Philos. Mag.* 13, 214–232. doi: 10.1080/14786440709463595

Razavi, B., O'Neill, W. E., and Paige, G. D. (2007). Auditory spatial perception dynamically realigns with changing eye position. *J. Neurosci.* 27, 10249–10258. doi: 10.1523/JNEUROSCI.0938-07.2007

Roder, B., Teder-Salejarvi, W., Sterr, A., Rosler, F., Hillyard, S. A., and Neville, H. J. (1999). Improved auditory spatial tuning in blind humans. *Nature* 400, 162–166. doi: 10.1038/22106

Savel, S. (2009). Individual differences and left/right asymmetries in auditory space perception. I. Localization of low-frequency sounds in free field. *Hear. Res.* 255, 142–154. doi: 10.1016/j.heares.2009.06.013

Shams, L., and Seitz, A. R. (2008). Benefits of multisensory learning. *Trends Cogn. Sci.* 12, 411–417. doi: 10.1016/j.tics.2008.07.006

Shaw, E. A., and Teranishi, R. (1968). Sound pressure generated in an external-ear replica and real human ears by a nearby point source. *J. Acoust. Soc. Am.* 44, 240–249. doi: 10.1121/1.1911059

Shaw, E. A. G. (1974). "The external ear," in *Handbook of Sensory Physiology*, eds W. D. Keidel and W. D. Neff (Berlin: Springer-Verlag), 455–490.

Shelton, B. R., and Searle, C. L. (1980). The influence of vision on the absolute identification of sound-source position. *Percept. Psychophys.* 28, 589–596. doi: 10.3758/bf03198830

Shinn-Cunningham, B. G., Durlach, N., and Held, R. M. (1998). Adapting to supernormal auditory localisation cues: bias and resolution. *J. Acoust. Soc. Am.* 103, 3656–3666. doi: 10.1121/1.423088

Shinn-Cunningham, B. G., Kopco, N., and Martin, T. J. (2005). Localizing nearby sound sources in a classroom: binaural room impulse responses. *J. Acoust. Soc. Am.* 117, 3100–3115. doi: 10.1121/1.1872572

Shinn-Cunningham, B. G., Santarelli, S., and Kopco, N. (2000). Tori of confusion: binaural localization cues for sources within reach of a listener. *J. Acoust. Soc. Am.* 107, 1627–1636. doi: 10.1121/1.428447

Slattery, W. H., and Middlebrooks, J. C. (1994). Monaural sound localization: acute verses chronic unilateral impairment. *Hear. Res.* 75, 38–46.

Strait, D. L., and Kraus, N. (2014). Biological impact of auditory expertise across the life span: musicians as a model of auditory learning. *Hear. Res.* 308, 109–121. doi: 10.1016/j.heares.2013.08.004

Van Wanrooij, M. M., and Van Opstal, A. J. (2005). Relearning sound localization with a new ear. *J. Neurosci.* 25, 5413–5424. doi: 10.1523/jneurosci.0850-05.2005

Van Wanrooij, M. M., and Van Opstal, A. J. (2007). Sound localization under perturbed binaural hearing. *J. Neurophysiol.* 97, 715–726. doi: 10.1152/jn.00260.2006

Wenzel, E. M., Arruda, M., Kistler, D. J., and Wightman, F. L. (1993). Localization using non-individulaized head-related transfer functions. *J. Acoust. Soc. Am.* 94, 111–123.

Wightman, F. L., and Kistler, D. J. (1999). Resolution of front-back ambiguity in spatial hearing by listener and source movement. *J. Acoust. Soc. Am.* 105, 2841–2853. doi: 10.1121/1.426899

Woods, T. M., and Recanzone, G. H. (2004). Visually induced plasticity of auditory spatial perception in macaques. *Curr. Biol.* 14, 1559–1564. doi: 10.1016/j.cub.2004.08.059

Wright, B. A., and Zhang, Y. (2006). A review of learning with normal and altered sound-localization cues in human adults. *Int. J. Audiol.* 45 Suppl. 1, S92–S98. doi: 10.1080/14992020600783004

Zahorik, P., Bangayan, P., Sundareswaran, V., Wang, K., and Tam, C. (2006). Perceptual recalibration in human sound localization: learning to remediate front-back reversals. *J. Acoust. Soc. Am.* 120, 343–359. doi: 10.1121/1.2208429

Zwiers, M. P., Van Opstal, A. J., and Paige, G. D. (2003). Plasticity in human sound localization induced by compressed spatial vision. *Nat. Neurosci.* 6, 175–181. doi: 10.1038/nn999

17

Impact of hearing protection devices on sound localization performance

Véronique Zimpfer[1]* and David Sarafian[2]

[1] French-German Research Institute of Saint-Louis (ISL), Acoustics and Protection of Soldier Group, Saint-Louis, France
[2] Institut de Recherche Biomédicale des Armées, Département Action et Cognition en Situation Opérationnelle, Brétigny sur Orge, France

***Correspondence:**
Véronique Zimpfer, French-German Research Institute of Saint-Louis (ISL), 5 rue du Général Cassagnou, BP 70034, 68 301 Saint-Louis, France
e-mail: veronique.zimpfer@isl.eu*

Hearing Protection Devices (HPDs) can protect the ear against loud potentially damaging sounds while allowing lower-level sounds such as speech to be perceived. However, the impact of these devices on the ability to localize sound sources is not well known. To address this question, we propose two different methods: one behavioral and one dealing with acoustical measurements. For the behavioral method, sound localization performance was measured with, and without, HPDs on 20 listeners. Five HPDs, including both passive (non-linear attenuation) and three active (talk-through) systems were evaluated. The results showed a significant increase in localization errors, especially front-back and up-down confusions relative to the "naked ear" test condition for all of the systems tested, especially for the talk-through headphone system. For the acoustic measurement method, Head-Related Transfer Functions (HRTFs) were measured on an artificial head both without, and with the HPDs in place. The effects of the HPDs on the spectral cues for the localization of different sound sources in the horizontal plane were analyzed. Alterations of the Interaural Spectral Difference (ISD) cues were identified, which could explain the observed increase in front-back confusions caused by the talk-through headphone protectors.

Keywords: sound localization, HRTF, hearing protection device, spectral cues, behavioral method

INTRODUCTION

Hearing protectors are traditionally divided into two categories: protectors in which the attenuation is constant and does not depend on the sound level, and protectors in which attenuation depends on the sound level. Only the latter allow users to communicate and to perceive sounds in the environment. This category can be further divided into two types:

- passive-protection systems, such as non-linear-attenuation earplugs. This type of protector is usually very effective for protection against impulse noise as the attenuation increases with the increasing peak pressure level of the sound. Non-linear-attenuation earplugs usually include a sound path with acoustic impedance depending on the particle velocity. For instance, it may consist of a cylindrical cavity perforated at either end, which is inserted into an earplug. The acoustic impedance of this cavity is related to its viscous resistance, which has a non-linear component proportional to the particle velocity (Dancer and Hamery, 1998);
- active protection systems such as electronic "talk-through" systems. In these systems, sound is recorded using an external microphone and played back at an appropriate level via a miniature loudspeaker placed inside the Hearing Protection Device (HPD) close to the listener's ear. The gain is reduced as the sound level increases.

Protectors in which the attenuation depends on the sound level protect the ear against loud, impulsive noise while allowing an almost unaltered perception of faint or moderate level sounds. These systems facilitate oral communication. However, their impact on the sound-localization performance is not well known. However, the ability to localize danger (warning sounds) may be vital and is therefore important, even when using HPDs.

In order to localize sound sources, listeners make use of various cues. These cues result from two physical phenomena, which occur as the sound propagates from its source to the listener's eardrum: reflections, which are added to the direct sound, and absorption. The resulting cues provide information concerning the distance of the source from the listener (Mershon and King, 1975; Zahorik et al., 2005). Moreover, acoustic effects introduced by the listener's body (including, in particular, the pinna, head, and torso) result in differences between the sounds received by the left ear and the right ear which are used to determine the angle of incidence of sounds (Blauert, 1983; Wightman and Kistler, 1992; Wightman, 1999; Cheng and Wakefield, 2001). In particular, interaural time differences (ITDs) and interaural level differences (ILDs) are used to localize sound sources to within a cone of confusion (Blauert, 1983; Hartmann, 1999; Carlile et al., 2005). However, ITDs and ILDs do not allow the listener to determine the elevation of the source. To perceive this elevation, listeners must make use of their implicit knowledge of the acoustic effects of their body on incoming sounds.

A previous study by Hofmann et al. (1998) found that the insertion of a mold into the ear canal can have an impact on the listeners' ability to perceive the elevation of sound sources. Simpson et al. (2005) found modification in localization performance with linear HPDs in which the attenuation did not depend on the sound level. Lukas and Ahroon (2006) found degradation in localization performance with non-linear HPDs. To extend the findings of the previous studies (Lukas), we included active HPDs (talk-through system) in the present investigation. Sharon et al. (2007) showed a decreased performance in sound localization with a communication headset. (Gardner and Gardner, 1973) demonstrated that sound localization performance decreases with pinnae cavity occlusion. As described by Nicol (2010), many studies assess the sound localization performance in the horizontal plane which corresponds to the audiovisual horizon. But soldiers wearing HPDs move at all heights of the urban zone (for example, at the top of buildings) and need to localize sound also in the vertical plane. This is why we are interested in sound localization performance in azimuth and elevation. The goal of the present study was to investigate whether, and how, sound localization performance in azimuth and elevation is modified using active or passive hearing protection systems in which the attenuation depends on the sound level (e.g., Zimpfer et al., 2012). This sound localization performance was estimated using a psychophysical task method on different listeners. In the second part of the study, an analysis of the impact of the HPDs on the cues of the HRTFs was performed. This section highlights the distortion caused by the protection devices on the HRTFs.

The present study provides in particular some new contributions about localization performances in azimuth and elevation with level dependant HPD, and about a novel method using an artificial head to estimate localization performances with the same HPD.

BEHAVIORAL EXPERIMENT

MATERIALS AND METHODS

In order to quantify the influence of hearing protectors on sound localization performance, we measured the latter with and without hearing protectors in a group of listeners.

Listeners

Twenty listeners (10 males, 10 females, aged 24–51, mean age = 33.5 ± 7 years) participated in the study. All the listeners had normal hearing, defined as age-compensated pure-tone hearing thresholds of less than 20 dB HL at octave frequencies between 250 and 8000 Hz (ANSI S3.6-2004). Listeners were also checked by otoscopy for abnormal cerumen build-up (corresponding to more than 1/8 of occlusion) inside the ear canal prior to the experiment. In compliance with the guidelines of the declaration of Helsinki and of the Huriet law regulating biomedical research on human subjects in France, the listeners provided written informed consent prior to their inclusion in the study. The listeners were paid (50€) for their participation.

Hearing protection device

Five HPDs (four earplugs and one earmuff)—two passive protectors (non-linear system) and three active protectors (talk-through system)—were tested (as shown in **Figure 1**):

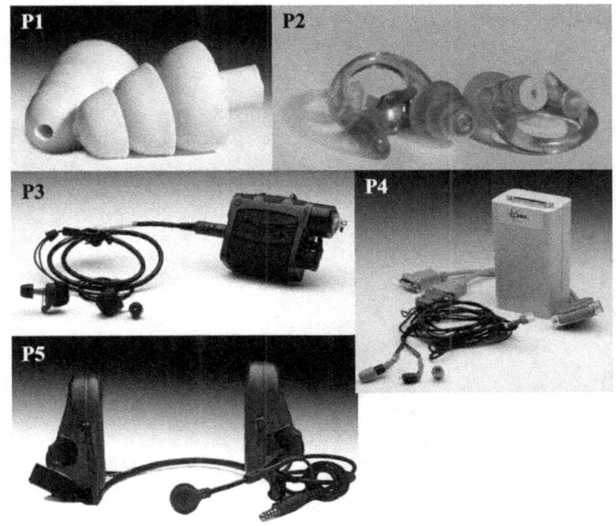

FIGURE 1 | Different HPDs tested in this study (see text for details).

- P1 is a commercial polymer earplug including an "ISL non-linear filter" with triple-flange design fit (3 sizes of earpieces).
- P2 is another polymer earplug including a Hocks-Noise-Braker® non-linear filter, with triple-flange design fit (3 sizes of earpieces).
- P3 is a commercial active earplug with a talk-through system and with modifiable foam tips (3 sizes).
- P4 is an ISL prototype earplug active talk-through system with modifiable foam tips (3 sizes).
- P5 is a commercial active earmuff with a talk-through system.

All the talk-through systems (earplug or earmuff) operate with two external microphones (one for each ear). For the three active systems, the tests were only carried out with the system in talk-through mode "ON," which allowed a very moderate attenuation to be obtained in a quiet environment (under 70 dB of noise).

Apparatus

In the center of a semi-anechoic chamber (polyhedron-shaped with a trapezoidal base (6 × 5.6 × 4.8 × 5 and 5.2 m high) with a carpet floor, eight loudspeakers were placed at the vertices of a cube having an edge dimension of 4 m. The background noise was measured with a Brüel and Kjaer type 4179 microphone and was in compliance with the ISO 4869-1: 1990 background sound level specifications. Listeners were individually seated on a chair placed in an elevated position (at an elevation of about 2 m, **Figure 2**) with the head placed in the center of this cube. They held a ball-shaped device with eight buttons on its surface, with each button corresponding to one speaker. The task of the listener was to press the button corresponding to the speaker which they identified as being the origin of the sound that was played to them. The number of correct responses and the test duration was recorded. This apparatus offers a 12.5% chance of having correct responses.

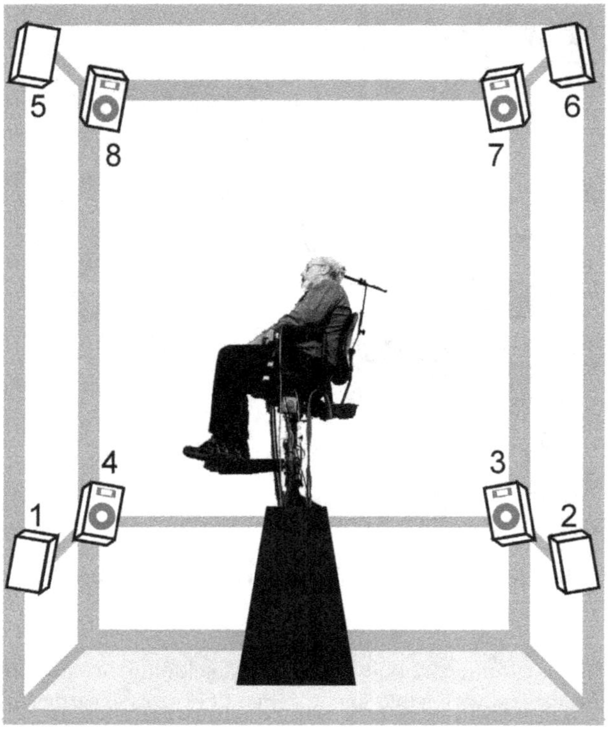

FIGURE 2 | Setup for sound-localization testing.

Auditory stimuli

On each trial, one of the eight loudspeakers emitted a brief signal; a 230 ms burst of wideband noise (see Butler and Planert, 1976). The acoustic stimuli were generated digitally at a 48 kHz sampling rate using a real-time processor (RX8; Tucker-Davis Technologies) with eight digital-to-analog converters (DACs). The output of each DAC was attenuated (PA5; Tucker-Davis Technologies) and routed to the corresponding loudspeaker via an amplifier (D-75A; Crown). The frequency response of each loudspeaker was equalized to provide the same acoustic signal at the listener's head location. The level of the signal (measured in the center of the cuboid speaker array) was set to 60 dB (SPL, lin.) for measurements without hearing protection and at 65 dB (SPL, lin.) for measurements with hearing protectors. In both cases, the stimulus was perfectly audible to all of the listeners. Indeed, with these noise levels, the different HPDs show no attenuation or only a very moderate one. To verify that the noise level was high enough, intelligibility tests using word lists were conducted with and without HPDs on each listener. These intelligibility tests were performed in the same anechoic chamber as the localization tests. The words were reproduced at the same level (65 dB) by one of the loudspeakers placed in front of the subject. During a test the subject had to recognize 15 words consisting of three phonemes. The rate of intelligibility was estimated by counting the number of correct phonemes (45 phonemes per test). The result of the intelligibility test was excellent with a rate of success of about 98% without and with HPDs. This proved that the sound level selected was sufficient for audibility.

Table 1 | Testing orders for days 2–4.

	Day 2				Day 3				Day 4			
1	P1	P2	P3	P4	P5	N	P1	P2	P3	P4	P5	N
2	P2	P3	P4	P5	P1	P2	P3	N	P4	P5	P1	N
3	P3	P4	P5	P1	P2	P3	N	P4	P5	P1	P2	N
4	P4	P5	P1	P2	P3	P4	P5	N	P1	P2	P3	N
5	P5	P1	P2	P3	P4	P5	N	P1	P2	P3	P4	N

The numbers (1–5) in the first column indicate different testing orders for the different HPDs (P1–P5). Each entry corresponds to one test session. Entries labeled "N" (for "None") indicate test sessions during which listeners were tested with naked ears. The five testing orders of HPDS were a circular permutation of the listeners, so the testing order 1 was assigned to listeners 1, 6, 11, and 16 were assigned testing order 1, and so forth.

Procedure

Prior to the experiment proper, listeners participated in three practice sessions, the goal of which was to acquaint them with the experimental apparatus and the task. During each practice session, eight sounds were presented sequentially to the listeners, each sound coming, in random order, from one of the eight loudspeakers. The listener's task was to identify the loudspeaker that emitted the sound. The purpose of these practice sessions was to reduce the training effect during the actual sessions.

During the actual experiment, the listeners participated in 13 test sessions. For three of these the listeners did not wear an HPDs; for the other 10 sessions, listeners wore HPDs (two test sessions for each HPD). The interest of these repeated sessions was to increase the reliability of the scores by averaging. During each of these sessions, 80 sounds (10 sounds per loudspeaker) were presented sequentially, in random order, to the listeners. The task was the same as during the practice sessions. To limit fatigue, sessions were separated by mandatory breaks of 10–15 min each, and listeners did not perform no more than four sessions per day. Four sessions with breaks lasted for about 50 min. Accordingly, the testing of each listener spanned 4 days. On the first day, otoscopic examination, and pure-tone audiometry tests were performed, after which the listener participated in three practice sessions and then in the first test sessions, without an HPD. Our intent was to begin and to finish with a session without HPDs in order to check the stability of the listener's localization performance. On the second day, each listener participated in four test sessions involving four different HPDs. On the third day, the listener performed three test sessions with different HPDs, and one test session without HPDs. On the fourth day, the listener performed three test sessions with different HPDs and finally, a session without HPDs. In order to avoid the effects of the order of testing of the different HPDs, a circular permutation of the listeners was arranged (see **Table 1** for details). The entire experiment spanned 4 weeks.

In an attempt to provide the best possible fit for each listener, the size of the earpiece was selected on an individual basis, except for P5 (earmuff). Pictures of ears wearing the earpieces were taken in order to check the suitable insertion of each HPD throughout the tests. For the device labeled P3, the tightness of the fit was evaluated using an active (acoustic) system, which "beeped"

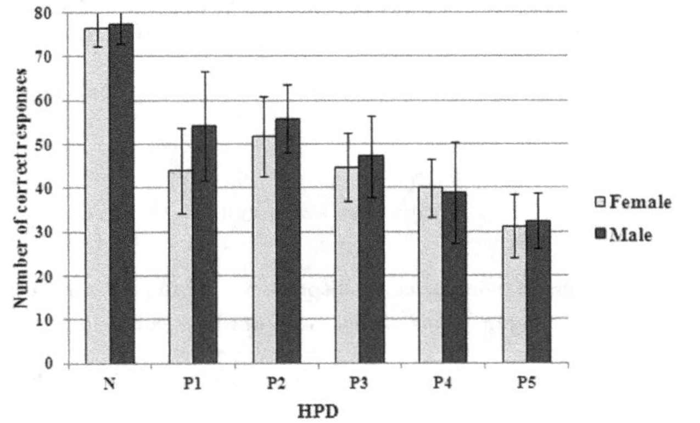

FIGURE 3 | Mean number of correct responses (for one session of 80 sounds) in the localization task for the different test conditions. N: no HPD; P1–P5: for different HPDs. Error bars show ±1 standard deviation of the mean across listeners in the gender group considered (male or female).

every minute if the fit was not sufficiently tight. For four of the 20 listeners, a tight fit could not be obtained, regardless of which of the three available earpiece sizes was used. Therefore, these four listeners could not be tested with this device, and the mean results reported in paragraph 2.2 for P3 are based on the results from 16 listeners only (8 females and 8 males); for all the other HPDs, the mean results reported in the following section are based on 20 listeners.

RESULTS

For each hearing condition (N, P1–P5), we compared the two or three sessions which were realized. We observed the same mean number of correct responses for all listeners between the sessions with the same hearing condition. The differences between the sessions are not significant. For the following analyses, we represented the average between the sessions of same hearing condition.

Figure 3 shows the mean number of correct scores for each of the conditions tested in the localization task. The numbers of correct responses measured while the listeners were using HPDs (P1–P5) were always lower than those measured while the listeners were not wearing HPDs (N).

Without HPDs, the number of correct responses was analyzed using the analysis of variance (ANOVA) method with repeated measurements performed on one factor, i.e., the loudspeaker (eight positions). The results showed that the positions of the loudspeakers had no significant effect [$F_{(7,\ 152)} = 1.3$; $p = 0.254$]. The positions of the loudspeakers did not have a marked effect on sound localization performance.

The duration of each session (80 sounds) was recorded. Without the HPDs, the mean duration of a session was 215 s with a standard deviation of 17 s. On the contrary, with the HPDs this mean duration was 245 s with a standard deviation of 45 s. We noted an increase of the mean duration of a session as well as the standard deviation when the listener wears a hearing protection. An Analysis ANOVA showed a difference very significant ($p < 0.001$) between different hearing configuration (without or with HPDs). For the following analyses, the duration effect was not taken into account.

Table 2 | Results of pairwise comparisons covering the different test conditions, including the no-HPD (N) condition and each of the five HPD conditions (P1–P5) for 16 listeners.

	N	P1	P2	P3	P4
P1	$p < 0.001$				
P2	$p < 0.001$	$p = 0.306$			
P3	$p < 0.001$	$p = 0.990$	$p = 0.0799$		
P4	$p < 0.001$	$p = 0.019$	$p < 0.001$	$p = 0.108$	
P5	$p < 0.001$	$p < 0.001$	$p < 0.001$	$p < 0.001$	$p = 0.319$

The mean individual number of correct responses, which was obtained by averaging the number of correct scores covering all the test conditions for each listener, ranged from 39 (/80) to 59 (/80). The standard deviations of these previous scores varied widely according to the different test conditions for each listener and ranged from 12 to 29. On the whole, no significant differences between the listeners were found [$F_{(19,\ 100)} = 0.41, p = 0.98$]. No main gender effect was detected ($p > 0.3$ for all hearing conditions), contrary to the lower performance of women in the spatial analysis of auditory scenes as described by Lewald and Hausmann (2013). Statistically, our scores did not depend on the listener effect.

The data (number of correct responses) were analyzed using a Two-Way repeated-measure analysis of variance (ANOVA). The results showed the significant main effect of the test condition factor (six levels: N, and P1 through P5; $p < 0.001$).

We chose to perform Two-Way ANOVA tests with software "R" only on the 16 listeners on whom the five HPDs were tested. Prior to this stage, the means of repetition were transformed by the function asin(sqrt(x)). The Mauchly sphericity test was significant with $p = 0.040$. So we applied the Greenhouse-Geisser correction which yielded a new value $F_{(2.9,\ 10.6)} = 68.33$ with $p < 0.001$. This correction did not change the significance of the first results. The test of effect size gave $\eta^2 = 0.85$ which corresponds to a high effect with a $f_{cohen} > 0.40$. The multiple comparisons of means (Tukey Contrasts) test were performed. **Table 2** gives the p-value of the planned pairwise comparisons. It shows significant differences between the sessions without HPDs and with all the HPDs. It shows no significant differences between P1, P2, and P3 and between P4 and P5. The lack of a statistically significant difference between conditions P1 and P2 may be related to the fact that these two protectors were of the same type (passive HPD). We can conclude from it that the active systems yielded lower scores (53 and 40% correct) than passive systems (63% correct). Besides, the active earmuff system yielded the lowest score (40% correct). The differences in average performance between the three types of HPDs (passive earplug, active earplug and active earmuff) were highly significant ($p < 0.001$), whatever the comparisons (passive earplug vs. active earplug, passive earplug vs. active earmuff and active earplug vs. active earmuff).

Figure 4 shows for one session (80 sounds) the mean number of different types of localization errors for each test condition. The

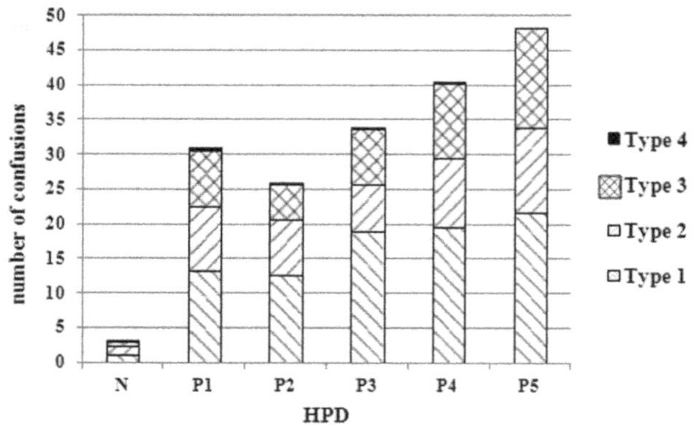

FIGURE 4 | Mean number of confusions (for one session of 80 sounds) for each test condition. The different types of confusions are color-coded as follows. Type 1: up-down; Type 2: front-back; Type 3: combination of up-down and front-back; Type 4: combination of up-down, front-back, and left-right.

Table 3 | Two-Way (test condition) repeated-measure analysis of variance (ANOVA) results for different types of confusion.

Confusion	ANOVA analysis
Up-down	$[F_{(5,\ 110)} = 20.36;\ p < 0.001]$
Front-back	$[F_{(5,\ 110)} = 13.65;\ p < 0.001]$
Up-down + front-back	$[F_{(5,\ 110)} = 19.4;\ p < 0.001]$
Left-right	$[F_{(5,\ 110)} = 0.97;\ p = 0.439]$

most common types of errors were up-down confusions, followed by front-back confusions. These two types of confusions also occurred frequently in combination. Left-right confusions were rare and, when they did occur, they were almost always associated with up-down or front-back confusions. This is why they were grouped with the latter two types of confusions in this analysis. For these (left-right) confusions, the differences between the different conditions were not statistically significant (**Table 3**). For all the other types of confusions (i.e., front-back and up-down), highly significant differences were observed. For up-down confusions, pairwise comparisons between the different types of HPDs showed significant differences between all the test conditions, except for active earplugs vs. active earmuffs (**Table 4**); passive earplugs were found to produce fewer up-down confusions than active systems (earplugs or earmuffs). For front-back confusions, the planned pairwise comparisons showed significant differences between all the test conditions, except for passive earplugs vs. active earplugs (**Table 5**). The same remark can be made regarding front-back and up-down confusions (**Table 6**). No statistically significant difference could be found between passive earplugs and active earplugs, except for the elevation error. Whatever the confusion (up-down, front-back, and left-right) the difference between without HPD and with each HPD is significant.

DISCUSSION

The results of this study show that HPDs have a significant detrimental impact on sound localization performance. This was the

Table 4 | Results of pairwise comparisons between the different test conditions for different types of HPDs for up-down confusions.

	N	Passive earplug	Active earplug
Passive earplug	$p < 0.001$		
Active earplug	$P < 0.001$	$p = 0.003$	
Active earmuff	$p < 0.001$	$P < 0.0001$	$p = 0.200$

Table 5 | Results of pairwise comparisons between the different test conditions for different types of HPDs for front-back confusions.

	N	Passive earplug	Active earplug
Passive earplug	$p < 0.001$		
Active earplug	$P < 0.001$	$p = 0.0928$	
Active earmuff	$p < 0.001$	$p = 0.008$	$P < 0.001$

Table 6 | Results of pairwise comparisons between the different test conditions for different types of HPDs for combined up-down and front-back confusions.

	N	Passive earplug	Active earplug
Passive earplug	$p < 0.001$		
Active earplug	$p < 0.001$	$p = 0.176$	
Active earmuff	$p < 0.001$	$p < 0.001$	$p < 0.001$

case of all the systems tested in this study, including the passive earplugs, the active earplugs, and the active earmuff. The latter system caused the largest deterioration in sound-localization performance: the mean number of correct responses was 32 vs. the mean number of correct responses for the "naked ear" test condition which was 77. The percent-correct localization score obtained with this device (40%) was significantly lower than the scores achieved with any of the other devices tested in this study, including the other two active HPDs (earplugs). Passive earplugs were found to have the smallest impact on sound-localization performance, with an average score of 51 (/80), which still corresponds to a decrease of about 26 correct responses, compared to the "naked ear" condition. The scores for the two passive earplug systems tested here did not differ statistically. However, the score obtained with one of these two passive earplugs was also not significantly different from that measured with one of the two active earplugs. Another important observation was that HPDs increased both the front-back and up-down confusions. In particular, active systems distort the up-down localization perception. Front-back confusions are usually more detrimental than up-down confusions in real-life situations, as sounds of interest are usually located around, rather than above or below, the listener. Lastly, very few left-right confusions were observed and, when such confusions did occur, they were often accompanied by front-back or up-down confusions. These rare left-right confusions may be possibly due to a moment's inattention on the part of the listeners.

The detrimental effects of HPDs on sound-localization performance observed in this study can be explained by the fact that HPDs alter, or remove, cues used by listeners for localizing sounds, especially in the front-back and up-down dimensions. In particular, earplugs modify ear-canal resonances, which are known to introduce useful cues for sound localization in the form of spectral peaks and dips (Batteau, 1967; Hofmann et al., 1998). Earmuffs alter spectral cues introduced by the pinna, which may explain why the earmuff-based protection system (P5) was found to be the most detrimental to sound-localization performance. Many localization confusions with active earmuff may be due to the fact that the pinna are hidden (Batteau, 1967; Hofman and van Opstal, 2003).

ACOUSTIC MEASUREMENT

HRTFs provide a representation of the spectral modifications introduced by the listener's morphology (in particular, the torso, the head, and the pinna). These modifications can be determined by comparing the spectra of the recordings of a broadband noise (presented in the free field) at the entrance to the ear canal or close to the listener's eardrum, and the spectra of the recordings of the same signal obtained using a microphone placed at the location of the listener's head, in the listener's absence (Butler and Belendiuk, 1977; Blauert, 1983; Wightman and Kistler, 1989; Andéol et al., 2011).

MATERIALS AND METHODS

To obtain information on the effects of the HPDs on the spectral cues for sound localization, we measured and compared the HRTFs using an artificial head in the horizontal plane without, and with, the HPDs in place. However, due to physical (volume and shape) constraints, the microphone used to measure the HRTFs could not be placed close to the listener's eardrum at the same time as an earplug. To solve the problem mentioned in Materials and methods, the HRTFs were measured using an artificial head built at ISL (Parmentier et al., 2000).

Hearing protection device

We used the same five HPDs as in the behavioral experiment.

Apparatus

The artificial head used is equipped with an IEC 711 compatible ear simulator (B&K 4157) in which the measured acoustic signal is close to that measured at a real eardrum. The outer ear and the ear canal are modeled using HeadAcoustics® materials. The artificial head was used to measure HRTFs without an HPD, and then with each of the HPDs. The measurements were performed in an audiometric cabin. Inside the cabin (2.6 × 4 × 2.2 m), the walls were covered with sound-absorbing material and the floor with a carpet.

Sound source

The sound source (loudspeaker) used for these measurements was located in the horizontal plane of the head. The distance between the loudspeaker and the artificial head was equal to 1.5 m. The 800 samples of HRTFs were recorded using the swept sine function with logarithmic steps [100 Hz–20 kHz]. The sound source level was fixed to 70 dB SPL, in order to prevent the active HPD from attenuating the sound as in the behavioral method.

Procedure

Measurements were performed in the horizontal plane for eight different orientations of the head (with respect to the sound source), spanning 360° in steps of 45°, and for each ear simultaneous (left and right). In the first orientation the head faces the source, which corresponds to the 0° angle. The sound source is fixed and the head is rotated to perform the measurements. For each orientation two measurements have been realized. After each measure, the HPD has been taken off and put back on the artificial ear. In order to avoid the parameter of the measurement chain, the reference measurement has been performed at the center of artificial head without the head. The HRTFs presented are the average of the two measurements. A comparison of the results of the acoustic measurement method with those of the previously mentioned psychophysical method cannot be strictly made. Indeed, the two methods do not analyze the same sound sources.

RESULTS

Figure 5 shows the HRTFs measured in the right ear, without an HPD and with the P5 device in place, for the eight orientations of the artificial head. It illustrates the effect of the head orientation on the HRTFs without the HPD in place. Similar figures were obtained on the left ear. In particular on the higher graph of **Figure 5**, it can be noted that as the orientation of the head with respect to the sound source varied from 0 to 315°, the sound power above 400 Hz initially increased, then decreased, thus reflecting the position of the right ear with respect to the source. Systematic variations in sound power as a function of the head orientation can also be observed at lower frequencies, down to about 400 Hz (Shaw, 1974). These orientation-dependent level variations in sound power levels at the eardrum correspond to the ILD which listeners potentially use to localize sound sources in the horizontal plane. The lower graph of **Figure 5** shows that, with the P5 device in place, the HRTF in the 400 Hz–5 kHz frequency range varies only very little as a function of the head orientation (except for two orientations 225 and 270°). We can even note that for the 0 and 45° head orientations the HRTF curves are similar until 5 kHz. Eight curves of HRTF obtained with P5 are very different from those obtained without hearing protection (cf. **Figure 5**). This device also highlighted a small difference between the right and the left ears which may be due to the fact that this earmuff-based HPD was less symmetric than the others; in particular, as can be seen in **Figure 1**, this device featured a speech microphone only on the left side. The markedly reduced head-shadow effect produced by the earmuff of the HPD type suggests that listeners had to rely primarily on the ITD for left-right localization.

To obtain information about the relationship between the effects of HPDs on HRTFs and some possible front-back confusions, we were interested in HRTFs for the orientations of 45 and 135°. These two orientations correspond to front-right and back-right source locations, respectively. Specifically, we computed the Interaural Spectral Difference (ISD) which is the differences between the HRTFs measured in the left and right ears, for each of the two orientations. This was done for naked ears and for each HPD separately. The results, which are shown in **Figure 6**,

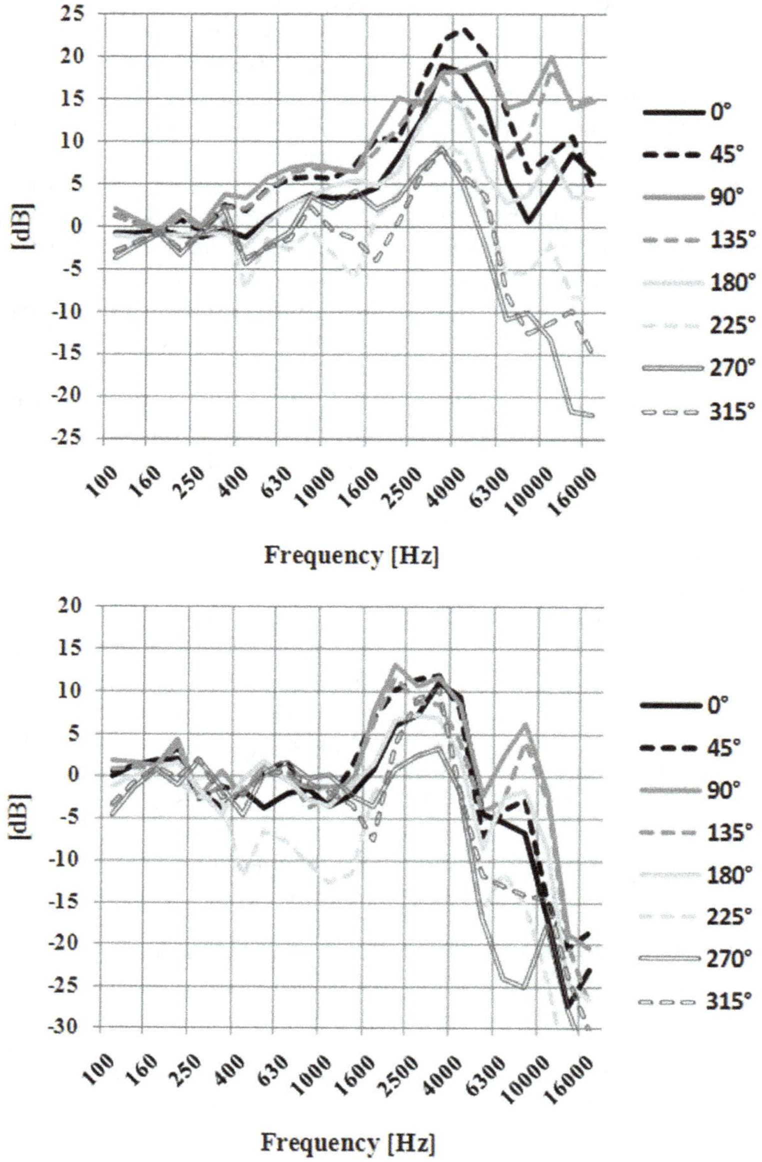

FIGURE 5 | HRTFs measured in the right ear, without an HPD in place at the top and with P5 in place at the bottom, for the eight orientations of the artificial head with respect to the noise source. Different types of lines correspond to different orientations.

illustrate the ISD cues that may have been available to the listeners for distinguishing between the front and back sources, for each HPD.

DISCUSSION ABOUT FRONT-BACK CONFUSION

It must be noted that, for the no-HPD condition (N), differences (up to 5 dB) between the ISD curves corresponding to the two orientations were observed over a wide range of frequencies (above approximately 500 Hz). Such differences provide a potential basis for the ability of listeners to distinguish between front and back locations. Differences between the two curves were also observed for the measurements performed with the HPDs in place. However, the magnitude and shape of these differences differed largely, depending on the type of HPD. This can be most easily seen in **Figure 7**, which shows the differences between the 45 and 135° ISD curves for the different HPDs, all superimposed on the same plot. It can be noticed that the ISD difference curves most similar to the reference (no-HPD) curve corresponded to P1, P2, and P3; for P4, and even more so for P5, large deviations from the reference curve were observed. This observation was confirmed quantitatively by comparing the mean of squared differences between the ISD difference curve for the naked ear and the ISD difference curves for each HPD, over the 0.5–10 kHz range (**Table 7**); the mean of squared difference was largest for P5. This indicates that the normal (naked-ear) pattern of the ISD cues for front-back distinctions was more severely altered by P5 than by the other HPDs. **Table 7** shows the impact of HPDs on the HRTFs and the ISD cues.

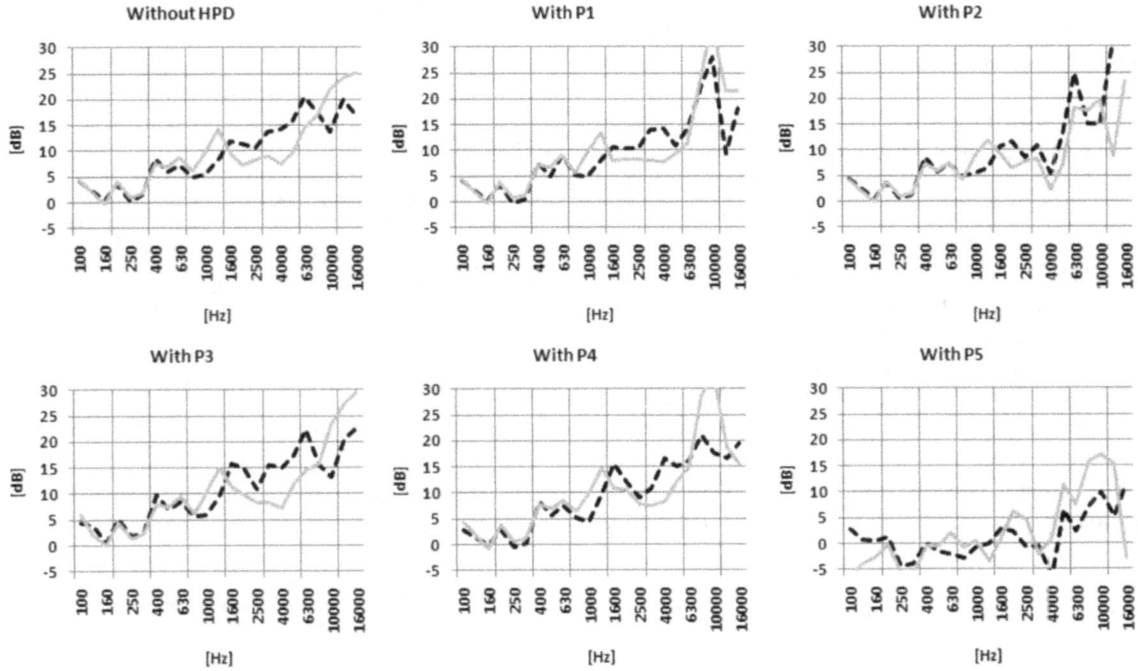

FIGURE 6 | The Interaural Spectral Difference (ISD) for head orientations of 45 (black, dashed line) and 135° (gray, solid line). The different panels correspond to different HPDs, or to the no-HPD condition (upper-left panel).

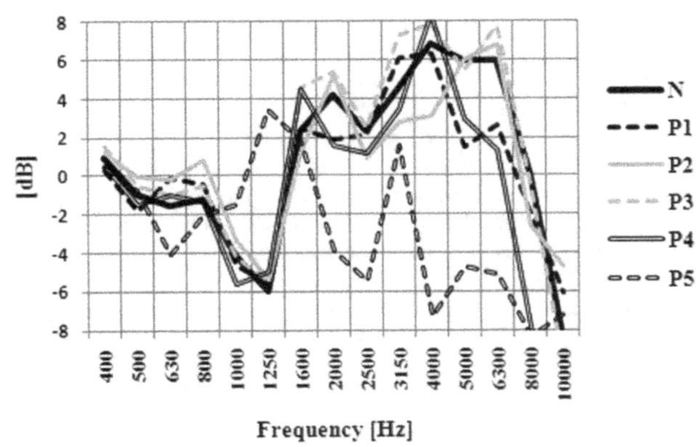

FIGURE 7 | Differences in the ISD cues between the 45 and 135° orientation for the right ear.

As indicated in **Table 7**, the pattern of the ISD cues with respect to the distinction between the 45 and 135° orientations was the least altered by P3. Thus, the lowest proportion of front-back confusions was observed for P3, P2, and P1. For these three protectors, the differences between the ILD cues with and without hearing protection were the lowest. We could suppose that with these three HPDs the front-back confusions will be the lowest. Moreover, the information provided by **Figure 7** and **Table 7** also goes some way toward explaining the pattern of possible front-back confusions. We can note similarities between the two methods by comparing **Figure 4** (behavioral method) with **Table 7** (acoustic measurement method). Indeed, the three HPDs that are associated with the smallest mean of squared differences in **Table 7**, i.e., P1, P2, and P3 are the same three HPDs that were found to yield the smallest proportions of front-back confusions during the experiment. Besides, the worst result was obtained for the P5 protector for both methods (behavioral method and mean squared difference approach). These similarities between the two methods should be verified in future.

Table 7 | Mean of squared difference between ISD-difference curves for the five HPDs (Figure 7).

	P1	P2	P3	P4	P5
Mean of squared difference (dB^2)	4.05	3.81	1.74	12.24	57.90

DISCUSSION AND PERSPECTIVES

The results of this study demonstrated the significant impact of the HPDs on sound-localization performance. The impact was more or less marked, depending on the type of HPD. It was less important for passive earplugs than for active systems. The decrease in sound-localization performance was the highest for the earmuff-based active system tested here. A larger number of localization errors, and especially, up-down confusions, were observed with active systems than with passive earplugs. However, front-back confusions were almost as numerous for passive earplugs (P1 and P2) as for one of the active earplug systems (P3). When comparing the physical dimensions of the different earplug devices with their results with respect to the localization performance, we note that the localization performance may possibly depend on the distance of the sound-pickup-point to the entrance of the ear canal.

Comparisons between the HRTFs measured with and without the HPDs provided some information about the origin of the decrease in localization performance in the horizontal plane due to HPDs. Specifically, by comparing the pattern of ILD cues used to distinguish between the 45 (front right) and 135° (back right) locations, we found that this pattern was more severely altered by P5 than by any of the other HPDs tested in this study. Moreover, this analysis showed that P1, P2, and P3 had a smaller impact on ISD cues than P4 and P5. These observations seem to correlate with the fact that localization performance was less degraded by P1, P2, and P3 than by P4 and P5. However, this correlation is, at the moment, more or less speculation, as it has to be confirmed by a new set of experiments conducted, with an identical setup for the measurement of HRTFs and the determination of the localization performance.

A limitation of the present study is due to the fact that HRTFs with HPDs (earplug) could not be measured in the human participant's ears. Ideally, HRTFs should have been measured while the participants were wearing the HPDs, for each HPD. Such measurements could not be performed due to the physical impossibility of fitting the HPD and the recording microphone into the ear canal. This is why HRTFs were measured using the artificial head. We are aware that this is not an ideal arrangement, and that future studies should try to resolve the technical difficulties associated with HRTF measurements in human participants wearing HPDs.

It is important to note that the HRTF measurements performed on an artificial head have shown spectral alterations caused by HPDs, which may explain the increase in front-back confusions observed for some HPDs. Once the measurement system is in place, HRTF measurements on an artificial head are less time-consuming than psychophysical tests which usually require multiple participants (in order to average out interindividual variability) and many stimulus presentations per participant. We have to demonstrate that the classification of the localization performance based on the HRTFs can be compared to the classification based on the psychophysical measurements. In this case, HRTF measurements using an artificial head may provide a fast(er) method for estimating the impact of HPDs on sound-localization performance. Specific alterations of the HRTF leading to particular errors in localization and measurement reproducibility could be interesting tracks for a next experiment. A limitation of this approach, however, is that it is based on a standard artificial head; it can only be used to predict average performance. HPDs may have a different impact on localization performance for different individuals, depending on morphological specificities (e.g., ear canal and/or pinna morphology) as well as on the quality of the fit. This poses an interesting challenge for future efforts to develop HRTF-based methods of predicting sound localization performance with HPDs.

ACKNOWLEDGMENT

The author thanks the two anonymous reviewers, and also K. Buck, P. Naz (ISL) and Christophe Micheyl (University of Minnesota) for their comments on this manuscript.

REFERENCES

Andéol, G., Guillaume, A., Micheyl, C., Savel, S., Pellieux, L., and Moulin, A. (2011). Auditory efferents facilitate sound localization in noise in humans. *J. Neurosci.* 31, 6759–6763. doi: 10.1523/JNEUROSCI.0248-11.2011

Batteau, D. W. (1967). The role of pinna in human localization. *Proc. R. Soc. Lond. B* 168, 158–180. doi: 10.1098/rspb.1967.0058

Blauert, J. (1983). *Spatial Hearing: The Psychophysics of Human Sound Localization*. Cambridge, MA: MIT Press.

Butler, R. A., and Belendiuk, K. (1977). Spectral cues utilized in the localization of sound in the median sagittal plane. *J. Acoust. Soc. Am.* 61, 1264–1269. doi: 10.1121/1.381427

Butler, R. A., and Planert, N. (1976). The influence of stimulus band-width on localization of sound in space. *Percept. Psychophys.* 19, 103–108. doi: 10.3758/BF03199393

Carlile, S., Martin, R., and McAnally, K. (2005). Spectral information in sound localisation. *Int. Rev. Neurobiol.* 70, 399–434. doi: 10.1016/S70074-7742(05)70012-X

Cheng, C. I., and Wakefield, G. H. (2001). Introduction to Head Related Transfer Functions (HRTF's). Representation of HRTF's in time, frequency and space. *J. Audio Eng. Soc.* 49, 231–249. doi: 10.1162/01489260152815297

Dancer, A., and Hamery, P. (1998). "Nonlinear hearing protection devices," in *National Hearing Conservation Association - NHCA-Meeting* (Albuquerque, NM).

Gardner, M. B., and Gardner, R. S. (1973). Problem of localization in the median plane: effect of pinna cavity occlusion. *J. Acoust. Am. Soc.* 53, 400–408. doi: 10.1121/1.1913336

Hartmann, W. M. (1999). How we localize sound. *Phys. Today* 52, 24–29. doi: 10.1063/1.882727

Hofman, P. M., and van Opstal, A. J. (2003). Binaural weighting of pinna cues in human sound localization. *Exp. Brain Res.* 148, 458–470. doi: 10.1007/s00221-002-1320-5

Hofman, P. M., Van Riswick, J. G. A., and Van Opstal, A. J. (1998). Relearning sound localization with new ears. *Nat. Neurosci.* 1, 417–421. doi: 10.1038/1633

Lewald, J., and Hausmann, M. (2013). Effects of sex and age on auditory spatial scene analysis. *Hear. Res.* 299, 46–52. doi: 10.1016/j.heares.2013.02.005

Lukas, K. B., and Ahroon, W. A. (2006). Free-field sound localization with non-linear hearing protection devices. *J. Acoust. Soc. Am.* 120, 3080–3081. doi: 10.1121/1.4787423

Mershon, D. H., and King, L. E. (1975). Intensity and reverberation as factors in the auditory perception of egocentric distance. *Percept. Psychophys.* 18, 409–415. doi: 10.3758/BF03204113

Nicol, R. (2010). *Binaural Technology. AES Monograph.* New York, NY: Audio Engineering Society.

Parmentier, G., Dancer, A., Buck, K., Kronengerger, G., and Beck, C. (2000). Artificial Head (ATF) for evaluation of hearing protectors. *Acustica* 86, 847–852.

Sharon, M. A., Tsang, S., and Boyne, S. (2007). Sound localization with communications headsets: comparison of passive and active systems. *Noise Health* 9, 101–107. doi: 10.4103/1463-1741.37426

Shaw, E. A. G. (1974). Transformation of sound pressure level from the free field to the eardrum in the horizontal plane. *J. Aeoust. Soc. Am.* 56, 1848–1861. doi: 10.1121/1.1903522

Simpson, B. D., Bolia, R., Mckinley, R., and Brungart, D. (2005). The impact of hearing protection on sound localization and orienting behavior. *Hum. Fact.* 47, 188–198. doi: 10.1518/0018720053653866

Wightman, F. (1999). Resolution of front back ambiguity in spatial hearing by listener and source movement. *J. Acoust. Soc. Am.* 105, 2841–1853. doi: 10.1121/1.426899

Wightman, F., and Kistler, D. J. (1989). Headphone simulation of freefielld listening: i stimulus synthesis. *J. Acoust. Soc. Am.* 85, 858–867. doi: 10.1121/1.397557

Wightman, F., and Kistler, D. J. (1992). The dominant role of low-frequency interaural time differences in sound localization. *J. Acoust. Soc. Am.* 91, 1648–1166. doi: 10.1121/1.402445

Zahorik, P., Brungart, D. S., and Bronkhorst, A. W. (2005). Auditory distance perception in humans: a summary of past and present resarch. *Acta Acust. united Ac.* 91, 409–420.

Zimpfer, V., Sarafian, D., and Hamery, P. (2012). "Spatial localization of sound with hearing protection devices allowing speech communication," in *Proceeding of the Annual IOA Meeting and The 11th SFA Meeting* (Nantes), 5.

18

Relating age and hearing loss to monaural, bilateral and binaural temporal sensitivity[1]

Frederick J. Gallun[1,2]*, Garnett P. McMillan[1,3], Michelle R. Molis[1,2], Sean D. Kampel[1], Serena M. Dann[1] and Dawn L. Konrad-Martin[1,2]

[1] National Center for Rehabilitative Auditory Research, Department of Veterans Affairs, Portland VA Medical Center, Portland, OR, USA
[2] Otolaryngology/Head and Neck Surgery, Oregon Health and Science University, Portland, OR, USA
[3] Department of Public Health and Preventive Medicine, Oregon Health and Science University, Portland, OR, USA

***Correspondence:**
Frederick J. Gallun, VA RR&D National Center for Rehabilitative Auditory Research, Portland VA Medical Center, 3710 SW US Veterans Hospital Road (NCRAR), Portland, OR 97207, USA
e-mail: frederick.gallun@va.gov

Older listeners are more likely than younger listeners to have difficulties in making temporal discriminations among auditory stimuli presented to one or both ears. In addition, the performance of older listeners is often observed to be more variable than that of younger listeners. The aim of this work was to relate age and hearing loss to temporal processing ability in a group of younger and older listeners with a range of hearing thresholds. Seventy-eight listeners were tested on a set of three temporal discrimination tasks (monaural gap discrimination, bilateral gap discrimination, and binaural discrimination of interaural differences in time). To examine the role of temporal fine structure in these tasks, four types of brief stimuli were used: tone bursts, broad-frequency chirps with rising or falling frequency contours, and random-phase noise bursts. Between-subject group analyses conducted separately for each task revealed substantial increases in temporal thresholds for the older listeners across all three tasks, regardless of stimulus type, as well as significant correlations among the performance of individual listeners across most combinations of tasks and stimuli. Differences in performance were associated with the stimuli in the monaural and binaural tasks, but not the bilateral task. Temporal fine structure differences among the stimuli had the greatest impact on monaural thresholds. Threshold estimate values across all tasks and stimuli did not show any greater variability for the older listeners as compared to the younger listeners. A linear mixed model applied to the data suggested that age and hearing loss are independent factors responsible for temporal processing ability, thus supporting the increasingly accepted hypothesis that temporal processing can be impaired for older compared to younger listeners with similar hearing and/or amounts of hearing loss.

Keywords: aging, hearing loss, gap discrimination, monaural, binaural

INTRODUCTION

It has been shown that older listeners often do more poorly at detecting or discriminating temporal differences imposed on stimuli at the various time scales relevant to speech understanding (e.g., Ross et al., 2007; Fitzgibbons and Gordon-Salant, 2010; Ruggles et al., 2011; Moore et al., 2012). One area that has received substantial attention recently is sensitivity to extremely rapid changes in acoustical information over time, sometimes referred to as "temporal fine structure" (TFS) (Moore, 2014), and a number of studies have shown that TFS sensitivity is impaired in older listeners (e.g., Durlach et al., 1981; Moore et al., 1992; Dubno et al., 2002, 2008; Ross et al., 2007; Strelcyk and Dau, 2009; Grose and Mamo, 2010; Ruggles et al., 2011; Hopkins and Moore, 2011). In addition, there are a large number of studies that have looked at performance differences between older and younger listeners at longer time scales sometimes associated with "envelope" processing (see, for example, Gordon-Salant and Fitzgibbons, 1999; Roberts and Lister, 2004; Lister and Roberts, 2005; Ajith and Sangamanatha, 2011). One persistent difficulty in studies of the impacts of aging on both TFS and envelope processing is the confounding of age and hearing loss due to the prevalence of age-related hearing loss in the samples tested, especially given the extensive evidence that cochlear damage reduces sensitivity to temporal information (e.g., Buss et al., 2004; Lorenzi et al., 2006; Henry and Heinz, 2012; reviewed in Moore, 2014). Thus, the common occurrence of age-related hearing loss complicates the interpretation of the impacts of age on temporal processing for the majority of published studies, especially if one considers the possibility that even relatively small changes in hearing could have substantial impacts on temporal processing ability (e.g., Takahashi and Bacon, 1992; He et al., 2008; Ruggles et al., 2011).

While there are studies that have shown that aging can impact both TFS (e.g., He et al., 2008; Moore et al., 2012; King et al.,

[1]Portions of this research were presented at the 2012 Midwinter Meeting of the Association for Research in Otolaryngology, San Diego, CA and the 2014 American Auditory Society Meeting, Scottsdale, AZ.

2014) and envelope processing (e.g., Ajith and Sangamanatha, 2011) independent of hearing loss, there are two other issues that make it difficult to draw as strong conclusions as we might like about the role of aging on temporal processing from the literature. The first is that there are few examples of studies that have examined how aging affects performance in the same listeners across multiple tasks and multiple stimuli, which raises the possibility that the deficits observed may not generalize to other stimuli and to the sorts of real world situations with which we are most concerned. Hopkins and Moore (2011) reported on one of the few studies that has examined TFS sensitivity and aging using multiple tests. In that study, they found significant impacts of age on TFS processing (but not frequency selectivity) as well as a modest but significant relationship between two different TFS tests.

The second issue that could make it difficult to draw strong inferences about the effects of aging on temporal processing is the fact that studies of aging and temporal sensitivity routinely have found that as a group older listeners are much more variable than are younger listeners, regardless of the task examined and the stimuli used. Although the source of this variation is not well understood, it has been hypothesized that small variations in hearing thresholds (in or near the "normal" range) are associated with larger suprathreshold discrimination difficulties (e.g., Ruggles et al., 2011). If this is the case, then one possibility is that deficits in suprathreshold discrimination are proportional to hearing loss, and thus groups of listeners who appear to all have "normal" hearing could actually vary in ability due to slight changes in hearing sensitivity. An alternative hypothesis is that older listeners are more variable in their basic ability to perform psychophysical tasks, due to cognitive difficulties commonly associated with aging, such as declines in working memory and decreased speed of processing (e.g., Schneider et al., 2010). A third hypothesis is that age-related changes at the level of the brainstem and its auditory nerve input could degrade the temporal information available at these and all later stages of processing (e.g., Helfert et al., 1999; Wang et al., 2009; Sergeyenko et al., 2013). While these central-auditory changes might be correlated to some extent with hearing loss, they may represent sources of additional variability in temporal processing performance.

To test these various hypotheses, and to generally learn more about the temporal processing abilities of older listeners, three temporal discrimination tasks were investigated in a large group of listeners varying in age and with normal hearing ranging to moderate hearing loss, using a variety of stimuli varying in TFS. There were two main goals of the experiments. The first was to determine whether or not performance was limited for the older listeners across all tasks and stimuli, or whether there were some tasks or stimuli for which performance was preserved. This was assessed by examining both the group differences in performance and the correlations in performance across the tasks and stimuli. In order to examine the importance of sensitivity to TFS, both in the various tasks and across listener groups, four stimuli were developed (described in detail below). All were 4 ms in total duration and shared a similar onset/offset envelope, but the frequency content and/or phase relationships of the stimulus components were varied in a manner that was hypothesized to change the pattern and timing of the activity on the basilar membrane and thus, presumably, on the auditory nerve as well. It was hypothesized that if listeners were sensitive only to the envelope cues, then all four stimuli would produce similar thresholds and performance for the four stimuli would be highly correlated for a given task. Futhermore, it was hypothesized that older listeners might obtain less benefit from the rising-frequency chirps due to increased temporal jitter at the level of the auditory nerve, which would reduce the ability to take advantage of a stimulus designed to create synchronous activity across many auditory nerve fibers.

The second main goal of the study was to use a statistical model to distinguish the effects of age on performance from the effects of hearing loss. This was facilitated by recruiting a large number of listeners with a range of ages, all with relatively good hearing thresholds. If the effects of age were due primarily to small changes in hearing thresholds, then the model would be expected to account for performance primarily based on hearing thresholds with little independent contributions of aging.

To reduce potential acoustic cues unrelated to temporal processing that can be introduced when a narrowband signal is perturbed in time (e.g., Leshowitz and Wightman, 1971; Schneider et al., 1994), the stimuli for each task always consisted of two brief pulses presented in either a standard configuration, which had the smallest gap possible given the constraints of the envelope ramps, or a comparison (or target) configuration, which had a larger gap (see below for details). This also had the advantage of making the psychophysical tasks very similar in that the same stimuli were presented and the task was to discriminate the standard "no gap" condition from the comparison "gap" condition. While this does not ensure that the same internal processes are used, it does eliminate potential confounds such as grouping or pitch cues that might be present in one task but not another if very different stimuli were used. A within-subjects design using similar stimuli also has the advantage that cognitive factors related to general task performance and memory for signal information (such as those identified by Neher et al., 2011) would be more likely to have equal influence on all measures than if the tests involved very different tasks or different groups of listeners.

The first task was the discrimination of the duration of temporal gaps in pairs of monaurally-presented stimuli. Previous research on monaural gap detection and duration discrimination (reviewed in Fitzgibbons and Gordon-Salant, 2010) has been fairly inconclusive, owing in large part to the variability among older listeners and the influence of various stimulus factors such as bandwidth and duration. For example, Moore et al. (1992) found substantially increased gap detection thresholds for two or three of their older listeners, but many of the older listeners had gap detection thresholds that were within the normal range. Similarly, Roberts and Lister (2004; Lister and Roberts, 2005) found that while gap detection thresholds were significantly higher for their older listeners, the difference between the younger and older listeners was fairly modest when the gap occurred between two stimuli of the same frequency rather than when the gap occurred between two stimuli differing in frequency. Fitzgibbons and Gordon-Salant (2010) suggest that variability in performance across a group of older listeners is more common when gaps are inserted into long-duration stimuli.

The second task was bilateral gap discrimination. The pairs of stimuli were almost identical to those used in the monaural gap discrimination task, with the crucial difference that the first stimulus in the pair was presented to the left ear and the second stimulus was presented to the right ear. This stimulus induces what has been termed the "precedence effect" (Wallach et al., 1949) or the "law of the first wavefront" (Blauert, 1997), whereby at small delays a listener hears only a single sound coming from the location of the first sound—in this case the left ear. The percept is entirely lateralized to the left ear for very short delays and then eventually becomes more centrally lateralized before finally breaking apart into two different stimuli (for a full description, see Stecker and Gallun, 2012). Roberts and Lister (2004; Lister and Roberts, 2005) found that the ability to detect a gap was much greater than in the monaural condition for all listeners and that the bilateral presentation revealed a greater difference between older and younger listeners than did the monaural. The number of listeners tested in those studies (24) was small enough, however, that some of the trends apparent in the data failed to reach statistical significance. By recruiting a larger group of listeners and limiting the amount of hearing loss, it was hoped that stronger relationships among tasks could be examined. Crucially, it was anticipated that the potential similarity (or dissimilarity) of the mechanisms underlying the monaural and bilateral gap discrimination tasks might be revealed by correlating performance within individual listeners—an analysis that failed to produce conclusive results for Lister and Roberts (2005).

The final task was a binaural discrimination task, in which the same stimuli were used, but presentation was synchronized across ears such that only a single stimulus was perceived, with the task now being the discirimination of diotic standard vs. a target that had an interaural difference in time ("ITD") imposed on both the envelope (onset and offset) and TFS (ongoing) portions of the stimulus. For young normal-hearing listeners, diotic presentation produces a single fused percept located in the center of the head. For the comparison stimulus, the onset of the stimulus presented to the right ear was delayed in time. This ITD produces the percept of a single stimulus located to the left of the center of the head. This task is similar to the "TFS-LF" (temporal fine structure with a low-frequency stimulus) task described by Hopkins and Moore (2010, 2011) in that it relies upon binaural differences. It has been well established that while hearing loss and/or aging are quite likely to reduce ITD thresholds (e.g., Durlach et al., 1981; Buus et al., 1984; Smoski and Trahiotis, 1986; Gabriel et al., 1992; Koehnke et al., 1995; Lacher-Fougère and Demany, 2005; Moore et al., 2012; King et al., 2014), very little is known about the relationships of monaural and binaural thresholds, or the correlation with bilateral gap discrimination using a precedence-like stimulus.

By testing a large group of listeners on a range of tests that probe the auditory system's temporal resolution abilities at a range of time scales, it was anticipated that stronger conclusions could be drawn regarding the effects of aging separate from hearing loss, as well as the importance of factors underpinning monaural temporal sensitivity for processing involving binaural brainstem mechanisms, such as ITD sensitivity.

EXPERIMENTAL METHODS

OVERVIEW

Two very similar experiments were conducted over two to three test sessions, using largely identical methods but a range of different stimuli. Seventy-eight listeners participated in the first experiment and 65 of those returned for the second experiment. For ease of comparison, the methods, results, and discussion of the two experiments are presented together in the sections below.

LISTENERS

Seventy-eight adults aged 18–75 years participated in this study. For initial analyses, the participants were divided into a "younger" group ($n = 37$; 18–44 yrs; average ("avg") 29.0 years, standard deviation ("SD"), of 7.1 years) and an "older" group ($n = 41$; 45–75 years; avg of 58.7 years, SD of 8.4 yrs). Average hearing thresholds were between 8 and 20 dB HL for octave and half-octave audiometric frequencies between 250 and 8000 Hz, with SD at each frequency of 6–20 dB HL. Audiometric data are shown in **Figure 1** for the younger and older listeners. The younger listeners had pure-tone averages of the frequencies 500, 1000, 2000, and 4000 Hz (PTAs) of 6.3 dB HL in the left ear (SD of 5.1 dB HL) and 6.9 dB HL in the right ear (SD of 4.4 dB HL). The older listeners had PTAs of 17.2 dB HL in the left ear (SD of 8.6 dB HL) and 16.8 dB HL in the right ear (SD of 7.9 dB HL). No listeners had sensorineural hearing losses greater than 40 dB HL at frequencies below 1000 Hz or greater than 60 dB HL at frequencies between 1000 and 4000 Hz. Comparisons of air and bone conduction audiometric thresholds, along with immittance results confirmed the sensorineural nature of the hearing losses. The difference in PTAs across ears was similar for the younger (avg of 2.7 dB, SD of 2.0 dB) and older listeners (avg of 4.1 dB, SD of 3.4 dB). The greatest difference in the younger group was 8.75 dB and the greatest difference in the older group was 15 dB. While PTAs described above demonstrate that the hearing thresholds of most listeners were in or near the "normal" range, it is still the case that some moderate losses were present, especially at higher frequencies, and, more importantly, that age and hearing loss were covarying in this data set. Consequently, a statistical model was applied to the data to allow these two factors to be further distinguished. All subjects provided written informed consent prior to participation and were paid per session. The procedures were approved and overseen by the Portland VA Medical Center's Institutional Review Board.

Sixty-five of the listeners returned for testing on a second experiment. Twenty-eight returned from the younger group (avg age of 29.0 yrs, SD of 7.5) and 37 returned from the older group (avg age of 58.19 years, SD of 8.0). The younger listeners had PTAs of 6.3 dB HL in the left ear (SD of 5.0 dB HL) and 6.9 dB HL in the right ear (SD of 4.5 dB HL). The older listeners had PTAs of 17.6 dB HL in the left ear (SD of 9.0 dB HL) and 17.0 dB HL in the right ear (SD of 8.2 dB HL). The avg difference in PTAs across ears for the younger listeners was 2.2 dB (SD of 1.5 dB) and the avg difference for the older listeners was 4.2 dB (SD of 3.5 dB). The greatest difference in the younger group was 6.25 dB and the greatest difference in the older group was 15 dB. The data from Experiment Two were also entered into the statistical model in order to better distinguish the effects of age and hearing loss.

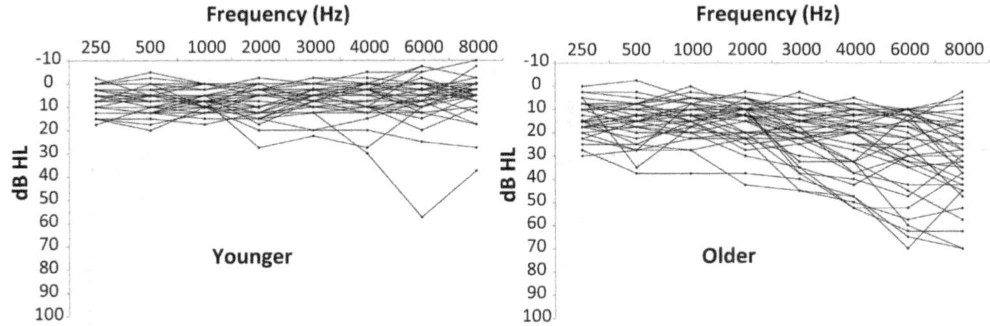

FIGURE 1 | Audiometric data for younger (left panel) and older (right panel) participants. See text for details.

STIMULI

Tasks (described below in Procedures) were each conducted using one of four different types of stimuli (shown in **Figure 2**). **Figure 2A** shows the temporal and spectral representations of the "tone burst" stimulus, which consisted of a 2 kHz pure tone multiplied by a 4-ms Gaussian envelope. The frequency spread of this stimulus was fairly narrow (50 dB down at 1 and 3 kHz) and the amplitude was near zero outside of the region from 0.75 ms to 3.5 ms. **Figure 2B** shows the "chirp" stimulus, which was based on the rising-frequency glide stimulus developed by Dau et al. (2000) in an attempt to invert the timing of the cochlear traveling wave and thus stimulate the entire basilar membrane simultaneously. In order to reduce the differences in audibility across listeners, the high-frequency portion of the original stimulus was truncated, resulting in a signal with maximum energy at about 2 kHz, and little energy (50 dB down) by 10 kHz. Substantial energy was still present at the lower frequencies, however (approximately 10 dB down at 20 Hz and 4 kHz).

To address some of the issues associated with comparing such different stimuli, two further stimuli were developed, on which a subset of the listeners were tested in the second experiment. The "reverse chirp" is shown in **Figure 2C**, and it can be seen that the spectrum is identical to that of the chirp stimulus, but the temporal waveform is reversed. The "noise chirp," for which the energy was the same as for the chirp, but the phases of the components were randomized, is shown in **Figure 2D**. This signal was created by transforming the chirp into a frequency domain representation by Fast-Fourier Transform (FFT, Matlab; Mathworks, Natick, MA), randomizing the phase values, and then performing an inverse transform (IFFT, Matlab). As the waveforms created in this way were influenced substantially by the randomization process, a new waveform was generated on each trial, although the same waveform was used throughout the entire trial. Thus for each trial a single waveform was generated and then was used multiple times (i.e., on either side of the gap and in each interval).

PROCEDURES

Single stimulus detection

In order to establish true detectability of the stimuli used in the temporal discrimination experiments, all listeners first performed a single stimulus detection task for the "tone burst" stimulus and the "chirp" stimulus (described above in "Stimuli"). Thresholds were obtained for both ears by employing a four-interval (two-cue, two-alternative) forced-choice procedure in which the target was silence and the level of the standard was adaptively varied using a two-down, one-up procedure (Levitt, 1971). On each trial, four temporal intervals were presented (each marked visually), three of which contained the standard stimulus and one of which contained silence. On each trial, listeners were presented with an array of four vertically-aligned boxes, each of which was illuminated during one of the four listening intervals. The first and last intervals always contained the standard stimulus, as did either the second or third interval. The remaining interval (either the second or the third) contained the target (silence) and the task of the listener was to use the computer mouse to click on the box that had been illuminated while the target was presented. Listeners were provided with trial-by-trial feedback.

Standard stimuli were presented at a starting level of 70 dB peSPL, which is defined as the peak equivalent SPL, or the peak level of a pure tone at a given dB SPL (in this case 70 dB SPL). Because of the very short duration of the signals, the root-mean-square (RMS) level is a poor descriptor of signal level, so peak level (peSPL) was used instead. The initial level was changed by 5 dB on each of the first three reversals and then changed by 1 dB for the remaining six reversals, after which the levels at which those six reversals had occurred were averaged and that average was the estimated threshold. Levels were not allowed to fall below 0 dB or exceed 95 dB peSPL. Tracks hitting these upper or lower limits simply resulted in repeated presentations of the limiting values. This rarely occurred. The thresholds obtained in this single stimulus detection task were all below the levels used in the temporal discrimination tasks, which established that all stimuli were audible (i.e., discriminable from silence) in the discrimination tasks and provided a measure of hearing threshold that was specific to these stimuli. In addition, the detection task served to familiarize the listeners both with the four-interval procedure and with the stimuli.

Discrimination tasks

Following the detection task, three discrimination tasks were conducted in fixed order: monaural gap discrimination, bilateral gap discrimination, and ITD discrimination. All stimuli in the remaining experiments were presented at a level of 85 dB peSPL. In Experiment 1, each task was conducted with both the tone

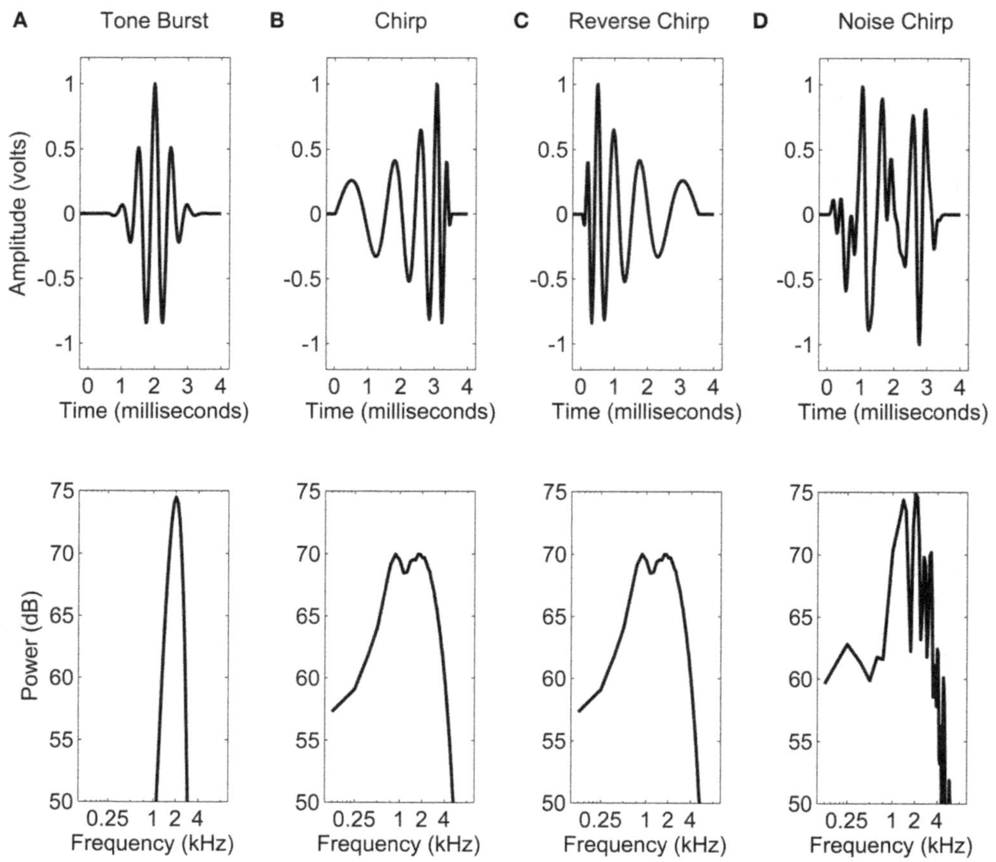

FIGURE 2 | Time waveforms (upper panels) and frequency spectra (lower panels) for the four stimulus types used. See text for details: **(A)** Tone burst; **(B)** Chirp; **(C)** Reverse chirp; and **(D)** Noise chirp.

burst and the chirp stimulus, and the order in which the two stimuli were tested for each task was assigned randomly for each listener. The sequence of three tasks was then repeated, yielding two measures on each of the three tasks for both stimuli. All subjects completed the full set of tasks for both stimuli in no more than two test sessions. Those who needed to return for a second session were given a practice run of all three tasks to remind them of the tasks and the stimuli. Testing on the reversed chirp and noise chirp took place on a subsequent session (Experiment 2), on which a subset of the tasks were tested and the tone and original chirp were re-tested as well.

All three discrimination tasks employed the same four-interval (two-cue, two-alternative) forced-choice procedure used in the detection task, but for the discrimination tasks the stimulus dimension being tested was temporal delay, which was adaptively varied using a two-down, one-up procedure (Levitt, 1971) with logarithmically-spaced intervals in time. Having been trained with the detection task, in which the target interval was easily identified (it being the interval that had both and auditory and a visual stimulus), listeners had no difficulty following these instructions and understanding the display.

Monaural gap discrimination

In this task, which was conducted independently for the left and right ears, the standard stimulus was two signals of the same type presented sequentially with no additional gap. Due to the need to ramp the signals on and off to control the frequency content (Leshowitz and Wightman, 1971), the signals all contained brief silent intervals at the beginning and end of the nominal durations. Consequently, there was a change in energy (a "gap") even in the standard stimulus. The target stimulus, therefore, was defined as the stimulus with the longer gap.

Target gap durations were initially set at 4 ms and were increased or decreased according to a two-down, one-up adjustment rule with adjustments occurring on a log scale. The first three reversals resulted in adjustments of five log units (i.e., from 4 ms up to 5.65 ms or down to 2.83 ms), while the remaining six reversals resulted in adjustments of one log unit (i.e., from 4 ms up to 4.28 ms or down to 3.73 ms). The geometric mean of the last six reversals was used as the threshold estimate. No delays smaller than 0.06 ms or greater than 128 ms were allowed to be presented.

Bilateral gap discrimination ("precedence threshold")

In this task, which can also be considered a "precedence" threshold, the standard and targets were a pair of stimuli identical to those used in the monaural gap discrimination task, but were presented sequentially at the two ears rather than sequentially to the same ear. First, the left-ear signal was presented, and immediately afterwards, the right-ear stimulus was presented. The target stimulus also consisted of a pair of bilateral signals presented first to the left ear and then to the right ear, but an additional delay was inserted between the offset at the left ear and the onset at the right ear. The initial delay was 4 ms, which should produce a percept of two signals in young, normally hearing listeners, and the duration was adaptively varied using the same stepping and averaging rules as for the monaural gap discrimination task. No delays smaller than 0.06 ms or greater than 128 ms were presented.

Interaural time difference (ITD) discrimination. In the final task, the standard stimulus was presented as a single diotic (identical onset and offset times at the two ears) waveform, thus producing a percept centered in the middle of the listener's head. The target stimulus was delayed in onset and offset at the right ear, producing interaural differences in time of onset, time of offset, and ongoing time differences all favoring the left ear. This should have produced a shift in perceived location toward the left ear (Blauert, 1997). The initial delay was set to 610 μs (0.61 ms), which is near the physiological limit of the time delays that the human head can produce, and the first three reversals resulted in changes of 5 log units (i.e., up from 0.61 ms to 0.91 ms or down to 0.41 ms) while the remaining six reversals resulted in changes of 1 log unit (i.e., up from 0.61 ms to 0.66 ms or down to 0.56 ms). The geometric mean of the last six reversal delays was taken as threshold. No delays smaller than 0.0048 ms (4.8 μs) or greater than 34 ms were presented.

RESULTS

SINGLE STIMULUS DETECTION

Average single stimulus detection thresholds for the tone burst and chirp stimuli were significantly different for the younger and older listeners. Average thresholds for both stimuli across groups are shown in **Table 1**. Thresholds averaged across the left and right ears are shown as a function of age for both stimuli in **Figure 3**. Results of a repeated-measures ANOVA performed on thresholds averaged between ears with stimulus as a within-subjects factor and age group as a between-subject factor is shown in **Table 4**, where it can be seen that age group was a significant factor and accounted for 31% of the variance, while stimulus type was also significant and accounted for 14% of the variance. **Table 1** shows that, while statistically significant, the differences between groups and between stimuli were fairly small (no greater than 8 dB at most) relative to the 20–25 dB threshold differences typically used to distinguish normal from impaired hearing.

MONAURAL GAP DISCRIMINATION

Monaural gap discrimination thresholds were calculated by taking the geometric mean of all of the values at which reversals occurred from all of the adaptive tracks obtained for each listener across all sessions tested. **Figures 4A,B** show the left and right ear discrimination thresholds as a function of age group and stimulus type. Average values, standard deviations, and 95% confidence intervals for the mean values are reported in **Table 2**. For comparison, binaural and bilateral discrimination thresholds are also shown in **Figures 4C,D**, with corresponding descriptive statistics shown in **Table 3**.

For the 78 subjects tested on the chirp and tone burst, a repeated-measures ANOVA conducted on the log-transformed

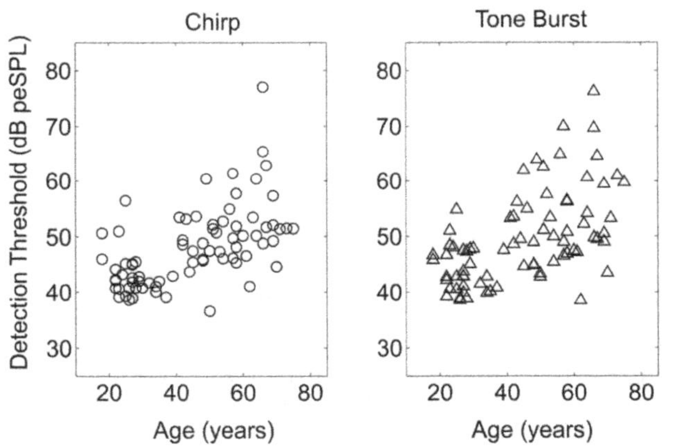

FIGURE 3 | Single stimulus detection thresholds plotted as a function of age of the listener for the Chirp and Tone Burst stimuli. Thresholds plotted are the average of the thresholds for the left and right ears.

Table 1 | Summary data for the single stimulus detection task, transformed from logarithmic values where appropriate, for ease of comparison with previously published data.

Stimulus	Ear	Age group	*n*	Single stimulus mean detection threshold (dB)	95% confidence interval for mean		Range
					Lower	Upper	
Tone burst	Left	Younger	37	45.17	43.03	47.30	4.27
		Older	41	54.24	51.20	57.29	6.09
	Right	Younger	37	44.85	43.36	46.35	2.99
		Older	41	52.95	50.23	55.66	5.42
Chirp	Left	Younger	37	43.55	41.80	45.29	3.49
		Older	41	51.27	48.60	53.94	5.34
	Right	Younger	37	44.03	42.36	45.71	3.35
		Older	41	51.80	49.74	53.86	4.11

Range (log) indicates the range of logarithmic values prior to transformation.

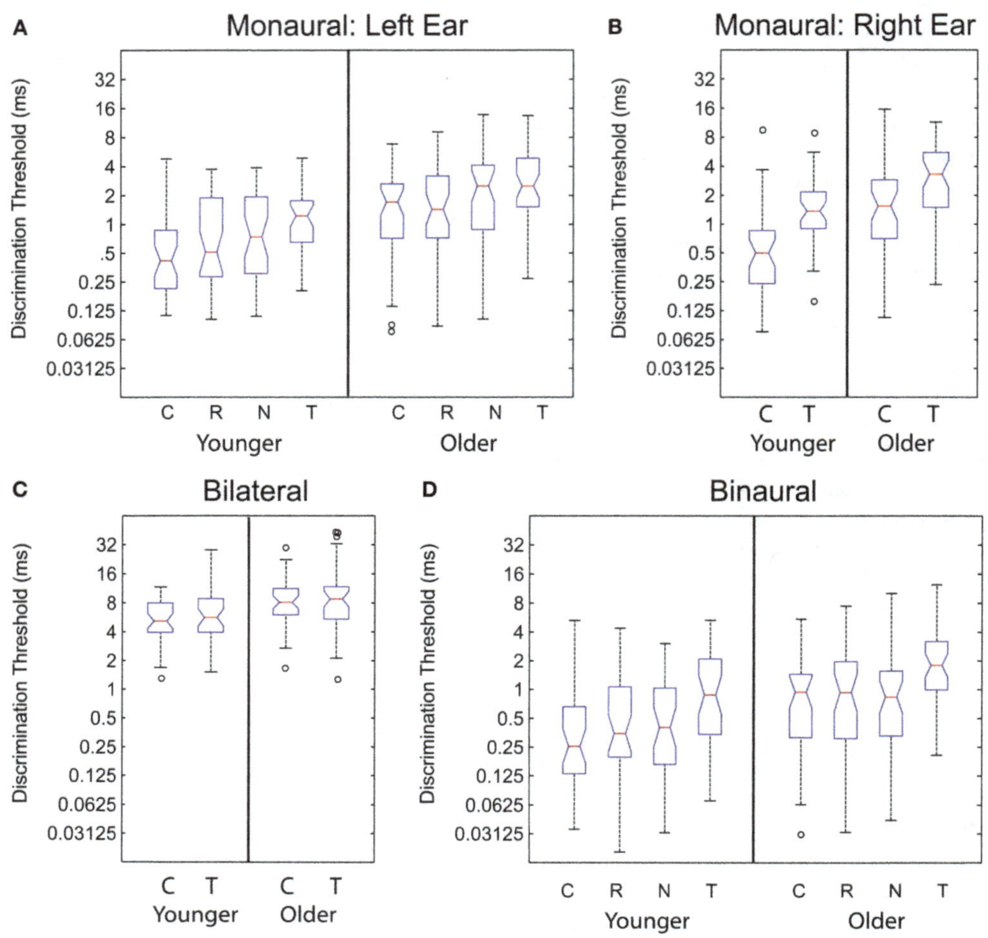

FIGURE 4 | Monaural (Panels A,B), bilateral (Panel C), and binaural (Panel D) discrimination thresholds plotted for the younger and older listeners as a function of stimulus type. C, Chirp; R, Reverse Chirp; N, Noise Chirp; T, Tone Burst. See text for details.

thresholds averaged across ears revealed a significant effect of stimulus and age group, but no significant interaction. Partial Eta Squared was used as a measure of variance explained, and stimulus accounted for 53%, while age accounted for 25%. The full set of statistical analyses is reported in **Table 4**.

For the 65 listeners tested on the reverse chirp and noise chirp stimuli in Experiment 2, only the left ear was tested. Average thresholds for the two age groups are shown in **Table 2** and the results of a repeated-measures ANOVA conducted on the chirp, reversed chirp, and noise chirp stimuli, with age group again added as a between-subjects factor, are shown in **Table 4**, in which results are pooled across both experiments. A significant effect of stimulus was obtained as well as a significant effect of age group, while again the interaction was not significant. The proportion of the variance accounted for by stimulus type was 10%, while age group accounted for 17%. A within-subjects contrast analysis of the three stimulus types revealed that thresholds on the original chirp were lower than for the reverse chirp, both of which were lower than for the noise chirp [$F_{(1, 63)} = 11.20$, $p < 0.01$], with this difference in stimulus type accounting for 15% of the variance in thresholds.

Discussion and conclusions

Results with the tone and chirp revealed that monaural gap discrimination thresholds were significantly higher for the older listeners. The discrimination thresholds are similar to those found by Schneider et al. (1994), although differences in the way the gap duration is described in that report make direct comparisons difficult. Thresholds in this study and in Schneider et al. (1994) are substantially lower than in many other reports, presumably due to the use of very brief stimuli. Further evidence that stimulus characteristics can have a substantial impact on performance was provided by the significantly lower thresholds for the chirp than for the tone burst for both the younger and older listeners. While this difference could be attributed to the broader bandwidth of the chirp, it was also possible that there was actual improvement in temporal performance due to the greater temporal synchrony at the level of the basilar membrane that is the result of the time-alignment of the stimulation for the rising-frequency chirp (see Dau et al., 2000 for a full discussion). The second experiment was developed to test this question, and to ask whether or not the younger listeners were more sensitive to this temporal synchrony. The results

Table 2 | Summary data for the monaural gap discrimination task, transformed from logarithmic values for ease of comparison with previously published data.

Stimulus	Ear	Age group	*n*	Monaural gap discrimination threshold (ms)	95% confidence interval for mean		Range	Range (log)
					Lower	Upper		
Tone burst	Left	Younger	37	1.11	0.85	1.44	0.59	0.75
		Older	41	2.57	1.98	3.34	1.36	0.76
	Right	Younger	37	1.29	0.98	1.69	0.71	0.78
		Older	41	2.83	2.16	3.72	1.56	0.79
Chirp	Left	Younger	37	0.46	0.34	0.63	0.29	0.89
		Older	41	1.28	0.89	1.83	0.94	1.04
	Right	Younger	37	0.50	0.35	0.72	0.37	1.04
		Older	41	1.51	1.07	2.13	1.06	0.99
Reversed chirp	Left	Younger	28	0.59	0.38	0.91	0.53	1.25
		Older	37	1.41	0.97	2.04	1.07	1.08
Noise chirp	Left	Younger	28	0.73	0.47	1.12	0.65	1.25
		Older	37	1.84	1.24	2.74	1.50	1.14

Range (log) indicates the range of logarithmic values prior to transformation.

Table 3 | Summary data for the bilateral and binaural discrimination tasks, transformed from logarithmic values where appropriate for ease of comparison with previously published data.

Stimulus	Task	Age group	*n*	Threshold (ms)	95% confidence interval for mean		Range	Range (log)
					Lower	Upper		
Tone burst	Bilateral	Younger	37	6.11	4.79	7.78	2.99	0.70
		Older	41	8.55	6.46	11.31	4.84	0.81
Chirp	Bilateral	Younger	37	5.05	4.18	6.10	1.92	0.55
		Older	41	8.11	6.76	9.73	2.97	0.53
Tone burst	Binaural	Younger	37	0.87	0.61	1.26	0.65	1.05
		Older	41	1.70	1.28	2.28	1.00	0.83
Chirp	Binaural	Younger	37	0.31	0.21	0.45	0.24	1.09
		Older	41	0.72	0.50	1.04	0.54	1.06
Reversed chirp	Binaural	Younger	28	0.39	0.24	0.65	0.41	1.45
		Older	37	0.74	0.47	1.16	0.69	1.30
Noise chirp	Binaural	Younger	28	0.37	0.23	0.59	0.35	1.33
		Older	37	0.74	0.49	1.13	0.64	1.21

Range (log) indicates the range of logarithmic values prior to transformation.

of the second experiment suggest that the timing of component frequencies reaching their characteristic frequency places at the level of the basilar membrane was important (i.e., best performance was achieved when each place was stimulated at about the same time), but that randomization of the component phases was more detrimental than reversing the component phase delays. Although reversing the timing should have substantially decreased the synchrony across auditory nerve fibers, the similar discrimination thresholds for original (rising frequency) and reversed (falling frequency) chirps suggest that the tone burst was less effective than the chirp primarily due to reduced bandwidth. The increased thresholds for the noise chirp relative to the rising and falling chirps suggest that listeners were using the temporal fine structure of the chirp itself to perform the discrimination, which would explain why randomizing the fine structure across trials would hurt performance. This is additional evidence against the use of a tonotopic ("place") cue, which would have been present regardless of the timing of the peaks in the waveform.

In order to examine the effect of age on variability, the range of values observed in the two age groups can be compared in **Table 2**. The column titled "Range" expresses the values in terms of linear units, while the column titled "Range (log)" shows the variation in log units. It is immediately apparent that a potential issue with comparing variability across these two groups differing in temporal discrimination thresholds is

Table 4 | Results of repeated-measures ANOVAs comparing the Tone vs. Chirp and Chirp vs. Reversed Chirp vs. Noise Chirp stimuli.

Task	Effect type	Source	Degrees of freedom	*F*	*p*-value	Partial eta squared
Single stimulus detection (Tone vs. Chirp)	Within-subjects	**Stimulus**	1,76	12.422	0.001	0.140
		Stimulus × Age group	1,76	0.811	0.371	0.011
	Between-subjects	**Age group**	1,76	33.740	0.000	0.307
Monaural gap discrimination (Tone vs. Chirp)	Within-subjects	**Stimulus**	1,76	87.568	0.000	0.535
		Stimulus × Age group	1,76	2.034	0.158	0.026
	Between-subjects	**Age group**	1,76	25.793	0.000	0.253
Monaural gap discrimination (Chirp vs. Reversed chirp vs. Noise chirp)	Within-subjects	**Stimulus**	2,126	7.443	0.001	0.106
		Stimulus × Age group	2,126	0.233	0.793	0.004
	Between-subjects	**Age group**	1,63	12.979	0.001	0.171
Bilateral gap discrimination (Tone vs. Chirp)	Within-subjects	Stimulus	1,76	1.599	0.210	0.021
		Stimulus × Age group	1,76	0.515	0.475	0.007
	Between-subjects	**Age group**	1,76	10.061	0.002	0.117
Binaural ITD discrimination (Tone vs. Chirp)	Within-subjects	**Stimulus**	1,76	96.198	0.000	0.559
		Stimulus × Age group	1,76	0.809	0.371	0.011
	Between-subjects	**Age group**	1,76	11.358	0.001	0.130
Binaural ITD discrimination (Chirp vs. Reversed chirp vs. Noise chirp)	Within-subjects	Stimulus	2,126	0.391	0.677	0.006
		Stimulus × Age group	2,126	0.423	0.656	0.007
	Between-subjects	**Age group**	1,63	5.859	0.018	0.085

Greenhouse-Geisser corrections for violations of the assumption of sphericity were conducted for the effect of stimulus, but the results were unchanged. Proportion of variance explained is estimated by the value of partial eta squared. Statistically significant sources of variance are indicated in bold.

that on a linear scale the ranges appear to differ by a factor of two to three, while on a log scale the ranges appear quite similar. For the same reason that the perception of amplitude is usually described using the logarithmic scale of decibels, it is appropriate to consider the perception of time on a logarithmic scale (see, for example, Saberi, 1995); as such, it seems likely that at least some of the increased variability previously observed for older listeners may have been due to the use of a linear scale in cases where a log scale would have been more appropriate.

BILATERAL GAP DISCRIMINATION

Listeners in the first experiment were tested on bilateral gap discrimination with the regular chirp and the tone burst stimulus. Thresholds for a given stimulus were again calculated as the geometric mean of all reversals from all of the adaptive tracks obtained for each listener across all sessions tested. Panel C of **Figure 4** shows the bilateral gap thresholds as a function of stimulus type and age group. Average threshold values are reported in **Table 3**. **Table 4** presents the results of a repeated-measures ANOVA conducted on the log-transformed bilateral gap thresholds, which did not show a significant effect of stimulus type but did show a significant effect of the between-subject factor of age group. The interaction was not significant. Age group accounted for 12% of the variance. As was observed for the monaural thresholds, the increased variability apparent on a linear scale was drastically reduced when the range of values was considered in logarithmic units.

Discussion and conclusions

This experiment revealed a significant effect of age group on bilateral gap discrimination. While a number of studies have examined the how age influences perception of precedence-type stimuli (e.g., Schneider et al., 1994; Roberts and Lister, 2004; Lister and Roberts, 2005), most have presented pairs of binaural stimuli rather than pairs of monaural stimuli. The design employed here reduces the potential influence of binaural sensitivity on the perception of precedence stimuli, but the greater perceived difference in position of the leading and lagging sounds may have interacted with the age effect, making direct comparisons with previous work more difficult. Schneider et al. (1994) found the delay at which the percept of two stimuli changed from a single sound to two sounds occurred at 6.6 ms for younger listeners and 7.0 ms for older listeners, but the variation in thresholds in both groups was very high. Similarly, Roberts and Lister (2004), found performance that was better than that observed in this study and that the non-significant age effect was in the opposite direction, with thresholds of 4.3 ms for younger listeners with normal hearing and 3.5 ms for older listeners with normal hearing. The number of subjects tested in those two studies was much lower than the number tested here; and so, it seems possible that neither of the previous studies had the statistical power to reveal effects between groups. In addition, it does not appear that logarithmic transformations were applied to the data before averaging, which would also have increased variability in the data, thus making it more difficult to observe differences that may have actually existed between the older and younger listener groups.

BINAURAL ITD DISCRIMINATION

Binaural ITD thresholds were calculated based on the geometric mean of all the reversals from all of the adaptive tracks obtained for each listener across all sessions tested. Mean data are shown in **Table 3** and displayed in **Figure 4D**, which shows the binaural discrimination thresholds as a function of age group for the four stimuli tested in Experiments 1 and 2. In **Table 4**, results of a repeated-measures ANOVA are shown. The effects of stimulus and age group were statistically significant and accounted for 56 and 13% of the variance, respectively. The interaction was not significant. The range of values observed for the younger listeners was similar to that for the older listeners when the log-transformed values were considered. For the 65 subjects tested on the additional chirp stimuli, a repeated-measures ANOVA comparing the original chirp, reversed chirp, and noise chirp failed to show a significant effect of stimulus type. The effect of age group was significant and accounted for 8.5% of the variance. The interaction was not significant. As with all of the other measures, the increased variability in thresholds for the older listeners was only present when the linear thresholds were considered.

Discussion and conclusions

These data augment the established observation that the binaural sensitivity of older listeners is degraded relative to that of younger listeners (e.g., Moore et al., 2012) by extending the finding to additional stimulus types. Most notably, unlike the monaural gap discrimination thresholds, there were no reliable differences among the three chirp stimuli, while thresholds were substantially lower for all three chirp stimuli relative to the tone burst. This suggests that for this task the energy of the chirp stimuli was playing a larger role in determining threshold than was the specific phase of the component frequencies. In particular, it seems likely that listeners were relying upon the low-frequency components of the stimuli, where the binaural information is strongest, and where the tone burst differs most from the chirps. The similarity across the chirp thresholds in the binaural discrimination task, but not in the monaural task, is consistent with the hypothesis that the information underlying the monaural judgment relates more strongly to the relative timing of the auditory nerve firings across fibers than does the binaural judgment, because performance on the monaural task was enhanced when activity on the basilar membrane would have stimulated the various frequency-tuned auditory nerve fibers at the same time, but performance on the binaural task was not. This is consistent with what is known about the inputs to the binaural system, which depend on cochlear nucleus processing to convey the information about the relative times at which stimuli are arriving at the two ears (reviewed in Stecker and Gallun, 2012) and so are less likely to be comparing information across auditory nerve fibers tuned to different frequencies.

GENERAL DISCUSSION

A primary goal of this study was to determine whether or not performance was limited for the older listeners across all tasks and stimuli, or whether there were some tasks or stimuli for which performance was preserved. A related goal was to examine the degree to which performances on all three tasks were correlated. This would indicate the degree to which performance was influenced by shared mechanisms such as cognitive declines associated with aging or shared peripheral or central auditory functioning. In many cases, performance measured on the various tasks with the various stimuli for an individual listener were reliably related to each other. Correlations across stimuli and tasks, as well as with age, are shown in **Table 5**. Correlations greater than 0.449 are significant after Bonferroni correction for multiple comparisons. The clearest result is the strong relationship among the three chirp stimuli for the monaural and binaural tasks (correlations of 0.79–0.87 for all combinations). This indicates a high test-retest reliability of the measures and suggests the maximum correlation that may be expected if the two tasks were drawing on very similar resources. The lower correlations between the chirp stimuli and the tone burst stimulus for the monaural gap task (values of 0.59–0.69) provide additional support for the conclusion that the monaural gap discrimination task is sensitive to the temporal fine structure of the stimulus. Fairly high correlations between the tone burst and the chirps for the binaural task (values of 0.72–0.80) suggest that the binaural task may be more strongly related to integrity of the binaural processing system *per se* and thus less influenced by stimulus factors.

High correlations between the monaural and binaural tasks suggest that there may be substantial overlap between the resources or neural elements contributing to these tasks. However, the finding that performance on the monaural task was more strongly influenced by differences in the temporal fine structure of the stimuli than was performance on the binaural task may reveal an important difference in resources required for these tasks. In particular, this finding is suggestive of a mechanism of TFS sensitivity that is present for the monaural task but not for the binaural task. Further support for a distinction between the neural resources supporting the two tasks comes from the modeling results (described below), which indicated a much stronger relationship between hearing loss and thresholds for the binaural than for the monaural task and, conversely, a greater impact of age on the monaural than on the binaural task.

While bilateral gap discrimination was reliably related to performance on both the monaural and binaural tasks, the range of correlations (values of 0.16–0.49) was substantially lower than the range of correlations between the monaural and binaural tasks (values of 0.46–0.64) and, in most cases, failed to reach statistical significance after correction for multiple comparisons. Even those that did reach significance failed to account for more than 10–15% of the variance. However, cognitive factors associated with aging still may have contributed to performances on these tasks and cannot be ruled out as potential influences. Furthermore, while the within-subjects design and the use of similar task demands was intended to reduce central influences, it is also the case that the three tasks may have relied upon very different decision processes, which would necessarily influence the results.

The second main goal of this study was to determine the degree to which the listener-specific factors that influence TFS sensitivity can be predicted by information about age and/or hearing loss. This issue is addressed by asking how much of the observed age effects depend on age alone and how much on concomitant

Table 5 | Correlations across stimuli and tasks, as well as with age.

		Monaural gap discrimination			
		Tone burst	**Chirp**	**Reversed chirp**	**Noise chirp**
Age		**0.516**	**0.524**	*0.398*	*0.384*
Single stimulus detection	Tone burst	**0.422**	**0.421**	*0.436*	*0.445*
	Chirp	**0.483**	**0.470**	*0.298*	*0.387*
Monaural gap discrimination	Tone burst		**0.691**	**0.572**	**0.591**
	Chirp			**0.857**	**0.793**
	Reversed chirp				**0.846**
Bilateral gap discrimination	Tone burst	**0.442**	*0.277*	0.207	0.160
	Chirp	**0.417**	**0.490**	*0.316*	*0.340*
		Bilateral gap discrimination		**Single stimulus detection**	
		Tone burst	**Chirp**	**Tone burst**	**Chirp**
Age		0.159	*0.374*	**0.512**	**0.535**
Single stimulus detection	Tone burst	*0.278*	*0.395*		**0.808**
	Chirp	*0.305*	*0.341*		
Bilateral gap discrimination	Chirp	*0.350*			
		Binaural ITD discrimination			
		Tone burst	**Chirp**	**Reversed chirp**	**Noise chirp**
Age		*0.403*	*0.381*	*0.287*	*0.311*
Single stimulus detection	Tone burst	**0.455**	*0.311*	*0.308*	*0.356*
	Chirp	*0.410*	*0.394*	*0.348*	*0.421*
Monaural gap discrimination	Tone burst	**0.488**	**0.587**	**0.503**	**0.495**
	Chirp	**0.569**	**0.627**	**0.509**	**0.636**
	Reversed chirp	**0.562**	**0.581**	**0.465**	**0.616**
	Noise chirp	**0.557**	**0.600**	**0.515**	**0.625**
Bilateral gap discrimination	Tone burst	*0.396*	**0.448**	*0.344*	*0.355*
	Chirp	**0.423**	*0.383*	*0.325*	*0.349*
Binaural ITD discrimination	Tone burst		**0.725**	**0.747**	**0.806**
	Chirp			**0.867**	**0.806**
	Reversed chirp				**0.857**

For ease of comparison, only left ear values are shown for monaural tasks, but relationships were similar for the two ears. Seventeen different values were entered into the correlation matrix from which the values shown below are drawn (four tasks, two to four stimuli, left and right ears for the monaural tests, and age). Using the Bonferroni adjustment for multiple comparisons (p-value/number of comparisons) indicates that the p-value for significance used should be 0.00018, rather than 0.05. For the reversed chirp and noise chirp stimuli ($n = 65$), all correlations above 0.245 (6% of variance accounted for) are significant at the $p < 0.05$ level, while only those above 0.449 (20% of variance) are significant at the $p < 0.00018$ level. For the tone burst and chirp stimuli ($n = 78$), all correlations above 0.230 (5% of variance) are significant at the $p < 0.05$ level, while only those above 0.412 (17% of variance) are significant at the $p < 0.00018$ level. Significant correlations ($p < 0.00018$) are indicated in bold type. Marginally significant correlations ($p < 0.05$) are indicated by italics.

hearing loss. The raw correlations are poor sources of information on this point due to the high correlations between age and single stimulus detection thresholds (correlations of 0.51–0.54). As performance on the various tasks was never correlated with age or hearing greater than 0.54, these raw correlations cannot be used to associate task performance with just a single listener factor. To address the issue of multiple potential predictors, a more sophisticated statistical analysis is required.

A partial correlation, in which the effects of one factor are "partialled out" to allow an estimate of the impact of the other, could be used to distinguish the impacts of age and hearing loss on the various task (e.g., Hopkins and Moore, 2011). While this would provide a parsimonious summary of the relationships between age, hearing loss, and test performance, there are several difficulties with this approach. Most importantly, each task is considered independently based on the average performance across all of the threshold measurements. This reduces the number of samples available and removes the ability to take into account the overarching ability of an individual listener to perform a psychophysical task. In addition, while the relationships can be specified, the exact changes in threshold that are associated with increasing age and hearing loss are not easily communicated. To avoid the limitations of the partial correlation approach, a linear mixed model was developed into which age and single stimulus detection threshold were entered as independent variables and thresholds were modeled for all three of the discrimination tasks. An important feature of this approach is the inclusion of a listener-specific random intercept to account for variability in each listener's ability to perform the tasks, independent of age and hearing loss. The model predictions, shown in **Table 6** and illustrated in **Figure 5**, are estimates of the percentage change in threshold (in log units) as a function of every 10% increase in single stimulus detection threshold for the tone stimulus (top panel) and the chirp stimulus (bottom panel). The gray lines represent

Table 6 | Results of a linear mixed model predicting changes in threshold on the three tasks as a function of age and single stimulus detection thresholds.

	Monaural			Binaural			Bilateral		
	Value (%)	Lower limit (%)	Upper limit (%)	Value (%)	Lower limit (%)	Upper limit (%)	Value (%)	Lower limit (%)	Upper limit (%)
% INCREASE IN THRESHOLD FOR EVERY 10 YEARS OF AGE									
Tone burst	31.3	18.2	45.8	15.1	−0.8	33.6	0.9	−11.3	14.8
Chirp	39.4	20.3	61.5	21.1	0.3	46.2	10.0	−0.1	21.1
Reversed chirp	28.3	5.8	55.7	17.6	−6.9	48.7	.	.	.
Noise chirp	21.6	−0.1	48.1	16.1	−5.7	43.0	.	.	.
% INCREASE IN THRESHOLD WITH 10% INCREASE IN SINGLE STIMULUS DETECTION THRESHOLD									
Tone burst	5.4	−3.5	15.1	23.0	7.3	41.0	13.7	0.9	28.0
Chirp	10.2	−2.8	24.9	21.2	−1.3	48.9	9.4	−1.5	21.6
Reversed chirp	14.1	−7.0	39.9	21.0	−5.9	55.7	.	.	.
Noise chirp	27.9	3.9	57.5	29.2	3.3	61.6	.	.	.

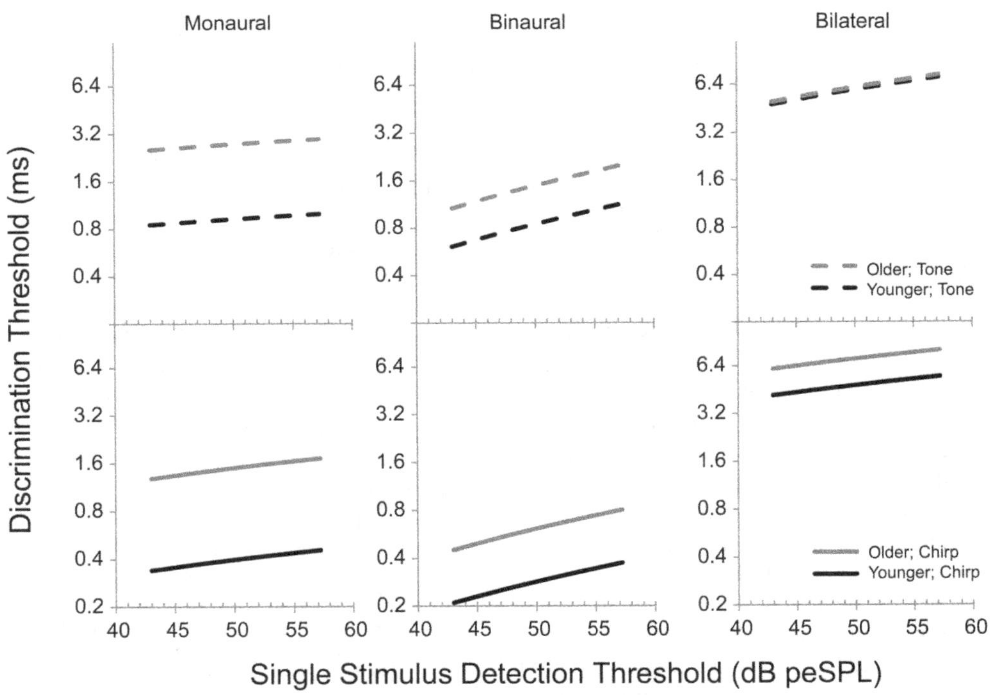

FIGURE 5 | Model predictions of discrimination thresholds as a function of age and single stimulus detection threshold. All predictions are based on increases in threshold relative to a listener who is 20 years old with thresholds based on the lower limits of estimate of the mean for each value (see **Table 1** for values). The black lines ("Younger") indicate the changes in discrimination threshold that would occur for various hypothetical listeners each of whom is 20 years old but vary in detection threshold. The gray lines ("Older") indicate the thresholds for a hypothetical 60 year old listener. The dashed lines ("Tone") in the top panel illustrate the estimates for the Tone Burst stimulus, while the solid lines ("Chirp") in the lower panels illustrated the estimates for the Chirp stimulus. See **Table 6** for the values used to calculate the changes in threshold as a function of increases in age and detection threshold.

the predicted effects of single stimulus detection threshold on performance in the three discrimination tasks for a hypothetical listener who is 60 years old, while the black lines represent the changes in threshold that would occur for a listener who is 20 years old. While tempting, it should be remembered that it is not appropriate to compare the size of the age effects to those of the hearing loss effects, because it does not make sense to assume, for example, that 10 years of age and 10 dB of hearing loss are in some way equivalent. It is appropriate, however, to ask the degree to which age or hearing loss has an equivalent effect on various tasks. The slope values and differences in the vertical locations of the lines were calculated directly from the values shown in **Table 6**. In order to examine the effect of age graphically, one should observe the difference in the vertical location of the black and gray lines. If the lines are on top of each other, there is no effect of age. To examine the effect of hearing loss graphically, one should observe the slope of the lines. If the line is flat, there is no effect of hearing loss (as measured in the single stimulus detection task). Note that the model did not specify a significant interaction between age and hearing loss, and so the lines in each panel are always parallel.

When analyzed in this manner, two trends are immediately apparent from the model predictions. First, age and hearing loss are each independently associated with changes in performance on nearly all of the tasks. The exception is the effect of age on the bilateral gap discrimination task with the tone burst stimulus, where the estimated effect size is only 0.9% (as indicated by the very small separation between the lines). For all other tasks, the predicted performance changes in discrimination threshold are all between 9.4 and 39.4% for every 10 years of difference in the ages of the participants or 10% difference in detection thresholds. The second clear trend from the modeling is that age appears to have a greater impact on monaural than on binaural performance (the lines are separated more substantially in the first vertical column of panels than in the second), while hearing loss has a greater influence on binaural than on monaural thresholds (the slopes of the lines are greater in the second vertical column of panels than in the first). Age appears to result in smaller changes to performance on the bilateral task than with the other two tasks (the lines are very close together in the third vertical column of panels), while hearing loss seems to result in similarly sized changes in performance for the monaural and bilateral tasks (the slopes are similar in the first and third vertical columns of panels).

Unfortunately, substantial amounts of the variability in performance across listeners was unrelated to either age or hearing, reducing the power of the predictive function for determining the expected temporal performance of an individual based solely on these two factors. Recent evidence shows that age-related changes in the temporal responses of neurons within the cochlear nucleus and inferior colliculus result from the loss of auditory nerve inputs to the brainstem (Helfert et al., 1999; Wang et al., 2009), which can occur as a consequence of exposure to noise (Kujawa and Liberman, 2006) even when noise exposures produce only temporary threshold shifts and no hair cell damage (Kujawa and Liberman, 2009). Ongoing research is aimed at determining the extent to which the remaining variability can be accounted for by auditory nerve fiber loss using non-invasive measures of auditory nerve survival in the same subjects.

SUMMARY

Group analyses revealed substantial increases in temporal discrimination thresholds for the older listeners, regardless of stimulus type and across all three tasks. Significant correlations were observed among all three tasks, but the correlations were relatively weak between the bilateral task and the other two, suggesting that the bilateral gap task was drawing upon a unique pool of neural processing elements, in addition to being limited by hearing thresholds and, potentially, by an overall decrease in cognitive function associated with aging.

The findings reported here have important implications for any future work examining TFS sensitivity by using a binaural task, such as that employed by Hopkins and Moore (2011). In particular, researchers using such a task will need to consider the possibility that, while both monaural and binaural tasks rely upon TFS, the specific processing needed for binaural tasks may not be directly related to the processing used in even a very similar monaural task. This issue is particularly relevant for those researchers interested in probing the role of TFS in speech understanding in complex auditory environments. Finally, it is important to note that, given the fairly low correlations observed across some of the tasks and stimuli, it is not obvious that real-world performance (which was not tested here) would be accurately predicted for an individual if that prediction were based only on performance with artificial stimuli or with tasks not strongly related to those performed in real-world environments.

ACKNOWLEDGMENTS

This research was supported by the Department of Veterans Affairs Rehabilitation Research and Development (VA RR&D) Service [Merit Award C7450R, Career Development Awards C4963W (Gallun) and C6116W (Molis), and Career Development Transition Award C7113N (Konrad-Martin)]. The work was supported with resources and the use of facilities at VA RR&D National Center for Rehabilitative Auditory Research, which is located at the Portland VA Medical Center. We are extremely grateful to the many participants who volunteered their time and ears to make this work possible. The code used to create the chirp stimuli was modified from original Matlab functions generously provided by Dr. Torsten Dau. The contents of this article are the private views of the authors and should not be assumed to represent the views of the Department of Veterans Affairs or the United States Government.

REFERENCES

Ajith, K. U., and Sangamanatha, A. V. (2011). Temporal processing abilities across different age groups. *J. Am. Acad. Audiol.* 22, 5–12. doi: 10.3766/jaaa.22.1.2

Blauert, J. (1997). *Spatial Hearing: the Psychophysics of Human Sound Localization, Rev. Edn.* Cambridge, MA: MIT Press.

Buss, E., Hall, J. W. 3rd., and Grose, J. H. (2004). Temporal fine-structure cues to speech and pure tone modulation in observers with sensorineural hearing loss. *Ear Hear.* 25, 242–250. doi: 10.1097/01.AUD.0000130796.73809.09

Buus, S., Scharf, B., and Florentine, M. (1984). Lateralization and frequency selectivity in normal and impaired hearing. *J. Acoust. Soc. Am.* 76, 77–86. doi: 10.1121/1.391010

Dau, T., Wegner, O., Mellert, V., and Kollmeier, B. (2000). Auditory brainstem responses with optimized chirp signals compensating basilar-membrane dispersion. *J. Acoust. Soc. Am.* 107, 1530–1540. doi: 10.1121/1.428438

Dubno, J. R., Ahlstrom, J. B., and Horwitz, A. R. (2002). Spectral contributions to the benefit from spatial separation of speech and noise. *J. Speech Lang. Hear. Res.* 45, 1297–1310. doi: 10.1044/1092-4388(2002/104)

Dubno, J. R., Ahlstrom, J. B., and Horwitz, A. R. (2008). Binaural advantage for younger and older adults with normal hearing. *J. Speech Lang. Hear. Res.* 51, 539–556. doi: 10.1044/1092-4388(2008/039)

Durlach, N. I., Thompson, C. L., and Colburn, H. S. (1981). Binaural interaction in impaired listeners. A review of past research. *Audiology* 20, 181–211. doi: 10.3109/00206098109072694

Fitzgibbons, P. J., and Gordon-Salant, S. (2010). "Behavioral studies with aging humans: hearing sensitivity and psychoacoustics," in *The Aging Auditory System*, eds S. Gordon-Salant, R. D. Frisina, R. R. Fay, and A. Popper (New York, NY: Springer), 111–134.

Gabriel, K. J., Koehnke, J., and Colburn, H. S. (1992). Frequency dependence of binaural performance in listeners with impaired binaural hearing. *J. Acoust. Soc. Am.* 91, 336–347. doi: 10.1121/1.402776

Gordon-Salant, S., and Fitzgibbons, P. J. (1999). Profile of Auditory temporal processing in older listeners. *J. Speech Lang. Hear. Res.* 42, 300–311.

Grose, J. H., and Mamo, S. K. (2010). Processing of as a function of age. *Ear Hear.* 31, 755–760. doi: 10.1097/AUD.0b013e3181e627e7

He, N. J., Mills, J. H., Ahlstrom, J. B., and Dubno, J. R. (2008). Age-related differences in the temporal modulation transfer function with pure-tone carriers. *J. Acoust. Soc. Am.* 124, 3841–3849. doi: 10.1121/1.2998779

Helfert, R. H., Sommer, T. J., Meeks, J., Hofstetter, P., and Hughes, L. F. (1999). Age-related synaptic changes in the central nucleus of the inferior colliculus of Fischer-344 rats. *J. Comp. Neurol.* 406, 285–298. doi: 10.1002/(SICI)1096-9861(19990412)406:3<285::AID-CNE1>3.0.CO;2-P

Henry, K. S., and Heinz, M. G. (2012). Diminished temporal coding with sensorineural hearing loss emerges in background noise. *Nat. Neurosci.* 15, 1362–1364. doi: 10.1038/nn.3216

Hopkins, K., and Moore, B. C. J. (2010). The importance of temporal fine structure information in speech at different spectral regions for normal-hearing and hearing-impaired subjects. *J. Acoust. Soc. Am.* 127, 1595–1608. doi: 10.1121/1.3293003

Hopkins, K., and Moore, B. C. J. (2011). The effects of age and cochlear hearing loss on temporal fine structure sensitivity, frequency selectivity, and speech reception in noise. *J. Acoust. Soc. Am.* 130, 334–349. doi: 10.1121/1.3585848

King, A., Hopkins, K., and Plack, C. J. (2014). The effects of age and hearing loss on interaural phase difference discrimination. *J. Acoust. Soc. Am.* 135, 342–351. doi: 10.1121/1.4838995

Koehnke, J., Culotta, C. P., Hawley, M. L., and Colburn, H. S. (1995). Effects of reference interaural time and intensity differences on binaural performance in listeners with normal and impaired hearing. *Ear Hear.* 16, 331–353. doi: 10.1097/00003446-199508000-00001

Kujawa, S. G., and Liberman, M. C. (2006). Acceleration of age-related hearing loss by early noise exposure: evidence of a misspent youth. *J. Neurosci.* 26, 2115–2123. doi: 10.1523/JNEUROSCI.4985-05.2006

Kujawa, S. G., and Liberman, M. C. (2009). Adding insult to injury: cochlear nerve degeneration after "temporary" noise-induced hearing loss. *J. Neurosci.* 29, 14077–14085. doi: 10.1523/JNEUROSCI.2845-09.2009

Lacher-Fougère, S., and Demany, L. (2005). Consequences of cochlear damage for the detection of interaural phase differences. *J. Acoust. Soc. Am.* 118, 2519–2526. doi: 10.1121/1.2032747

Leshowitz, B., and Wightman, F. L. (1971). On-frequency masking with continuous sinusoids. *J. Acoust. Soc. Am.* 49(Pt 2), 1180–1190. doi: 10.1121/1.1912480

Levitt, H. (1971). Transformed up-down methods in psychoacoustics. *J. Acoust. Soc. Am.* 49, 467–477. doi: 10.1121/1.1912375

Lister, J. J., and Roberts, R. A. (2005). Effects of age and hearing loss on gap detection and the precedence effect: narrow-band stimuli. *J. Speech Lang. Hear. Res.* 48, 482–493. doi: 10.1044/1092-4388(2005/033)

Lorenzi, C., Gilbert, G., Carn, H., Garnier, S., and Moore, B. C. J. (2006). Speech perception problems of the hearing impaired reflect inability to use temporal fine structure. *Proc. Natl. Acad. Sci. U.S.A.* 103, 18866–18869. doi: 10.1073/pnas.0607364103

Moore, B. C. J. (2014). *Auditory Processing of Temporal Fine Structure: Effects of Age and Hearing Loss*. Singapore: World Scientific.

Moore, B. C. J., Glasberg, B. R., Stoev, M., Füllgrabe, C., and Hopkins, K. (2012). The influence of age and high-frequency hearing loss on sensitivity to temporal fine structure at low frequencies. *J. Acoust. Soc. Am.* 131, 1003–1006. doi: 10.1121/1.3672808

Moore, B. C. J., Peters, R. W., and Glasberg, B. R. (1992). Detection of temporal gaps in sinusoids by elderly subjects with and without hearing loss. *J. Acoust. Soc. Am.* 92(Pt 1), 1923–1932. doi: 10.1121/1.405240

Neher, T., Laugesen, S., Jensen, N. S., and Kragelund, L. (2011). Can basic auditory and cognitive measures predict hearing-impaired listeners' localization and spatial speech recognition abilities? *J. Acoust. Soc. Am.* 130, 1542–1558. doi: 10.1121/1.3608122

Roberts, R. A., and Lister, J. J. (2004). Effects of age and hearing loss on gap detection and the precedence effect: narrow-band stimuli. *J. Speech Lang. Hear. Res.* 47, 965–978. doi: 10.1044/1092-4388(2004/071)

Ross, B., Fujioka, T., Tremblay, K. L., and Picton, T. W. (2007). Aging in binaural hearing begins in mid-life: evidence from cortical auditory-evoked responses to changes in interaural phase. *J. Neurosci.* 27, 11172–11178. doi: 10.1523/JNEUROSCI.1813-07.2007

Ruggles, D., Bharadwaj, H., and Shinn-Cunningham, B. G. (2011). Normal hearing is not enough to guarantee robust encoding of suprathreshold features important in everyday communication. *Proc. Natl. Acad. Sci. U.S.A.* 108, 15516–15521. doi: 10.1073/pnas.1108912108

Saberi, K. (1995). Some considerations on the use of adaptive methods for estimating interaural–delay thresholds. *J. Acoust. Soc. Am.* 98, 1803–1806. doi: 10.1121/1.413379

Schneider, B. A., Pichora-Fuller, K., and Daneman, M. (2010). "Effects of senescent changes in audition and cognition on spoken language comprehension," in *The Aging Auditory System*, eds S. Gordon-Salant, R. D. Frisina, R. R. Fay, and A. Popper (New York, NY: Springer), 167–210.

Schneider, B. A., Pichora-Fuller, M. K., Kowalchuk, D., and Lamb, M. (1994). Gap detection and the precedence effect in young and old adults. *J. Acoust. Soc. Am.* 95, 980–991. doi: 10.1121/1.408403

Sergeyenko, Y., Lall, K., Liberman, M. C., and Kujawa, S. G. (2013). Age-related cochlear synaptopathy: an early-onset contributor to auditory functional decline. *J. Neurosci.* 33, 13686–13694. doi: 10.1523/JNEUROSCI.1783-13.2013

Smoski, W. J., and Trahiotis, C. (1986). Discrimination of interaural temporal disparities by normal-hearing listeners and listeners with high frequency sensorineural hearing loss. *J. Acoust. Soc. Am.* 79, 1541–1547. doi: 10.1121/1.393680

Stecker, G. C., and Gallun, F. J. (2012). "Binaural hearing, sound localization, and spatial hearing," in *Translational Perspectives in Auditory Neuroscience: Normal Aspects of Hearing*, Chapter 14, eds K. L. Tremblay and R. F. Burkard (San Diego, CA: Plural Publishing, Inc.), 383–434

Strelcyk, O., and Dau, T. (2009). Relations between frequency selectivity, temporal fine-structure processing, and speech reception in impaired hearing. *J. Acoust. Soc. Am.* 125, 3328–3345. doi: 10.1121/1.3097469

Takahashi, G. A., and Bacon, S. P. (1992). Modulation detection, modulation masking, and speech understanding in noise in the Elderly. *J. Speech Lang. Hear. Res.* 35, 1410–1421.

Wallach, H., Newman, E. B., and Rosenzweig, M. R. (1949). The precedence effect in sound localization. *Am. J. Psychol.* 62, 315–336. doi: 10.2307/1418275

Wang, H., Turner, J. G., Ling, L., Parrish, J. L., Hughes, L. F., and Caspary, D. M. (2009). Age-related changes in glycine receptor subunit composition and binding in dorsal cochlear nucleus. *Neuroscience* 160, 227–239. doi: 10.1016/j.neuroscience.2009.01.079

19

A review on auditory space adaptations to altered head-related cues

Catarina Mendonça**

Department of Signal Processing and Acoustics, School of Electrical Engineering, Aalto University, Espoo, Finland

***Correspondence:**
Catarina Mendonça, Department of Signal Processing and Acoustics, School of Electrical Engineering, Aalto University, Otakaari 5, 02150 Espoo, Finland
e-mail: catarina.hiipakka@aalto.fi

In this article we present a review of current literature on adaptations to altered head-related auditory localization cues. Localization cues can be altered through ear blocks, ear molds, electronic hearing devices, and altered head-related transfer functions (HRTFs). Three main methods have been used to induce auditory space adaptation: sound exposure, training with feedback, and explicit training. Adaptations induced by training, rather than exposure, are consistently faster. Studies on localization with altered head-related cues have reported poor initial localization, but improved accuracy and discriminability with training. Also, studies that displaced the auditory space by altering cue values reported adaptations in perceived source position to compensate for such displacements. Auditory space adaptations can last for a few months even without further contact with the learned cues. In most studies, localization with the subject's own unaltered cues remained intact despite the adaptation to a second set of cues. Generalization is observed from trained to untrained sound source positions, but there is mixed evidence regarding cross-frequency generalization. Multiple brain areas might be involved in auditory space adaptation processes, but the auditory cortex (AC) may play a critical role. Auditory space plasticity may involve context-dependent cue reweighting.

Keywords: localization, recalibration, learning, training, generalization

OVERVIEW

It is nowadays well accepted that there is great plasticity in the sensory systems. Sensory plasticity was once thought to be limited to early stages of life (Parks et al., 2004). However, it is now well established that it is a lifelong process (Gilbert et al., 2001), and plasticity in the auditory domain is no exception (Rauschecker, 1999). Analyzing how humans adapt to changes in auditory localization cues is an increasingly relevant topic. There are nowadays a growing number of technologies in the field of hearing that impact auditory space cues. Cochlear implants greatly disrupt cues (Rosen et al., 1999), since spectral information is displaced in the auditory nerve and binaural cues are changed. Adaptation processes are also observed in hearing loss (for a review see Keating and King, 2013), and may impact how subjects adapt to new hearing aids. Hearing aids themselves affect auditory cues and require substantial adaptation. But even normal listeners face the challenges of adapting to altered spatial cues, as more and more sound systems resort to sound spatialization technologies that replace individual cues.

Auditory localization cues are individualized, since they are mostly a product of the interaction between sound waves and the body, namely the head. When head features change, so do the localization cues. Auditory localization cues are classified as either binaural or monaural cues (Middlebrooks and Green, 1991; Blauert, 1997). Binaural cues are principally linked with localization in the horizontal plane (left-right), whereas monaural cues are more highly weighted in the vertical plane (top-down) and in front-back distinctions. Binaural cues are obtained by comparing the sound input to each ear. This input varies in frequency, but most importantly in time of arrival and level. Differences in time of arrival at each ear are called interaural time differences (ITD) and differences in level are called interaural level differences (ILD). Monaural cues are those cues that could be obtained by a single ear. They consist of the level at each frequency, and are frequently called spectral cues. All these elements have been manipulated, often together, in studies on adaptation to altered head-related auditory space cues. The purpose of this review is to provide an overview on such studies.

Articles in this field have analyzed such processes using different nomenclature. Here we refer to auditory space as the localization of auditory events, therefore this concept refers to the relation between an auditory scene and how it is perceived in the space domain. The concepts of learning, adaptation and recalibration have been used almost interchangeably in this field. Learning can be described as a more explicit change, the subject can be aware of the adaptation process. Adaptation can be described as any change, resulting from accommodation to altered cues. Auditory space recalibration implies that the change is not only local, but a general adaptation in the direction of restoring the perceptual accuracy. In this paper we most often use the concept of adaptation.

The scope of this review has been limited to adaptation processes due to changes in head-related cues. We made this selection due to the fact that there is limited evidence that humans improve localization accuracy when trained in normal, unaltered cues. Some studies report a modest improvement, while other show no effects (for a review see Wright and Zhang, 2006). Due to addressing only studies using altered head-related cues, several relevant studies using altered environment or altered audiovisual correspondences are not reported. There is also a focus on normal-listeners, since most studies focus on this population. However, most of the data reported here applies to impaired listeners and many studies simulate hearing loss adaptation processes. Finally, we put great emphasis on studies with human subjects, but we also approach animal studies, namely when analyzing the neurophysiological correlates of adaptation to altered sound localization cues.

The studies reported here have been conducted over decades, and range considerably in methods and nomenclature. This is partly due to the fact that there are contributions from fields as different as medicine, biology, psychology, and engineering. This review attempts to organize and uniformize concepts regarding methods and results. Finally, an overview is presented over proposed and potential explanations of the underlying adaptation processes. Data are presented according to the following structure: overview of methods to induce adaptation; general adaptation results; adaptation aftereffects; neurophysiological correlates; underlying processes; and concluding remarks.

METHODS TO INDUCE AUDITORY SPACE ADAPTATION

NATURE OF LOCALIZATION CUE MANIPULATION

A way of testing the human adaptations to altered head-related localization cues is to artificially produce a change to such cues. Here we present an overview of methods used to produce such changes. Clinical studies and methods that have never shown potential to induce adaptation have been left out. One such example is ear swapping (Young, 1928; Hofman et al., 2002). Presenting subjects with switched binaural input has been implemented for periods as long as 30 weeks, but adaptation has never been found.

Ear blocks

The most common method for auditory cue manipulation in human studies has been the use of unilateral blocks, in which one ear is plugged with a sound attenuating earplug. This method has also been used to simulate conductive hearing loss and analyze adaptation effects. The main effect of the ear block is to produce a sound level attenuation, and therefore alter ILDs, but ITDs are also changed. However, the ear blocks do not affect exclusively binaural cues, since they can produce frequency dependent attenuation (Kumpik et al., 2010). This approach has been implemented in animals (King et al., 2001; Kacelnik et al., 2006) and in humans. In humans, it can be placed intermittently or in long-term. When long-term blocks are applied, subjects return to their daily activities and receive consistent natural feedback from the cue perturbation during a given period of time (Bauer et al., 1966; Florentine, 1976; McPartland et al., 1997). When intermittent, blocks are applied only during the test sessions, and removed between sessions (Musicant and Butler, 1980; Butler, 1987 Strelnikov et al., 2011).

Ear molds

In this method, wearable molds are fitted to the subjects' pinnae, to induce anatomical changes to the outer ear. Sound frequency levels (spectral cues) are therefore altered for each source position. There have been three studies resorting to this technique in normal-hearing humans. In a study by Hofman et al. (1998), four subjects wore molds in both ears for a period of up to 6 weeks. These molds disturbed the direction-depending spectral shaping of the outer ear without producing sound attenuation. In another study, van Wanrooij and van Opstal (2005) applied a similar mold but only to one of the ears, thus creating only a partial spectral perturbation. Carlile et al. (2013) applied small ear molds to both ears, filling 40 percent of the outer ear. Subjects wore them for 10 days, during all waking hours.

Electronic hearing devices

Hearing devices, like hearing aids, containing an external microphone and an internal speaker, have also been used to alter the head-related auditory localization cues. This method is technically more demanding, but allows more manipulations and greater control over the cue changes. Two studies have implemented this technique on normal hearing humans. Javer and Schwarz (1995) introduced a constant time delay to one ear, producing an azimuth shift of 66° to the sound image. Held (1955) used two matched hearing devices and displaced the microphones by 20° in azimuth.

Altered head-related transfer functions

Sound localization cues are produced by one's own body and its interactions with sound waves. It is possible to synthesize sounds that include such cues through the use of head-related transfer functions (HRTFs). These functions consist of the impulse response and its Fourier transform between a sound source position and a listener's ear canal entrance (Wightman and Kistler, 1988; Gardner and Martin, 1994). The stimuli are most often synthesized by convolving the sound of interest with the impulse response corresponding to the desired sound source position. Because subjects vary greatly in their anatomy, so do the HRTFs. Therefore, for good localization, it is necessary to use individualized HRTFs. On the other hand, the use of non-individualized or altered HRTFs poses an opportunity to learn how humans can adapt and learn to localize with someone else's localization cues.

Shinn-Cunningham et al. (1998a,b) altered the HRTFs such that they displaced the filters laterally, away from the center, thus creating "supernormal" cues for frontal source discrimination. Zahorik et al. (2006) used a head-mounted display to present subjects with an audiovisual virtual world, rendered in real-time though head-tracking and using non-individualized HRTF-based sounds. Mendonça et al. (2012, 2013) trained subjects to localize with non-individualized HRTFs, analyzing generalization patterns and long-term effects. Parseihian and Katz (2012) compared adaptation to individual HRTFs, with adaptation to more or less altered HRTFs. By controlling the amount of change of the localization cues, they could analyze its impact on adaptation processes. Majdak et al. (2013) trained subjects in localizing HRTF-based sounds that were either warped in frequency or band-limited.

Audiovisual discrepancy

Although it is not within the scope of this review, auditory space adaptation through displaced visual and auditory information should be mentioned. In such approach, there is no alteration of the head-related sound localization cues. Instead, visual spatial information is shifted in order to become misaligned with auditory spatial information. Many studies have looked into this cross-modal adaptation effect. In animals, it is common to apply a long-term prism that displaces the visual information by a few degree (for a review, see King, 2009). In humans, visual information has been shown to induce fast auditory localization shifts in an effect called the ventriloquism aftereffect (e.g., Recanzone, 1998; Lewald, 2002; Kopčo et al., 2009). In the ventriloquism effect, the perceived position of a sound is realigned with that of a visual source when both are presented concomitantly, but in different positions. In its aftereffect, a shift of perceived auditory position is still observed, even after the visual information is removed. This effect reveals the impressive dominance of vision in human space perception. However, visual information is not necessary for auditory adaptation and it can even be less efficient than other methods (Kacelnik et al., 2006; Strelnikov et al., 2011; Carlile and Blackman, 2014).

TRAINING PARADIGMS

The methods used to induce adaptation to the altered head-related auditory localization cues are presented in this section. Methods were organized into three subgroups that vary mostly in intentionality. In sound exposure, subjects learn implicitly, without necessarily being aware of the adaptation process. In training with feedback, subjects are aware of the adaptation process and follow a specific training program. In active learning, subjects are actively and engaged in the learning task, and can learn implicitly or explicitly. Despite being presented separately, the methods are not mutually exclusive. There have been a few studies using several methods at once (see Section Adaptation by training).

Sound exposure

Training by sound exposure involves introducing a change to the head-related localization cues and allowing subjects to spontaneously adapt by listening to the altered sounds. Studies on humans and animals with congenital hearing impairment fit in this category. Also, in animal studies, chronic changes can be applied to the ears and then tested over time (e.g., King et al., 2001; Kacelnik et al., 2006). In this paradigm, subjects learn implicitly by continuous multisensory feedback. Since in this method subjects are allowed to move freely, there is continuous motor and visual feedback, allowing for rich feedback that replaces training. Some studies in this paradigm consist of a pre-test, exposure period, and a final post-test (e.g., Held, 1955). But most commonly, there are also regular tests during the exposure period, to analyze the adaptation pattern. Sound exposure paradigms can be separated into two different classes: long-term exposure and intermittent exposure.

In long-term exposure, experimenters apply the change to the localization cues, and then subjects use them continuously until the end of the experiment. Florentine (1976) had subjects wear a long-term unilateral block for a period of either 5, 22, 27, or 101 days for each of the four test subjects, respectively. van Wanrooij and van Opstal (2005) applied a long-term (9–49 days) monaural spectral perturbation. Held (1955) applied electronic hearing devices to his subjects for 8 h and allowed them to carry on with normal daily activities. In Hofman et al. (1998) subjects wore molds for up to 6 weeks and were tested regularly. Bauer et al. (1966) applied a long-term ear block for 65–67 h (Experiment 1) and had frequent tests to monitor evolution. Javer and Schwarz (1995) had their normal hearing subjects wear hearing aids during all waking hours for 3–5 days. McPartland et al. (1997) had the subjects wear an ear block over a period of 1week. They implemented tests before, during, and after the week of blocking. Carlile and Blackman (2014) applied binaural ear molds to subjects for a period of up to 60 days, until adaptation plateaued. Subjects wore the mold during all waking hours of the day. They were tested before the mold fitting, regularly during the adaptation period, and after mold removal.

In intermittent exposure, subjects only contact with the altered sound localization cues during the experimental sessions, and keep their natural hearing between sessions. Musicant and Butler (1980) blocked the right ear canal of eight participants, only during the test sessions. In one of their experiments, Shinn-Cunningham et al. (1998a,b) also exposed their subjects to altered sounds only during the experimental sessions.

Training with feedback

As in other paradigms, training with feedback most often includes a pre-test, the training process, and a post-test. The typical training process consists of sound localization tasks followed by a feedback, either classifying the response as right or wrong (response feedback) or specifying the true location of the stimulus (positional feedback).

In humans, response feedback is often presented in the form of a symbol or word. Butler (1987) trained subjects in an azimuth localization task. There was always response feedback, in the form of a word "correct" or "incorrect." Irving and Moore (2011) implemented training sessions in which subjects had to localize sounds produced by an array of speakers. After response, there was feedback in the form of a green or red light, for *correct* or *incorrect* respectively. In training paradigms with positional feedback, after the subject points to the perceived auditory source position in space, the correct location is displayed. Bauer et al. (1966) had long-term unilateral plug combined with training (Experiment 2). Response feedback consisted of replaying the sound, combined with light flash, at the correct source location after the answer. Zahorik et al. (2006) trained subjects in sound localization and provided positional feedback by presenting, after each response, an audiovisual stimulus revealing the source position. Shinn-Cunningham et al. (1998a,b) presented positional feedback after each localization answer. This feedback consisted of a light flash at the correct location. Majdak et al. (2013) had an extensive feedback program. After response, a visual marker was displayed at the correct stimulus position. Subjects were required to find the source and point at it. Then, subjects returned to the original position, and the same sound was presented again, this time with the visual marker on. Subjects, again, had to find and point at the stimulus. Strelnikov et al. (2011) compared training methods. One group had only sound exposure; the second group had response feedback, with the presentation of the words "correct" and "incorrect" after response; and a third had positional feedback, with the presentation concomitant light and sound. Some researchers combined sound exposure, positional feedback and response feedback (Kumpik et al., 2010; Carlile et al., 2013). In these studies, the training sessions indicated not only the position of the stimulus, but also the magnitude of the response error.

Active learning

In this training type, subjects are actively engaged in the activity leading to auditory space adaptation. There are no predefined stimulus presentations or predetermined feedback. Stimulation is mostly a result of the subjects' own actions. However, unlike in sound exposure, there are specific sessions designed to accelerate the adaptation.

Parseihian and Katz (2012) used an implicit training method. The authors trained subjects in a virtual auditory environment. There was a game-like scenario in which subjects explored and localized auditory stimuli with a hand held tracked ball. While exploring, the subjects would hear an auditory virtual sound corresponding in space and time to the tracked ball. Though this perception-action coupling, the new HRTF-base sounds were learned.

Mendonça et al. (2012, 2013) used an explicit training method. They presented the subjects with an interface where they could select any of three to five source positions to be learned and play them freely. They were particularly encouraged to compare the differences between sounds. Subjects learned by actively studying the sounds. Play buttons were displayed in an array representing the source positions. Subjects had 5 min to complete the task. After the explicit learning phase, they went on to a phase of training with positional feedback, until all reached a criterion of 80 percent correct answers.

EFFECTS OF AUDITORY SPACE ADAPTATION

Effects found in auditory space adaptation studies are presented in two subsections, organized by training paradigms. The data presented focus on training length and adaptation found in studies with human subjects. Unfortunately, there is great variability across studies on the type of adaptation reported. Some studies reported results in terms of amount of stimulus needed to compensate for differences, some in terms of shift in auditory space (shifts in centroids), front-back confusions, polar/elevation/vertical angular error, lateral/azimuth/horizontal angle error, overall localization error, or even percentage of correct responses. Many studies also failed to provide clear numbers, reporting mostly statistical significances. As a consequence, comparisons across studies are somewhat difficult to achieve. Therefore, data are presented mostly regarding if adaptation effects were or not found, and what was the nature of such effects.

ADAPTATION BY SOUND EXPOSURE

Most studies using sound exposure used monaural blocks or ear molds to induce wearable cue changes. They then analyzed the evolution of subjects' localization abilities over time.

Adaptations in the horizontal plane have been reported in a number of studies altering mostly binaural cues, either by applying a unilateral block, or by changing binaural cues though a hearing aid. In a seminal work, Florentine (1976) applied a unilateral block to subjects. Subjects were tested daily for the first week and then every 48 h for the remaining time. There was also a pre-test and several post-tests upon plug removal. Test stimuli were pure tones a several frequencies. The adaptation period lasted for 27–101 days, but the author reported that, after 4–10 days of long-term use of a unilateral earplug (sound exposure), there was already a partial adaptation in centering auditory image. McPartland et al. (1997) had 6 subjects wear an ear block for 1 week. They tested their subjects with a pure tone localization task, during and after plugging. Four subjects revealed no change in lateralization during or after, while two subjects revealed effects during plugging. These results do not necessarily mean that subjects did not adapt. An alternative explanation would be that subjects adapted to every-day sounds, but could not extract horizontal localization cues from single frequency stimuli.

Held (1955) presented his subjects with sounds displaced in azimuth by 20° through an electronic hearing device and allowed them to experience these sounds freely for 8 h. To assess adaptation effects, the author tested subjects in an anechoic room prior to and after exposure. In the post-tests there was a displacement of auditory space halfway in the direction of the sound shift. Javer and Schwarz (1995) used binaural insert hearing aids to apply a constant time delay to one ear, thus altering the ITD. Subjects did not wear the device during the night. The shift produced after insertion was of approximately 66°. Tests were conducted in an anechoic chamber, where subjects had to localize sounds without feedback. Tests took place before device insertion and then at several intervals. Within hours of exposure, the displacement was reduced. The localization went on normalizing in subsequent days, but was never fully complete. Slattery and Middlebrooks (1994) used normal listening subjects and patients with congenital unilateral deafness. They applied a monaural plug to a group of normal listeners for a period of 24 h. The plug caused a prominent lateral displacement by an average of 30.9° toward the side of the open ear. Conversely, the patients had a considerable ability to localize, except for two patients that had a pattern very similar to the plugged group. After the 24-h period there was a slight trend toward improvement, with a reduction of 4.53° in lateral error, but there was great inter-subject variability, and therefore these differences were not significant. We hypothesize that this result may be due to the short exposure period used, having in mind that no specific training was used and that sound exposure studies usually last longer.

Musicant and Butler (1980) used intermittent exposure, by blocking the ear canal of participants in short localization sessions. They exposed the subjects only during testing sessions, and without any feedback. In a first test, they were exposed to 60 trials of broadband train bursts in a sound localization task. Then subjects performed only one trial per day, in a total of 60 trials. Finally, there was a post-test, similar to the first test. A second group skipped the pre-test. They showed that those subjects that had the first test had significantly lower errors in the 60 single trial sessions, than those without the first test. They also showed that, even without feedback, adaptation is possible, if enough exposure is provided.

Studies that analyzed adaptation in the vertical plane induced more prominent changes to the spectral localization cues, namely through the fitting of ear molds. Hofman et al. (1998) fitted molds to both ears of four subjects. Subjects were tested in elevation localization prior to fitting, and then regularly until plug removal. After mold insertion, localization in elevation was immediately impaired. During 23–39 days, subjects wore the plug at all time. Elevation localization was steadily reacquired throughout the experiment. van Wanrooij and van Opstal (2005) applied spectral perturbation only to one ear, by fitting an ear mold, and analyzed adaptations during a period of 9–49 days in elevation localization. Seven out of twelve subjects regained accuracy in elevation. The remaining five listeners varied in performance recovery. Subjects that were less perturbed in auditory cues were the ones that revealed less adaptation. Carlile and Blackman (2014) looked into adaptations inside and outside the visual field. They applied ear molds for 28–62 days (average 40.5 days), during all waking hours. Subjects completed two blocks of localization test at least twice a week, until performance gains plateaued. Subjects were also tested before insertion, immediately after, immediately before removal, after removal, and with the mold again 1 week after removal. Results were reported mostly in terms of front-back confusions. Front-back confusions were elevated immediately after mold insertion, but were gradually reduced during the adaptation period. Immediately after mold removal localization performance was found to overlap the baseline performance measured immediately before insertion. The patterns of adaptation were very similar both within and outside the visual field, showing that auditory space adaptations are not dependent on visual cues.

In sum, exposure to altered head-related localization cues seems to lead to gradual adaptations of auditory space. Time, stimuli and degree of cue change seem to affect the adaptation patterns.

ADAPTATION BY TRAINING

Bauer et al. (1966) were among the first authors to implement a specific training paradigm to induce adaptation in auditory space. With continuous usage of a monaural earplug (sound exposure), they obtained stabilization of localization improvement after 65–67 h. But when they added training with positional feedback, they found that improvement stabilization was obtained much faster, 5–8 h after start. Butler (1987) plugged subjects in one ear and administered training in five sessions, over a period of 2 weeks. He provided training with response feedback for sound sources varying in azimuth around the midline. After training, the displacement induced by the block was reduced.

Several authors implementing auditory space training programs compared feedback types. In Shinn-Cunningham et al. (1998a,b), subjects trained in with "supernormal" HRTFs gradually increased their lateralization resolution. Different experiments were conducted and there were two training paradigms. Half the subjects had training with positional feedback, while the others had speeded exposure to audiovisual pairs (positional feedback). Nevertheless, both groups showed a gradual adaptation to the altered cues. Strelnikov et al. (2011) applied intermittent unilateral ear blocks and trained subjects over five days, in one training session per day. There were three training groups: one with only sound exposure; one with positional feedback, where light and sound were presented simultaneously; and one with response feedback where after response subjects were told if response was correct or incorrect. Feedback was provided in only half of the trials. They found that improvement in azimuth localization upon plugging was obtained in both feedback conditions, but not in the sound exposure condition. Improvement was best for the group with positional feedback. Improvement with positional feedback was observed for all spatial regions, while improvement with response feedback was mostly in peripheral visual regions. Carlile et al. (2013) applied binaural ear molds for 10 days and compared training methods. All subjects had long-term exposure to the altered cues, since they wore the molds during all waking hours for the whole adaptation period. Additionally, there were four training conditions: only sound exposure; positional feedback in the form of a light indicating the sound source; positional and response feedback in the form of light and also sounds pulsing at a rate proportional to response error, subjects were also allowed to move their heads and explore the response feedback; same as the previous, but within a lit room. Training sessions were administered for 1 h daily. After the adaptation period, localization improvements, in terms of front-back confusions and elevation accuracy, were found in all combined training groups, but not in the no feedback group. The groups trained with positional and response feedback had significantly better results than the group trained only with positional feedback. The results in the no feedback group may be due to the short adaptation period used, since most studies with sound exposure last approximately twice as long (see next Section, Training type and Length). Nevertheless, it is quite surprising that the group with visual positional training did not reveal better results.

Other than comparing feedback types, some studies have implemented mixed training approaches. When trained to localize with altered HRTFs having rich multisensory and positional feedback, subjects reduced their front-back localization reversals after only two 30 min training sessions (Zahorik et al., 2006). In that study, participants were stimulated through a head-mounted display, in a virtual reality environment rendered in real-time as a function of subjects' movement. Therefore, in addition to the training with positional feedback, there was motor, visual, and auditory feedback by sound exposure. Localization accuracy was initially poor with frequent front-back reversals for five of six subjects. There was a general benefit of the training sessions, although the benefit was only observed on the front-back dimension. The richness of this training program might have contributed to the observed effects in such small amount of time. Mendonça et al. (2012, 2013) used an active learning paradigm with non-individualized HRTF-based stimuli. During the training session, subjects had to learn only a small sample of 3–5 sounds. In that session, subjects received explicit training for a period of 5 min, followed by training with positional feedback. All subjects reached the criterion of 80 percent accuracy in localizing the four/five selected sounds in less than 20 min. After this training procedure with selected sounds, there was an overall reduction of localization error in all other tested source positions, both in azimuth and elevation.

Irving and Moore (2011) also had a mixed training approach, combining both sound exposure and training with feedback. The authors compared participants with unilateral plugs and unplugged participants. All subjects had training prior to plugging (c.f. Section Adaptations to task, procedure, or auditory space?). Subjects that were plugged wore the plugs for 5 days. There were daily training sessions, lasting 45–60 min each, with response feedback. Stimuli were broadband noise bursts presented in the horizontal plane, 360° around the subjects. Despite the initial training, there was a large degree of inter-listener variability. Unplugged subjects improved slightly but significantly in localization until the last session. For subjects trained with unilateral earplugs, there was a steady growth of accuracy after the initial impairment.

Many questions remain open regarding the implementation of specific training procedures for auditory space adaptation. The type of feedback is only one of the many parameters that should be analyzed. The timing and duration of the training sessions, the selection of stimuli to use, and their relation to the degree to which auditory space cues have been changed are relevant questions that remain largely unexplored.

Kumpik et al. (2010) compared the timing and amount of training. Subjects were trained in localizing with a monaural earplug. Training consisted in positional and response feedback. One group did all training in 1 day, another did the same amount of training over a period of seven to 8 days, while a third group trained a larger number of trials over 8 days. Some subjects were trained in localizing sounds with constant flat spectrum, while others were trained in sounds with varying spectrum. Only subjects that were trained over 1week with predictable spectrum sounds showed adaptation by reducing the number of incorrect responses. This study revealed the benefit of spreading training in time, other than concentrating all training in a long session. Also, authors concluded that reliable spectral cues are needed for auditory space plasticity.

Parseihian and Katz (2012) compared directly the adaptation to different levels of head-related cue change. They trained and tested their subjects with HRTF-based sounds. The training task was a game-like scenario where blindfolded subjects could move freely. The interaction with the virtual world was through a hand-held position-tracked ball and sounds were spatialized at the hand position. Half subjects did all the training in 1day, while the other half had training sessions distributed over 3 consecutive days. There were three groups: one that trained in localizing with their own HRTFs; another that trained in localizing with non-individualized HRTFs that were close to their own, and another trained in very different HRTFs. Training sessions were three blocks of 12 min each. After the training sessions, the localization tests took place. No feedback was provided at that stage. Authors found that the group using individualized auralization started with, and kept, better localization results than the remaining groups. The greatest gain in performance was found after the first training session. Groups with only one training session had no significant improvement, but groups trained in 3 days did. Most of the improvement was found in decrease of vertical error. A slight improvement was found in horizontal error, in groups with good HRTFs (close to their own), but not bad. This revealed that possibly adaptation processes take longer when greater changes are applied.

Majdak et al. (2013) also compared different levels of cue change. They used a spherical virtual audiovisual environment with HRTF-based sounds. Subjects were trained with visual feedback 2 h per day, for 21 days. Prior to and after training, subjects were tested in localization of sounds with the original individualized HRTFs, and with low-passed, frequency warped, and band-limited versions of those HRTFs. Then they were trained in either the warped sounds or the band-limited sounds. Training was effective for both groups. However, those subjects that trained with frequency warped sounds started with much higher errors and never localized as well as subjects trained in band-limited sounds. Even after training, localization was not as good as with the subjects' original HRTFs. Results pointed out that subjects can easily adapt to narrower stimulation bands, which can be observed in hearing loss. Distortion of the frequency cues impact more auditory localization and lead to potentially longer adaptation processes.

In sum, implementing specific training paradigms or combined approaches seems to be highly effective, and thus a promising approach to induce auditory recalibration. Methods vary greatly, and different feedback modalities lead to different adaptation processes. It seems that the success of the training program depends on the nature of the task and feedback provided. Active learning may be a promising way to enhance adaptation. Also, combining approaches and providing sensory-motor engagement may provide for better learning conditions. Greater cue changes seem to lead to longer adaptation periods. On the other hand, several training sessions may be preferable to the use of intensive one-day training sessions.

TRAINING TYPE AND LENGTH

In this section we take a closer look into the various training types and associated effectiveness in terms of adaptation time. **Table 1** presents a summary of studies on adult humans with normal listening. All these studies applied a change in localization cues and analyzed adaptation effects. Overall, auditory adaptation studies in humans vary greatly in length, from 10–20 min (Mendonça et al., 2012, 2013), to 27–101 days (Florentine, 1976). To obtain an estimate of average training length per study type, we computed local averages for studies in which length was itself variable. Two studies were not considered, due to having very irregular training methods (Musicant and Butler, 1980; Irving and Moore, 2011). Only methods that produced effects were considered.

We calculated that sound exposure studies lasted on average 20 days ($SD = 22.4$ days). Studies using training with feedback (both types) lasted an average of 18.8 h, ($SD = 14.9$ h). The active learning studies lasted an average of 22 min ($SD = 12.12$ min). Comparing training with positional feedback and training with response feedback, we find that training with positional feedback studies had longer adaptation periods: average 13.8 h against 5 h in studies with response feedback. Regarding two studies that mixed training with feedback and simple exposure (Kumpik et al., 2010; Irving and Moore, 2011; Carlile et al., 2013) the average training duration was 7.5 h ($SD = 2.5$ h).

Table 1 | Summary of studies on auditory space adaptation with normal-hearing human listeners.

Source	Type of cue change	Auditory stimuli	Type of training	Duration of training	Adaptation effects	After effects
Held, 1955	Long-term hearing aid	Bandpassed noise	Sound exposure	8 h	Partial	–
Bauer et al., 1966	Long-term monaural block	Broadband noise	Sound exposure	65–67 h	Yes	Back to pre-plug levels
			Exposure, training with positional feedback (V)	5–8 h	Yes	Back to pre-plug levels
Florentine, 1976	Long-term monaural block	Pure tones	Sound exposure	27–101 days	Yes	Adaptation 7–15 days after removal
Musicant and Butler, 1980	Inttermittent monaural block	Bandpassed noise	Exposure without feedback	1 h + 1 trial/day over 60 days	Yes	–
				1 trial/day over 60 days	No	–
Butler, 1987	Inttermittent monaural block	Bandpassed noise	Training with response feedback (R/W)	1 h*5 (2 weeks)	Yes	Adaptation 2–2.5 months after training
Slattery and Middlebrooks, 1994	Long-term monaural block	Broadband noise	Sound exposure	24 h	No	–
Javer and Schwarz, 1995	Long-term hearing device	Bandpassed and broadband noise	Sound exposure	3–5 days	Yes	–
McPartland et al., 1997	Long-term monaural block	Pure tones	Sound exposure	1 week	Partial	–
Hofman et al., 1998	Long-term binaural ear mold	Broadband noise	Sound exposure	23–39 days	Yes	Back to pre-plug levels
Shinn-Cunningham et al., 1998a,b	Inttermittent altered HRTFs	Click trains	Training with positional feedback (V) (AVM); sound exposure	2 h*8 (2–6 weeks)	Yes	–
van Wanrooij and van Opstal, 2005	Long-term monaural mold	Bandpassed and broadband noise	Sound exposure 9–49 days	Partial (elevation)	Back to pre-plug levels soon after	
Zahorik et al., 2006	Inttermittent altered HRTFs	Bandpassed noise	Training with positional feedback (AV)	1 h*2	Yes	Effects lated over 4 months
Kumpik et al., 2010	Intermittent monaural ear block	Broadband noise	Training with positional (V) and response feedback(R/W)	1 day	No	Back to pre-plug levels
				~1 h *7–8 days	Yes	
Strelnikov et al., 2011	Intermittent monaural ear block	Broadband noise	Sound exposure	1 h*5 days	No	–
			Training with positional feedback (AV)		Yes	
			Training response feedback (R/W)		Yes	

(Continued)

Table 1 | Continued

Source	Type of cue change	Auditory stimuli	Type of training	Duration of training	Adaptation effects	After effects
Irving and Moore, 2011	Long-term monaural block	Broadband noise	Sound exposure; Training with response feedback (R/W)	5 days exposure; 5 h training	Yes	Immediately back to pre-plug levels
Mendonça et al., 2012	Inttermittent altered HRTFs	Broadband noise	Sound exposure (static)	10 blocks (1 h)	No	–
			Explicit training; Training with positional feedback (V)	10–20 min	Yes	–
Parseihian and Katz, 2012	Intermittent altered HRTFs	Broadband noise	Implicit training (AM)	3*12 min	Yes	–
Majdak et al., 2013	Intermittent altered HRTFs	Broadband noise	Training with positional feedback (V)	2 h*21 days	Yes	Same results 1 day later
Carlile et al., 2013	Long-term binaural ear mold	Broadband noise	Sound exposure	10 days	No	–
			Sound exposure; Training with positional feedback (V)	10 days, 10 h training	Yes	
			Sound exposure; Training with positional (AVM) and response feedback (level)	10 days, 10 h training	Yes	
Mendonça et al., 2013	Inttermittent altered HRTFs	Broadband noise and speech	Explicit training, training with positional feedback (V)	10–20 min	Yes	Effects lasted over 1 month
Carlile and Blackman, 2014	Binaural ear mold	Broadband noise	Sound exposure	28–62 days (average 40.5 days)	Yes	Back to pre-mold levels upon removal; adaptation still one

Acronyms stand for sensory modality of feedback: V, Visual; AV, Audiovisual; AM, Audiomotor; AVM, Audiovisual motor; R/W, Right/Wrong; Level, Level of response error.

There is therefore a clear benefit of training with feedback, comparing with sound exposure, and of active learning comparing to any other method. However, the number of studies using active learning is still too small to draw significant conclusions. Similarly, adaptation times reveal that response feedback can be associated to faster training processes than positional feedback, but differences are small and there are not enough studies to draw such comparisons in a conclusive way. Studies using training with positional feedback resorted mostly to visual, audiovisual and audiovisual motor information as feedback, while response feedback studies used words, colors, or pulsed sounds. It would be expected that the former feedback types, richer in spatial information, could lead to better adaptations. On the other hand, more symbolic feedback types may require the recruitment of additional attentional and memory resources, which are crucial for learning. Further studies are required to draw clear conclusions on the most efficient stimuli and methods to induce adaptations.

ADAPTATIONS TO TASK, PROCEDURE, OR AUDITORY SPACE?

It may be argued that improvements in localization accuracy observed in these studies are the result of a task, or procedure learning, instead of actual auditory space adaptations. There isn't enough research to understand and predict how much of the adaptation effects can be accounted by task or procedure learning. Here we refer to task learning as a process in which the subject becomes acquainted with the stimuli and the judgment type, a cognitive adaptation which includes establishing an internal criterion for the decision on the stimuli. By procedure learning we mean the adaptation to the interface and response type. It comprises optimizing the process of perceiving-deciding-responding. Unfortunately, these processes are very task- and subject-specific, so there is no good rule to predict the extent of their effects or how long they take. Psychophysical studies with human subjects usually include a very short practice block before starting the data collection. This has been used in some auditory space learning experiments (e.g., Strelnikov et al., 2011). Alternatively, some authors have resorted to longer preliminary training blocks with the subject's unaltered cues.

Slattery and Middlebrooks (1994) provided all subjects with two brief training sessions to familiarize them with the testing procedure, before applying monaural plugs. In the first training session, a light would turn on over the speaker that displayed the sound. This procedure was repeated 15 times. In the second session the loudspeaker light only appeared after the subjects answered by localizing the sound. Kumpik et al. (2010) trained subjects in localizing broadband noise stimuli prior to applying monaural earplugs. Subjects were trained until they reached 85 percent correct answers, which could take up to 6 days. Interestingly, only the group trained in localizing these same sounds after plugging revealed significant adaptations, but the authors never debated the potential role of the preliminary training on the final results. Irving and Moore (2011) had one of the longest, most comprehensive preliminary training programs. They started by training participants with unaltered cues for 4 days. Then, half participants wore a plug for 5 days, while others did not. Carlile et al. (2013) and Carlile and Blackman (2014) trained their subjects in the testing procedure before applying changes to the ears. The procedure included pointing with the nose at the perceived sound source after stimulus offset. After the answer, a light was presented over the loudspeaker that presented the stimulus; then, noise bursts were displayed from that speaker at a rate inversely proportional to the pointing error. Subjects were therefore trained in pointing to the perceived position with greater accuracy. There were 150–200 training trials altogether.

A few concerns can be raised in an approach in which subjects are first trained on their own cues and only then on the altered cues. Auditory training may have unknown effects. It can increase plasticity and improve the success of subsequent adaptation processes (Linkenhoker and Knudsen, 2002). Alternatively, it can increase strangeness when cue alteration is first applied, artificially raising the initial error levels. Indeed, if subjects have just been trained in a task with specific cues, they may exhibit initial enhanced errors solely due to expectations of particular cue arrangements. Unfortunately, no studies exist comparing pre-test adaptation procedures.

In an ingenious approach, Majdak et al. (2013) trained subjects in the procedure, without affecting the baseline sound localization results. They had a preliminary training session, where subjects learned to identify the visual target and point at it. No sounds were presented during this session. This way, subjects became acquainted with the task, interface, and improved response precision, presumably without affecting the performance on the auditory task. One common way to separate localization improvement from mere task training effects is to have different tasks and setups for the training and testing sessions (e.g., Mendonça et al., 2013). In such cases, much like in the training by sound exposure, the improvement in the localization task cannot be attributed to successive training. However, even in such cases, there is cumulative experience in the testing procedure itself. The only way to account for this effect is to have a control group (e.g., Irving and Moore, 2011) that undergoes the testing without the training. In this case, the differences between groups can clearly be attributed to adaptation to the new cues, rather than adaptation to task and procedure.

ADAPTATION AFTEREFFECTS

DURABILITY

To analyze the adaptation aftereffects in the time domain, we must look separately into studies that implemented long-term cue changes and intermittent changes. Studies that implemented long-term changes looked into hearing and localization upon the removal of such changes. There are conflicting results at this level.

Florentine (1976) reported a post-experimental effect of 7–15 days after removing the unilateral blocks. Subjects still required an imbalance of channel loudness to perceive the auditory image as centered. Since this was an exceptionally long study (27–101 days), we hypothesize that the long-term unilateral mold induced some hearing loss to the blocked ear. This is in line with other findings showing that temporary conductive hearing loss leads to a binaural hearing impairment that lasts beyond the duration of the impairment (for a review, see Moore et al., 2001). No other study implementing long-term monaural blocks obtained such an effect, but no other occluded the ear for such a long period. Irving and Moore (2011) observed that, upon removal of the block, subjects localized again exactly as they did before insertion. Bauer et al. (1966) also tested localization shift after plug removal. In one experiment subjects wore plugs for 65–67 h. In the other experiment, for 5–7 and had additional training with feedback. Post-plug shifts were modest or neglectable, compatible with assumption that subjects went back to their natural auditory map. Held (1955) reported that, upon removal of the hearing device, subjects were localizing like they did in the pre-test. Hofman et al. (1998) found that, after removal of binaural molds, localization in elevation was close to the original levels. In a similar way, van Wanrooij and van Opstal (2005), Kumpik et al. (2010), and Carlile and Blackman (2014) found that soon after restoring the subjects' ears localization abilities were at the same level as before the adaptation period. On the other hand, in Carlile and Blackman (2014), 1 week after removal, when the mold was reapplied, localization was similar to that obtained at the end of the adaptation period, demonstrating that the learned cue-to-space relationships were still available.

In experiments that applied only intermittent changes, similar enduring results were obtained. In Butler (1987), the subjects only wore the earplug during training sessions. They trained for five sessions, over a period of 2 weeks. Adaptation was retained for a period of 2–2.5 months. Zahorik et al. (2006) tested their subjects 4 days and 4 months after training. Benefits in localization accuracy were still found 4 months later. Mendonça et al. (2013) tested their subjects 1 h, 1 day, 1week, and 1 month after training. Effects of training were still observed 1 month after training. Implications of these finding are discussed in Section Underlying Processes.

GENERALIZATION

In perceptual learning, there are well known effects of specificity to trained attribute, position, orientation and context (Gilbert et al., 2001). Generalization occurs when the training-induced perceptual adaptation is found not only in the trained stimuli or task, but also in others. Generalization mechanisms are found in auditory learning, but they vary with task and stimuli, and are often limited to sound frequency (for a review, see Wright and Zhang, 2009). In auditory space learning with altered localization cues, findings are also often contradictory.

As already referred in Section Effects of Auditory Space Adaptation, Butler (1987) found that spatial adaptation was specific to trained cue spectrum, On the other hand, Zahorik et al. (2006) found that, after training, subjects improved in localizing not only the trained auditory source positions, but also other, untrained sources. A similar result was obtained by Mendonça et al. (2012). Mendonça et al. (2013) looked deeper into auditory space generalization patterns. They found that subjects trained in localizing sources varying exclusively in the vertical plane became better in localizing sources varying in the horizontal plane, and vice-versa. Subjects trained in localizing speech became better in localizing broadband noise, and vice versa. However, there was a benefit in training with broadband noise leading to improved learning and generalization levels. Finally, subjects were trained in only four stimuli positions, but revealed improvements in all subsequently tested positions. These results reveal the potential of using simplified training approaches to induce fast adaptations through generalization.

NEUROPHYSIOLOGICAL CORRELATES

There is great plasticity in the neural circuits that process sensory information (Rauschecker, 1999). It is most relevant during infancy, as the body grows, but it is maintained in the adult brain (King et al., 2000, 2011). Learning produces changes in the brain, which can take the form of increases in dendritic length, spine density, synapse formation, increased glial activity, or altered metabolic activity (Kolb and Whishaw, 1998). It is natural to assume that auditory space adaptation processes take place in the auditory pathway, where space is processed. However, since there is no full understanding on how space is encoded at higher instances of the human brain, there are also many open questions on the substrates of the adaptation processes. Furthermore, there seems to be substantial difference among species on this matter.

The localization process starts with the extraction of direction-dependent cues in the brainstem (e.g., King et al., 2001), early in the auditory pathway. Interestingly, the olivocochlear system, involved in the descending control of the cochlea, has been shown to be unnecessary for accurate auditory localization, but it is involved in relearning auditory space during unilateral conductive hearing loss (Irving et al., 2011). ITD and ILD are predominantly, but not only, processed in the medial superior olive and lateral superior olive respectively (Moore et al., 2010) and these nuclei project to the central nucleus of the inferior colliculus (IC). The IC also receives input from the contra-lateral dorsal cochlear nucleus, where monaural spectral cues seem to be processed (Yu and Young, 1997; Zatorre et al., 2002). There are multiple feedback loops between the auditory cortex (AC) and IC (Huffman and Henson, 1990; Oliver, 2005), and therefore the IC also receives massive descending projection from the AC (Maeder et al., 2001).

INFERIOR AND SUPERIOR COLLICULI

The IC is a midbrain nucleus of the ascending pathway (Maeder et al., 2001). It projects to the superior colliculus (SC) (Oliver and Huerta, 1992; King et al., 1998a). The SC has a topographical organization, where stimuli from different points in space activate different areas. It is mostly visual in the upper layer and multisensory in the lower layers (King and Palmer, 1983; Middlebrooks and Knudsen, 1984; King and Hutchings, 1987). So it has been proposed that there is a topographically aligned visual and auditory map in the SC (King and Palmer, 1983; Middlebrooks and Knudsen, 1984; King and Hutchings, 1987). This hypothesis has large support in several species, but remains open in primates.

Studies on animals raised with sensory impairment show that the map of auditory space in the SC is shaped during the development of both auditory and visual systems (King et al., 2000). In the barn owl, adaptation processes have been well documented. Plasticity at the level of the external nucleus of the IC is largely responsible for the frequency-dependent adjustments in ITD tuning that are observed in the optic tectum of owls raised with spectacles (Gold and Knudsen, 2000). The optic tectum is the homolog of the SC in the barn owl and contains mutually aligned neural maps of auditory and visual space (Brainard and Knudsen, 1993). There is a point-to-point projection from the optic tectum to the IC (Hyde and Knudsen, 2000). Therefore, this anatomical organization contributes to the visual calibration of the auditory space map at the IC (Brainard and Knudsen, 1993; Feldman and Knudsen, 1997; Hyde and Knudsen, 2000). In ferrets, the auditory spatial map is not as well organized, but activity in superficial layers of the SC is thought to play a role in the alignment of the topographical arrangement of the IC (King et al., 1996, 1998b). The SC in the mammal has many multisensory neurons in the deeper layers, thought to be responsible for a unified impression of the world, that activate selectively according to spatiotemporal constraints (Stein and Meredith, 1993). The upper layers of the SC are exclusively visual and are innervated by topographically organized projections from the retina and the visual cortex (Huerta and Harting, 1984). Therefore, despite a different organization at the IC, it is still reasonable to assume that the interactions between IC and SC might be related to auditory space adaptation in humans. This adaptation process would mostly be relative to visual and tactile spatial feedback.

THE CORTEX

In humans, both the AC and the posterior parietal cortex are involved in auditory localization (Griffiths et al., 1996; Zatorre et al., 2002). The parietal cortex is possibly involved in cross-correlating between auditory localization and head movement information (Rauschecker, 1999). The AC is key for auditory localization, since temporal lobe damage can lead to impaired auditory localization (Masterton, 1997; Clarke et al., 2000; King et al., 2011). The AC receives binaural inputs that are tuned to sound frequency, and it is organized in a tonotopic way. Preferred sound azimuths appear to be clustered across the AC (Imig et al., 1990; Rauschecker, 1999; Tian et al., 2001). The posterior AC responds to sounds that vary in spatial distribution, but only when multiple stimuli are presented together, implicating this cortical system in the disambiguation of overlapping auditory sources (Zatorre et al., 2002). It has been suggested that the sound localization mechanism based on spectral cues assumes a flat spectrum and compares the incoming sound with the acquired HRTF templates (Blauert, 1997). Therefore, regarding frequency-dependent cues, it would be more economical to adapt the spectral coding of sound localization by means of cortical plasticity (Rauschecker, 1999). Recent evidence revealed that the AC is involved in mammal auditory space adaptations. Nodal et al. (2012) reversibly deactivated different cortical areas of ferrets over a few weeks. The orientation of the animals to sounds was not affected by silencing any region of the AC, but the experience-dependent plasticity was. After plugging one ear, the localization recovery was not as complete in animals with the AC deactivated, compared to control animals. Also, selectively deactivating the cholinergic nucleus basalis that projects to the AC affects not only auditory localization, but also impairs experience-dependent auditory space adaptations (Leach et al., 2013). Additionally, the corticocollicular pathway, from the cortex to the IC, plays a crucial role in learning-induced auditory space plasticity of mammals. When these neurons were selectively killed in ferrets, the recovery in auditory localization after occlusion of one ear was impaired (Bajo et al., 2010). Keating et al. (2013) showed that the role of the AC in auditory space plasticity involves a reweighting of different spatial cues. Ferrets reared with unilateral plugs alternated with periods of normal hearing relied more on monaural cues than animals raised with normal hearing. This change in behavior was accompanied by changes in neuronal responses in the primary AC. However, this reweighting disappeared in periods of normal hearing, revealing that this type of adaptation is context-dependent.

UNDERLYING PROCESSES

In this section we attempt to bring together neurophysiological evidence and psychophysical data. We are still far from understanding the neuronal and cognitive mechanisms underlying auditory space adaptation processes. Keating and King (2013) proposed that adaptation may be achieved either by learning a new relationship between altered cues and points in space or by changing the way different cues are integrated in the brain. The former would consist of a cue remapping process, potentially involving structural changes in the brain, like the ones observed in the barn owl. The latter could involve a cue reweighting process. Cue processing would remain the same, but a different decision rule, regarding the corresponding position in space, would be applied. In a similar way, Shinn-Cunningham (2001) proposed that the auditory system is optimized for computing spatial location from normal spatial cues and short-term training cannot influence how spatial position is computed internally, but only how spatial percepts are associated to exocentric space. There is some evidence supporting the existence of cue reweighting processes in humans (Kumpik et al., 2010). This evidence pointed to the fact that, if such mechanisms were to exist, they should be context-dependent. In different contexts, different cue combination rules could be used.

As reported above, in most studies on the adaptation to a long-term cue change, such as fitting an earplug or mold, upon removal of the change subjects readily returned to localizing as they did before. An interpretation of these data is that subjects developed a new cue combination rule, between cues and perceived position. In these cases, the previous combination rule was not altered, and instead a new one was created for that new context. In a similar way, subjects that had intermittent training improved in localizing with the altered cues, while using their natural cue integration between experimental sessions. This continuous improvement of a second cue combination rule can only be explained if both rules were developed in parallel, and used one in each context.

van Wanrooij and van Opstal (2005) found that subjects that were less perturbed by a monaural ear mold improved less than subjects that had to deal with greater differences. The authors suggested that adaptation to spectral cue manipulations depends on the correlation between the new and the old cue combinations. In this case, before adaptation, there would be an analysis to correlate the perceived space and some form of feedback. If relevant differences were found, adaptation would take place.

All these findings point out that the brain might be able to develop and use different cue combination rules in parallel. This feature, despite computationally demanding, might be evolutionarily optimal. In real-world situations, not only the anatomy, but also the contexts, change considerably over time. The acoustic cues in a classroom or in a supermarket, for instance, are markedly different. But crucially, each context may remain stable over time (Keating and King, 2013).

A hypothetical process of continuous calibration and creation of new cue combination rules is proposed in **Figure 1**. First, the direction-dependent cues are extracted from the auditory stimulus in the brainstem. These cues then are combined and the source position is estimated, having in mind the contexts and quality of the cues. It is unclear where this process could take place in the brain, but it is likely that the AC plays a special role. Crucial to this process is the continuous feedback, provided by concomitant visual and motor cues. As approached in this review, this feedback can also take the form of a response feedback or direct specification of where the sound should be perceived. The cross-correlation between the auditory source percept and the perceived source position from other senses, namely vision, most likely requires the activity of the SC. However, it may be arguable that in cases of active learning or training with feedback, other cortical areas may also be involved. We propose that with each localization process there is a loop of confirmation or rejection of the cue combination mechanisms. It is precisely from this loop that auditory space adaptation can occur.

CONCLUDING REMARKS

Understanding how humans adapt to altered head-related auditory cues is a topic of growing relevance. Firstly, such adaptation processes should be acknowledged. There is a general lack of understanding on how humans deal with hearing loss, hearing surgery, hearing aids, and new hearing technologies. There is accumulated evidence that subjects will adapt to changes in the head-related localization cues. If provided with enough time to adapt, with several days of continuous exposure, subjects will change how they localize. This applies, for instance, to hearing impaired people that preserve their localization abilities, despite interaural sensitivity imbalances (e.g., Keating and King, 2013).

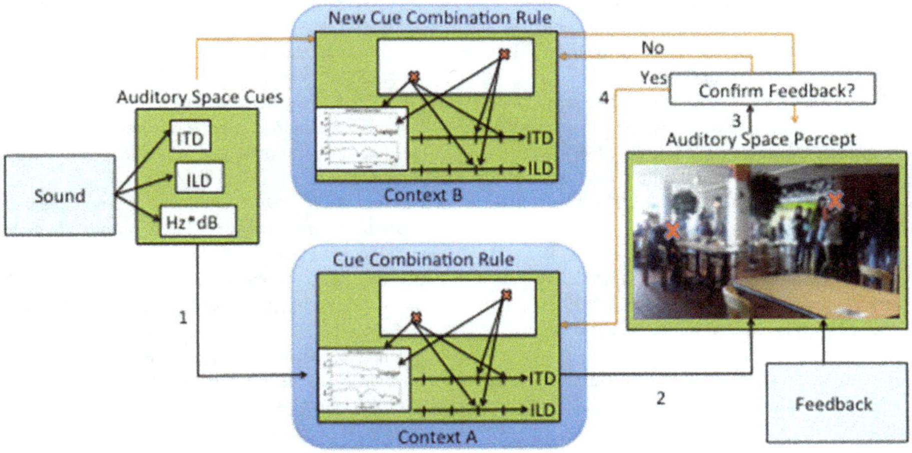

FIGURE 1 | Illustration of a hypothetical process of auditory adaptation through continuous sensory experience. First the input sound is decomposed into auditory space cues, then (1) a correspondence is established between the cues and a point in perceptual space. After a correspondence is established (2) a percept is formed. Perceiving auditory sources in space is most often accompanied by feedback. The feedback is compared to the auditory space percept (3). If no differences are found, then there is further tuning of the original cue combination rule. If the feedback is substantially different from the percept, then a new cue combination rule is created.

On the other hand, assessing new devices or interventions when subjects first experience them may lead to discouraging results, since time is crucial for adaptation. Here we have demonstrated that subjects can also adapt to cue alterations in a short period of time. For that, training programs can be devised to boost the adaptation. Such training programs can use either feedback or active learning, but we found that active learning or combined programs may lead to faster adaptations.

Auditory space learning is an ongoing lifelong process. We proposed that most likely humans are able to represent several auditory cue combination rules at once. This useful skill will allow subjects to adapt to new hearing devices and contexts, and switch between them without experiencing localization disruption. It might ultimately become useful in assistive technologies using augmented reality, where both virtual cues and natural cues are present at the same time. If confirmed, this finding opens perspectives for a future in hearing assistance that accounts for, and integrates, auditory adaptation processes.

ACKNOWLEDGMENTS

This project was funded by the Academy of Finland, project Audiovisual Space (#13266239). We thank the anonymous reviewers for the thorough analysis and insightful comments on previous versions of this manuscript.

REFERENCES

Bajo, V. M., Nodal, F. R., Moore, D. R., and King, A. J. (2010). The descending corticocollicular pathway mediates learning-induced auditory plasticity. *Nat. Neurosci.* 13, 253–260. doi: 10.1038/nn.2466

Bauer, R., Matuzsa, J., and Blackmer, R. (1966). Noise localization after unilateral attenuation. *J. Acoust. Soc. Am.* 40, 441–444. doi: 10.1121/1.1910093

Blauert, J. (1997). *Spatial Hearing: the Psychophysics of Human Sound Localization.* Cambridge, MA: MIT Press.

Brainard, M. S., and Knudsen, E. I. (1993). Experience-dependent plasticity in the Inferior Colliculus: a site for visual calibration of the neural representation of auditory space in the barn owl. *J. Neurosci.* 13, 4589–4680.

Butler, R. A. (1987). An analysis of monaural displacement of sound in space. *Percept. Psychophys.* 41, 1–7. doi: 10.3758/BF03208206

Carlile, S., Balachandar, K., and Kelly, H. (2013). Accommodating to new ears: the effects of sensory-motor feedback. *J. Acoust. Soc. Am.* 135, 2002–2011. doi: 10.1121/1.4868369

Carlile, S., and Blackman, T. (2014). Relearning auditory spectral cues for locations inside and outside the visual field. *J. Assoc. Res. Otolaryngol.* 15, 249–263. doi: 10.1007/s10162-013-0429-5

Clarke, S., Bellmann, A., Meuli, R. A., Assal, G., and Steck, A. J. (2000). Auditory agnosia and auditory spatial deficits following left hemispheric lesions: evidence for distinct processing pathways. *Neuropsychologia* 38, 797–807. doi: 10.1016/S0028-3932(99)00141-4

Feldman, D. E., and Knudsen, E. I. (1997). An anatomical basis for visual calibration of the auditory space map in the barn owl's mid brain. *J. Neurosci.* 17, 6820–6837.

Florentine, M. (1976). Relation between lateralization and loudness in asymmetrical hearing losses. *J. Am. Audiol. Soc.* 1, 243–251.

Gardner, B., and Martin, K. (1994). HRTF measurements of a KEMAR dummy-head microphone. *Mass. Inst. Technol.* 280, 1–7.

Gilbert, C. D., Sigman, M., and Crist, R. E. (2001). The neural basis of perceptual learning. *Neuron* 31, 681–697. doi: 10.1016/S0896-6273(01)00424-X

Gold, J. I., and Knudsen, E. I. (2000). A site for auditory experience-dependent plasticity in the neural representation of auditory space in the barn owl's inferior colliculus. *J. Neurosci.* 20, 3469–3486.

Griffiths, T. D., Rees, A., Witton, C., Shakir, R. A. A., Henning, G. B., and Green, G. G. (1996). Evidence for a sound movement area in the human cerebral cortex. *Nature* 383, 425–427. doi: 10.1038/383425a0

Held, R. (1955). Shifts in binaural localization after prolonged exposures to atypical combinations of stimuli. *Am. J. Psychol.* 68, 526–548. doi: 10.2307/1418782

Hofman, P. M., van Riswick, J. G. A., and van Opstal, A. J. (1998). Relearning sound localization with new ears. *Nat. Neurosci.* 1, 417–421. doi: 10.1038/1633

Hofman, P. M., Vlamig, M. S. M. G., Termeer, P. J. J., and van Opstal, A. J. (2002). A method to induce swapped binaural hearing. *J. Neurosci. Methods* 113, 167–179. doi: 10.1016/S0165-0270(01)00490-3

Huerta, M. F., and Harting, J. K. (1984). "The mammalian superior colliculus: studies of its morphology and connections," in *Comparative Neurology of the Optic Tectum*, ed H. Vanegas (New York, NY: Plenum), 687–773. doi: 10.1007/978-1-4899-5376-6_18

Huffman, R. F., and Henson, O. W. Jr. (1990). The descending auditory pathway and acusticomotor systems: the connection with the inferior colliculus. *Brain Res. Rev.* 15, 295–323. doi: 10.1016/0165-0173(90)90005-9

Hyde, P. S., and Knudsen, E. I. (2000). Topographic projection from the optic tectum to the auditory space map in the inferior colliculus of the barn owl. *J. Comp. Neurol.* 421, 146–160. doi: 10.1002/(SICI)1096-9861(20000529)421:2%3C146::AID-CNE2%3E3.0.CO;2-5

Imig, T. J., Irons, W. A., and Samson, F. R. (1990). Single-unit selectivity to azimuthal direction and sound pressure level of noise bursts in cat high-frequency primary auditory cortex. *J. Neurophysiol.* 63, 1448–1466.

Irving, S., and Moore, D. R. (2011). Training sound localization in normal hearing listeners with and without a unilateral ear plug. *Hear. Res.* 280, 100–108. doi: 10.1016/j.heares.2011.04.020

Irving, S., Moore, D. R., Liberman, M. C. I., and Summer, C. J. (2011). Olivocochlear efferent control in sound localization and experience-dependent learning. *J. Neurosci.* 31, 2493–2501. doi: 10.1523/JNEUROSCI.2679-10.2011

Javer, A. F., and Schwarz, D. W. (1995). Plasticity in human directional hearing. *J. Otolaryngol.* 24, 111–117.

Kacelnik, O., Nodal, F. R., Parson, C. H., and King, A. J. (2006). Training-induced plasticity of auditory localization in adult mammals. *PLoS Biol.* 4:e71. doi: 10.1371/journal.pbio.0040071

Keating, P., Dahmen, J. C., and King, A. J. (2013). Context-specific reweighting of auditory spatial cues following altered experience during development. *Curr. Biol.* 23, 1291–1299. doi: 10.1016/j.cub.2013.05.045

Keating, P., and King, A. J. (2013). Developmental plasticity of spatial hearing following asymmetric hearing loss: context-dependent cue integration and its clinical implications. *Front. Syst. Neurosci.* 7:123. doi: 10.3389/fnsys.2013.00123

King, A. J. (2009). Visual influences on auditory spatial hearing. *Philos. Trans. R. Soc. B* 364, 331–339. doi: 10.1098/rstb.2008.0230

King, A. J., Dahmen, J. C., Keating, P., Leach, N. D., Nodal, F. R., and Bajo, V. M. (2011). Neural circuits underlying adaptation and learning in the perception of auditory space. *Biobehav. Rev.* 35, 2129–2139. doi: 10.1016/j.neubiorev.2011.03.008

King, A. J., and Hutchings, M. E. (1987). Spatial response properties of acoustically responsive neurons in the superior colliculus of a ferret: a map of auditory space. *J. Neurophysiol.* 75, 596–624.

King, A. J., Jiang, Z. D., and Moore, D. R. (1998a). Auditory brainstem projections to the ferret superior colliculus: anatomical contribution to the neural coding of sound azimuth. *J. Comp. Neurol.* 390, 342–365.

King, A. J., Kacelnik, O., Mrsic-Flogel, T. D., Schnupp, J. W., Parsons, C. H., and Moore, D. R. (2001). How plastic is spatial hearing? *Audiol. Neurotol.* 6, 182–186. doi: 10.1159/000046829

King, A. J., and Palmer, A. R. (1983). Cells responsive to free-field auditory stimuli in the guinea-pig superior colliculus: distribution and response properties. *J. Physiol.* 342, 361–381.

King, A. J., Parsons, C. H., and Moore, D. R. (2000). Plasticity in the neural coding of auditory space in the mammalian brain. *Proc. Nat. Acad. Sci. U.S.A.* 97, 11821–11828. doi: 10.1073/pnas.97.22.11821

King, A. J., Schnupp, J. W. H., Carlile, S., Smith, A. L., and Thompson, I. D. (1996). Chapter 24 The development of topographically aligned maps of the visual and auditory space in the superior colliculus. *Progr. Brain Res.* 112, 335–350. doi: 10.1016/S0079-6123(08)63340-3

King, A. J., Schupp, J. W. H., and Thompson, I. D. (1998b). Signals from the superficial layers of the superior colliculus enable the development of the auditory space map in the deeper layers. *J. Neurosci.* 18, 9394–9408.

Kolb, B., and Whishaw, I. Q. (1998). Brain plasticity and behavior. *Annu. Rev. Psychol.* 43, 43–64. doi: 10.1146/annurev.psych.49.1.43

Kopčo, N., Lin, I. F., Shinn-Cunningham, B. G., and Groh, J. M. (2009). Reference frame of the ventriloquism aftereffect. *J. Neurosci.* 29, 13809–13814. doi: 10.1523/JNEUROSCI.2783-09.2009

Kumpik, D. P., Kacelnik, O., and King, A. J. (2010). Adaptive reweighting of auditory localization cues in response to chronic unilateral earplugging in humans. *J. Neurosci.* 30, 4883–4894. doi: 10.1523/JNEUROSCI.5488-09.2010

Leach, N. D., Nodal, F. R., Cordery, P. M., King, A. J., and Bajo, V. M. (2013). Cortical cholinergic input is required for normal auditory perception and experience-dependent plasticity in adult ferrets. *J. Neurosci.* 33, 6659–6671. doi: 10.1523/JNEUROSCI.5039-12.2013

Lewald, J. (2002). Rapid adaptation to auditory-visual spatial disparity. *Learn. Mem.* 9, 268–278. doi: 10.1101/lm.51402

Linkenhoker, B. A., and Knudsen, E. I. (2002). Incremental training increases the plasticity of the auditory space map in adult barn owls. *Nature.* 419, 293–296. doi: 10.1038/nature01002

Maeder, P. P., Meuli, R. A., Adriani, M., Bellman, A., Fornari, E., Thiran, J. P., et al. (2001). Distinct pathways involved in sound recognition and localization: a human fMRI study. *Neuroimage* 14, 802–816. doi: 10.1006/nimg.2001.0888

Majdak, P., Walder, T., and Labak, B. (2013). Effect of long-term training on sound localization performance with spectrally warped and band-limited head-related transfer functions. *J. Acoust. Soc. Am.*134, 2148–2159. doi: 10.1121/1.4816543

Masterton, R. B. (1997). "Role of the mammalian forebrain in hearing," in *Acoustical Signal Processing in the Central Auditory System*, ed J. Syka (New York, NY: Plenum Press), 1–17. doi: 10.1007/978-1-4419-8712-9_1

McPartland, J. L., Culling, J. F., and Moore, D. R. (1997). Changes in lateralization and loudness judgments during one week of unilateral ear plugging. *Hear. Res.* 113, 163–172. doi: 10.1016/S0378-5955(97)00142-1

Mendonça, C., Campos, G., Dias, P., and Santos, J. A. (2013). Learning auditory space: Generalization and long-term effects. *PLoS ONE* 8:e77900. doi: 10.1371/journal.pone.0077900

Mendonça, C., Campos, G., Dias, P., Vieira, J., Ferreira, J. P., and Santos, J. A. (2012). On the improvement of localization accuracy with non-individualized HRFT-based sounds. *J. Audio Eng. Soc.* 60, 1–10.

Middlebrooks, J. C., and Green, D. M. (1991). Sound localization by human listeners. *Annu. Rev. Psychol.* 42, 135–159. doi: 10.1146/annurev.ps.42.020191.001031

Middlebrooks, J. C., and Knudsen, E. I. (1984). A neural code for auditory space in the cat's superior colliculus. *J. Neurosci.* 4, 2621–2634.

Moore, D. R., Fuchs, P. A., Rees, A., Palmer, A., and Plack, C. J. (eds.). (2010). *The Oxford Handbook of Auditory Science: the Auditory Brain* (Vol. 2). Oxford: Oxford University Press.

Moore, D. R., Hogan, S. C., Kacelnik, O., Parsons, C. H., Rose, M. M., and King, A. J. (2001). Auditory learning as a cause and treatment of central dysfunction. *Audiol. Neurotol.* 6, 216–220. doi: 10.1159/000046836

Musicant, A. D., and Butler, R. A. (1980). Monaural localization: An analysis of practice effects. *Percept. Psychophys.* 28, 236–240. doi: 10.3758/BF03204379

Nodal, F. R., Bajo, V. M., and King, A. J. (2012). Plasticity of spatial hearing: behavioral effects of cortical inactivation. *J. Physiol.* 590, 3965–3986. doi: 10.1113/jphysiol.2011.222828

Oliver, D. L. (2005). "Neuronal organization in the inferior colliculus," in *The Inferior Colliculus*, eds J. A. Winer and C. E. Schneider (New York, NY: Springer), 69–114. doi: 10.1007/0-387-27083-3_2

Oliver, D. L., and Huerta, M. F. (1992). "Inferior and superior colliculi," in *The Mammalian Auditory Pathway: Neuroanatomy*, eds D. B. Webster, A. N. Popper, and R. R. Fay (New York, NY: Springer), 168–221. doi: 10.1007/978-1-4612-4416-5_5

Parks, T. N., Rubel, E. W., Popper, A. N., and Fay, R. R. (2004). *Plasticity in the Auditory System*. New York, NY: Springer. doi: 10.1007/978-1-4757-4219-0

Parseihian, G., and Katz, B. F. G. (2012). Rapid head-related transfer function adaptation using virtual auditory environment. *J. Acoust. Soc. Am.* 131, 2948–2957. doi: 10.1121/1.3687448

Rauschecker, J. P. (1999). Auditory cortical plasticity; A comparison with other sensory systems. *Trends Neurosci.* 22, 74–80. doi: 10.1016/S0166-2236(98)01303-4

Recanzone, G. H. (1998). Rapidly induced auditory plasticity: the ventriloquism aftereffect. *Proc. Nat. Acad. Sci. U.S.A.* 95, 869–875. doi: 10.1073/pnas.95.3.869

Rosen, S., Faulkner, A., and Wilkinson, L. (1999). Adaptation by normal listeners to upward spectral shifts of speech: Implications for cochlear implants. *J. Acoust. Soc, Am.* 106, 3629–3636. doi: 10.1121/1.428215

Shinn-Cunningham, B. (2001). Models of plasticity in spatial auditory processing. *Audiol. Neurotol.* 6, 187–191. doi: 10.1159/000046830

Shinn-Cunningham, B. G., Durlach, N. J., and Held, R. M. (1998a). Adapting to supernormal auditory localization cues. I. Bias and resolution. *J. Acoust. Soc. Am.* 103, 3656–3666. doi: 10.1121/1.423088

Shinn-Cunningham, B. G., Durlach, N. J., and Held, R. M. (1998b). Adapting to supernormal auditory localization cues. II. Constraints and adaptation of mean response. *J. Acoust. Soc. Am.* 103, 3667–3676. doi: 10.1121/1.423107

Slattery, W. H., and Middlebrooks, J. C. (1994). Monaural sound localization: acute versus chronic unilateral impairment. *Hear. Res.* 75, 38–46. doi: 10.1016/0378-5955(94)90053-1

Stein, B. E., and Meredith, M. A. (1993). *The Merging of the Senses*. Cambridge, MA: MIT Press.

Strelnikov, K., Rosito, M., and Barrone, P. (2011). Effect of audiovisual training on monaural spatial hearing in horizontal plane. *PLoS ONE* 6:e18344. doi: 10.1371/journal.pone.0018344

Tian, B., Reser, D., Durham, A., Kustov, A., and Rauschecker, J. P. (2001). Functional specialization in rhesus monkey auditory cortex. *Science* 292, 290–293. doi: 10.1126/science.1058911

van Wanrooij, M. M., and van Opstal, A. J. (2005). Relearning sound localization with a new ear. *J. Neurosci.* 25, 5413–5424. doi: 10.1523/JNEUROSCI.0850-05.2005

Wightman, F. L., and Kistler, D. J. (1988). Headphone simulation of free-field listening I: Stimulus synthesis. *J. Acoust. Soc. Am.* 85, 858–867. doi: 10.1121/1.397557

Wright, B. A., and Zhang, Y. (2006). A review of hearing with normal and altered sound-localization cues in human adults. *Int. J. Audiol.* 45(Suppl. 1), s92–s98. doi: 10.1080/14992020600783004

Wright, B. A., and Zhang, Y. (2009). A review of the generalization of auditory learning. *Philos. Trans. R. Soc. B* 364, 301–311. doi: 10.1098/rstb.2008.0262

Young, P. T. (1928). Auditory localization with acoustical transposition of the ears. *J. Exp. Psychol.* 11, 399–429. doi: 10.1037/h0073089

Yu, J. J., and Young, E. D. (1997). Linear and non-linear pathways of spectral information transmission in the cochlear nucleus. *Proc. Nat. Acad. Sci. U.S.A.* 97, 11780–11786. doi: 10.1073/pnas.97.22.11780

Zahorik, P., Bangayan, P., Sundareswaran, V., Wang, K., and Tam, C. (2006). Perceptual recalibration in human sound localization: Learning to remediated front-back reversals. *J. Acoust. Soc. Am.* 120, 343–359. doi: 10.1121/1.2208429

Zatorre, R. J., Bouffard, M., Ahad, P., and Belin, P. (2002). Where is "where" in the human auditory cortex? *Nat. Neurosci.* 5, 905–909. doi: 10.1038/nn904

20

Perception and coding of high-frequency spectral notches: potential implications for sound localization

***Ana Alves-Pinto*[1*†], *Alan R. Palmer*[2] *and Enrique A. Lopez-Poveda*[3]**

[1] *Klinikum rechts der Isar, Technische Universität München, Munich, Germany*
[2] *Medical Research Council Institute of Hearing Research, University Park, Nottingham, UK*
[3] *Departamento de Cirugía, Facultad de Medicina, Instituto de Neurociencias de Castilla y León, Instituto de Investigación Biomédica de Salamanca, Universidad de Salamanca, Salamanca, Spain*

***Correspondence:**
Ana Alves-Pinto, Research Unit of the Buhl–Strohmaier Foundation for Pediatric Neuro-Orthopaedics and Cerebral Palsy, Klinikum rechts der Isar, Technische Universität München, Ismaninger Strasse 22, 81675 Munich, Germany
e-mail: alvespinto.ana@gmail.com

†Present address:
Ana Alves-Pinto, Research Unit of the Buhl–Strohmaier Foundation for Pediatric Neuro-Orthopaedics and Cerebral Palsy, Klinikum rechts der Isar, Technische Universität München, Munich, Germany

The interaction of sound waves with the human pinna introduces high-frequency notches (5–10 kHz) in the stimulus spectrum that are thought to be useful for vertical sound localization. A common view is that these notches are encoded as rate profiles in the auditory nerve (AN). Here, we review previously published psychoacoustical evidence in humans and computer-model simulations of inner hair cell responses to noises with and without high-frequency spectral notches that dispute this view. We also present new recordings from guinea pig AN and "ideal observer" analyses of these recordings that suggest that discrimination between noises with and without high-frequency spectral notches is probably based on the information carried in the temporal pattern of AN discharges. The exact nature of the neural code involved remains nevertheless uncertain: computer model simulations suggest that high-frequency spectral notches are encoded in spike timing patterns that may be operant in the 4–7 kHz frequency regime, while "ideal observer" analysis of experimental neural responses suggest that an effective cue for high-frequency spectral discrimination may be based on sampling rates of spike arrivals of AN fibers using non-overlapping time binwidths of between 4 and 9 ms. Neural responses show that sensitivity to high-frequency notches is greatest for fibers with low and medium spontaneous rates than for fibers with high spontaneous rates. Based on this evidence, we conjecture that inter-subject variability at high-frequency spectral notch detection and, consequently, at vertical sound localization may partly reflect individual differences in the available number of functional medium- and low-spontaneous-rate fibers.

Keywords: auditory nerve, rate profile, phase-locking, temporal profile, head-related transfer function, HRTF

INTRODUCTION

The ridges and cavities of the outer ear alter the spectra of sounds that enter the ear canal, mainly (but not only) attenuating energy at high frequencies, such that notches are introduced into the spectra (Shaw and Teranishi, 1968; Lopez-Poveda and Meddis, 1996). These notches are thought useful for judging the vertical location of sound sources (Hebrank and Wright, 1974; Butler and Belendiuk, 1977; Butler and Humanski, 1992; Carlile et al., 2005). In particular, the human pinna introduces a notch whose center frequency increases gradually from around 6.5 to 10 kHz as the vertical location of the sound source moves from $-40°$ to $+60°$ relative to the horizontal plane (for a review see, e.g., Lopez-Poveda, 1996). The bandwidth (BW) of this notch at its 5-dB-down frequencies ranges from $\sim$1 kHz at $-40°$ elevation to $\sim$4 kHz at $+10°$ elevation (Shaw and Teranishi, 1968; Chapter 4 in Lopez-Poveda, 1996). The ability to use these notches for localizing sounds must depend ultimately on the quality of their representation in the auditory nerve (AN), as the nerve is the only path of transmission of acoustic information from the peripheral to the central auditory system[1]. Understanding the nature of the neuronal code underlying the representation of high-frequency spectral notches is therefore pertinent to understanding how sound elevation is perceived. The aim of the present study is to review existing evidence and shed new light on the nature of this code.

The spectrum of a sound may be encoded in the AN activity in at least two ways: in the average discharge rate across fibers tuned to different frequencies (a *rate profile*), and/or in the timing of spikes from fibers tuned to different frequencies. These two mechanisms, however, may not be available for encoding all the temporal and spectral characteristics of a sound. AN fibers can fire in synchrony with a particular phase of the stimulus waveform, a property called "phase-locking," and this enables them to encode the periodicities of the stimulus waveform in the timing of their spikes. However, as the stimulus frequency increases beyond several kHz, and its period becomes comparable to the variability of synaptic transmission, the jitter of ensuing spike timings degrades the quality of the spectral information. This limits the

[1] 90–95% of the population of spiral ganglion neurons comprise type I cells. These are connected to the inner hair cells and encode most auditory information. The rest 5–10% of the population consist of type II afferents that are connected to outer hair cells. Their role in auditory coding remains unclear but they are likely involved in the regulation of the operating point of the "cochlear amplifier" (Pickles, 1988; Jagger and Housley, 2003; Ashmore et al., 2010).

range of stimulus frequencies that can be encoded in the spiking times of individual fibers (Johnson, 1980; Palmer and Russell, 1986). In other words, this makes the encoding of high-frequency components in the phase-locking of individual fibers ineffective (Delgutte and Kiang, 1984a; Rice et al., 1995; Lopez-Poveda, 2005). Phase locking starts to roll-off at roughly 2 kHz. The frequency beyond which its degradation significantly impacts on spike statistics varies across species, being generally acknowledged to lie at 4 kHz for the guinea-pig (Palmer and Russell, 1986). If a similar 4 kHz phase-locking limit ocurred for humans (and this issue is currently being debated, e.g., Moore and Sek, 2009), then one might presume that the high-frequency spectral notches in the 4–9 kHz range must be encoded via firing rate profiles (Poon and Brugge, 1993; Rice et al., 1995). Here, we present strong evidence that undermines this view.

The question of how high frequency spectral notches are encoded in the AN can be approached by simply testing the hypothesis that they are encoded as AN rate profiles. If this were the case, then the internal, AN representation, and consequently the perception, of high-frequency spectral notches should deteriorate at high sound levels due, firstly, to the broadening of the fibers' frequency response at high levels (Rose et al., 1971), and, secondly, to the saturation of the discharge rate of the majority (~61%) of AN fibers (Rose et al., 1971; Sachs and Abbas, 1974; Evans and Palmer, 1980). While the remaining fibers have wider dynamic ranges (~50–60 dB; Sachs and Abbas, 1974; Evans and Palmer, 1980), only a small proportion of them remain unsaturated at high levels (Palmer and Evans, 1980).

We have previously tested the hypothesis that the internal representation of high-frequency spectral notches deteriorates with increasing sound level in a series of psychoacoustical and computational modeling studies. The results of these studies, reviewed here in the section 'Human psychophysics' and 'Computational simulation of inner hair cell receptor potentials evoked by flat-spectrum and notch noises' respectively, did not support the rate-profile code and rather pointed to alternative codes. The section 'Analysis of AN responses to flat-spectrum and notch noises' presents new data and analyses pertaining to AN activity elicited by stimuli identical to those used in our previous studies. This new set of physiological data also undermines the rate-profile code and rather suggests that the information required for discriminating between noises with different high-frequency spectra is carried in a temporal code. The combined evidence from this series of related psychoacoustical, computational modeling, and physiological studies will be discussed in the last section in terms of its implications for spatial hearing and for the across-listener variability in auditory-based spatial skills.

HUMAN PSYCHOPHYSICS

PSYCHOACOUSTICAL DISCRIMINATION BETWEEN FLAT-SPECTRUM AND NOTCH NOISES

Localization of impulsive sounds in the medial sagittal plane by human listeners deteriorates with increasing sound level up to about 70 dB SPL (Hartmann and Rakerd, 1993). This localization ability is believed to be mediated by the perception of high-frequency spectral notches generated by the filtering action of the human pinna (Hebrank and Wright, 1974; Butler and Belendiuk, 1977; Butler and Humanski, 1992; Carlile et al., 2005). Assuming that the perception of high-frequency spectral features is based on analyzing the AN rate profile then, as with vertical sound localization, the detection of high-frequency spectral notches should become increasingly more difficult as the sound level increases due to the saturation of the fiber firing rates. This hypothesis was tested *psychoacoustically* in humans by measuring the threshold notch depth necessary to discriminate between a flat-spectrum broadband noise and a similar noise with a spectral notch centered at 8 kHz (**Figure 1A**) at increasing noise levels, from 32 to 100 dB SPL (Alves-Pinto and Lopez-Poveda, 2005). If the hypothesis were true, then notch detection thresholds should increase, i.e., discrimination should become increasingly more difficult, with increasing noise level, as a result of the deterioration of the AN rate-profile representation of the spectral notch at high levels.

Surprisingly, however, threshold notch depth varied *non*-monotonically with level for most, but not all, listeners, increasing up to about 70–80 dB SPL and decreasing for higher levels (**Figure 1B**). The non-monotonic effect, when present, was comparable for notch BWs of 1, 2, and 4 kHz (see Figure 6 of Alves-Pinto and Lopez-Poveda, 2005), and for stimulus durations of 20 and 200 ms (see Figure 8 of Alves-Pinto and Lopez-Poveda, 2005), even though notch depth thresholds were generally higher for narrower notches and shorter stimuli. Stimulus rise times (2, 10, or 30 ms) did not affect notch depth thresholds at any of the levels tested (see Figure 7 of Alves-Pinto and Lopez-Poveda, 2005). These observations suggest that the non-monotonic shape of the threshold notch depth vs. level function is independent of stimulus duration and of the number of AN fibers that "see" a difference in energy between the two stimuli, that is, the fibers' with CFs within the notch frequency band.

Hence, the initial hypothesis of a monotonic increase in notch detection thresholds with increasing level was not supported by the experimental results, which rather suggested that the notch must be better represented internally at levels above and below around 70–80 dB SPL than at these mid-levels. This result prompted further research aimed at investigating the quality of the internal representation of the spectra of flat-spectrum and notch noises at increasing sound levels using diverse approaches: first, by comparing psychoacoustical masking patterns evoked by the two noises; second, by comparing computer simulations of the peripheral auditory system response to the two noises; and lastly, by analyses of direct AN fiber responses to the two noises.

PSYCHOACOUSTICAL MASKING-PATTERN REPRESENTATION OF HIGH-FREQUENCY SPECTRAL NOTCHES

The quality of the rate-profile representation of flat-spectrum and notch noises was assessed psychoacoustically by measuring the forward-masking patterns of the two noises (Alves-Pinto and Lopez-Poveda, 2008). A masking pattern is a graphical representation of the detection thresholds of masked probe tones as a

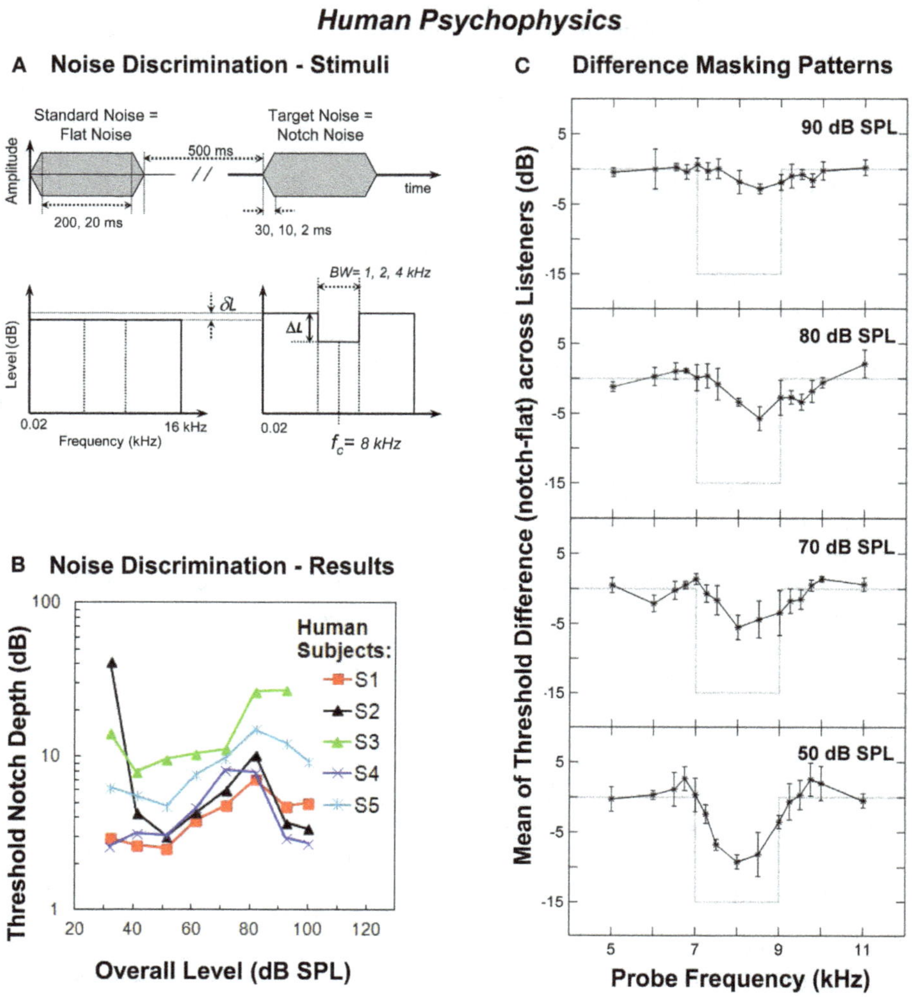

FIGURE 1 | Human psychophysics. (A) Schematic description of the waveforms and spectra of the flat-spectrum ("Standard Noise") and notch ("Target Noise") noises used in the noise discrimination experiment. The notch depth (ΔL) was defined as the difference in dB between the spectrum level in the notch and the reference spectrum level of the noise in the notch side bands. δL represents the reduction in spectrum level applied to the standard noise in order to make its overall level equal to that of the target noise. Also indicated are the values of stimulus duration, stimulus on/off time and the notch bandwidth (BW) tested in the experiments (adapted from Alves-Pinto and Lopez-Poveda, 2005). **(B)** Individual threshold notch depths for discriminating between the standard and target noises (panel **A**) as a function of overall stimulus level. The notch bandwidth was 2 kHz and the notch depth is in dB re the spectrum level in the notch side bands. Each symbol/color illustrates the results for a different listener (adapted from Alves-Pinto and Lopez-Poveda, 2005). **(C)** Differences between the masking patterns of the flat-spectrum and notch noise (notch—flat) at increasing masker levels averaged across listeners. Each panel illustrates the results for a different masker level, as indicated in the top-right corner of the panel. Error bars represent one standard deviation from the mean difference. Dotted lines illustrate the difference between the spectra of the two noises (adapted from Figure 8 of Alves-Pinto and Lopez-Poveda, 2008).

function of probe frequency. Psychoacoustical forward masking is thought to reflect (to a large extent) the incomplete recovery of AN fibers from previous stimulation and/or the persistence of neural (post-AN) activity (Oxenham, 2001; Meddis and O'Mard, 2005). Whatever the case, detection of a low-level tonal probe is likely mediated by the *average* discharge rate evoked by the probe in AN fibers with CFs similar to the frequency of the probe. When the probe is preceded by a masker sound, this rate almost certainly changes depending on the activity evoked by the masker in those same fibers (Harris and Dallos, 1979; Meddis and O'Mard, 2005). Hence, the activity evoked by the flat-spectrum noise on AN fibers with CFs within the notch band would be likely different from that evoked by the notch noise. This difference should be reflected as a difference in masked probe detection thresholds and, consequently, in the masking patterns produced by the two noises. Furthermore, by presenting the probe after the masker any potential interactions between the two stimuli (e.g., suppression, distortion, or beating effects) are minimized, thus favoring forward masking to psychoacoustically assess the quality of the internal representation of the two noises.

The forward masking pattern of the flat-spectrum/notch noises were obtained by measuring the masked threshold of detection of pure tones with frequencies covering the spectral region of the notch. They were measured for low (50 dB SPL), medium (70 and 80 dB SPL), and high (90 dB SPL) masker overall levels, to allow comparison with the non-monotonic effect of level in the main discrimination task (**Figure 1B**). The quality of the internal representation of the spectral notch was inferred from the difference between the masking patterns of the flat-spectrum and notch noises.

The spectral notch was clearly visible in the difference masking patterns at 50 dB SPL, less obvious at 70 and 80 dB SPL, and barely visible at 90 dB SPL (**Figure 1C**). The fact that the two masking patterns became more similar as the level increased from 50 to 80 dB SPL is consistent with the increase in discrimination threshold notch depth over the same level range (**Figure 1B**). Above 80 dB SPL, however, the difference between the two masking patterns continued to decrease (**Figure 1C**, upper panel) even though notch detection became easier (i.e., threshold notch depth generally decreased above around 80 dB SPL, **Figure 1B**). Insofar as a masking pattern is regarded as the psychoacoustical correlate of a neural excitation pattern, this result suggests that discrimination between the flat-spectrum and notch noises is, at least above 80 dB SPL, unlikely based on comparisons of the AN rate-profile representations of the noise spectra.

COMPUTATIONAL SIMULATION OF INNER HAIR CELL RECEPTOR POTENTIALS EVOKED BY FLAT-SPECTRUM AND NOTCH NOISES

The quality of the internal AN representation of high-frequency spectral notches must be limited by the signal processing that takes place before the AN. The inner hair cell (IHC) receptor potential is the driving potential of AN fibers' activity and therefore sets a limit on the quality of the representation of spectral information in the AN. It is possible, for example, that the excitation pattern representation of the stimulus spectrum degrades at high sound levels because saturation already occurs at the level of the IHC receptor potential (e.g., Russell and Sellick, 1978). For this reason, the quality of the representation of high-frequency spectral notches was assessed pre-AN by using a computational model of *receptor potential signals* generated by a bank of IHCs in response to flat-spectrum and notch noises (Lopez-Poveda et al., 2008). Assessing the quality of the representation high-frequency notches at the level of the receptor potential is advantageous also because the receptor potential is a deterministic, continuous signal that is easier to analyze than stochastic, discrete signals like AN spike trains.

The model included realistic cochlear mechanical level-dependent gain and tuning and a realistic IHC model (see Lopez-Poveda et al., 2008 for details). The model was evaluated in the time domain in response to both a flat-spectrum broadband noise and a noise with a 15-dB deep, 2-kHz wide, rectangular spectral notch centered at 7 kHz. The levels of the two noises were identical to those used in the psychoacoustical spectral discrimination task. The model output was a collection of receptor potential waveforms for a bank of IHCs with different CFs. The receptor potential waveforms were analyzed in two different ways: first, by plotting the root-mean-square (rms) receptor potential amplitude of each IHC as a function of the cell's CF—an *excitation pattern* representation (**Figure 2A**). This representation is akin to the AN rate profile representation of the stimulus spectrum, since the average discharge rate of an AN fiber is thought to be proportional to the rms receptor potential of its corresponding IHC (Cheatham and Dallos, 2001). The second analysis method involved: (1) applying a fast Fourier transform (FFT) to the receptor potential waveform of each IHC in the bank; and (2) adding all the resulting spectra, one per IHC, in the frequency domain to obtain a *population receptor potential FFT* representation of the stimulus spectrum (**Figure 2C**). This population response spectrum roughly reflects the total magnitude of phase-correlated response of the whole IHC population. In the real ear, each IHC would be actually innervated by several AN fibers, all of which would be driven by a common IHC receptor potential waveform. The FFT of an individual IHC receptor potential waveform represents an upper boundary to the temporal periodicities that could be encoded by the group of AN fibers innervating that IHC in their aggregated spike times. Likewise, the aggregated receptor potential FFTs for all IHCs represent an upper boundary to the periodicities that could be encoded by the population AN, hence providing a representation akin to the phase-locking representations in the AN (further details in Lopez-Poveda et al., 2008).

The results of the simulations showed that the quality of the IHC excitation pattern representation of the spectral notch (blue line in **Figure 2A**) degraded gradually with increasing stimulus intensity, a result clearly visible in the difference excitation patterns (**Figure 2B**). Differences between the two excitation patterns occurred for IHCs with CFs within or around the notch band only, with the largest difference occurring for the lowest intensity (40 dB SPL). By contrast, differences in the simulated IHC population receptor potential FFTs were smaller at mid intensities, around 60–80 dB SPL, than at lower and higher intensities (**Figures 2C,D**). Interestingly, significant differences occurred for frequencies outside the notch frequency band, particularly at the highest intensities (**Figure 2D**).

If psychoacoustical discrimination between the flat-spectrum and notch noise were determined by differences between the IHC representations of the flat-spectrum and notch noise spectra, then the simulations suggested that discrimination based on the excitation pattern should be increasingly more difficult with increasing level (**Figure 2B**), whilst discrimination based on the population receptor potential FFT should be easier below and above 70 dB SPL (**Figure 2D**). Only the latter is *qualitatively* consistent with the non-monotonic shape of the psychoacoustical threshold notch depth *vs.* level functions (**Figure 1B**).

What is the origin of the non-monotonic effect of level in the population receptor potential FFT? This issue was addressed by Lopez-Poveda et al. (2008). In short, they suggested that the gradual decrease in notch sensitivity up to 60–80 dB PSL is due to the cochlear mechanical compression whilst the improvement at high levels seemed to be due to IHC nonlinearities: at high sound levels, the flat-spectrum noise saturates the population IHC receptor potential more than does the notch noise and this would alter the spike patterns of AN fibers innervating a saturated IHC relative to

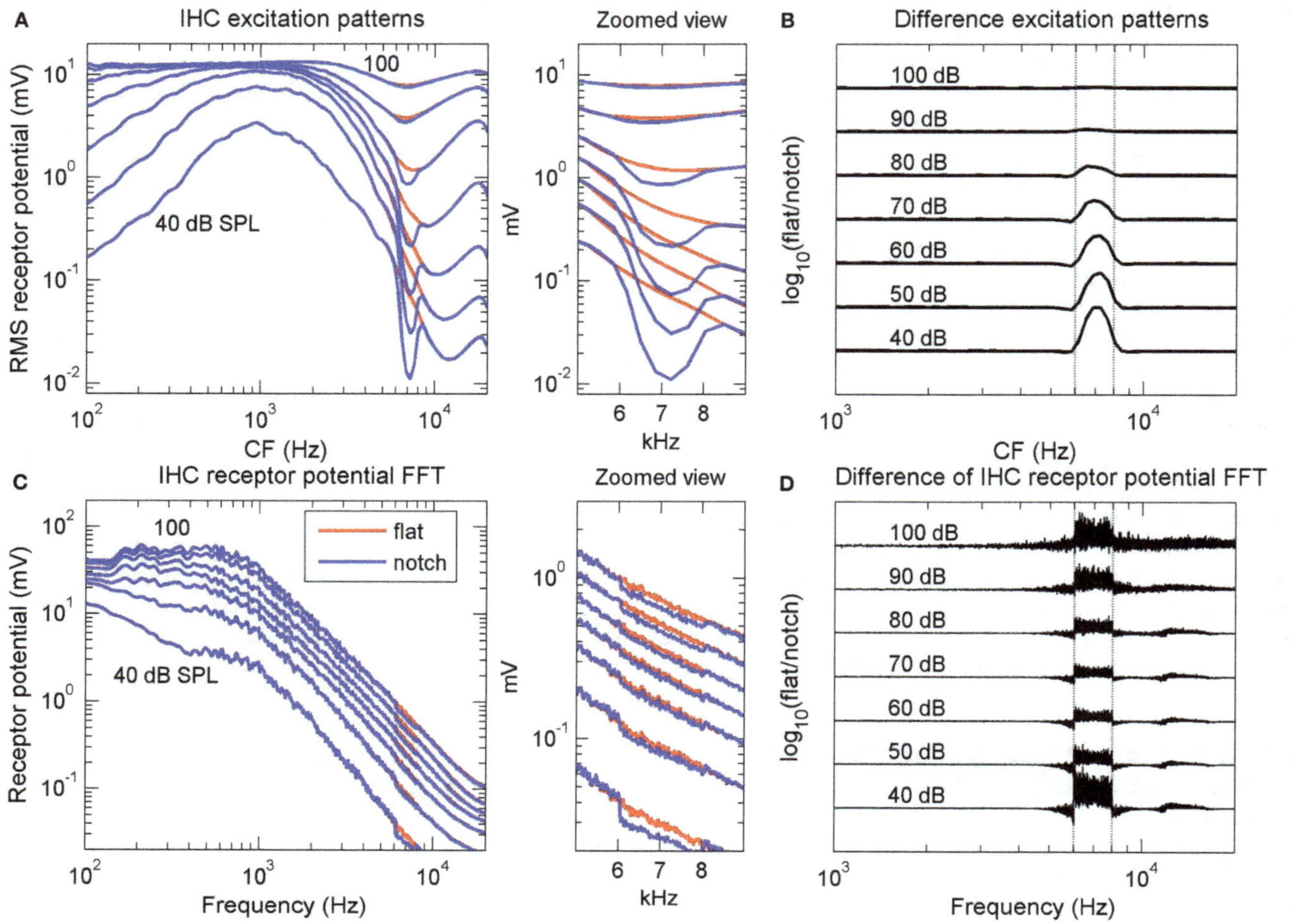

FIGURE 2 | Computational simulation of inner hair cell receptor potentials. Simulated IHC responses to broadband noises with a flat spectrum and with a 2-kHz wide, 15-dB spectral notch centered at 7 kHz. The noise duration was longer than that used in the psychoacoustical experiments (0.5 vs. 0.2 s) to obtain "smoother" responses. **(A)** IHC excitation pattern representation of the flat-spectrum (red) and notch noises (blue). Each curve illustrates the average (rms) receptor potential of each IHC as a function of the cell's CF, for a different stimulus level, from 40 to 100 dB SPL, as indicated by the numbers next to each trace. **(B)** Difference excitation patterns (in dB) normalized to the maximum value across CFs and intensities. The numbers next to each trace indicate stimulus intensity in dB SPL. **(C)** Spectra of the IHC receptor potential representation of the two noises for the same stimulus levels as in **(A)**. Each curve depicts the frequency-wise summed spectra of individual IHC receptor potential spectra (see main text). **(D)** Difference receptor potential FFT (in dB) normalized to the maximum value across frequencies and intensities. In **(B,D)**, the curves have been arbitrarily displaced vertically for convenience. Vertical dotted lines in **(B,D)** indicate the notch frequency band. The middle panels illustrate zoomed views of panels **(A,C)** over the frequency range of the spectral notch.

those innervating a non-saturated IHC (see Lopez-Poveda et al., 2008 for a detailed explanation).

Even though the model may not perfectly simulate the human IHC response (Lopez-Poveda et al., 2008), the simulations suggested two important aspects about the nature of the code underlying the psychoacoustical discrimination between flat-spectrum and notch noises. First, that the quality of the IHC excitation pattern representation of the spectral notch decreased gradually with increasing sound level (**Figure 2B**) means that the quality of the AN rate profile must necessarily decrease with increasing intensity, regardless of the type of AN fiber. This undermines the suggestion that the peak in the behavioral threshold notch depth *vs.* level function (**Figure 1B**) reflects the transition between the dynamic ranges of AN fibers with low and high thresholds, according to which the notch would be encoded in the activity of low-threshold (or high-spontaneous rate, HSR) fibers at low to mid-levels and on that of high-threshold (or low-spontaneous rate, LSR) fibers at high noise levels (Alves-Pinto et al., 2005).

Second, the similarity between the effects of intensity on the difference IHC receptor potential FFT (**Figure 2D**) and the threshold notch depths for spectral discrimination (**Figure 1B**) suggests that high-frequency spectral discrimination could be based on comparisons of internal representations of the spectra obtained by precise analysis of the *timing* of AN spikes. The actual mechanism that would allow the central auditory system to extract such a representation is uncertain (see below), but the model simulations suggested that it could be similar in effect to a Fourier transform of the spike trains (Young and Sachs, 1979). This would imply that useful frequency information is actually encoded in the timing of AN discharges even at stimulus frequencies at which phase-locking is significantly diminished (>4 kHz; Palmer and Russell, 1986). A similar conjecture has been put forward by a modeling study on the limits of human auditory perception of single tones (Heinz et al., 2001). Heinz et al. suggested that psychoacoustical frequency difference limens are consistent with frequency information being encoded in the discharge times of AN fibers for frequencies up to 10 kHz. This has been supported by recent physiological studies that have shown that detectable phase-locking can occur for frequencies as high as 14 kHz (Recio-Spinoso et al., 2005).

Inspired by this, further insight about the neuronal code responsible for the internal representation of high-frequency spectral notches and for the main psychoacoustical discrimination results was sought by directly measuring the activity of AN fibers in response to the flat-spectrum and notch noises used in the psychoacoustical and simulation experiments. These new data are described in the following section.

ANALYSIS OF AUDITORY NERVE RESPONSES TO FLAT-SPECTRUM AND NOTCH NOISES

RATIONALE

The quality of the internal representation of the high-frequency spectral notch at the level of the AN was assessed physiologically by directly recording the activity of guinea-pig AN fibers in response to stimuli like those used in the main psychoacoustical study. Following the evidence from the psychoacoustical and simulation studies (reviewed above), analyses of neuronal activity included an evaluation of the representation of the spectral notch in the average rate profile, but also in the temporal pattern of ANfiber discharges. For the latter, we could not apply the FFT analysis that we had used to analyze IHC receptor potential simulations because of (1) the discrete nature of the AN spike trains, (2) the short duration of the recording interval (110 ms), and (3) the limited number of recorded AN units. Instead, we used an "ideal observer" analysis (see below).

METHODS

Physiological recordings

Recordings from AN fibers of anaesthetized guinea pig were made using the methods described in Palmer et al. (1986). Data were collected from 163 fibers (from 18 animals) with CFs between 0.9 and 19 kHz, a CF range sufficient to cover the relevant spectral content of the stimulus. Fifty three of the 163 fibers had spontaneous rates less than 18 spikes/s, i.e., had low-to-medium spontaneous rates, a proportion consistent with the distribution of the different types of fibers in the guinea pig in terms of spontaneous rate and threshold levels (Yates, 1991).

Stimuli

AN fibers were stimulated with bursts of broadband (0.02–16 kHz) noise similar to those used in the psychoacoustical and simulation experiments. Two types of noises were used: one had a flat spectrum; the other was similar except for a frequency region centered at 7 kHz where it had a rectangular spectral notch (**Figure 1A**). The spectrum level in the notch band was 0 (i.e., flat spectrum), 3, 6, 9, 15, 21, or 27 dB below the spectrum level outside the notch band. Notch BWs of 2 and 4 kHz were used. Stimuli were presented for overall levels ranging from 40 to 100 dB SPL in 10-dB steps. Noise bursts had a total duration of 110 ms, including a 10-ms rise time; no fall ramp was applied. A different stimulus condition, defined by the notch depth and the overall sound level of the stimulus, was presented every 880 ms. Conditions were presented in random order.

The noise bursts were generated as described in the related behavioral study (Alves-Pinto and Lopez-Poveda, 2005). A single noise token was generated in the digital domain for each notch depth and used for repeated measures of AN responses at all levels (i.e., the noise was "frozen"). The noise bursts used in the present study were shorter (110 ms *vs.* 220 ms) and the notch center frequency was lower (7 kHz *vs.* 8 kHz) than those used in the related psychoacoustical study. Despite these differences, the fundamental characteristics of the stimuli remained the same: in both cases the notch frequency band was beyond the cut-off frequency of phase-locking (~4 kHz according to Palmer and Russell, 1986), and the stimulus duration was longer than the fast-adaptation period of AN fibers (~30 ms according to Westerman and Smith, 1984).

Rate profile analysis of auditory nerve responses

In this analysis a subpopulation of 106 fibers, for which at least 5 and typically 10 complete spike trains were recorded for all stimulus conditions tested, was used. The mean discharge rate was calculated over the whole stimulus duration (110 ms). Raw rate profiles are uninformative of the spectral content of the stimulus due to the large across-fiber variability in spontaneous and saturated rates (Rice et al., 1995). To account for the rate variability across fibers, normalized rate profiles (varying from 0 to 1) were used instead. The normalization was done as follows (Rice et al., 1995): $R_{norm} = (R - SR)/(R_{max} - SR)$, where R is the average discharge rate of the fiber, SR its spontaneous rate, and R_{max} its maximum discharge rate. Here, SR and R_{max} were estimated as the average discharge rates for a flat-spectrum noise stimulus of 40 and 100 dB SPL, respectively. Due to the small number of fibers with low-to-medium spontaneous rates (31 fibers only), reliable rate profiles for separate fiber type groups could not be obtained. Instead, the whole unit sample was used to properly sample the frequency range of interest in a rate profile. In the related behavioral task (Psychoacoustical discrimination between flat-spectrum and notch noises), subjects were asked to discriminate between a flat-spectrum noise and a noise with a spectral notch. Therefore, difference rate profiles for the two stimuli were also calculated as they provide a more relevant neural correlate of psychoacoustical performance than do normalized rate profiles. All rate profiles were smoothed by applying a running average calculated over 1/3rd-octave-band intervals.

"Ideal observer" analysis of auditory nerve responses

The psychoacoustical threshold notch depth for discriminating between a flat-spectrum and a notch noise, $\Delta\alpha$, was predicted from the responses collected for the sample of AN fibers according to the following equation (Siebert, 1970; Heinz et al., 2001):

$$\Delta\alpha = \left\{ \sum_i \int_0^T \frac{1}{r_i(t,\alpha)} \left[\frac{\partial r_i(t,\alpha)}{\partial \alpha} \right]^2 dt \right\}^{-0.5}, \quad (1)$$

where t denotes time, T denotes the stimulus duration, and $r_i(t, \alpha)$ the instantaneous discharge rate of the i-th fiber in response to the stimulus with notch depth α. The term in square brackets determines the change in instantaneous discharge rate $r_i(t, \alpha)$ of the i-th fiber at a given time instant, t, as a result of a change, $\partial\alpha$, in the stimulus condition. This term is squared to make positive and negative changes equally relevant. This change is then divided by the fiber's "instantaneous" discharge rate $r_i(t, \alpha)$, a sort of "normalization" procedure that takes into account the fiber's particular physiological characteristics. This is important because, for example, whilst a change of 1 spike/s may be meaningless for an HSR fiber, it may represent a huge change for a LSR fiber whose average discharge rate can be below 1 spike/s. The relative change in discharge rate is summed [integral in Equation (1)] throughout the stimulus duration, T, providing a measure of the overall sensitivity of this i-th fiber to a change $\partial\alpha$ in the stimulus. These individual sensitivities are then summed across fibers to obtain a measure of the ability of the *sample* of fibers to indicate a change in the stimulus conditions through a change in discharge rate of any of the fibers.

Given the discrete nature of the recorded AN responses and the limited number of stimulus conditions tested, a discrete version of the above equation was adopted for the current analysis:

$$\Delta\alpha = \left\{ \sum_i \sum_{k=1}^{nbins} s_{i,k} \right\}^{-0.5} \quad (2a)$$

where $s_{i,k}$is the *sensitivity* of the i-th fiber over the k-th time bin and is defined as follows:

$$s_{i,k} = \frac{1}{r_i(\Delta t_k, 0)} \cdot \left[\frac{r_i(\Delta t_k, 0) - r_i(\Delta t_k, 3)}{3 - 0} \right]^2 \cdot \Delta t_k \quad (2b)$$

where k is the index for the time bins considered in the analysis. The "instantaneous" discharge rate is replaced in Equation (2b) by the average discharge rate within a time interval (time bin) of duration Δt. $r_i(\Delta t_k,\ 0)$ is then the average discharge rate in the k-th time bin in response to the flat-spectrum noise (notch depth = 0 dB), and $r_i(t_k,\ 3)$ the average discharge rate in response to the 3-dB-deep notch noise. This was the smallest notch depth for which AN responses were recorded, and so it was assumed analogous to the incremental change $\partial\alpha$ of the stimulus parameter in Equation (1). Hence, the relative change in average discharge rate in each time bin, between responses to flat-spectrum and 3-dB-deep notch noises, was calculated for each fiber and added across time bins and across fibers.

Figure 3 illustrates example post-stimulus time histograms elicited by the flat-spectrum noise (filled bars) and the 3-dB notch noise (open bars) for two *individual* fibers: an HSR fiber (blue bars; CF = 3.6 Hz) and an LSR fiber (red bars; CF = 6.9 Hz) fiber. The discharge rate scale is on the left y-axis. Each stimulus typically elicits different discharge rates in each time bin (**Figure 3A**). This difference in discharge rate is the basis for the sensitivity of that single fiber to the two different stimuli. The sensitivity in each time bin was calculated using Equation (2b) and is represented by the blue squares (HSR) and red triangles (LSR) in **Figures 3A,B** (referred to the log-scale on the right y-axis). When similar discharge rates are evoked by the two stimuli the fiber is unable to distinguish between the two simply based on the rate difference information, and consequently its sensitivity becomes zero (missing symbols in some bins in **Figure 3A**). Summation of all these sensitivities across bins yields an overall measure of sensitivity at a given level for that individual fiber and consequently to an individual sensitivity (or its inverse, a discrimination threshold estimate) *vs.* level function for that fiber (**Figures 3C,D**). The sensitivity also depends on the binwidth [Equation (2b)]. Assessing the discharge rate using longer time bins (**Figure 3B**; responses are for the same two fibers represented in **Figure 3A**, only the binwidth for computation of the discharge rate is different) produces different patterns of discharge and consequently produces different sensitivities and discrimination thresholds (**Figures 3C,D**; notice the different scales in the right y-axis).

It becomes evident that this analysis is designed to detect the maximum relative change in discharge rate available throughout the stimulus duration and throughout the population of fibers and that it optimizes the information that each fiber can convey in its response toward the detection of a change in the stimulus, hence the term "ideal observer" analysis. The information carried in the variance of firing rate in each time bin counts and, in this sense, this "ideal observer" analysis contrasts with the average rate profile analysis that disregards any rate fluctuations in time and considers only the information conveyed in the overall discharge rate of the fibers assessed throughout the whole stimulus duration.

Equation (1) was derived on assumption that the occurrence of AN spikes follows a Poisson distribution, that is, that spikes occur at times that are independent of each other. Furthermore, in using Equation (1) to predict psychoacoustical discrimination thresholds, the implicit assumption is made that the listener can make optimal use of every bit of information available in the activity of the population of fibers, as explained above. Although neither of these two assumptions apply here (Siebert, 1965, 1968, 1970), we assumed that the error in using Equation (2) for predicting the psychoacoustical thresholds is comparable for all sound levels, and hence that Equation (2) serves to qualitatively predict how threshold notch depths change with sound level, as reported in the related psychoacoustical study (Alves-Pinto and Lopez-Poveda, 2005).

$\Delta\alpha$ was computed for different time bin durations, Δt, from 0.333 to 110 ms. For Δts that were not submultiples of the stimulus duration, the last bin, that had a different duration from the other bins, was eliminated from the sum in Equation (2a). Eliminated bins were no longer than 2 ms. When Δt is set to the stimulus duration, the resulting $\Delta\alpha$ corresponds to performance

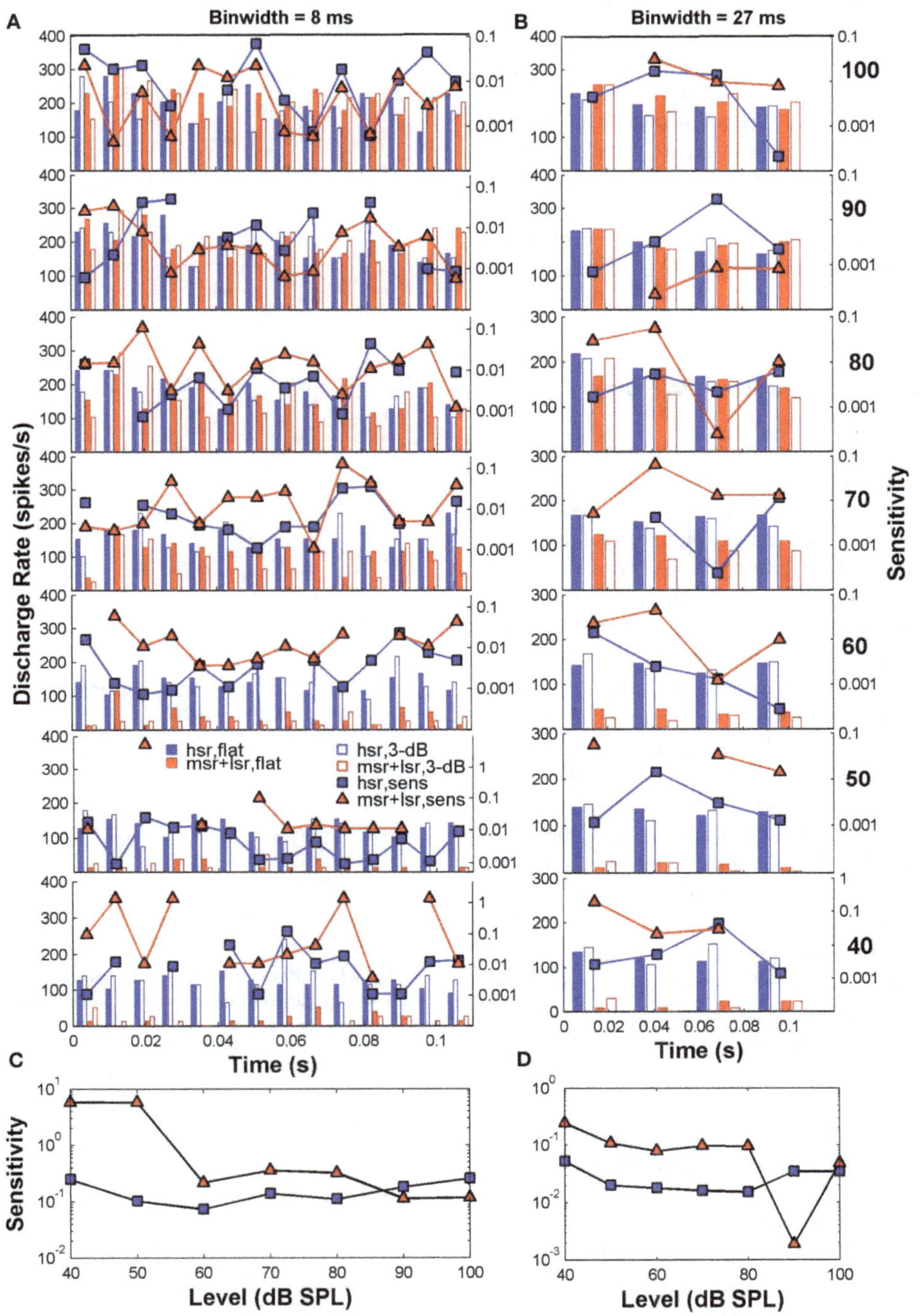

FIGURE 3 | Auditory nerve data: example post-stimulus time histograms (PSTHs; scale on the left y-axis) and related sensitivity (scale on the right y-axis) for one HSR fiber (blue bars and squares: CF = 3.6 Hz, SR = 111 spikes/s, 10 repeats/stimulus) and one LSR fiber (red bars and triangles: CF = 6.9 Hz, SR = 11.2 spikes/s, 10 repeats/stimulus). **(A)** PSTHs calculated for time binwidths of 8 ms. **(B)** PSTHs calculated for a binwidth of 27 ms. In each panel, filled and open blue bars illustrate the PSTHs for the HSR fiber when stimulated with a flat-spectrum and 3-dB-deep notch noise, respectively. Filled and open red bars illustrate corresponding PSTHs for the LSR fiber. Each row illustrates results for a different stimulus level as indicated by the bold numbers on the right part of the figure (in dB SPL). Also represented in each panel is the fiber's sensitivity in each time bin (log-scale on the right y-axis) for each of the two fibers (blue squares for the HSR fiber; red triangles for the LSR fiber; one symbol per bin). Sensitivity was calculated using Equation (2b) and yields a measure of a fiber's ability to discriminate between the two stimuli through a change in the discharge rate evoked by them, in different time bins. Missing symbols indicate bins for which the two stimuli elicited identical discharge rates, hence sensitivity became zero. **(C)** Overall sensitivity as a function of stimulus level for each of the fibers represented in panel **(A)**. Overall sensitivity for a given level was obtained by summing all the sensitivities across all bins for that level [Equation (2a)], represented by the symbols in the corresponding panel **(A)**. Blue squares and red triangles illustrate the sensitivity *vs.* level function for the HSR and LSR fibers, respectively. **(D)** The same as in C but for time binwidths of 27 ms. Overall sensitivity for each fiber was obtained by summing all the sensitivities at the corresponding level in panel **(B)**. The results presented in all panels are based on the responses of the same two AN fibers. For each fiber, different sensitivities within each time bin (panels **A,B**) produce different sensitivity *vs.* level functions (panels **C,D**).

based on a rate-profile code only. $\Delta\alpha$ becomes unrealistically equal to zero when the discharge rate of any fiber is equal to zero for any bin (no bar for the 3-dB notch noise at some of the time bins in **Figure 3A**). To prevent this artifactual result, a small, arbitrary constant of 0.1 spikes/s was added to the measured discharge rate in all bins of all fibers. The actual value of this constant did not alter results significantly. The results presented are based on the results of the group of 163 fibers for which at least 5 and typically 10 repeats were recorded for a flat-spectrum noise and for a notch depth of 3 dB at each of the different sound levels tested.

RESULTS

AN rate profiles do not explain psychoacoustical noise discrimination as a function of level

First, we tested whether psychoacoustical spectral discrimination could be accounted for using only the AN rate-profile representation of the stimulus spectrum. A simple visual analysis of both normalized and difference rate profiles (**Figures 4A,B**) revealed a lower discharge rate for those fibers with CFs around the frequency band of the notch, with deeper notches eliciting lower discharge rates at mid-levels. This would suggest that AN rate-profile comparisons constitute a reasonable physiological basis for psychoacoustical discrimination of high-frequency spectra. However, a closer look disproves this suggestion: the absolute rate difference was largest for overall levels around 60–80 dB SPL. This implies that discrimination should be easiest around these levels, in clear contrast with the actual psychoacoustical results (**Figure 1B**). Noticeably, the notch is still observed in the difference rate profiles at very high levels (upper panels in **Figure 4B**), provided that the notch is sufficiently deep (notch depth $\geq$ 9 dB). While at first sight this may seem inconsistent with the deterioration of the rate-profile representation of the notch due to the broadening of fibers' tuning, rate profiles are "noisy" and indeed the discrimination information available in the rate profile decreases gradually with increasing level beyond 80 dB SPL, as shown in the next section.

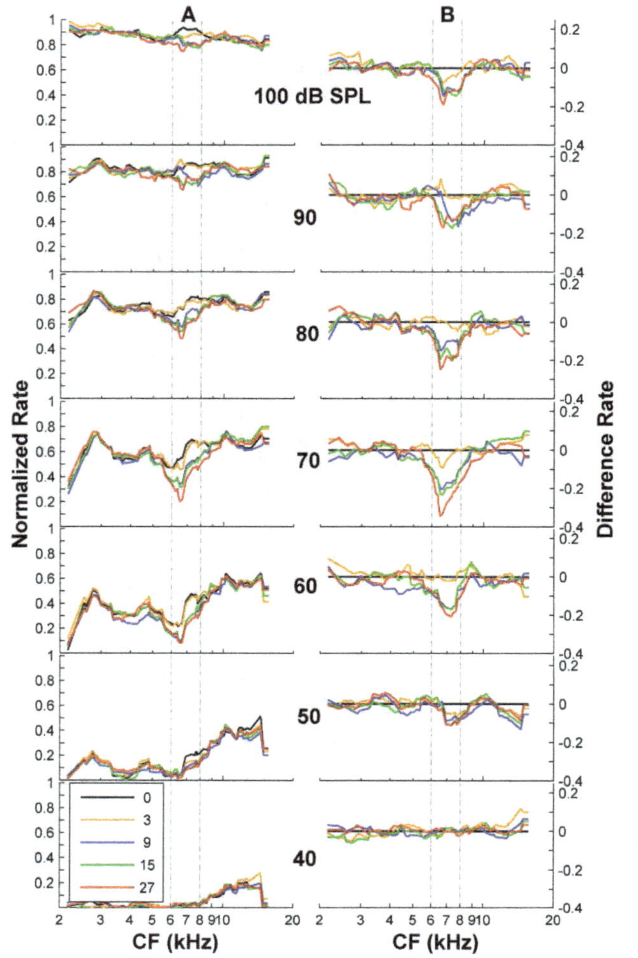

FIGURE 4 | Auditory nerve data: rate profiles for different overall noise levels and for different notch depths. (A) Normalized rate profiles. Each curve is for a different notch depth (in dB), as indicated by the inset. **(B)** Difference between the rate profiles for the flat-spectrum and the notched noises. The numbers in the inset denote notch depths in dB re spectrum level of the notch side bands. Vertical dashed lines illustrate the frequency band of the spectral notch.

Population d′ estimates based on rate profiles are inconsistent with psychoacoustical threshold notch depth vs. level functions

The above conclusion was confirmed by a signal-detection-theory *d*-prime (d') analysis of the physiological responses (Green and Swets, 1966; Shackleton et al., 2003). The "internal decision variable" in the psychoacoustical task was assumed to be proportional to the difference in firing rate between the flat-spectrum and notch conditions, assessed relative to the intrinsic variability in AN activity (the same stimulus token was used for all measurements for a given condition; hence, the variability in the responses arises exclusively from the stochastic nature of AN firing). A d' for the population of AN fibers was calculated for all conditions as the square root of the sum of the squared-d' values for individual AN fibers (Viemeister, 1988). This population d' was compared with the psychoacoustical thresholds previously measured using a 3-alternative, forced-choice paradigm (Alves-Pinto and Lopez-Poveda, 2005). The relation between the AN population-d' and the psychoacoustical threshold estimates did not need to be direct because, for example, as it is calculated, the population-d' increases with the number of fibers in the sample. Nevertheless, the population-d' provides a reasonable way of assessing, at least qualitatively, the expected perceptual performance based on intrinsically variable AN rate-profile information as a function of stimulus level.

The results (**Figure 5**) confirmed the insight gained from the visual analysis of the rate profiles (**Figure 4**) in terms of the effect of level. AN population-d' values were highest (hence discrimination thresholds would be lowest), at levels around 70–80 dB SPL for virtually all notch depths (**Figure 5**), in clear contradiction with the perceptual results (**Figure 1B**), which suggested that d' should be lowest around 80 dB SPL. In agreement with the evidence from the psychoacoustical and computer simulation studies (reviewed above), it can be, therefore, concluded that discrimination between auditory stimuli with different high-frequency spectral characteristics cannot be based on comparisons of their corresponding AN rate-profile representations.

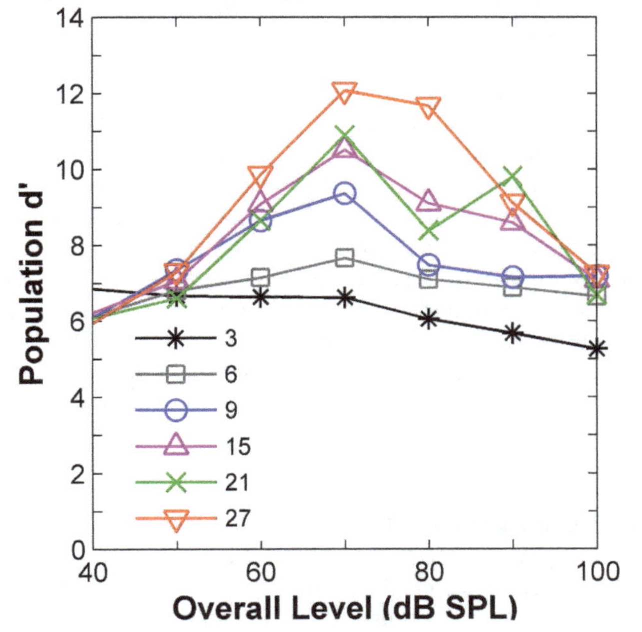

FIGURE 5 | Auditory nerve data: population *d'* as a function of the noise overall level. The numbers in the inset indicate notch depths in dB re spectrum level of the notch side bands.

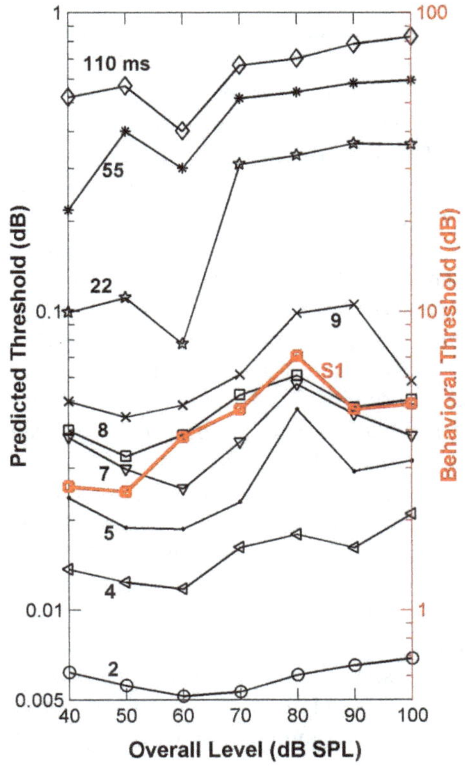

FIGURE 6 | Auditory nerve data: psychoacoustically observed notch-depth thresholds *vs.* "ideal observer" predictions from neural data. Psychoacoustical (red squares, right ordinate axis) thresholds as a function of noise level for an example listener (S1; **Figure 1B**). Predicted thresholds (open symbols, left ordinate axis) were obtained using an "ideal observer" type of analysis of physiological AN responses [Equations (2a) and (2b)]. Different curves illustrate predicted thresholds when AN activity is analyzed over non-overlapping time binwidths of different durations, as indicated by the numbers next to each trace (in ms; adapted from Figure 1 of Lopez-Poveda et al., 2007).

Predicted performance based on the analysis of auditory nerve responses by an "ideal observer"

The "ideal observer" analysis (Siebert, 1970; Heinz et al., 2001) is based on comparisons of discharge rates evoked by the two different stimuli (in this case a flat-spectrum noise and a noise with a 3-dB notch) computed in short non-overlapping time bins (**Figure 3**). This comparison between discharge rates was made for each single fiber and for each time bin of the fiber's PSTH (**Figures 3A,B**). Differences in discharge rate elicited by the two stimuli (filled *vs.* open bars in **Figure 3A**) vary across time bins with the sensitivity in each bin contributing additively to the overall sensitivity of each single fiber to the two stimuli (symbols in **Figures 3A,B**). By sensitivity we mean the ability of a fiber to discriminate between the flat-spectrum and the notch noises based on differences in discharge rate in each time bin elicited by the two stimuli [Equation (2b)]. This means that short-term differences in discharge rates evoked by the two stimuli, or equivalently, that temporal information, may also contribute discrimination information. Of course, different degrees of temporal information may be gained by sampling the instantaneous discharge rate in non-overlapping time bins of different durations; the shorter the time bin, the more precise the timing information, the greater the discrimination capability of the system, and the lower the discrimination thresholds. This was indeed found to be the case. For any given sound level, the predicted threshold notch depths decreased with shortening the sampling time bin (**Figure 6**). In absolute terms, however, the predicted thresholds were about two orders of magnitude lower than the behavioral ones (**Figure 6**). This mismatch likely reflects the pooling of information that occurs as different auditory inputs converge into higher nuclei in the auditory system. It may also reflect differences in cochlear processing between humans and guinea pigs, and/or that humans do not operate as optimal spectral discriminators, as others have suggested (Siebert, 1965, 1968, 1970; Delgutte, 1996; Heinz et al., 2001). Otherwise observed (psychoacoustical) and predicted (neural) absolute thresholds should match.

Monitoring nerve activity in shorter time bins of 4–9 ms predicted the level effect observed psychoacoustically

Remarkably, the *shape* of the predicted threshold notch depth *vs.* level functions varied greatly depending on the time binwidth. Only for time binwidths within the range from 4 to 9 ms were the predicted functions non-monotonic with a peak at or around 80 dB SPL, thus resembling the *shape* of most psychoacoustical functions (**Figure 1B**, and open red squares in **Figure 6**). This suggests that an effective cue for high-frequency spectral discrimination may be based on sampling rates of spike arrivals of AN fibers using non-overlapping time binwidths of between 4 and 9 ms (**Figure 6**).

To confirm this optimal analysis time binwidth, Kendall's τ non-parametric correlation coefficient (Press et al., 1992) was used to quantify the degree of correlation between the *shapes* of the predicted functions for different time binwidths and the observed functions for each one of five listeners (S1–S5, for which discrimination between flat-spectrum and a 2-kHz wide notch noise was tested) considered in the psychoacoustical study (**Figure 1B**). The actual degree of correlation varied considerably across listeners (not shown), but the highest correlations always occurred for a time binwidths between 7 and 9 ms. The mean value across subjects was approximately 8 ms (**Figure 7D**).

The notch depth threshold values predicted by the "ideal observer" analysis of AN fiber responses shown in **Figure 6** were derived from the responses of the population of 163 AN fibers to the flat-spectrum and 3-dB notch noises. Analysis of individual fiber's sensitivity as a function of CF revealed that not all fibers contributed equally to the overall population sensitivity (**Figure 7**). Individual sensitivities for a binwidth of 8 ms showed that fibers with CF away from the notch band can contribute significantly to the population sensitivity (**Figure 7A**). Furthermore, the sub-populations of fibers with the highest sensitivities, therefore determinant to the discrimination threshold, also varied depending upon the analysis binwidth (compare **Figures 7A–C**).

The "ideal observer" analysis for a time binwidth equal to the stimulus duration (110 ms) disregards any temporal information. Hence, it was another way of testing the rate-profile code hypothesis. The shape of the associated predicted function (diamonds in **Figure 6**) clearly differed from that of the psychoacoustical function (red squares in **Figure 6**). Threshold notch depths were smallest for low-level sounds and gradually increased with increasing the sound level. Not surprisingly this shape resembles the curve that would be obtained by inverting the population-d' *vs.* level function for a notch depth of 3 dB (**Figure 5**). Therefore, this analysis also indicates that the rate-profile is unlikely to provide the basis for high-frequency spectral discrimination.

Selective use of different fiber types does not account for the psychoacoustical discrimination as a function of level

The possibility exists that the non-monotonic shape of the behavioral threshold notch depth *vs.* level functions could reflect the existence of only two fiber types with different thresholds and dynamic ranges in the human AN, with the peak in the behavioral function occurring at the transition sound level between the dynamic ranges of the HSR and LSR fibers (Alves-Pinto and Lopez-Poveda, 2005). This mechanism has been put forward as one way that the AN handles information over a much wider range of sound levels than the dynamic range of its individual fibers; that is, as a solution for the dynamic range problem of hearing (Viemeister, 1988; Delgutte, 1996).

This conjecture was tested here by applying the "ideal observer" analysis to two groups of AN fibers, with units classified according to spontaneous rate as HSR or LSR+MSR when their spontaneous rate was higher or lower than 18 spikes/s, respectively (Liberman, 1978). The resulting HSR and LSR+MSR groups contained 110 and 53 fibers, respectively. The mean optimal time binwidth of 8 ms (**Figure 7D**) was used.

Predicted threshold notch depth *vs.* level functions differed for the two groups (**Figure 8**). Nevertheless, predicted thresholds at low sound levels were lower for the LSR+MSR group than for the HSR group. This means that LSR+MSR fibers are more sensitive to spectral changes at low sound levels than are HSR fibers. Most important is, perhaps, that the predicted functions were almost identical for the LSR+MSR group and for the combined HSR+LSR+MSR sample, and that both their shapes were highly correlated with the shape of the perceptual discrimination functions (**Figure 1B**). This suggests that LSR+MSR fibers may be more significant to high-frequency spectral discrimination than are HSR fibers at all sound levels tested. This result indicates that the non-monotonic shape of the behavioral discrimination functions is unlikely to reflect a transition between the dynamic ranges of the two fiber types.

The effect of stimulus duration

In the psychoacoustical discrimination study, it was observed that threshold notch depths for discrimination were on average 2.5 times larger for a short (20-ms duration) than for a long (220 ms) stimulus, and that this ratio was approximately constant across sound levels (Alves-Pinto and Lopez-Poveda, 2005). In other words, the effect of level was independent of stimulus duration. The ideal observer analysis was therefore used to predict the behavioral thresholds for stimulus durations of 110 and 20 ms. A time binwidth of 5 ms was used in this case for convenience because it is a submultiple of these two stimulus durations.

The resulting predicted thresholds were higher for the short than for the long stimulus (**Figure 9**). Moreover, the ratio between the two values (red squares in **Figure 9**) was similar across levels and on average equal to 2.8. These results match well with those from the main psychoacoustical study (Alves-Pinto and Lopez-Poveda, 2005). This match reveals that the "ideal observer" analysis provides a reasonable account of the behavioral discrimination thresholds based on the *relative* neural information available for the short and long stimuli. In the context of the present analysis, we would suggest that higher thresholds resulted from having fewer time bins in which to assess differences between the neural responses to the two stimuli.

DISCUSSION OF EXPERIMENTAL NEURAL FINDINGS

We have shown that psychoacoustical discrimination between auditory broadband stimuli with and without high-frequency spectral notches is uncorrelated with the differences in the overall AN rate-profile representations of their spectra. Although the spectral notch is visible in the rate-profile for all sound levels above 50 dB SPL provided it is sufficiently deep (**Figure 4B**), the effect of level on the quality of that neuronal representation does not match, and therefore is unlikely to explain, the effect of level in the behavioral notch discrimination thresholds. Altogether, the present neural results are inconsistent with the view that high-frequency spectral features are encoded in the AN average-rate profile (e.g., Rice et al., 1995), and support the inferences made from the related human masking patterns (**Figure 1C**) and computational modeling studies (**Figure 2**). The

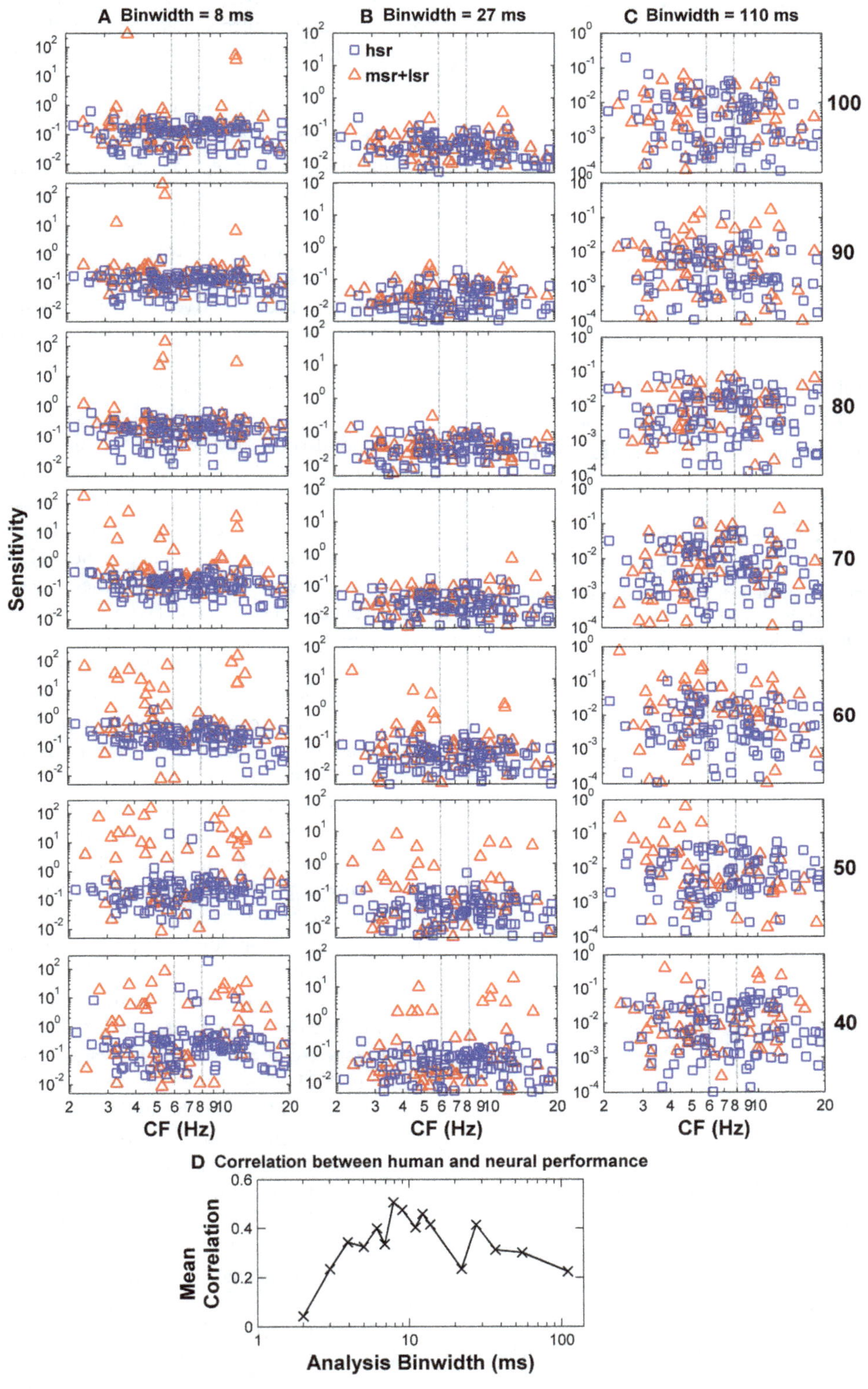

FIGURE 7 | Auditory nerve data: individual AN fiber sensitivity as a function of fiber's CF. Sensitivity values for HSR and LSR fibers are illustrated by blue squares and red triangles, respectively. Sensitivity was calculated for three different time binwidths: 8 ms **(A)**, 27 ms **(B)**, and 110 ms **(C)**. Notice the different sensitivity scales used for the different binwidths. Stimulus level increases from the bottom to the top panel as indicated by the numbers on the right side of the figure (in units of dB SPL). Individual sensitivity values varied with stimulus level and with binwidth, with the highest sensitivity values occurring for different subgroups of fibers for different levels and binwidths. **(D)** Kendall's Tau non-parametric correlation between the *shape* of individual behavioral notch-depth thresholds (**Figure 1B**) and "ideal observer" neural predictions for different analysis time binwidths (black symbols in **Figure 6**). The figure illustrates the mean correlation coefficient values across five participants (**Figure 1B**).

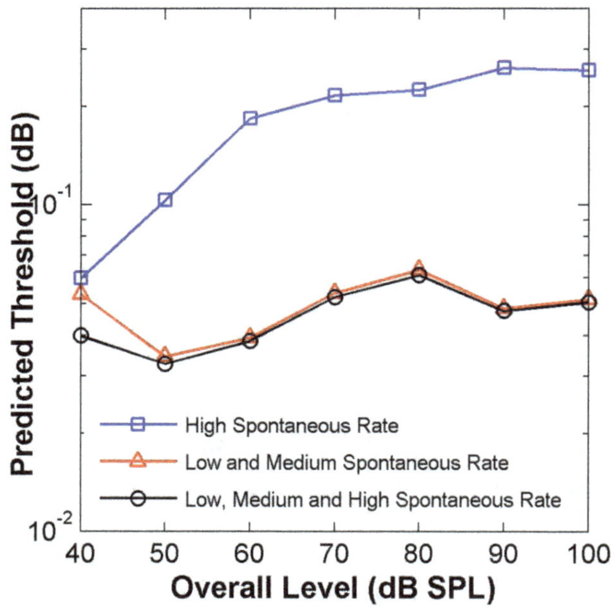

FIGURE 8 | Auditory nerve data: predicted threshold notch depth *vs.* level functions from an "ideal observer" analysis of neural responses from different fiber types, as indicated in the legend. Predictions are for an analysis time window of 8 ms.

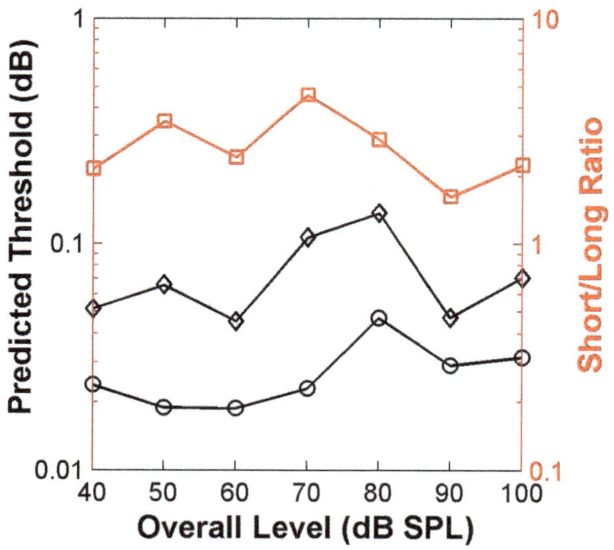

FIGURE 9 | Auditory nerve data: threshold notch depth *vs.* level functions predicted by an "ideal-observer" analysis of neural responses for noise bursts with different duration: 20 ms (diamonds) and 110 ms (circles). Red squares (right ordinate axis) illustrate the ratio between predicted thresholds for the long and short stimuli.

present AN results support a combined rate-time code instead. The nature of the code is uncertain, but the present analysis suggests that information decoding requires sampling the discharge rate of the fiber population in time binwidths of approximately between 4 and 9 ms. Unfortunately the number of stimulus repeats used here for the physiological experiments was insufficient to draw reliable conclusions and further experimental evidence is still necessary to confirm the present conclusions, to dismiss the rate profile as the only encoding strategy for high frequency features, and to elucidate the nature of the rate-time code underlying high-frequency spectral discrimination.

Differences in neuronal processing between humans and guinea pigs may have contributed to the mismatch between the psychoacoustical and the neural results in terms of level dependence of rate-profile derived discrimination thresholds. Also the anesthetic may have had an effect on neuronal responses. Both of these factors would have however also affected the correspondence between psychoacoustic and neural results based on the "ideal-observer" analysis. Nevertheless, the idea that some form of temporal code may be used for high-frequency spectral discrimination is not new and agrees with evidence from other independent studies in a number of aspects. It has been put forward, for example, to explain the limits of human auditory frequency discrimination for single tones (Heinz et al., 2001) and for the sensitivity to the spectral fine-structure of sounds in the high-frequency range (> 4 kHz; e.g., Moore and Sek, 2009). The results presented here support this principle. Furthermore, the present neural results extend the validity of the principle to spectral discrimination of broadband *aperiodic* stimuli (which is a more natural type of auditory task than pure tone discrimination) and reveal the existence of an optimal decoding time binwidth of 8 ms.

What is the nature of the temporal code? We have no definite answer, only conjectures. Any AN fiber is effectively driven by a half-wave rectified, low-pass filtered version of the basilar membrane response waveform at its corresponding place in the cochlea. With broadband noise stimulation, this response can be described as a randomly amplitude-modulated carrier with a carrier frequency near the fiber's CF. The range of modulation frequencies is limited by the BW of the cochlear filter (Louage et al., 2004) or the cut-off of phase locking. The BW of basilar membrane responses increases with increasing sound level (Robles and Ruggero, 2001). Therefore, the range of modulation frequencies as well as the phase of the basilar membrane response waveform both depend on sound level. AN fibers can phase-lock to the envelope of basilar membrane excitation even at high levels, when their discharge rate is at saturation (Cooper et al., 1993). Given that fibers with CFs near the notch frequency surely "see" a different level than those with CFs well away from it, it is therefore, possible that spectral discrimination be based on detecting either the range of modulation frequencies or the phase differences implicit in AN spike trains (or both). In other words, the auditory system might be treating a spectral discrimination task as an envelope discrimination task; the envelope being that of the signals coming from different cochlear channels. An envelope-based discrimination code would be consistent with the found optimal time binwidth of 4–9 ms.

That said, however, any difference in the envelopes evoked by the flat-spectrum and notch noises should show up in the aggregated FFTs of the simulated IHC receptor potential waveforms;

that is, they should show up in **Figures 2C,D**. Admittedly, some differences between the FFTs for the two noises did indeed occur for frequencies below 100 Hz (not shown in **Figures 2C** or **2D**) but they were almost negligible and much smaller than the differences in the notch frequency band highlighted in **Figure 2D**. Insofar as **Figure 2C** represents an upper limit to the periodicities that can be represented via phase locking in the AN-fiber population by the "volley principle" (Wever, 1949), **Figure 2C** suggests that the fine-time structure of AN activity would be a stronger cue for high-frequency spectral notch discrimination than the information available through synchronized responses to the envelopes. Unfortunately, gathering spectral information from the timings of spikes for spectral components around 7 kHz would require analyzing spike trains with very short binwidths, of 0.14 ms, and to avoid artifactual results [i.e., very high sensitivity due to close-to-zero discharge rate, Equations (1) and (2b)], this would require having many more repeats for each fiber than we have measured. For this reason, we could not confirm or reject this hypothesis using the available data. In summary, further experimental evidence is still necessary to clarify the nature of the temporal code.

The present neural results support the "multiple-looks" model for auditory long-term temporal integration: the decrease in threshold with increases in the stimulus duration. Such temporal integration does not actually involve integrating stimulus energy (or correspondingly accumulating nerve spikes) over time, but is more consistent with a model whereby "multiple-looks" of the output envelopes from auditory filters are taken in non-overlapping time windows of about 5–10 ms of duration (Viemeister and Wakefield, 1991). The "looks" would be stored in memory and accessed selectively for further processing and decision making. This model was proposed to account for behavioral observations, but has lacked physiological support to date. The present physiological results are consistent with such a model and even the range of optimal time binwidths found here (4–9 ms) matches the duration of the time windows proposed in the "multiple-looks" model.

The present physiological results are also consistent with explanations proposed for the so-called "dynamic range problem" of hearing. This refers to the apparent mismatch between the wide range of sound levels over which good intensity discrimination can be shown and the dynamic range of most AN fibers (Viemeister, 1988; Delgutte, 1996; Moore, 2003). Several different mechanisms are likely to contribute, but none of them seems to be critical or to fully explain the various behavioral results (Delgutte, 1996). Some models indicate that an appropriate combination of information from only a *few* AN fibers can account for intensity discrimination thresholds, even at high intensities (Delgutte, 1987; Viemeister, 1988). Further, they indicate that the activity of LSR fibers determines behavioral performance at high sound levels (Viemeister, 1988). The present study concerns a different perceptual task, but the results provide experimental support to those ideas. Here it was observed that only a handful of highly-sensitive fibers sufficed to produce the observed improvement in discrimination at very high sound levels (> 80 dB SPL) (**Figures 1B, 6**). Furthermore, the subpopulation of LSR+MSR fibers appears to convey enough information to account for most of the psychoacoustical thresholds (**Figures 7, 8**). Interestingly, this was true over the whole range of sound levels that were used.

Some questions remain. First, the "ideal observer" predictions showed that performance could improve substantially if the discharge rate of AN fibers were sampled in time binwidths shorter than 8 ms (**Figure 6**). This is true even allowing for the fact that humans do not operate as optimal discriminators, hence the two-order-of-magnitude difference between psychoacoustical and predicted thresholds. That is, it seems as though humans are not using all the information available in the AN. On the other hand, the value of 8-ms for the optimal time binwidth does not seem coincidental. It matches well with the conclusions from the "multiple-looks" model. Furthermore, there is also indirect evidence that visual information is processed in time windows of comparable durations (Van Rullen and Thorpe, 2001). The question is what does it mean? One possibility is that it relates to the time constant of cochlear nucleus neurons specialized in spectral-notch or spectral-edge detection (Reiss et al., 1995; Zheng and Voigt, 2006).

Second, the amount of perceptually-relevant information for high-frequency spectral discrimination was shown to be less for sound levels around 80 dB SPL than for lower or higher levels. This still needs explaining. The results presented here demonstrate that it is unrelated to having two fiber populations with different thresholds and dynamic ranges. It is possible that spectral representation of the notch in the BM excitation pattern may be compromised at mid-levels due to cochlear mechanical compression (see Lopez-Poveda et al., 2008).

POTENTIAL IMPLICATIONS FOR UNDERSTANDING ACROSS-LISTENER VARIABILITY IN SOUND LOCALIZATION

SPECTRAL-NOTCH CUES VARY ACROSS LISTENERS

It has been long thought that high-frequency spectral notches in the head-related transfer function (HRTF) are important cues for human (vertical) sound localization (e.g., Butler and Belendiuk, 1977; Butler and Humanski, 1992). On the other hand, the depth and the BW of HRTF notches vary widely across listeners [(see, for instance, Shaw (1982) or Chapter 3 in Lopez-Poveda, 1996)], probably reflecting differences in ears' shape and size across listeners (Lopez-Poveda and Meddis, 1996). Furthermore, we have shown that notch depth at discrimination threshold varies widely across listeners (**Figure 1B**) and depends on the notch BW as well on stimulus level and duration (Alves-Pinto and Lopez-Poveda, 2005). Assuming that behavioral discrimination between flat-spectrum and notch noises is based on the quality of the internal representation of the notches, then, in light of the present evidence, sound localization accuracy should vary across listeners, should be more precise for long than for short stimuli and for levels below 60–70 dB SPL than for levels around 70–80 dB SPL and this is indeed the case (Hartmann and Rakerd, 1993; Macpherson and Middlebrooks, 2000; Vliegen and Van Opstal, 2004; Macpherson and Sabin, 2013). Furthermore, vertical localization accuracy should improve for levels higher than about 80 dB SPL, although this remains to be tested.

In any case, the ability of listeners to actually use high-frequency HRTF notches as sound localization cues must depend on a complex combination of their level of performance in notch detection tasks, the shape of their ears, and the characteristics of the stimulus (duration and level).

POTENTIAL VARIABILITY ASSOCIATED TO NEURAL ENCODING OF SPECTRAL FEATURES

Performance in high-frequency notch detection tasks, and hence in spatial localization involving detection of these spectral features, will ultimately depend on the quality of the representation of the spectral notch in the AN. The evidence provided here suggests that high-frequency spectral information may be encoded in the temporal pattern of AN discharges, analyzed over time binwidths 4–9 ms long. Studies on the temporal aspects of spectral processing in sound localization also reported that information about the spectrum level of a cochlear filter can only be reliably obtained when the signal from that filter is integrated over a time window of about 5 ms (Jin, 2001), a duration similar to that estimated from the "ideal observer" analysis of AN fibers' responses (**Figure 7D**).

Spectral notch encoding based on the temporal patterns of discharge of AN fibers is likely to be more susceptible to variability than encoding based on the long-term average discharge rate. Spikes occur stochastically in time and spike counts for constant stimuli are likely to vary from time bin to time bin. Variations in the number of spikes have a larger effect in a small than in a larger time window, making any changes that are not stimulus related to more strongly affect the quality of the information encoded in the spike pattern. This higher susceptibility to variability could partly contribute to the large variability in the detection of spectral notches across listeners observed here.

Finally, discrimination thresholds derived from the "ideal observer" analysis of responses of LSR and MSR fibers were comparable to those derived using all fibers, including HSR fibers (**Figure 8**). This suggests that LSR and MSR fibers, despite their being a smaller population, are more sensitive to high-frequency spectral differences than are HSR fibers at all levels and so that LSR and MSR fibers could be key for detecting high-frequency spectral notches. Furthermore, it suggests that high-frequency notch discrimination would be probably impaired by damage and/or loss of these more sensitive fibers. According to a recent report (Furman et al., 2013), noise exposure selectively damages LSR fibers without altering audiometric thresholds. It has been suggested that this significantly impairs hearing in noise (Lopez-Poveda and Barrios, 2013). It is possible, therefore, that different audiometrically normal listeners may suffer from different degrees of (hidden) LSR fiber loss, depending on their individual histories of noise exposure and/or genetic sensitivity to noise, which would lead to variable performance in spectral discrimination tasks and, consequently, to variable performance in spatial localization involving the detection of high-frequency spectral notches. Further research is required to test this conjecture.

CONCLUSIONS

For most listeners, high-frequency spectral notch detection becomes gradually more difficult with increasing level up to 70–80 dB SPL and improves at higher levels. However, across-listener variability is high and depends both on the stimulus characteristics (duration and level) and on the notch BW.

Psychoacoustical, modeling, and physiological results consistently suggest that the non-monotonic effect of level on notch detection is inconsistent with the notch being encoded in the rate profile of AN fibers only and support, instead, that the temporal pattern of AN discharges monitored in time binwidths of 4–9 ms of duration conveys encoding relevant information. Physiological data suggest that LSR fibers are key to notch encoding.

The present evidence suggests that high-frequency spectral notch detection, and consequently, also vertical sound localization accuracy, requires information carried in the temporal characteristics of AN activity, particularly, by the available number of low and medium spontaneous rate fibers. The number of fibers likely varies substantially across individuals, which might contribute to across-listener variability in sound localization.

ACKNOWLEDGMENTS

Experimental work supported by the Spanish Fondo de Investigaciones Sanitarias (grants PI02/0343 and G03/203) and by European Regional Development Funds to Enrique A. Lopez-Poveda. The preparation of this paper was supported by the Spanish Ministry of Innovation and Competitiveness to Enrique A. Lopez-Poveda (grant BFU2012-39544-C02).

REFERENCES

Alves-Pinto, A., and Lopez-Poveda, E. A. (2005). Detection of high-frequency spectral notches as a function of level. *J. Acoust. Soc. Am.* 118, 2458–2469. doi: 10.1121/1.2032067

Alves-Pinto, A., and Lopez-Poveda, E. A. (2008). Psychophysical assessment of the level-dependent representation of high-frequency spectral notches in the peripheral auditory system. *J. Acoust. Soc. Am.* 124, 409–421. doi: 10.1121/1.2920957

Alves-Pinto, A., Lopez-Poveda, E. A., and Palmer, A. R. (2005). "Auditory nerve encoding of high-frequency spectral information," in *Interplay Between Natural and Artificial Computation (IWINAC)*, eds J. Mira and J. R. Álvarez (Berlin; Heidelberg: Springer-Verlag), 223–232.

Ashmore, J., Avan, P., Brownell, W. E., Dallos, P., Dierkes, K., Fettiplace, R., et al. (2010). The remarkable cochlear amplifier. *Hear. Res.* 266, 1–17. doi: 10.1016/j.heares.2010.05.001

Butler, R. A., and Belendiuk, K. (1977). Spectral cues utilized in the localization of sound in the median sagittal plane. *J. Acoust. Soc. Am.* 61, 1264–1269. doi: 10.1121/1.381427

Butler, R. A., and Humanski, R. A. (1992). Localization of sound in the vertical plane with and without high-frequency spectral cues. *Percept. Psychophys.* 51, 182–186. doi: 10.3758/BF03212242

Carlile, S., Martin, R., and McAnally, K. (2005). Spectral information in sound localization. *Int. Rev. Neurobiol.* 70, 399–434. doi: 10.1016/S0074-7742(05)70012-X

Cheatham M. A., and Dallos P. (2001). Inner hair cell response patterns: implications for low-frequency hearing. *J. Acoust. Soc. Am.* 110, 2034–2044. doi: 10.1121/1.1397357

Cooper, N. P., Robertson, D., and Yates, G. K. (1993). Cochlear nerve-fiber responses to amplitude-modulated stimuli - variations with spontaneous rate and other response characteristics. *J. Neurophysiol.* 70, 370–386.

Delgutte B. (1987). "Peripheral auditory processing of speech information: implications from a physiological study of intensity discrimination," in *The Psychophysics of Speech Perception*, Vol. 39, ed M. E. H. Schouten (Dordrecht: Nijhoff), 333–353.

Delgutte, B. (1996). "Physiological models for basic auditory percepts," in *Auditory Computation*, eds H. L. Hawkins, T. A. McMullen, A. N. Popper and R. R. Fay (New York, NY: Springer-Verlag), 157–220.

Delgutte, B., and Kiang, N. Y. (1984a). Speech coding in the auditory nerve: III. Voiceless fricative consonants. *J. Acoust. Soc. Am.* 75, 887–896. doi: 10.1121/1.390598

Evans, E. F., and Palmer, A. R. (1980). Relationship between the dynamic range of cochlear nerve fibres and their spontaneous activity. *Exp. Brain Res.* 40, 115–118. doi: 10.1007/BF00236671

Furman, A. C., Kujawa, S. G., and Liberman, M. C. (2013). Noise-induced cochlear neuropathy is selective for fibers with low spontaneous rates. *J. Neurophysiol.* 110, 577–586. doi: 10.1152/jn.00164.2013

Green, D. M., and Swets, J. A. (1966). *Signal Detection Theory and Psychophysics.* New York, NY: John Wiley and Sons, Inc.

Harris, D. M., and Dallos, P. (1979). Forward masking of auditory nerve fiber responses. *J. Acoust. Soc. Am.* 42, 1083–1107.

Hartmann, W. M., and Rakerd, B. (1993). Auditory spectral discrimination and the localization of clicks in the sagittal plane. *J. Acoust. Soc. Am.* 94, 2083–2092. doi: 10.1121/1.407481

Hebrank, J., and Wright, D. (1974). Spectral cues used in the localization of sound sources on the median plane. *J. Acoust. Soc. Am.* 56, 1829–1834. doi: 10.1121/1.1903520

Heinz, M. G., Colburn, H. S., and Carney, L. H. (2001). Evaluating auditory performance limits: i. one-parameter discrimination using a computational model for the auditory nerve. *Neural Comput.* 13, 2273–2316. doi: 10.1162/089976601750541804

Jagger, D. J., and Housley, G. D. (2003). Membrane properties of type II spiral ganglion neurons identified in a neonatal rat cochlear slice. *J. Physiol.* 552, 525–533. doi: 10.1111/j.1469-7793.2003.00525.x

Jin, C. T. (2001). *Spectral Analysis and Resolving Spatial Ambiguities in Human Sound Localization.* University of Sidney.

Johnson, D. H. (1980). The relationship between spike rate and synchrony in responses of auditory-nerve fibers to single tones. *J. Acoust. Soc. Am.* 68, 1115–1122. doi: 10.1121/1.384982

Liberman, M. C. (1978). Auditory-nerve response from cats raised in a low-noise chamber. *J. Acoust. Soc. Am.* 63, 442–455. doi: 10.1121/1.381736

Lopez-Poveda, E. A. (1996). *The Physical Origin and Physiological Coding of Pinna-Based Spectral Cues.* Loughborough: Loughborough University.

Lopez-Poveda, E. A. (2005). "Spectral processing by the peripheral auditory system," in *International Review in Neurobiology,* eds M. Malmierca and D. R. F. Irvine (Elsevier Academic Press), 7–48.

Lopez-Poveda, E. A., Alves-Pinto, A., and Palmer, A. R. (2007) "Psychophysical and physiological assessment of the representation of high-frequency spectral notches in the auditory nerve," in *Hearing: From Sensory Processing to Perception,* eds B. Kollmeier, G. Klump, V. Hohmann, U. Langemann, M. Mauermann, S. Uppenkamp, and J. Verhey (Heidelberg: Springer-Verlag), 51–59.

Lopez-Poveda, E. A., Alves-Pinto, A., Palmer, A. R., and Eustaquio-Martin, A. (2008). Rate versus time representation of high-frequency spectral notches in the peripheral auditory system: a computational modeling study. *Neurocomputing* 71, 693–703. doi: 10.1016/j.neucom.2007.07.030

Lopez-Poveda, E. A., and Barrios, P. (2013). Perception of stochastically undersampled sound waveforms: a model of auditory deafferentation. *Front. Neurosci.* 7:124. doi: 10.3389/fnins.2013.00124

Lopez-Poveda, E. A., and Meddis, R. (1996). A physical model of sound diffraction and reflections in the human concha. *J. Acoust. Soc. Am.* 100, 3248–3259. doi: 10.1121/1.417208

Louage, D. H. G., Van Der Heijden, M., and Joris, P. X. (2004). Temporal properties of responses to broadband noise in the auditory nerve. *J. Neurophysiol.* 91, 2051–2065. doi: 10.1152/jn.00816.2003

Macpherson, E. A., and Middlebrooks, J. C. (2000). Localization of brief sounds: effects of level and background noise. *J. Acoust. Soc. Am.* 108, 1834–1848. doi: 10.1121/1.1310196

Macpherson, E. A., and Sabin, A. T. (2013). Vertical-plane sound localization with distorted spectral cues. *Hear. Res.* 306, 76–92. doi: 10.1016/j.heares.2013.09.007

Meddis, R., and O'Mard, L. P. (2005). A computer model of the auditory-nerve response to forward-masking stimuli. *J. Acoust. Soc. Am.* 117, 3787–3798. doi: 10.1121/1.1893426

Moore, B. C. J. (2003). *An Introduction to the Psychology of Hearing.* London: Academic Press.

Moore, B. C. J., and Sek, A. (2009). Sensitivity of the human auditory system to temporal fine structure at high frequencies. *J. Acoust. Soc. Am.* 125, 3186–3193. doi: 10.1121/1.3106525

Oxenham, A. J. (2001). Forward masking: adaptation or integration? *J. Acoust. Soc. Am.* 109, 732–741. doi: 10.1121/1.1336501

Palmer, A. R., and Evans, E. F. (1980). Cochlear fibre rate-intensity functions: no evidence for basilar membrane nonlinearities. *Hear. Res.* 2, 319–326. doi: 10.1016/0378-5955(80)90065-9

Palmer, A. R., and Russell, I. J. (1986). Phase-locking in the cochlear nerve of the guinea-pig and its relation to the receptor potential of inner hair-cells. *Hear. Res.* 21, 1–15. doi: 10.1016/0378-5955(86)90002-X

Palmer, A. R., Winter, I. M. and Darwin, C. J. (1986). The representation of steady-state vowel sounds in the temporal discharge patterns of guinea pig cochlear nerve. *J. Acoust. Soc. Am.* 79, 100–113.

Pickles, J. O. (1988). *An Introduction to the Physiology of Hearing.* San Diego: Academic Press.

Poon, P. W., and Brugge, J. F. (1993). Sensitivity of auditory nerve fibers to spectral notches. *J. Neurophysiol.* 70, 655–666.

Press, W. H., Teukolsky, S. A., Vetterling, W. T., and Flannery, B. P. (1992). *Numerical Recipes in C: the Art of Scientific Computing.* New York, NY: Cambridge University Press.

Recio-Spinoso, A., Temchin, A. N., Van Dijk, P., Fan, Y. H., and Ruggero, M. A. (2005). Wiener-kernel analysis of responses to noise of chinchilla auditory-nerve fibers. *J. Neurophysiol.* 93, 3615–3634. doi: 10.1152/jn.00882.2004

Reiss, J. J., Young, E. D., and Spirou, G. A. (1995). Spectral edge sensitivity in neural circuits of the dorsal cochlear nucleus. *J. Acoust. Soc. Am.* 97, 1764–1776.

Rice, J. J., Young, E. D., and Spirou, G. A. (1995). Auditory-nerve encoding of pinna-based spectral cues: rate representation of high-frequency stimuli. *J. Acoust. Soc. Am.* 97, 1764–1776. doi: 10.1121/1.412053

Robles, L., and Ruggero, M. A. (2001). Mechanics of the mammalian cochlea. *Physiol. Rev.* 81, 1305–1352.

Rose, J. E., Hind, J. E., Anderson, D. J., and Brugge, J. F. (1971). Some effects of stimulus intensity on response of auditory nerve fibers in the squirrel monkey. *J. Neurophysiol.* 34, 685–699.

Russell, I. J., and Sellick, P. M. (1978). Intracellular studies of hair cells in the mammalian cochlea. *J. Physiol.* 284, 261–290.

Sachs, M. B., and Abbas, P. J. (1974). Rate versus level functions for auditory-nerve fibers in cats: tone-burst stimuli. *J. Acoust. Soc. Am.* 56, 1835–1847. doi: 10.1121/1.1903521

Shackleton, T. M., Skottun, B. C., Arnott, R. H. and Palmer, A. R. (2003). Interaural time difference discrimination thresholds for single neurons in the inferior colliculus of guinea pigs. *J. Neurosci.* 23, 716–724.

Shaw, E. A. G. (1982). "External ear response and sound localization," in *Localization of Sound: Theory and Applications,* ed R. W. Gatehouse (Groton, CT: Amphora), 30–41.

Shaw, E. A., and Teranishi, R. (1968). Sound pressure generated in an external-ear replica and real human ears by a nearby point source. *J. Acoust. Soc. Am.* 44, 240–249. doi: 10.1121/1.1911059

Siebert, W. M. (1965). Some implications of stochastic behaviour of primary auditory neurons. *Kybernetik* 2, 206. doi: 10.1007/BF00306416

Siebert, W. M. (1968). "Stimulus transformation in the peripheral auditory system," in *Recognizing Patterns,* eds P. A. Kolers and M. Eden (Cambridge: MA: MIT Press), 104–133.

Siebert, W. M. (1970). Frequency discrimination in the auditory system: place or periodic mechanisms. *Proc. IEEE.* 58, 723–730. doi: 10.1109/PROC.1970.7727

Van Rullen, R., and Thorpe, S. J. (2001). Rate coding versus temporal order coding: What the retinal ganglion cells tell the visual cortex. *Neural Comput.* 13, 1255–1283. doi: 10.1162/08997660152002852

Viemeister, N. F. (1988). Intensity coding and the dynamic-range problem. *Hear. Res.* 34, 267–274. doi: 10.1016/0378-5955(88)90007-X

Viemeister, N. F., and Wakefield, G. H. (1991). Temporal integration and multiple looks. *J. Acoust. Soc. Am.* 90, 858–865. doi: 10.1121/1.401953

Vliegen, J., and Van Opstal, A. J. (2004). The influence of duration and level on human sound localization. *J. Acoust. Soc. Am.* 115, 1705–1713. doi: 10.1121/1.1687423

Westerman, L. A., and Smith, R. L. (1984). Rapid and short-term adaptation in auditory nerve responses. *Hear. Res.* 15, 249–260. doi: 10.1016/0378-5955(84)90032-7

Wever, E. G. (1949). *Theory of Hearing.* New York, NY: Wiley.

Yates, G. K. (1991). Auditory-nerve spontaneous rates vary predictably with threshold. *Hear. Res.* 57, 249–260. doi: 10.1016/0378-5955(91)90074-J

Young, E. D., and Sachs, M. B. (1979). Representation of steady-state vowels in the temporal aspects of the discharge patterns of populations of auditory-nerve fibers. *J. Acoust. Soc. Am.* 66, 1381–1403. doi: 10.1121/1.383532

Zheng, X. H., and Voigt, H. F. (2006). A modeling study of notch noise responses of type III units in the gerbil dorsal cochlear nucleus. *Ann. Biomed. Eng.* 34, 697–708. doi: 10.1007/s10439-005-9073-5

Permissions

All chapters in this book were first published by Frontiers; hereby published with permission under the Creative Commons Attribution License or equivalent. Every chapter published in this book has been scrutinized by our experts. Their significance has been extensively debated. The topics covered herein carry significant findings which will fuel the growth of the discipline. They may even be implemented as practical applications or may be referred to as a beginning point for another development.

The contributors of this book come from diverse backgrounds, making this book a truly international effort. This book will bring forth new frontiers with its revolutionizing research information and detailed analysis of the nascent developments around the world.

We would like to thank all the contributing authors for lending their expertise to make the book truly unique. They have played a crucial role in the development of this book. Without their invaluable contributions this book wouldn't have been possible. They have made vital efforts to compile up to date information on the varied aspects of this subject to make this book a valuable addition to the collection of many professionals and students.

This book was conceptualized with the vision of imparting up-to-date information and advanced data in this field. To ensure the same, a matchless editorial board was set up. Every individual on the board went through rigorous rounds of assessment to prove their worth. After which they invested a large part of their time researching and compiling the most relevant data for our readers.

The editorial board has been involved in producing this book since its inception. They have spent rigorous hours researching and exploring the diverse topics which have resulted in the successful publishing of this book. They have passed on their knowledge of decades through this book. To expedite this challenging task, the publisher supported the team at every step. A small team of assistant editors was also appointed to further simplify the editing procedure and attain best results for the readers.

Apart from the editorial board, the designing team has also invested a significant amount of their time in understanding the subject and creating the most relevant covers. They scrutinized every image to scout for the most suitable representation of the subject and create an appropriate cover for the book.

The publishing team has been an ardent support to the editorial, designing and production team. Their endless efforts to recruit the best for this project, has resulted in the accomplishment of this book. They are a veteran in the field of academics and their pool of knowledge is as vast as their experience in printing. Their expertise and guidance has proved useful at every step. Their uncompromising quality standards have made this book an exceptional effort. Their encouragement from time to time has been an inspiration for everyone.

The publisher and the editorial board hope that this book will prove to be a valuable piece of knowledge for researchers, students, practitioners and scholars across the globe.

List of Contributors

William M. Hartmann and Eric J. Macaulay
Psychoacoustics Laboratory, Department of Physics and Astronomy, Michigan State University, East Lansing, MI, USA

Paul W. Anderson
Department of Psychological and Brain Sciences, University of Louisville, Louisville, KY, USA

Pavel Zahorik
Department of Psychological and Brain Sciences, University of Louisville, Louisville, KY, USA
Division of Communicative Disorders, Department of Surgery, School of Medicine, University of Louisville, Louisville, KY, USA

W. Owen Brimijoin and Michael A. Akeroyd
Scottish Section, Institute of Hearing Research, Medical Research Council/Chief Scientist Office, Glasgow, UK

Guillaume Andéol
Département Action et Cognition en Situation Opérationnelle, Institut de Recherche Biomédicale des Armées, Brétigny sur Orge, France

Sophie Savel
Laboratoire de Mécanique et d'Acoustique, Centre National de la Recherche Scientifique, UPR 7051, Equipe Sons, Aix-Marseille Université, Centrale Marseille, Marseille, France

Anne Guillaume
Laboratoire d'Accidentologie, de Biomécanique et d'Étude du Comportement Humain, Nanterre, France

Gaëtan Parseihian and Brian F. G. Katz
Laboratoire de Mécanique et d'Informatique pour les Sciences de l'Ingénieur, LIMSI - CNRS, Universite Paris Sud, Orsay, France

Christophe Jouffrais
IRIT, CNRS, Université de Toulouse, Toulouse, France

Vanessa Tabry, Robert J. Zatorre and Patrice Voss
Department of Neurology and Neurosurgery, Montreal Neurological Institute, McGill University, Montreal, QC, Canada
International Laboratory for Brain, Music and Sound Research (BRAMS), Montreal, QC, Canada

Elvira Perez, Abby McCormack and Barrie A. Edmonds
NIHR Nottingham Hearing Biomedical Research Unit, School of Medicine, University of Nottingham, Nottingham, UK

Isabelle Viaud-Delmon and Olivier Warusfel
CNRS, UMR 9912, Sciences et Technologies de la Musique et du Son, Paris, France
Institut de Recherche et Coordination Acoustique/Musique, UMR 9912, Sciences et Technologies de la Musique et du Son, Paris, France
Sorbonne Universités, Université Pierre et Marie Curie, UMR 9912, Sciences et Technologies de la Musique et du Son, Paris, France

Atsushi Ochi
Human Information Science Laboratory, NTT Communication Science Laboratories, NTT Corporation, Atsugi, Japan
Department of Otolaryngology, Faculty of Medicine, University of Tokyo, Tokyo, Japan

Tatsuya Yamasoba
Department of Otolaryngology, Faculty of Medicine, University of Tokyo, Tokyo, Japan

Shigeto Furukawa
Human Information Science Laboratory, NTT Communication Science Laboratories, NTT Corporation, Atsugi, Japan

Ken I. McAnally and Russell L. Martin
Aerospace Division, Defence Science and Technology Organisation, Melbourne, VIC, Australia

Griffin D. Romigh and Brian D. Simpson
Air Force Research Laboratory, Dayton, OH, USA

Piotr Majdak, Robert Baumgartner and Bernhard Laback
Psychoacoustics and Experimental Audiology, Acoustics Research Institute, Austrian Academy of Sciences, Wien, Austria

Matthew G. Wisniewski
711th Human Performance Wing, U. S. Air Force Research Laboratory, Wright-Patterson Air Force Base, OH, USA
Department of Psychology, University at Buffalo, The State University of New York, Buffalo, NY, USA

Eduardo Mercado III and Barbara A. Church
Department of Psychology, University at Buffalo, The State University of New York, Buffalo, NY, USA

Klaus Gramann
Biological Psychology and Neuroergonomics, Berlin Institute of Technology, Berlin, Germany

Scott Makeig
Swartz Center for Computational Neuroscience, Institute for Neural Computation, University of California, San Diego, San Diego, CA, USA

Martijn J. H. Agterberg, Marc M. Van Wanrooij and Ad F. M. Snik
Department of Biophysics, Donders Institute for Brain, Cognition and Behaviour, Radboud University Nijmegen, Nijmegen, Netherlands
Department of Otorhinolaryngology, Donders Institute for Brain, Cognition and Behaviour, Radboud University Medical Center, Nijmegen, Netherlands

Myrthe K. S. Hol
Department of Otorhinolaryngology, Donders Institute for Brain, Cognition and Behaviour, Radboud University Medical Center, Nijmegen, Netherlands

A. John Van Opstal
Department of Otorhinolaryngology, Donders Institute for Brain, Cognition and Behaviour, Radboud University Medical Center, Nijmegen, Netherlands

Adriana A. Zekveld
Department of Behavioural Sciences and Learning, Linköping University, Linköping, Sweden
Linnaeus Centre for Hearing and Deafness Research, The Swedish Institute for Disability Research, Linköping and Örebro Universities, Linköping, Sweden
Section Audiology, Department of Otolaryngology-Head and Neck Surgery and EMGO Institute for Health and Care Research, VU University Medical Center, Amsterdam, Netherlands

Mary Rudner and Jerker Rönnberg
Department of Behavioural Sciences and Learning, Linköping University, Linköping, Sweden
Linnaeus Centre for Hearing and Deafness Research, The Swedish Institute for Disability Research, Linköping and Örebro Universities, Linköping, Sweden

Sophia E. Kramer and Johannes Lyzenga
Section Audiology, Department of Otolaryngology-Head and Neck Surgery and EMGO Institute for Health and Care Research, VU University Medical Center, Amsterdam, Netherlands

Simon Carlile
School of Medical Sciences and Bosch Institute, University of Sydney, Sydney, NSW, Australia

Véronique Zimpfer
French-German Research Institute of Saint-Louis (ISL), Acoustics and Protection of Soldier Group, Saint-Louis, France

David Sarafian
Institut de Recherche Biomédicale des Armées, Département Action et Cognition en Situation Opérationnelle, Brétigny sur Orge, France

Frederick J. Gallun, Michelle R. Molis and Dawn L. Konrad-Martin
National Center for Rehabilitative Auditory Research, Department of Veterans Affairs, Portland VA Medical Center, Portland, OR, USA
Otolaryngology/Head and Neck Surgery, Oregon Health and Science University, Portland, OR, USA

Garnett P. McMillan
National Center for Rehabilitative Auditory Research, Department of Veterans Affairs, Portland VA Medical Center, Portland, OR, USA
Department of Public Health and Preventive Medicine, Oregon Health and Science University, Portland, OR, USA

Sean D. Kampel and Serena M. Dann
National Center for Rehabilitative Auditory Research, Department of Veterans Affairs, Portland VA Medical Center, Portland, OR, USA

Catarina Mendonça
Department of Signal Processing and Acoustics, School of Electrical Engineering, Aalto University, Espoo, Finland

Ana Alves-Pinto
Klinikum rechts der Isar, Technische Universität München, Munich, Germany

Alan R. Palmer
Medical Research Council Institute of Hearing Research, University Park, Nottingham, UK

Enrique A. Lopez-Poveda
Departamento de Cirugía, Facultad de Medicina, Instituto de Neurociencias de Castilla y León, Instituto de Investigación Biomédica de Salamanca, Universidad de Salamanca, Salamanca, Spain

Index

www.ingramcontent.com/pod-product-compliance
Lightning Source LLC
LaVergne TN
LVHW082221200926
848484LV00008B/2285
* 9 7 9 8 8 8 7 4 0 4 6 3 9 *